Endometriosis and Adenomyosis

Engin Oral
Editor

Endometriosis and Adenomyosis

Global Perspectives Across the Lifespan

Springer

Editor
Engin Oral
Department of Obstetrics and Gynecology
Bezmialem Vakif University Medical Faculty
Istanbul, Turkey

ISBN 978-3-030-97235-6 ISBN 978-3-030-97236-3 (eBook)
https://doi.org/10.1007/978-3-030-97236-3

This Springer imprint is published by the registered company Springer Nature Switzerland AG
The registered company address is: Gewerbestrasse 11, 6330 Cham, Switzerland

Foreword

Every person in the world is likely to have their life touched in some way by endometriosis or adenomyosis, so wide ranging is the suffering of almost 200 million souls on our globe who currently endure the ravages of these diseases, for some, every single day of their lives. This wonderful book, *Endometriosis & Adenomyosis: Across the Lifespan – Global Aspects*, is in every regard global. It is a global revelation of all that we know about endometriosis and adenomyosis – and much that we are yet to fully comprehend – and a global journey of an endometriosis/adenomyosis sufferer's lifespan. This book is written by an author group that represents the giants of our globe in this field, and is skilfully crafted and weaved together by gifted editor Engin Oral for us to enjoy and to learn. Like you, I cannot wait to dive in.

Neil Johnson
Professor of Reproductive Health, Robinson Research Institute
Adelaide, SA, Australia

Gynaecologist and REI Subspecialist, Auckland Gynaecology Group and
Repromed, Auckland, New Zealand

NZ Representative and Executive Board Member, ASPIRE
Auckland, New Zealand

Past President, World Endometriosis Society
Vancouver, Canada

The original version of this chapter was revised to reflect a correction to Dr Hanan Alsalem's name which was misspelled in the initial publication as Hanan Amsalem. An erratum to this chapter can be found at https://doi.org/10.1007/978-3-030-97236-3_45

Foreword

Endometriosis as a disease has many faces. That might explain why it is called a chameleon. And once suspected or diagnosed, it is hard to estimate the extent of the disease; thus, it has been compared with an iceberg as a major part of the tumor is hiding under the surface.

Endometriosis is benign but infiltrating; even though infiltration rarely turns malignant, it is hormone dependent yet cannot be cured by hormones.

Hypotheses of its origin are multifold, and treatment options are very limited. Unfortunately, the interval from onset of symptoms to diagnosis of endometriosis on average takes years which is by far too long and effectively means suffering of predominantly young women in the prime years of their lives. In association with underdiagnosing and under treatment are negative impacts on performance at work, school and university, sexual life, family relationship, and social activities.

Once diagnosed, the dilemma continues as medical treatment of endometriosis often interferes with family planning for couples because most hormonal therapies exert contraceptive effects, often requiring assisted reproductive technologies. This is particularly true as in most developed countries couples desiring a child are beyond their thirties, which adds another fertility-reducing factor to endometriosis.

Following an often-unsuccessful medical treatment of endometriosis surgery remains the only choice for reducing pain and invasion into other organs. However, since the difficulty of surgery exponentially increases with the extent of the disease, severe stages of endometriosis and adenomyosis require experts not only for diagnosis but also for treatment.

The editor of this textbook, Prof. Engin Oral, has dedicated part of his life to increase awareness, understanding, and cognizance of medical specialists as well as the public about problems related to endometriosis. He has successfully motivated a group of renowned experts in the field of endometriosis and adenomyosis to compile this up-to-date manual. The careful reader will find a comprehensive collection of chapters which in total cover the entire field and allows for a holistic view on endometriosis and adenomyosis.

This book provides valuable information for anyone interested in in-depth knowledge regarding all aspects associated with endometriosis, offering practical application for daily practice.

Hans-Rudolf Tinneberg, MD, PhD
Frauenklinik Nordwest Krankenhaus
Frankfurt, Germany

Foreword

Endometriosis is among the most common gynecologic disorders associated with infertility and pelvic pain; therefore, it represents a major personal and public health concern. Pathogenesis of endometriosis and adenomyosis has puzzled researchers for more than a century and still remains one of the most enigmatic disorders in gynecology. In the last decade alone more than 5000 articles on endometriosis and adenomyosis appeared in the world scientific literature, many of them contradictory, reflecting our difficulties in deciphering this disorder.

More recently, the application of cellular and molecular biology techniques to the study of endometriosis allowed us to better understand the pathogenesis and pathophysiology of endometriosis and helped us to develop new therapeutic approaches. Major advances in the understanding of endometrial biology and simultaneous advances in surgical instrumentation are critical elements fueling the endometriosis/adenomyosis renaissance.

This book, edited by Professor Engin Oral, is designed to present both cellular and molecular aspects and clinical management of endometriosis and adenomyosis. It represents the culmination of the clinical experiences, basic research, and consensus opinions of experts in the field of endometriosis and adenomyosis. A diverse group of internationally recognized experts have come together to provide a detailed discussion of various aspects of endometriosis and adenomyosis. I would like to express my gratitude to Professor Oral for asking me to write a foreword to this book. Our interaction began in 1994 as a mentor, but he became eventually a very valuable colleague and a friend. As one of the international experts in endometriosis and adenomyosis, he has been a leader in the field, bringing awareness of these diseases to the public in general.

I do hope that this book will serve women, their physicians, and investigators well in the ongoing battle against this enigmatic disease.

Aydin Arici, MD
Professor of Obstetrics, Gynecology and Reproductive Sciences
Yale University School of Medicine
New Haven, CT, USA

Preface

Hello to all readers,

I think I was introduced to endometriosis, also known as "chocolate cyst" disease, while I was studying medicine at Istanbul Medical Faculty. At that time the name sounded a bit strange to me. Later, when I chose obstetrics and gynecology, we came across endometriosis patients at Istanbul University Cerrahpaşa Medical Faculty, but now when I look at it, little did we know about the disease itself. Patients were coming, saying "I have pain" or "I can't get pregnant," and sometimes we gave medical treatment, but mostly we performed surgery. The person who made me realize this disease is my dear mentor from the USA, one of the foreword writers of this book, Prof. Dr. Aydin Arici. When I was accepted as a postdoctoral fellow to Yale University Obstetrics and Gynecology Department of Reproductive Endocrinology and Infertility in 1995, I realized that Prof. Arici was dealing mainly with endometriosis patients. Thus, I joined his team and became acquainted with this disease. I never knew about the research aspect of the disease, but during my time at Yale, as a team, my friends and I, under the leadership of Aydın Arici and now deceased David Olive, conducted both research and clinical studies that had contributed to the literature. The first study we did was a clinical study, we looked at the effect of endometriosis on implantation, and when that study was accepted in the *F&S* journal, the head of the department at that time (Frederick Naftolin) and Aydın Arıcı sent me to the "Endometriosis 2000" meeting in May 1995, where important scientists were found. I attended this meeting with Aydın Arıcı. At that time, I had the opportunity to meet important people dealing with this issue in the USA, and this motivated me even more. For the next 2 years, I dealt almost exclusively with this disease both in the laboratory and clinics. I watched surgeries at Yale, had the opportunity to watch in vitro fertilization cases, and in the laboratory, we worked on molecules such as growth factors, cytokines in endometriosis tissue samples, and cell cultures. When I returned to Turkey, my goal was to "provide better solutions to people suffering from this disease." During this period, after becoming associate professor and professor, I had the chance to see many clinical cases at Istanbul University Cerrahpaşa Medical Faculty. The years progressed rapidly, and in 2009, I decided to establish an association that provides academic education on this disease as well as increases the awareness of it among the public. In retrospect, this was truly one of the best things I've ever done. The association, which we established with 14 people, has now become a recognized and respected association not only in Turkey but also throughout Europe and even worldwide. This is the 12th year of the association, and if they were asked in these 12 years "What did you work for the most? What did you spend most of your time on? My answer will probably be the Endometriosis and Adenomyosis Society. With this association, we primarily aimed to increase the knowledge and training of doctors on this subject. In the following years, we tried to increase the public's knowledge and awareness of the disease. In 2012, we held the second meeting of the "Asian Endometriosis and Adenomyosis Association" in Istanbul. The first took place in China and the second in Turkey under my presidency. Just 2 years later, in 2014, under my chairmanship, we held a meeting on deep endometriosis in Istanbul, where international experts gave lectures on both theoretical and surgical cases. In 2016, it was time to open our doors to Europe, and we were invited to Budapest for the meeting of the European Endometriosis Society, with the invitation of Dr. Tinneberg and Dr. Renner, founders of the "European Endometriosis Society." There, Dr. Taner Usta, who I've been always proud of as mentor and who is the current president of the Endometriosis and Adenomyosis Society, Turkey, and has been with me since almost the foundation of the association, and I were elected to the board of directors. In 2018, I became the elected president of the European Endometriosis Society, and during this period, we organized the annual meetings of the European Endometriosis Society in Vienna and Prague. In 2019, I was selected as a senior ambassador of the World Endometriosis Association. In 2020, we faced COVID facts and we still have been struggling to live under pandemic. As for the Endometriosis and Adenomyosis Association, we have mostly shifted our meetings online. Since the last 2 years, we have been having only online meetings, webinars, etc.

As for the story of this book (what you have read so far is the story of me and the association), the idea of this book was seeded when my dear friend Prof. Dr. Orhan Bukulmez introduced me to Kristoffer Springer from Springer Nature during ASRM 2019 meeting. After that meeting, Springer Nature officially invited me to edit an endometriosis book, and I gladly accepted this offer. Our aim in this book was to create a bedside classic that covers the basics of endometriosis and adenomyosis. When you see the chapters and topics, I think you will agree with me. This book is the result of the joint effort of 87 authors from 19 diffferent countries who contributed in teams to create the 44 chapters of this book. This book has been written by several experts on endometriosis from all over the world, but especially from Europe, who are the founders and/or members of the European Endometriosis Society. I thank them all one by one.

At the beginning of this book, I would like to thank dear Orhan Bukulmez (USA), who helped to determine the topics, and dear Ertan Saridogan (England), one of the most hardworking and reliable people I know, with whom I always work with pleasure.

During the writing and editing phase, two of my students, who also have chapters in this book, contributed more than me. My heartfelt thanks to my dear Nura Fitnat Topbas Selcuki (she has now started her PhD at Oxford University, Department of Women's and Reproductive Health) and dear Ezgi Darici (she will start the ESHRE Travelling Fellowship Universitair Ziekenhuis Brussels – Reproductive Endocrinology and Infertility clinical – research fellowship program in Belgium in February). Also, I would like to thank all the members of the board of directors of the European Endometriosis Association (Founding President: Hans-Rudolf Tinneberg; President: Harald Krentel; Treasurer: Stefan P Renner; and Board Members: Horace Roman, Caterina Exacoustos, and Attila Bokor).

Special thanks to Sangeetha Annaswamy, Shirly Christina, and Kristoffer Springer at Springer Nature.

Many thanks to Yale University lecturer Aydin Arici; Hans-Rudolf Tinneberg, founding president of the European Endometriosis Association; and Neil Johnson from New Zealand, former president of the World Endometriosis Association, who all kindly accepted my request to write for forewords to this book.

I would like to thank my wife and both my daughters for all the time I stole from my family, including my first day working on endometriosis and adenomyosis, and writing this book.

Last but not least, I hope this book will be a useful guide for all healthcare professionals, especially physicians, who work for the diagnosis and treatment of endometriosis and adenomyosis and who try to learn, try to help patients, and want to do research.

Best Regards,

Prof. Engin Oral, MD

Past President, Executive Board Member of European Endometriosis League

Senior Ambassador of World Endometriosis Society

Founder President, Executive Board Member of Endometriosis & Adenomyosis Association, Turkey

Istanbul, Turkey
November 2021

Engin Oral, MD

Contents

Contributors

Jason A. Abbott School of Women's and Children's Health, UNSW Sydney, Sydney, NSW, Australia

Maribel Acien Department of Obstetrics and Gynecology, San Juan University Hospital, Miguel Hernández University, Alicante, Spain

Sanjay K. Agarwal Fertility Services & Center for Endometriosis Research and Treatment, Department of Obstetrics, Gynecology & Reproductive Sciences, UC San Diego, La Jolla, CA, USA

Silvia Ajossa Department of Obstetrics and Gynecology, University of Cagliari, Policlinico Universitario Duilio Casula, Monserrato, Cagliari, Italy

Luis Juan Alcazar Department of Obstetrics and Gynecology, Clínica Universidad de Navarra, School of Medicine, University of Navarra, Pamplona, Spain

Hanan Alsalem Franco-European Multidisciplinary Endometriosis Institute (IFEMEndo), Clinique Tivoli-Ducos, Bordeaux, France

Stefano Angioni Department of Surgical Sciences, University of Cagliari, Cagliari, Italy

H. Paige Anglin Department of Obstetrics, Gynecology & Reproductive Sciences, UC San Diego, La Jolla, CA, USA

Jwal Banker Nova IVF Fertility, Ahmedabad, India

IVI, Madrid, Spain

Manish Banker Nova IVF Fertility, Ahmedabad, India

Fabio Barra Academic Unit of Obstetrics and Gynecology, IRCCS Ospedale Policlinico San Martino, Genoa, Italy

Department of Neurosciences, Rehabilitation, Ophthalmology, Genetics, Maternal and Child Health (DiNOGMI), University of Genoa, Genoa, Italy

Mohamed A. Bedaiwy Department of Obstetrics and Gynaecology, BC Women's Hospital and Health Center, Faculty of Medicine, The University of British Columbia, Vancouver, BC, Canada

Giuseppe Benagiano Department of Maternal and Child Health, Gynaecology and Urology, Sapienza University of Rome, Rome, Italy

Tudor Birsan Center for Endometriosis, Hospital St. John of God, Vienna, Austria

Atilla Bokor Department of Obstetrics and Gynecology, Semmelweis University, Budapest, Hungary

Elvira Bratila Department of Obstetrics Gynecology, "Carol Davila" University of Medicine and Pharmacy, Bucharest, Romania

Department of Obstetrics Gynecology, "Prof. Dr. Panait Sirbu" Clinical Obstetrics and Gynecology Hospital, Bucharest, Romania

Sara Clemenza Department of Experimental, Clinical and Biomedical Sciences, Careggi University Hospital, Florence, Italy

Ana Cobo IVI Madrid, Rey Juan Carlos University, Madrid, Spain

Elena Commodari Department of Educational Sciences, University of Catania, Catania, Italy

Henrique D'Allagnol IVI Madrid, Rey Juan Carlos University, Madrid, Spain

Maurizio Nicola D'Alterio Department of Surgical Sciences, University of Cagliari, Cagliari, Italy

Angelos Daniilidis School of Medicine, Aristotle University of Thessaloniki, 2nd Dept. OB-GYN, "Hippokration" Hospital, Thessaloniki, Greece

Ezgi Darici Department of Obstetrics Gynecology, İznik State Hospital, Bursa, Turkey

Caterina Exacoustos University of Rome "Tor Vergata", Department of Surgical Sciences, Obstetrics and Gynecological Unit, University Hospital of Tor Vergata, Rome, Italy

Simone Ferrero Academic Unit of Obstetrics and Gynecology, IRCCS Ospedale Policlinico San Martino, Genoa, Italy

Department of Neurosciences, Rehabilitation, Ophthalmology, Genetics, Maternal and Child Health (DiNOGMI), University of Genoa, Genoa, Italy

Warren G. Foster Department of Obstetrics and Gynecology and the School of Biomedical Engineering, McMaster University, Hamilton, ON, Canada

Juan Antonio Garcia-Velasco IVI, Madrid, Spain Rey Juan Carlos University, Madrid, Spain

Fabio Ghezzi Department of Obstetrics and Gynecology, "Filippo Del Ponte" Hospital, University of Insubria, Varese, Italy

Stefano Guerriero Department of Obstetrics and Gynecology, University of Cagliari, Policlinico Universitario Duilio Casula, Monserrato, Cagliari, Italy

Sun-Wei Guo Shanghai Obstetrics and Gynecology Hospital, Fudan University, Shanghai, China

Shanghai Key Laboratory of Female Reproductive Endocrine-Related Diseases, Fudan University, Shanghai, China

Marwan Habiba Department of Health Sciences, University of Leicester and University Hospitals of Leicester, Leicester, UK

Tasuku Harada Obstetrics and Gynecology, Tottori University, Yonago, Japan

Michael Hibner Arizona Center for Chronic Pelvic Pain, Scottsdale, AZ, USA

Yasushi Hirota Department of Obstetrics and Gynecology, Graduate School of Medicine, The University of Tokyo, Tokyo, Japan

Gernot Hudelist Scientific Endometriosis Foundation (Stiftung Endometrioseforschung/SEF), Westerstede, Germany

Department of Gynaecology, Center for Endometriosis, Hospital St. John of God, Vienna, Austria

Jörg Keckstein Endometriosis Clinic Dres. Keckstein, Villach, Austria

University Ulm, Ulm, Germany

Scientific Endometriosis Foundation (Stiftung Endometrioseforschung/SEF), Westerstede, Germany

Richard Wagner Strasse, Villach, Austria

Khaleque N. Khan Department of Obstetrics and Gynecology, The Clinical and Translational Research Center, Graduate School of Medical Science, Kyoto Prefectural University of Medicine, Kyoto, Japan

Shaheen Khazali Royal Holloway-University of London, London, UK

HCA The Lister Hospital, Centre for Endometriosis and Minimally Invasive Gynaecology (CEMIG), London, UK

Ludwig Kiesel Department of Gynecology and Obstetrics, University Hospital Münster (UKM), Münster, Germany

Graciela Kohls IVI Madrid, Rey Juan Carlos University, Madrid, Spain

Hiroaki Komatsu Obstetrics and Gynecology, Tottori University, Yonago, Japan

Harald Krentel Clinic of Gynecology, Obstetrics, Gynecological Oncology and Senology, Academic Teaching Hospital, Bethesda Hospital, Duisburg, Germany

Marina Kvaskoff Exposome and Heredity Team, Centre for Research in Epidemiology and Population Health, Inserm (French National Institute for Health and Medical Research), Villejuif, France

Antonio Simone Laganà Department of Obstetrics and Gynecology, "Filippo Del Ponte" Hospital, University of Insubria, Varese, Italy

Valentina Lucia La Rosa Department of Educational Sciences, University of Catania, Catania, Italy

Marc R. Laufer Division of Gynecology, Boston Children's Hospital, Boston, MA, USA

Center for Infertility and Reproductive Surgery, Brigham and Women's Hospital, Boston, MA, USA

Harvard Medical School, Boston, MA, USA

Quang Khoi Le Department of Gynecology and Obstetrics, University Hospital Münster (UKM), Münster, Germany

Tinya Lin Department of Obstetrics and Gynecology, The University of British Columbia, Vancouver, BC, Canada

Donatella Lippi Department of Experimental and Clinical Medicine, School of Sciences of Human Health, University of Florence, Florence, Italy

U. Leone Roberti Maggiore Gynecologic Oncology Unit, Fondazione IRCCS, Istituto Nazionale dei Tumori, Milano, Italy

Dan C. Martin School of Medicine, University of Tennessee Health Science Center, Memphis, TN, USA

Institutional Review Board, Virginia Commonwealth University, Richmond, VA, USA

Sylvia Mechsner Department of Gynecology, Endometriosis Unit Charité, Charité – University Hospital Berlin, Berlin, Germany

Gita D. Mishra School of Public Health, The University of Queensland, Brisbane, QLD, Australia

Stacey A. Missmer Department of Obstetrics, Gynecology, and Reproductive Biology, College of Human Medicine, Michigan State University, Grand Rapids, MI, USA

Michael D. Mueller Department of Gynecology and Gynecological Oncology, Inselspital, Bern University Hospital, Bern, Switzerland

Eleonora Musa Department of Obstetrics and Gynecology, University of Cagliari, Policlinico Universitario Duilio Casula, Monserrato, Cagliari, Italy

Manuela Neri Department of Obstetrics and Gynecology, University of Cagliari, Policlinico Universitario Duilio Casula, Monserrato, Cagliari, Italy

Konstantinos Nirgianakis Department of Gynecology and Gynecological Oncology, Inselspital, Bern University Hospital, Bern, Switzerland

Peter Oppelt Scientific Endometriosis Foundation (Stiftung Endometrioseforschung/SEF), Westerstede, Germany

Department of Gynecology, Obstetrics and Gynecological Endocrinology, Kepler University Hospital Linz, Johannes Kepler Universität Linz, Linz, Austria

Engin Oral Department of Obstetrics and Gynecology, Bezmialem Vakif University Medical Faculty, Istanbul, Turkey

Yutaka Osuga Department of Obstetrics and Gynecology, Graduate School of Medicine, The University of Tokyo, Tokyo, Japan

George Pados School of Medicine, Aristotle University of Thessaloniki, 1st Dept. OB-GYN, "Papageorgiou" Hospital, Thessaloniki, Greece

Centre for Endoscopic Surgery, "Diavalkaniko" Hospital, Thessaloniki, Greece

Mariachiara Pagliuca Department of Obstetrics and Gynecology, University of Cagliari, Policlinico Universitario Duilio Casula, Monserrato, Cagliari, Italy

Angela M. Pascual Department of Obstetrics, Gynecology, and Reproduction, Hospital Universitari Dexeus, Barcelona, Spain

Monica Pilloni Department of Obstetrics and Gynecology, University of Cagliari, Policlinico Universitario Duilio Casula, Monserrato, Cagliari, Italy

Nilufer Rahmioglu Wellcome Centre for Human Genetics, University of Oxford, Oxford, UK

Oxford Endometriosis Care Centre, Nuffield Department of Women's and Reproductive Health, John Radcliffe Hospital, University of Oxford, Oxford, UK

Stefan P. Renner Department of Gynecology and Obstetrics, Boeblingen Hospital, Sindelfingen–Boeblingen Clinics, Boeblingen, Germany

Horace Roman Franco-European Multidisciplinary Endometriosis Institute (IFEMEndo), Clinique Tivoli-Ducos, Bordeaux, France

Ingrid J. Rowlands School of Public Health, The University of Queensland, Brisbane, QLD, Australia

Luca Saba Department of Radiology, Azienda Ospedaliero Universitaria di Cagliari, Cagliari, Italy

Ertan Sarıdoğan Women's Health Division, University College London Hospital, London, UK

Institute for Women's Health, University College London, University College London Hospital, London, UK

Sebastian Daniel Schäfer Department of Gynecology and Obstetrics, University Hospital Münster (UKM), Münster, Germany

Rasmus Schmaedecker Department of Gynecology and Obstetrics, Martin Luther Krankenhaus, Berlin, Germany

Nura Fitnat Topbas Selcuki Department of Obstetrics and Gynecology, University of Health Sciences Turkey, Istanbul Sisli Hamidiye Etfal Training and Research Hospital, Istanbul, Turkey

Omar Shebl Kepler University Hospital Linz, Department of Obstetrics, Gynaecology and Gynaecological Endocrinology, Linz, Austria

Jessica Y. Shim Division of Gynecology, Boston Children's Hospital, Boston, MA, USA

Brintha Sivajohan Schulich School of Medicine & Dentistry, Western University, London, ON, Canada

Fuminori Taniguchi Obstetrics and Gynecology, Tottori University, Yonago, Japan

Tina Tellum Department of Gynaecology, Oslo University Hospital, Oslo, Norway

Carla Tomassetti University Hospitals Leuven, Department of Obstetrics and Gynaecology, Leuven University Fertility Center, Leuven, Belgium

KU Leuven, Faculty of Medicine, Department of Development and Regeneration, LEERM (Laboratory for Endometrium, Endometriosis and Reproductive Medicine), Leuven, Belgium

Uwe Andreas Ulrich Department of Gynecology and Obstetrics, Martin Luther Krankenhaus, Berlin, Germany

Taner Usta Acibadem Mehmet Ali Aydinlar University, Istanbul, Turkey

Endometriosis and Pelvic Pain Center, Department of Obstetrics and Gynecology, Acibadem Altunizade Hospital, Istanbul, Turkey

Silvia Vannuccini Department of Experimental, Clinical and Biomedical Sciences, Careggi University Hospital, Florence, Italy

Salvatore Giovanni Vitale Obstetrics and Gynecology Unit, Department of General Surgery and Medical Surgical Specialties, University of Catania, Catania, Italy

Ioannis Vlachodimitris Clinic of Gynecology, Obstetrics, Gynecological Oncology and Senology, Academic Teaching Hospital, Bethesda Hospital, Duisburg, Germany

Marie Vogel Department of Gynecology and Obstetrics, University Hospital Münster (UKM), Münster, Germany

Krina T. Zondervan Wellcome Centre for Human Genetics, University of Oxford, Oxford, UK

Oxford Endometriosis Care Centre, Nuffield Department of Women's and Reproductive Health, John Radcliffe Hospital, University of Oxford, Oxford, UK

Part I

Endometriosis: An Overview

A History of Endometriosis

1

Donatella Lippi, Marwan Habiba,
and Giuseppe Benagiano

Contents

D. Lippi
Department of Experimental and Clinical Medicine, School of Sciences of Human Health, University of Florence, Florence, Italy

M. Habiba (✉)
Department of Health Sciences, University of Leicester and University Hospitals of Leicester, Leicester, UK
e-mail: mah6@leicester.ac.uk

G. Benagiano
Department of Maternal and Child Health, Gynaecology and Urology, Sapienza University of Rome, Rome, Italy

E. Oral (ed.), *Endometriosis and Adenomyosis*,
https://doi.org/10.1007/978-3-030-97236-3_1

1.1 Introduction

Different accounts have been provided of the history of the condition we today call endometriosis. The use of different terminology may have contributed to the difficulty in tracing early literature describing the condition. Literature that did not contribute to progressive knowledge is more likely to be of interest to those concerned with understanding the dynamics of scientific progress, rather than those concerned with the evolution of our understanding of endometriosis. This is because endometriosis is a specific disease condition with characteristic histological features but without pathognomonic clinical features. Symptoms linked to endometriosis include cyclical pelvic pain and infertility which are common to range of other conditions. Endometriosis can also be asymptomatic. Thus, a history of endometriosis is necessarily distinct from a history of pelvic pain or infertility, as well as from a narrative of how medicine or society addressed affections or manifestations of diseases of women. A history specific to endometriosis needs to be based on clear evidence of the identification of the condition. The insistence on disease "identification" is necessary for there to be a history specific to endometriosis. We can find no reason in the literature to justify doubt about the existence of endometriosis in earlier human history. What did not happen until some 150 years ago was the recognition and description of a disease linked to characteristic histological features. Such description is essential for developing a classification and clinical correlates, and this is why it has been argued that when starting to draw a history of a disease, it is necessary to outline the specific methodological approach adopted [1].

We believe that the choice is between constructing a history of how symptoms that could be associated with endometriosis were addressed by societies over human history or, alternatively, constructing a history of the progress in recognizing the specific condition as revealed through descriptions in scientific papers that incorporated pathological features typical of the various phenotypes of endometriosis. In choosing between these two options, we must be aware that even today with the wide availability of modern imaging techniques (some of which, like magnetic resonance and elastography, look promising), it is considered impossible to arrive at a definitive diagnosis of superficial peritoneal disease without histological confirmation.

The first of these choices can be informative of the way science and society have progressed over time, but cannot constitute a history of the specific condition. It is for this reason that we opted for a historical account centered on the presently agreed definition of endometriosis as characterized by "the presence of functional endometrial-like tissue outside the uterus, but in the pelvic cavity, or even outside, with evidence that lesions are cellularly active, or have an effect on normal physiology" [2].

Broadening this approach, we argue that the history of endometriosis starts with the first description of "reddish/bluish" spots in the peritoneal cavity, chocolate cysts in the ovary, or rectovaginal nodules. It is perhaps surprising, but to our knowledge there is no account from older text that describes the macroscopic features of endometriosis. In 1999, Vincent J. Knapp [3] unearthed from the US National

Library of Medicine a number of old *dissertations* dating back to the seventeenth and the eighteenth centuries. These are purported to describe the characteristic clinical features of endometriosis linked to lesions that range from ulcers to inflammations of the uterus. Knapp expressed his conviction that already in 1690, Daniel Schrön [4] described ulcers on the peritoneum that were prominent in the bladder, the intestines, the broad ligament, and the outside of the uterus and the cervix. Although Schrön refers to these as inflammatory, Knapp prefered to interpret them as evidence of non-ovarian endometriosis. This is curious because Schrön described lesions that could become pus filled and that could form abscesses. Knapp also claims that in 1739 Crell [5] had described "ovarian endometriotic cysts" with the words: "*Tumorem fundo uteri externe adherentem describit.*" We have analyzed the texts he quoted in detail but concluded that, with the possible exception of the report by Crell, the other cases are not consistent with the macroscopic features of endometriosis [6].

More recently, Nezhat et al. [7] went further in their review of ancient texts. They adopted a broad view of representations of pelvic pain as being evidence of endometriosis even though menstrual pain was rarely ever chronicled. The depictions they gathered included of women who are unwell, or who were attended by medical personnel or by other healers of the time. Nezhat et al. interpreted a mention of "hysteria" as an indication of endometriosis. Despite the vast effort they expended, this approach does not focus on the characteristic symptom of cyclical pain and was only able to take account of the pathognomonic histological features when considering the contributions of authors from the mid-nineteenth century onward. We believe that when Nezhat et al. stated that they were "*filtering all histories and ancient reports through the lens of modern understandings*," they made the classic error of presuming a knowledge in ancient physicians that they simply could not have had.

To trace the beginning of its identification as a specific condition and not a description of symptoms that can only be loosely linked to endometriosis, we need to search for early microscopical descriptions of heterotopic endometrial cells and stroma. This will naturally be linked to developments in microscopy, the invention of the microtome, and the introduction of microscopic examination of excised tissues or organs. It is because of the importance of this paradigm that endometriosis has been referred to as a "modern disease" [8]; the adjective in no way implies that the condition did not exist in ancient times. It simply emphasizes the relatively recent recognition of the nature of the condition.

Roland Batt attempted to place the discovery of adenomyosis and endometriosis in the context of the prevailing scientific trends of the time of the first observations [9]. The approach is illuminating as it demonstrates the important influence of attitudes and circumstances on scientific progress. The narrative provided by Batt is as much a history of the evolution of histopathology in the late nineteenth century, as it is about endometriosis.

One final point is the idea of attributing the exclusivity of a scientific discovery should be demystified: almost 60 years ago, Clarke [10] argued against searching for "forerunners" or "anticipators" and viewed such an effort to be rooted in a concept of historical reversibility which destroys the very object of the history of science. This is especially true when discussing endometriosis, because of a heated debate, starting toward the end of the nineteenth century and ending only in 1920, on the nature of the *epithelial cells* found in the peritoneal cavity. For this reason, while it is apt to acknowledge the role of all those who contributed to the debate, emphasis should be made on contributions which eventually led to the identification of a hitherto unrecognized condition.

1.2 The Identification of Adenomyoma

The starting point when describing the events leading to the identification of the condition we call today endometriosis is one of nomenclature. Until the 1920s all *mucosal invasions of peritoneal organs*, including the myometrium, were referred to under the common name *adenomyoma*. This word was coined around the end of the nineteenth century: in 1896, both Cullen and von Recklinghausen described the presence of adenomyomas [11, 12]. They were followed by Pick [13] and Rolly [14, 15] in 1897. Further details of reports on adenomyomas, the findings by Carl Rokitansky [16], and the comprehensive definition of adenomyoma by Lockyer [17] are provided in Chap. 25.

Early investigators focussed on the nature of the "epithelial invasions" they observed, and up until the publication of two seminal articles by Thomas Cullen in 1903 and 1920 [18, 19], the majority of pathologists and gynecologists rejected the hypothesis that the glands were endometrial. As an example, in his early writings, von Recklinghausen [12] argued that adenomyomas were the result of displacement of Wolffian (mesonephric) remnants, and, as late as 1918, Lockyer wrote: *Nothing but the topography of the tumour, nothing but laborious research entailing the cutting of serial sections in great numbers, can settle the question as to the starting point of the glandular inclusions for many of the cases of adenomyoma* [17].

As mentioned, the clearest description of the morphological and clinical features of adenomyomas was made by Thomas Cullen. He collected 90 uteri with adenomyomas and described their various features; his specimens were from the myometrial wall (where he appreciated the continuity between eutopic endometrial glands and the nests in the myometrium), uterine horns, the subserosa, uterine ligaments, ovaries, and even the umbilicus. Cullen considered intrauterine and peritoneal "invasion" by endometrial cells as one disease; the adenomyoma [17].

1.3 Adenomyosis and Endometriosis

Once the endometrial nature of mucosal invasions of intraperitoneal organs became generally accepted, its two variants (intra- and extra-myometrial) came to be regarded as distinct entities.

In 1925, Oskar Frankl [20] described the anatomical features of what would later be named endometriosis interna to distinguish it from endometriosis externa (peritoneal, or deep lesions). He coined the expression *adenomyosis uteri*, which he chose in order to stress the absence of any inflammatory origin. He also specified the criteria for differentiating adenomyosis from adenomyoma (the various phenotypes of endometriosis).

In the same year in which Frankl published his seminal paper, Sampson introduced the term *endometriosis*, although he also utilized the term *implantation adenomyoma* [21]. His view was that the term Müllerian, as advocated by Bailey [22], would have been inclusive and correct, but he feared that it may imply an embryonic origin. He was also opposed to terms such as endometriomyoma, or endometrioma as advocated by Blair Bell [23].

Clements [24], who reconstructed the history of gynecological pathology in a series of articles, mentions that Sampson was not initially comfortable with the term and felt the necessity (as did Frankl [20] when advocating the term adenomyosis) to explain his choice of nomenclature. Then, in 1927, Sampson asserted the "birth of endometriosis" with the words: *The histologic study of the ectopic endometrial tissue in a direct or primary endometriosis (so-called adenomyoma of mucosal origin) shows that this tissue contains venous capillaries similar to those of the mucosa lining the uterine cavity* [25].

1.4 Identifying the Various Phenotypes of Endometriosis

It is probable that the first variant to be described of what we today call endometriosis is the affection of the ovaries. With few exceptions [26], this phenotype was not described under the name adenomyoma, and, from its early description, it was considered a separate entity. What is not clear is whether the endometrial nature and its implications were recognized in early descriptions of these lesions. In terms of priority, Roland Batt [9, 27] staunchly defended the view that Carl Rokitansky was the first to describe an ovarian endometrioma. However, Rokitansky's own contemporaries hardly acknowledged that he had described an ovarian endometrioma (or, more exactly, a "tarry or chocolate cyst of the ovary," or an "ovarian hematoma," or a "hemorrhagic cyst of the ovary" as they were variably described at the end of the nineteenth century). Batt [9] attempted to explain the reason for this neglect by arguing that Rokitansky utilized a personal definition of tumors, coining *sarcomas* for the *benign growths* and leaving for malignancies *"their ancient characteristic appellation cancer, carcinoma.*" When, in 1860, Rokitansky published his cases [16], he did that under the title *On the neoplasm of uterus glands, on uterine and ovarian sarcomas*, and there he described "*an ovarian cystosarcoma.*" A careful reading of the article leaves little doubt that Rokitansky identified epithelial structures in this tumor and considered these as endometrial in nature. However, the case in question was that of a 66-year-old woman who had a fist-sized ovarian tumor. The description may fit with what is now recognized as a serous or mucous multicystic lesion, but almost certainly not an endometrioma.

We found no reference to the work of Rokitansky in any of the articles published around the turn of the nineteenth century when discussing the presence of *hemorrhagic cysts* of the ovary. The explanation may rest in the simple fact that the features he described in the case of the ovary, irrespective of the terminology used, were too different from the *ovarian hematomas*, or *chocolate/tarry cysts* to be taken into consideration. Emge [28], who analyzed Rokitansky's work, reached the conclusion that he used the word sarcoma to indicate an abnormally active proliferation of the stroma; if so, abnormal and active proliferation of glandular tissue in a multicystic tumor of the ovary of a 66-year-old marasmic woman could hardly be suggestive of endometriosis.

1.4.1 The Ovarian Endometrioma

Leaving this controversy aside, the first unequivocal description of the presence of endometrial tissue within an ovary was that provided by Russel in 1899 [29] who presented a case in which, under the microscope, he observed a number of "*areas, which were an exact prototype of the uterine glands and interglandular connective tissue*." These glands "*were arranged as in normal uterine mucous membrane and opened into spaces, their epithelium being continuous with its lining membrane*." Of importance is that glands and interglandular connective tissue were occasionally surrounded by bundles of smooth muscle. This description is similar to the observation made by Hughesdon [30] in his report on endometriotic cysts. Hughesdon noted the presence of smooth muscle fibers surrounding the cysts. A similar observation was made recently by Fukunaga [31] and is likely to be related to smooth muscle metaplasia.

A few additional cases were published within a few years [32–41], and around 1920 researchers began to identify the lining of these cysts with the endometrium: Casler [38] reported on a woman who – after hysterectomy – "*consistently maintained that, at regular monthly intervals, she menstruated for a part of one day each month*." The author specified that the "*the entire cyst, or uterine cavity as it really is, is lined throughout by a single layer of tall columnar epithelium of the uterine type, and in places cilia can be made out*." It is noteworthy that Casler found "*interlacing bundles or columns of smooth muscle tissue*." It is possible that the repeated presence of muscular tissue convinced researchers that this was a variety of adenomyoma. Cullen [19] published three cases: the first featured a cyst with a *brownish membrane* and *an inner lining of cylindrical epithelium*; in the second, the right ovary looked like *a miniature uterine cavity*. In this latter case, the ovarian cyst was associated with a *widespread adenomyoma of the recto-vaginal septum*. Cullen interpreted this to indicate that *the uterine mucosa on the surface of the ovary was due to an overflow of the adenomyoma of the recto-vaginal septum*. The third case featured an ovary containing several cavities filled with partially coagulated blood.

In 1921, Donald [26] published a clear description of "ovarian adenomyomas" and observed that they contain endometrial stroma and smooth muscle, that the lining can exhibit changes similar to the endometrium and a decidual-like reaction in pregnancy. He noted a frequent association with lesions in the rectovaginal space, bilaterality, and that they are not malignant. Of interest is his comment that this type of cyst was long known to all gynecologists but that its true nature had only recently been discovered.

1.4.2 Deep Endometriotic Nodules

The work of Donald [26] seems to have established a connection between "ovarian adenomyomas" and lesions that we would call today deep endometriosis. In earlier days this type of pathology may have been described as posterior parametritis. Interestingly, reference to this condition exists in literature from the late nineteenth century [42, 43] and perhaps earlier, but it was not attributed to the presence of endometrial epithelium. In 1909, Meyer [44] established a link between these lesions and the one he called parametritis nodosa posterior. Subsequently, Eden and Lockyer [45] further described these lesions, drawing a distinction between this type of lesion which they refer to as adenomyoma and which does not lead to suppuration and other causes of pelvic cellulitis, which are mostly related to peripartum sepsis. Eden and Lockyer included in their paper a reproduction of the image published by Kleinhans [46] in 1904 of an adenomyoma affecting the so-called recto-genital septum. In his early work, Cullen [18] does not include description of disease affecting the pouch of Douglas, but this entity becomes a major focus of his article published in 1920 [19] where he credits Lockyer [47], with enabling him to recognize that his first cases belonged to this disease category. In his book of 1918, Lockyer [17] refers as the earliest description the two cases by Pfannenstiel [48] and one case by von Herff [49].

1.4.3 Superficial Peritoneal Lesions

The identification of peritoneal lesions seems to have occurred at the same time as that of "adenomyomas." These were initially reported as lesions of the organs covered by the peritoneum. The work of both Lockyer [17] and Cullen [19] included descriptions of lesions affecting extrauterine locations (e.g., the fallopian tubes, ovaries, round ligament). There is considerable debate in the early literature about the origin of these lesions. Iwanoff [50] proposed that they arise through metaplasia; others viewed the glands as derived from remnants of Gartner's duct. Meyer [44] held the view that the glands develop in response to a sequence of inflammation, induration, and epithelial hypertrophy and that the source of the epithelium is the overlying peritoneum. He also maintained that the surrounding mantle originates from original connective tissue that exhibited a response to inflammation. Lockyer concluded that it had not been proven that mature uterine mucosa provided any gland tissue for any extrauterine growth and maked a clear distinction between an origin from dystopic (congenital) or orthotopic (mature) mucosa [47].

1.5 The Work of Sampson

Today, the vast majority of investigators adopted the theory of retrograde menstruation favored by Sampson [25] to explain the pathogenesis of endometriosis. However, his contribution to the study of endometriosis preceded the enunciation of the theory that is commonly linked to his name. In 1921, Sampson [41] described 23 cases of "perforating hemorrhagic cysts of the ovary" which he also called chocolate cysts. The cysts varied in diameter from 1 to 9 cm; mostly they ranged from 2 to 4 cm. Sampson described the presence of a perforation on the lateral or on the free surface of the ovary and instances where ovarian lesions coexisted with lesions in the pouch of Douglas. He went on to suggest that the latter arise secondary to leakage of irritating content from the ovarian cysts. He speculated as to the origin of pelvic lesions outside the ovary and wrote: *The question naturally arises: In what way do the contents of the cyst or ovary cause the development of these adenomas? Is it due to some 'specific' irritant present in the cyst contents which stimulates the peritoneal 'endothelium', thus causing a metaplasia and the development of 'endometrial' tissue typical both in structure and in function? Some may assert that dormant 'endometrial' epithelium may be present in the tissues soiled by the contents of the cyst and this is stimulated to further growth. It seems to me that the condition found in many of these specimens is analogous to the implantation of ovarian papilloma or cancer on the peritoneal surface of the pelvis from the rupture of an ovarian tumor containing these growths.*

The theory of ovarian lesions as a source of pelvic affections has in the view of Bailey [22]: *revolutionized all pre-existing theories as to the etiology of pelvic growths of adenomyomatous nature by pointing out their obvious relationship to the so-called chocolate cysts found in the ovaries*. But Bailey, who performed serial sections of ovarian lesions, disagreed with Sampson's description [51], as he believed that a chocolate cysts is best described as a cavity and that such lesions don't form a cyst; rather, the invading endometrium erodes the ovary, and the mouth of the cavity becomes obstructed by adhesion to its surroundings. In addition, he did not accept the view of the ovary as an incubator, hot bed, or intermediary host in the development of pelvic implantation of adenomas of endometrial type. Bailey believed that there is no in-out perforation of the ovarian lesion, since these develop from outside the ovary. Bailey's view eventually prevailed, and the theory that endometriotic lesions on the cortex invade the ovary is today widely recognised [52]. It was only some 30 years later that Hughesdon [30] could demonstrate that in 90% of the cases, the wall of the cyst is made up of ovarian cortex and that its active invagination is followed by a more or less abortive attempt at creating a muscular wall. The end result is a pseudo-uterus, to which follows a more or less abortive attempt at a muscular wall.

In conclusion, it is through his work on "*adenomas of endometrial (Müllerian) type*" that Sampson focused attention on peritoneal endometriosis and, in 1927, enunciated the theory, still considered the most likely explanation, that *peritoneal endometriosis* is *due to the menstrual dissemination of endometrial tissue into the peritoneal cavity*. In subsequent years, a number of investigations provided evidence that added weight to his hypothesis.

References

1. Benagiano G, Brosens I. Who identified endometriosis? Fertil Steril. 2011;95:13–6.
2. Audebert A, Backstrom T, Barlow DH, Benagiano G, Brosens I, Bühler K, Donnez J, Evers JL, Pellicer A, Mettler L, et al. Endometriosis 1991: a discussion document. Hum Reprod. 1992;7:432–5.
3. Knapp VJ. How old is endometriosis? Late 17th- and 18th-century European descriptions of the disease. Fertil Steril. 1999;72:10–4.
4. Schrön D. Disputatio inauguralis medica de ulceribus uteri. Jena: Rudolf Wilhelm Crause, Literis Krebsianis; 1690. p. 6–17.
5. Crell J. Tumorem fundo uteri externe adhaerentem describit. Wittenberg: Typis; 1739. p. 5–8.
6. Benagiano G, Brosens I, Lippi D. The history of endometriosis. Gynecol Obstet Investig. 2014;78:1–9.
7. Nezhat C, Nezhat F, Nezhat C. Endometriosis: ancient disease, ancient treatments. Fertil Steril. 2012;98(6 Suppl):S1–62.
8. Brosens I, Benagiano G. Endometriosis, a modern syndrome. Indian J Med Res. 2011;133:581–93.
9. Batt RE. A history of endometriosis. London, Heidelberg: Springer; 2011.
10. Clark JT. The philosophy of science and the history of science. In: Clagett M, editor. Critical problems in the history of science. Madison: The University of Wisconsin Press; 1959. p. 103–40.
11. Cullen T. Adenomyoma of the round ligament. Johns Hopkins Hosp Bull. 1896;7:112–3.
12. von Recklinghausen F. Die Adenomyomata und Cystadenomata der Uterus und Tubenwandung: Ihre Abkunft von Resten des Wolffischen Körpers [*The adenomyomas and cystadenomas of the uterus and tube wall: their origin from remnants of the Wolffian body*]. Berlin: August Hirschwald Verlag; 1896.
13. Pick L. Ein neuer Typus des voluminösen paroophoralen Adenomyoms – zugleich über eine bisher nicht bekannte Geschwulst Form der Gebärmutter (Adenomyoma psammopapillare) und über totale Verdoppelung des Eileiters [*A new type of voluminous paroophoral adenomyomas – both on a previously unknown form of tumour of the uterus (adenomyoma psammopapillare) and a total doubling of the oviduct*]. Arch Gynakol. 1897;54:117–206.
14. Rolly F. Ueber einen Fall von Adenomyoma uteri mit Uebergang in Carcinom und Metastasenbildung. [*About a case of uterine adenomyoma with transition to carcinoma and metastasis*]. Archiv Pathol Anat Physiol Klinische Med. 1897;150:555–82.
15. Rolly F. Ueber einen Fall von Adenomyoma uteri etc. [*About a case of adenomyoma of the uterus, etc.*]. Virchows Arch. 1897;150:555.
16. Rokitansky C. Über Uterusdrüsen-Neubildung in Uterus- und Ovarial-Sarcomen. [*On the neoplasm of uterus glands on uterine and ovarian sarcomas*]. Zeitschr Gesellschaft der Aerzte in Wien. 1860;16:577–81.
17. Lockyer C. Fibroids and allied tumours (Myoma and Adenomyoma). London: Macmillan; 1918.
18. Cullen TS. Adeno-myome des uterus. Berlin: Verlag von August Hirschwald; 1903.
19. Cullen TS. The distribution of adenomyomata containing uterine mucosa. Arch Surg. 1920;1:215–83.
20. Frankl O. Adenomyosis uteri. Am J Obstet Gynecol. 1925;10:680–4.
21. Sampson JA. Inguinal endometriosis (often reported as endometrial tissue in the groin, adenomyoma in the groin, and adenomyoma of the round ligament). Am J Obstet Gynecol. 1925;10:462–503.
22. Bailey KV. The etiology, classification and life history of tumours of the ovary and other female pelvic organs containing aberrant Müllerian elements, with suggested nomenclature. J Obstet Gynaecol Br Emp. 1924;31:539–79.

relevant, albeit somewhat higher at 11%, but is largely dependent on the method of diagnosis [1]. The 10% prevalence estimate continues to prevail within the clinical, research and lay literature. However, estimates of prevalence and incidence of endometriosis across studies and countries paint a very inconsistent picture of the epidemiology of the disease. This chapter will review global estimates of the prevalence and incidence of endometriosis. In doing so, we discuss the wide variations in estimates according to the study design and geographical location of the research. We preface this chapter by discussing the challenges associated with diagnosing endometriosis, including the individual, social and healthcare determinants of receiving a diagnosis, and the consequences for estimating the epidemiology of endometriosis.

2.2 The Diagnosis of Endometriosis and the Dilemma for Epidemiology

A major challenge in studying the epidemiology of endometriosis is identifying women with the disease. Currently, the only method of definitively diagnosing endometriosis is via surgery followed by histological confirmation [2]. Historically, the surgical approach has been regarded as the 'gold standard' for the diagnosis of endometriosis, but even this method has its pitfalls leading some to argue that we haven't yet reached that gold standard [3]. Surgery relies on visual confirmation of the disease and depends on the skills and expertise of the operating surgeon. Even when surgery is supplemented with histology, the quality and size of the biopsy taken at the time of surgery influences the histological outcome [4]. Consequently, the surgical and histological diagnoses may not always be compatible.

Surgery to diagnose endometriosis is invasive and may not be necessary, desired or even geographically or financially possible for many women [5]. Owing to the problems with surgical diagnosis of endometriosis, there has been a recent shift in the diagnostic paradigm for endometriosis [6] away from the surgical approach, to recognise the value of the clinical diagnosis that prioritises women's symptoms [7]. Clinical practice has long supported the conservative treatment of endometriosis, with several professional bodies advocating for treatment of endometriosis prior to surgical confirmation [4, 6]. Early diagnosis is paramount to providing women with specialised, interdisciplinary care to maintain or improve quality of life. Yet tensions remain about best practice methods for diagnosing endometriosis [6, 8], amidst rapid advances in imaging of the disease [9], which has implications for estimating the epidemiology of the disease. Although improved diagnosis of endometriosis is vital, discussions about the diagnosis of endometriosis rarely address the broader social and healthcare disparities that often create insurmountable barriers for women to receive a diagnosis. The epidemiology of endometriosis will only be as good as the underlying sample population.

2.3 Individual, Social and Medical Determinants of an Endometriosis Diagnosis

In diagnosing endometriosis, the focus is largely on individuals within medical settings. Symptoms, scans and surgery often dictate who receives a diagnosis. The diagnosis of endometriosis is however more complex, incorporating an interconnecting web of social, healthcare, economic, cultural and political factors that determine who receives a diagnosis (see Fig. 2.1). Women often have to navigate their way through the multiple layers to receive a diagnosis, rendering a diagnosis of endometriosis inaccessible to many women. The challenges for women receiving a diagnosis have significant ramifications for estimating the epidemiology of the disease. Social and healthcare disparities have prevented an accurate picture of the epidemiology of endometriosis, by biasing estimates in favour of those who have financial and geographical access to healthcare [5].

2.3.1 Individual Determinants of Diagnosis

Age is an important determinant of endometriosis. Although peak incidence is between 30 and 34 years [1, 10], symptoms of endometriosis can emerge during adolescence following the onset of menarche. Lengthy diagnostic delays of between 7 and 12 years [11–13] mean that the vast majority of studies estimating the

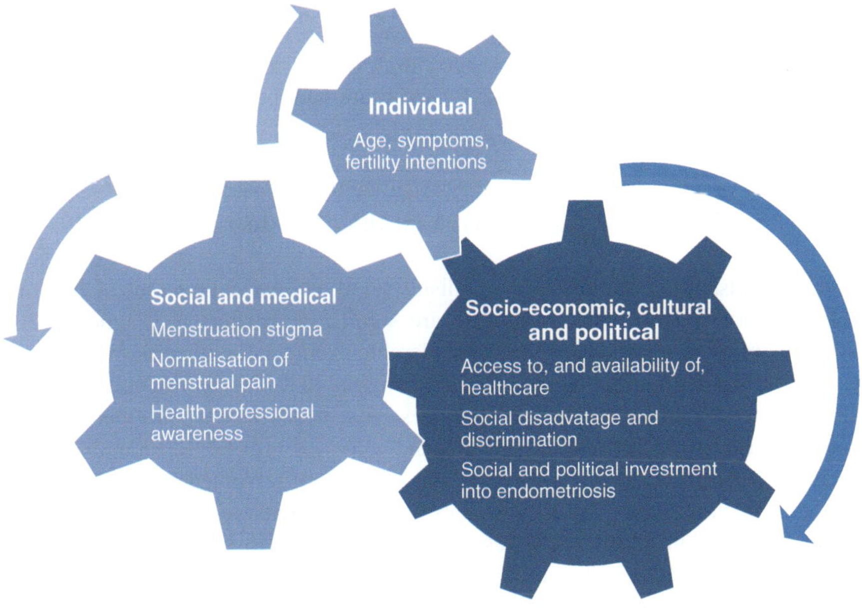

Fig. 2.1 Individual, social, medical, socio-economic, cultural and political factors that influence the diagnosis of endometriosis

prevalence of endometriosis are based on adult women presenting for surgery. Studies focusing on the prevalence and incidence of endometriosis in adolescents are limited but report high prevalence rates [14–16]. In a systematic review based on 15 studies largely from the USA, Janssen and colleagues reported that 62% of adolescents undergoing surgery for chronic pelvic pain or dysmenorrhea had endometriosis [16]. A more recent review of the literature identified only four new studies but reported similarly high prevalence rates [15]. The percentage of adolescents with endometriosis in this review varied from 36% to 100% [15]. These findings are largely due to the reliance on small, hospital-based samples of adolescents undergoing surgical investigation for chronic pelvic pain, at 'high risk' for endometriosis. Population-based studies of endometriosis in adolescents, which may be more representative of the population, are currently absent from the literature.

2.3.2 Symptoms

Endometriosis is often synonymous with severe period pain (dysmenorrhea), but there is a broad experience of symptoms including pain during sex, urination, defecation and gastrointestinal symptoms [2]. Women can report complex symptom combinations of varying severity throughout the menstrual cycle, although some women will remain asymptomatic. The unpredictability of symptoms and overlap with other conditions make it incredibly challenging to distinguish endometriosis from other conditions [17]. High rates of endometriosis among asymptomatic women with infertility suggest that infertility may be a potential marker of the disease [18]. Women's symptomatology is increasingly valued in the clinical diagnosis of endometriosis [6, 8]. Statistical algorithms for the diagnosis of endometriosis based on the common symptoms have been examined, but are not reliable enough to replace surgical methods of diagnosis [19].

2.3.3 Social and Medical Constructions of Endometriosis

The stigmatisation, normalisation and dismissal of women's symptoms of endometriosis in social and medical contexts are significant barriers to diagnosis [20]. Women are often socialised to feel considerable shame and embarrassment related to menstruation, described as 'menstruation stigma' [21, 22]. In most cultures, menstruation is constructed as a 'dirty' process that needs to be concealed and not socially discussed [22]. Some cultures and religions ascribe considerable taboo related to menstruation, such that girls and women are separated from the community during menstruation [23, 24]. These practices generate a culture of secrecy about normal, biological processes that are important to women's reproductive health. Consequently, across cultures, adolescents and women may have limited knowledge about what is and is not 'normal' regarding menstruation [25].

The normalisation of women's menstrual pain often contributes to diagnostic delay [11]. This may begin in the family context where mothers and sisters construct the pain of menstruation as a rite of passage, synonymous with being a 'woman'. Reassurance from family that menstrual pain is a normal part of 'womanhood' may discourage women from seeking support for pain or heavy bleeding, even when symptoms progress, further delaying diagnosis [21]. Unfortunately, when women do seek professional support, health professionals may similarly construct a discourse of women's menstrual pain as a normal, biological imperative. Qualitative research with women with endometriosis has extensively described how health professionals dismiss the severity of women's pain and symptoms as 'normal' [26, 27]. Women may feel stigmatised by health professionals who invalidate their experience by describing their symptoms as 'psychologically' constructed [28]. Women's attempts to manage the disease for years without professional guidance can disrupt their self-concept, intimate relationships and broader social lives [20, 26, 29]. The limited awareness of endometriosis among the social and medical community remains a significant challenge in the diagnosis and management of the disease. Long diagnostic delays for endometriosis creates bias by producing low incidence and prevalence rates, particularly among adolescent and among young women because of the difficulties accessing a diagnosis.

2.3.4 Socio-economic, Cultural and Political Context

A major challenge to the diagnosis of endometriosis is that socio-economic disparities often determine who receives a surgical diagnosis of endometriosis [5]. Women from socially disadvantaged backgrounds typically have poor access to health services and may be less likely to seek professional support, forming a barrier to diagnosis [30, 31]. As the diagnosis of endometriosis necessitates surgical confirmation, research is largely based on women attending hospital who have good access to healthcare [32]. Clinical stereotypes of women with endometriosis as 'white, lean, middle class, career-driven women' typify the bias in the research samples [32]. Women who are obese may face considerable difficulty receiving a diagnosis of surgically confirmed endometriosis due to social and medical reasons [33, 34]. A previous multi-country study of women with surgically confirmed endometriosis reported increasing diagnostic delays with increasing body mass index [33]. Evidence from a systematic review also suggests that ethnic disparities exist in the diagnosis of endometriosis, with Black women less likely to be diagnosed with endometriosis than White women [35]. These disparities sum up the long-standing inherent diagnostic biases in the research related to endometriosis.

Socio-economic disparities are inextricably linked to the political and cultural context in which individuals live. Political and cultural responses to endometriosis vary considerably across countries, but are constantly evolving, and have the potential to drive significant changes in prevalence and incidence rates for the disease. Greater political investment into endometriosis helps to build research, education and healthcare initiatives that improve care for women living with endometriosis. Endometriosis support groups in several high-income countries have been central to mobilising social and political awareness of the disease. Advocacy groups have voiced women's concerns, validated their pain and experiences and advocated for improved healthcare treatment and funding into endometriosis. The 2020 national inquiry into endometriosis in the UK reported an average of 8 years to diagnosis, suggesting there has been no reduction in diagnostic times for women in the last decade [36]. In Australia, decades of lobbying from endometriosis advocacy groups led to the initiation of the Federal Government's 2018 National Action Plan for Endometriosis [37]. Almost $13 million has been invested to improve social awareness, medical diagnosis and treatment and research [37].

The impact of increasing awareness of endometriosis and a focus on education can be positive, and has been reported to have an effect, with two Australian studies reporting a decrease in time to diagnosis to 4.9 and 6.4 years [38, 39]. More recently in the USA, lobbying from the Endometriosis Foundation of America generated increased federal research funding for endometriosis from $13 million in 2019 to $26 million in 2020 [40]. Increased international awareness of endometriosis will inevitably change what we know about the disease and its epidemiology. Countries that invest in ongoing surveillance of endometriosis by ensuring that high-quality data is collected will significantly expand knowledge on the aetiology and progression of the disease.

2.4 Epidemiology of Endometriosis

Epidemiology is concerned with identifying the distribution and determinants of disease in specific populations. Epidemiologists can examine the distribution of disease in different ways, often by estimating both the *incidence* and the *prevalence* of the disease. Incidence refers to the number of new cases identified in the population during a specific period. Prevalence refers to the total number of people affected with the disease at one time point or during a specific period [41]. The number of new cases of disease in the population (incidence) over time can provide an estimate of the total number of cases within the population during a period of time (prevalence). Prevalence and incidence are therefore complementary, but are two different frequency measures that cannot be used interchangeably. In comparing incidence and prevalence across studies, it can often be difficult even if the same disease definition is used [41]. Variations in study designs including the size and type of sample and the sources used to identify women with endometriosis can yield substantially different estimates.

2.4.1 Incidence

Annual incidence rates for endometriosis are largely based on studies using hospital or insurance claims databases and vary anywhere from 0.97 to 1.87 cases per 1000 person-years or 0.72 to 3.5 per 1000 women [42–46]. Variations in the historical timing of these studies that cannot account for changes to the clinical diagnosis and classification of endometriosis and the increased social and health professional

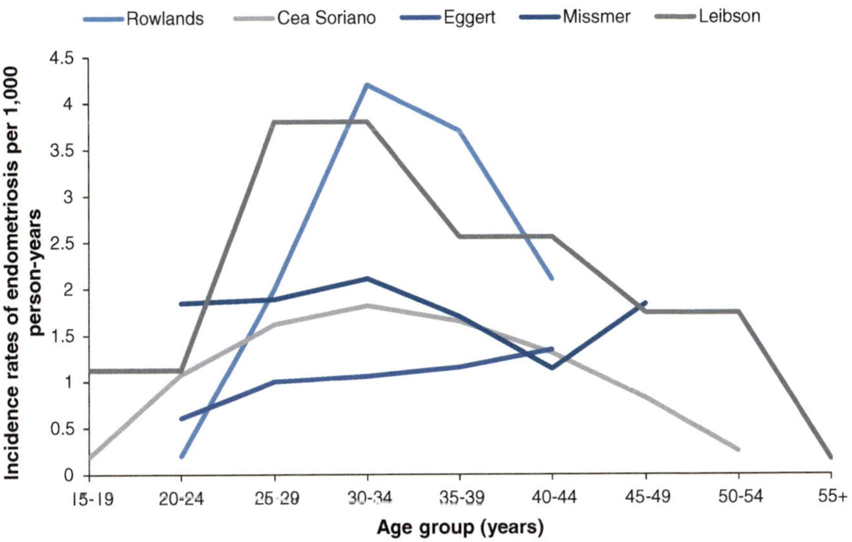

Fig. 2.2 Age-specific incidence rates of endometriosis across studies. Rowlands is based on national hospital discharge data from 2000 to 2018 [1]; Cea Soriano is based on medical records from multiple health databases from 2000 to 2010 [10]; Eggert is based on national hospital discharge data from 1990 to 2004 [47]; Missmer is based on national survey data during 1989–1999 [18]; Leibson is based on medical records from 1987 to 1999 [46]

awareness of the disease over time are likely to explain the heterogeneity in incidence rates.

Historically, endometriosis is characterised as a disease affecting women of 'reproductive age', with peaks in incidence often reported between the ages of 30 and 34 years (see Fig. 2.2). Peaks in incidence of endometriosis may reflect the timing of the first surgical diagnosis, which may be delayed due to social, medical and financial reasons or only prioritised when women experience problems becoming pregnant. Hysterectomy for the treatment of endometriosis may also contribute to peaks in incidence, but published data are lacking.

The natural incidence of the disease is limited due to the lack of longitudinal data available. However, endometriosis does occur in adolescents, with some reporting pain commencing at the time of menarche [2]. Menarche may be an important marker of onset, but inflammatory processes that give rise to endometriosis may begin from birth [48]. Life course data on endometriosis would significantly add to the evidence base.

2.4.2 Prevalence

2.4.2.1 Hospital/Clinic Samples

The literature related to the prevalence of endometriosis has historically relied on hospital-based samples of women attending surgery. These studies rely on small samples of women with underlying pathology and pain who are at 'high risk' of endometriosis. Prevalence in these studies range anywhere from 0.2% to 71.4% but was estimated to be 22.9% overall in a review of the literature [14]. The proportion of women with endometriosis was higher among women undergoing surgery for chronic pelvic pain (29.1%) and infertility (26.8%), and to a lesser extent a hysterectomy (15.6%), surgery for ovarian cancer (10.0%) and tubal sterilisation (5%) [14]. Studies based on women presenting for surgery often represent women with more severe forms of endometriosis, who may have better access to health services, which introduces selection bias into the study design. Estimates using small, clinical samples are therefore unlikely to translate well to the larger population of women living with endometriosis.

2.4.2.2 General Population Samples: Hospital Records/Insurance Claims Databases

To obtain larger, more nationally representative samples of women with endometriosis, several studies have used hospital records or insurance claims databases to identify women with disease, often via International Classification of Diseases (ICD) diagnostic coding. These studies offer a different perspective on the prevalence of endometriosis by looking at extent of the disease within larger samples, often at the population level. Relative to the hospital-based samples of women with endometriosis, prevalence rates tend to be lower in studies relying on hospital and insurance databases. A review of the literature estimated a 5% endometriosis prevalence rate among samples from hospital and insurance databases, but crude percentages ranged from 0.8% to 23.2% [14]. The availability of data in these studies ranged from 5 to 15 years [14]. However, some studies estimated prevalence at one time point during this period, known as 'point prevalence', often yielding low prevalence estimates. A point prevalence may underestimate the prevalence of endometriosis because the data only captures a select group of women diagnosed at a single point in time. Certain groups may be underestimated using this approach, including young women who may be less often referred for surgery, contributing to biased estimates. The alternative approach is to look at a 'cumulative' or 'period' prevalence for the population over the entire period available. Given the long diagnostic delays experienced by women with endometriosis, a period prevalence will be more robust than a point prevalence.

2.4.2.3 General Population Samples: Self-Reported Endometriosis

While the literature largely focuses on women with surgically confirmed endometriosis, there has been a recent shift in the diagnostic paradigm [6] to recognise the value of the clinical diagnosis and the importance of women's symptoms [7]. The prevalence of endometriosis in studies based on general population samples where endometriosis is largely self-reported ranges from 0.7% to 8.6%, with an estimated overall prevalence of 3.4% [14], which is only slightly higher than studies relying on endometriosis diagnoses from hospital or insurance databases. Most studies relying on women's self-reported endometriosis do not clinically confirm diagnoses of endometriosis, potentially limiting the validity of the studies. However, the value of these estimates from these studies lies in capturing women who are treated more conservatively, who cannot access or afford surgery or who decide against surgical intervention. These are most likely to be younger women, women from disadvantaged backgrounds and those residing outside of metropolitan areas where access to clinical expertise for endometriosis may be limited.

2.4.2.4 Geographical Variations in Prevalence

Global data on endometriosis are largely from high-income countries, with low-income countries underrepresented in the literature. The 2013 Global Burden of Diseases Study estimated the global prevalence of endometriosis was 4.8% during 2006 and 2013 [49] and more recently estimated a 3.0% decline in age-standardised rates from 2007 to 2017 [50]. A recent review of the literature during 1989 and 2019 identified 69 studies estimating the prevalence and incidence of endometriosis, with most originating in Europe (38%) followed by Asia (27%), North America (22%) and to a much lesser extent Africa (10%) [14]. Only two studies from Australia were identified [14]. Wide variations in the prevalence of endometriosis were reported both within and across regions, largely due to the methodological heterogeneity across the studies (see Fig. 2.3). The prevalence of endometriosis was highest for Asia at 20.7% but dropped to less than 1% when weighting by study sample size [14]. Moderately high prevalence rates were reported in the Americas (13.0%), followed by Europe (11.5%) and Africa (10.6%), with substantially lower rates reported in Australia (3.6%). A more recent estimate of endometriosis prevalence in

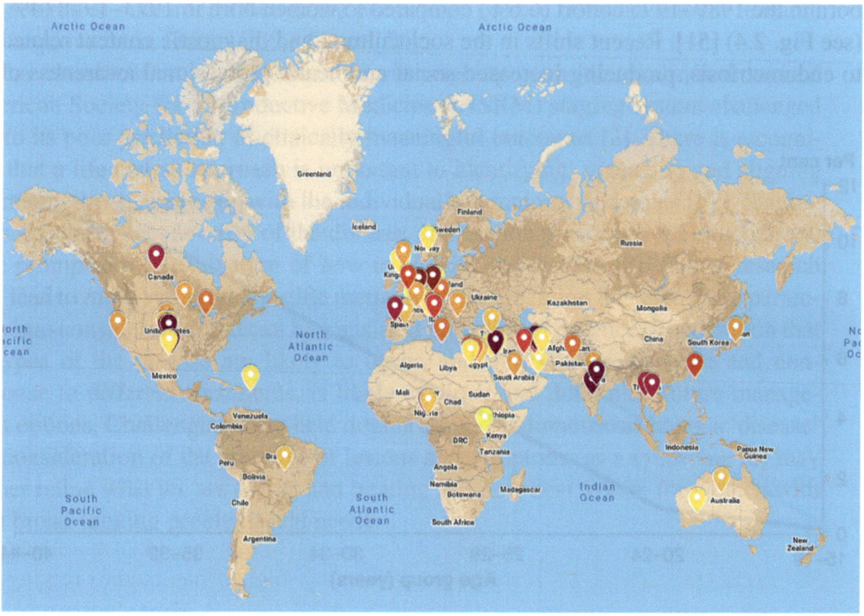

Fig. 2.3 Global geographic spread and variation in endometriosis prevalence [14]. Darker colours represent higher prevalence

speculated that the cysts could include histology of mucous membrane of the tube and papillary tumors of the ovary [15, 42].

Kossmann argued that not only was the tubal epithelium involved in production of Müllerian remnant cysts but also that these did not come from mature epithelial elements. Rather, they came from the germinal epithelium that developed into the tubes. This is an early understanding that it is differentiation rather than transdifferentiation that is the process of conversion from a normal Müllerian or non-Müllerian precursor (stem cell) to endometriosis. This implied that it was the differentiation of the germinal epithelium into endometriosis [15, 32, 33].

3.2.3 Müllerian Rests

The growth of endometriosis from Müllerian cellular rests was suggested as early as 1896 by Cullen, who discussed the striking resemblance of the glandular elements of adenomyomata (endometriosis) to those of the uterine mucosa. Cullen suggested that adenomyomata (endometriosis) may be an "abnormal embryonic deposit of a portion of Müller's duct" in or near the area of normal embryologic Müllerian development. This was reinforced in Russell's publication of endometriosis hidden within an ovary and behind adhesions in an otherwise normal ovary [15, 32].

Batt expanded Cullen's and Russell's [15, 32] observations into a theory of congenital Müllerianosis. Batt's Müllerianosis concluded that four congenital Müllerian diseases paralleled the four acquired diseases endometriosis, endosalpingiosis, adenomyosis, and endosalpingiosis [24]. Müllerianosis was due to tissue misplaced during organogenesis. The four acquired diseases of the same name were due to retrograde menstrual, venous, or lymphatic dissemination. Müllerianosis might also include organoid diseases such as accessory and cavitated uterine masses [43] and ovarian [44], broad ligament [44], inguinal [45], or rectal endomyometriosis [46]. As in endometriosis, there is a debate of whether these are one or two diseases and if either or both are congenital [47, 48].

Redwine focuses on endometriosis in his theory that began as Mülleriosis, not Müllerianosis, focusing on Müllerian rests and more recently expanded to Mülleriotic mesodermal disease to cover distal sites of endometriosis [35, 36, 49]. This converts his theory from an aberrant placement of Müllerian tissue during organogenesis to an in situ metaplasia theory. As mesoderm is the source not only of Müllerian tissue but also the endothelial vascular lining, then endometriosis can form by metaplasia anywhere in the body that has a vascular supply [35]. His Mülleriotic mesodermal disease theory concludes, with no data, that mesodermal derivatives can only develop into endometriosis if they are present at the end of organogenesis and cannot be disseminated after birth. He considers incisional endometriosis as a form of induced mesodermal metaplasia, not surgical transplantation.

3.2.4 Endometriosis as a Cell of Origin

Sampson suggested that pelvis endometriosis resulted from intra-abdominal spill of endometriotic tissue from the ovaries [50]. Transplantation of endometriosis at the time of surgery into the abdominal wall is not uncommon. Fragments of pelvic endometriosis are considered the source of this surgical transplantation [51].

3.2.5 Wolffian (Mesonephric) Duct Remnants

Batt cited von Recklinghausen as suggesting the displacement of Wolffian (mesonephric) duct remnants as a source of endometriosis in 1896 [52] (Batt 2011, p. 2708). Stevens described isolated small vaginal wall nodules with characters of diffuse adenomyoma of the uterus. He contended that a Wolffian origin was more than likely for the small adenomyoma than Müllerian origin [53].

3.2.6 Coelomic Metaplasia

Lockyer quotes Klages as considering coelomic metaplasia and inflammatory induction as early as 1912 [54]. Coelomic metaplasia is the differentiation of peritoneal, pleural, pericardial, or omental stem cells [23] into endometriosis. Coelomic metaplasia is based on a common mesothelial precursor of the Müllerian ducts and the coelomic surfaces that include the peritoneum, pleura, and pericardium in embryonic development [14, 23]. Novak concluded that the mucosa of the genital organs represented only varying modifications of coelomic epithelium, the primitive peritoneum, and could be responsible for endometriosis and endosalpingiosis. Novak's conclusions were a modification of Iwanoff, who concentrated on the uterine serosa, and Meyer, who considered metaplasia to be an inflammatory process. Novak rejected the inflammatory theory and replaced it with an unknown endocrine origin but understood that the theories were not facts [14, 55]. In 1968, Ridley summarized the possible initiating events as hormonal stimulation, inflammation, or biochemical or immunologic factors [14, 31]. The biochemical or immunologic products may be due to retrograde, venous, or lymphatic dissemination [31].

Although Ridley concluded that Iwanoff's and Meyer's theories of metaplasia of the coelomic epithelium, the primitive peritoneum, championed by Novak had its origin by evolution and not proof [14], recent markers suggest that metaplasia may be a factor in both female and male endometriosis [31, 34]. Although coelomic metaplasia may be an explanation for peritoneal and pleural endometriosis, it does not explain bowel or pulmonary parenchymal involvement [23].

3.2.7 Endometrium (Acquired Müllerian Disease)

Endometrium was first considered as the origin in 1921 [50]. The endometrium is one of the Müllerian derivatives that includes the uterus, tubes, and upper vagina. It was suggested as the cell of origin in retrograde [50, 56, 57], venous [58], and lymphatic [56] dissemination theories of acquired endometriosis. Those theories are covered later in this chapter.

3.2.8 Bone Marrow Stem Cells

Bone marrow-derived stem cells (BMDSCs) and possibly progenitor cells can migrate to the endometrium and incorporate and grow in endometriosis [2, 37]. BMDSCs can increase the growth of endometriosis in association with previous endometriotic lesions, particularly in the endometrial stromal cell population. Research suggests that endometrial cell proliferation results from stem cell-derived trophic factors that lead to the growth of endometriosis [59]. However, there is no current evidence that BMDSCs can cause de novo growth of endometriosis.

3.3 Methods of Dissemination

3.3.1 Retrograde Menstruation

Retrograde menstruation theory was first discussed by Sampson in 1921 at a meeting of the American Gynecologic Society. It is noted that near-duplicate versions were in *Archives of Surgery* [60] and *Transactions of the American Gynecological Society* [50]. The *Transactions* version includes "Two possible sources of the origin of these small tubules or cysts of endometrial type in the ovary present themselves: first, congenital, and second, acquired from the implantation of epithelium escaping from the tube during menstruation and its subsequent invasion of the ovary." It was later expanded into a full theory in 1927 [57]. Although Sampson proposed the retrograde menstruation theory, he also realized that this was inadequate to explain all endometriosis. He also published his venous dissemination study in 1927 [58] and multiple other possibilities in his lifetime [1]. Although he is sometimes only credited for retrograde flow, he also discussed that endometrium and endometriosis were different in "structure and in function" and this may have resulted from metaplasia [60]. Dr. Sampson also pointed out the inflammatory nature of endometriosis [61]. Like many of the study theory, he knew that theory was of secondary importance. The care of patients, the need to solve unsolved problems of endometriosis, and the acquisition of knowledge were primary [62].

The growth of autotransplants of the endometrium to produce endometriosis was confirmed in 1925 in animal models [63]. But the ability of a whole tissue endometrial fragments to pass through the tubes and to survive and grow was questioned

[27]. More recently, it has been realized that stem cells and not whole tissue fragments are likely the form of the cell of origin [2]. Even harvested stromal cells can be used to develop three-dimensional, in vitro, self-organizing cultures of epithelial cells called organoids. Organoids can be incorporated as in vitro models in drug and toxicity testing and disease modeling and substitutes for animal models [28–30].

3.3.2 Retrograde Menstruation Model

Sampson's theories did not explain all of the recent advances in science. To explain those, Wang et al. have suggested a retrograde menstruation model that would incorporate the molecular genetic findings, clonality immune surveillance concepts, chronic inflammation, receptors pathways, dysregulated inflammation–hormonal loop, and cancer-associated mutations associated with developing endometriosis [2].

3.3.3 Hematogenous/Venous Dissemination

Hematogenous dissemination of intrauterine contents into the vascular tree which was proposed by Sampson in 1918 is a concept to explain puerperal infection [64]. Sampson later expanded this to be a potential source of endometrium in endometriosis [58]. More recently, this has been suggested as a potential source of pulmonary and more distal endometriosis [65].

3.3.4 Lymphatic Dissemination

The presence of endometrial tissue and lymph nodes was published as early as 1906 by Taussig according to Javert. Taussig is said to have reported endometrial tissue in 1 of the 26 lymph nodes in dissection for cervical carcinoma [56]. Lymphatics have been suggested as a source of pulmonary [65] and abdominal wall endometriosis [51].

Lenz et al. examined immunophenotype in cases with and without node involvement and found that they were similar in the proliferative phase. They found strong nuclear estrogen receptor (ER) and progestogen receptor expression in more than 90% of endometrial glandular and stromal cells. In the late secretory phase, there was a significant decrease of ER expression only in cases without nodal involvement. There was a perineural spread with neural hypertrophy, hyperplasia, and involvement of the ganglia. Histologically and immunohistochemically, deep infiltrating endometriosis and lymph node endometriosis appear to be the same. The marked endometriosis-associated neural changes (endometriotic neuropathy) could be a cause of impaired function of the affected organs and a cause of pain [66].

3.3.5 Surgical Transplantation

Transplantation of endometriosis at the time of surgery into the abdominal wall is not uncommon. Fragments of pelvic endometriosis are considered the source of this surgical transplantation [51].

3.3.6 Embryonic Development

Müllerian rests can be disseminated during embryonic development due to deviation in Müllerian development. Signorile et al., using immunohistochemical stains for CD10 and cytokeratin 7, characterized fetal ectopic endometrium and demonstrated that it displays the morphological phenotype of the fetal endometrium. This was found in the area of the rectovaginal pouch and septum [67, 68]. This is the same area as type III deep infiltrating endometriosis that was considered as a possible embryonic rest by Koninckx and Martin [69]. Koninckx's image of a non-visualized example is associated with a flat pouch of Douglas and no discernable uterosacrals suggestive of a congenital anomaly [70].

3.3.7 Direct Extension

In 1916, Stevens noted adenomyomatous growths arising from the uterus and invading the rectum, sigmoid, and other parts. These could be traced by serial sections from the uterine mucous membrane to the growth [53]. Donnez et al. have concluded that adenomyosis externa is a retrocervical or retrouterine extension of adenomyosis to deep endometriotic nodules. They may also be the cause of deep anterior endometriosis (bladder adenomyotic nodules) [26]. Direct infiltration through the diaphragm after retrograde menstruation and intraperitoneal spread may be a source of pulmonary endometriosis [31].

3.4 Conclusion

Theories can be useful in education, guiding research, understanding concepts, postulating physiology, and discussing why therapy might work. However, theory can create a false narrative and should not be used to guide treatment. The inappropriate application of theory to guide medical care can result in the tomato effect or medical reversal.

A cell of origin is needed to begin any theory of endometriosis. That cell must be accompanied by a method of dissemination (metastasis) or in situ development during embryonic or fetal development or after birth; a force of stimulation, activation, or induction of the transition from a cell of origin to endometriosis; and mechanisms for growth to become endometriosis. Inactivation and clearance can potentially limit the growth.

Research should be directed at early events in the development of endometriosis to prevent the development of fibrosis, which may only respond to surgery or natural inactivation. Those early events include the dissemination of the cell of origin, activation, and growth. In the retrograde theory, this also includes attachment and infiltration. If endometriosis can be controlled or inactivated before it develops into deep infiltrating, ovarian, or severely adhesive disease, surgery may be avoided, or the degree of surgery that is needed may be decreased.

Early treatment could be aimed at inflammation, pain, activation of transformation, estrogenic stimulation, immune dysfunction, an overload of the immune system, comorbidities, decreasing delayed care, and quality of life. Although this chapter focuses on cells of origin and methods of dissemination, that is not meant to detract from research on activation, transition, and inactivation.

Declaring that surgery for early surgical diagnosis is needed based on tertiary or quaternary center data on women with a long delay to a diagnosis is not scientific. Data are needed on the results of early treatment of symptoms suggesting endometriosis or of surgical approaches in adolescents and adults with the delay interval documented to separate those treated early from those with delayed treatment. Before an early diagnosis is a reasonable goal, we need medical or surgical treatment protocols that are proven to work.

References

1. Martin DC. Endometriosis concepts and theories 2021. Available: https://www.danmartinmd.com/endoconcepts.html. Accessed 15 Jan 2021.
2. Wang Y, Nicholes K, Shih IM. The origin and pathogenesis of endometriosis. Annu Rev Pathol. 2020;15:71–95.
3. Knox B, Ong YC, Bakar MA, Grover SR. A longitudinal study of adolescent dysmenorrhoea into adulthood. Eur J Pediatr. 2019;178:1325–32.
4. Shafrir AL, Farland LV, Shah DK, Harris HR, Kvaskoff M, Zondervan K, Missmer SA. Risk for and consequences of endometriosis: a critical epidemiologic review. Best Pract Res Clin Obstet Gynaecol. 2018;51:1–5.
5. Staal AH, Van der Zanden M, Nap AW. Diagnostic delay of endometriosis in the Netherlands. Gynecol Obstet Investig. 2016;81:321–4.
6. Redwine DB. Conservative laparoscopic excision of endometriosis by sharp dissection: life table analysis of reoperation and persistent or recurrent disease. Fertil Steril. 1991;56:628–34.
7. Roman H, Merlot B, Forestier D, Noailles M, Magne E, Carteret T, Tuech JT, Martin DC. Nonvisualized palpable bowel endometriotic satellites. Hum Reprod. 2021;36(3):656–65.
8. Yeung P, Sinervo K, Winer W, Albee RB. Complete laparoscopic excision of endometriosis in teenagers: is postoperative hormonal suppression necessary? Fertil Steril. 2011;95:1909–12, 1912 e1.
9. Remorgida V, Ferrero S, Fulcheri E, Ragni N, Martin DC. Bowel endometriosis: presentation, diagnosis, and treatment. Obstet Gynecol Surv. 2007;62:461–70.
10. Remorgida V, Ragni N, Ferrero S, Anserini P, Torelli P, Fulcheri E. How complete is full thickness disc resection of bowel endometriotic lesions? A prospective surgical and histological study. Hum Reprod. 2005;20:2317–20.
11. Badescu A, Roman H, Aziz M, Puscasiu L, Molnar C, Huet E, Sabourin JC, Stolnicu S. Mapping of bowel occult microscopic endometriosis implants surrounding deep endometriosis nodules infiltrating the bowel. Fertil Steril. 2016;105:430–4. e26.

12. Pandiyan N, Surya P, Khan SD, Pandiyan R. Early diagnosis of endometriosis – quo Vadis? Chettinad Health City Med. 2015;4:68–9.
13. Sampson JA. Inguinal endometriosis (often reported as endometrial tissue in the groin, adenomyoma in the groin, and adenomyoma of the round ligament). Am J Obstet Gynecol. 1925;10:462–503.
14. Ridley JH. The histogenesis of endometriosis: a review of facts and fancies. Obstet Gynecol Surv. 1968;23:1–35.
15. Russell WW. Aberrant portions of the Mullerian duct found in an ovary. Johns Hopkins Hosp Bul. 1899;94,95,96:8–10.
16. Waldeyer. Die epithelialen Eierstocksgeschwülste, insbesondere die Kystome. Arch Gynakol. 1870;1:252–316.
17. Goodwin JS, Goodwin JM. The tomato effect. Rejection of highly efficacious therapies. JAMA. 1984;251:2387–90.
18. Karnaky KJ. The use of stilbestrol for endometriosis; preliminary report. South Med J. 1948;41:1109–11.
19. Prasad V, Cifu A, Ioannidis JP. Reversals of established medical practices: evidence to abandon ship. JAMA. 2012;307:37–8.
20. Ottolina J, Schimberni M, Makieva S, Bartiromo L, Fazia T, Bernardinelli L, Vigano P, Candiani M, Gentilini D. Early-life factors, in-utero exposures and endometriosis risk: a meta-analysis. Reprod Biomed Online. 2020;41:279–89.
21. Zondervan KT, Becker CM, Missmer SA. Endometriosis. N Engl J Med. 2020;382:1244–56.
22. Veurink M, Koster M, Berg LT. The history of DES, lessons to be learned. Pharm World Sci. 2005;27:139–43.
23. Ganshina IV. Serous cavities of coelomic origin as possible organs of the immune system. Part 1. Biol Bull Rev. 2016;6:497–504.
24. Batt RE, Yeh J. Mullerianosis: four developmental (embryonic) mullerian diseases. Reprod Sci. 2013;20:1030–7.
25. Batt R, Mitwally MF. Endometriosis from thelarche to midteens: pathogenesis and prognosis, prevention and pedagogy. J Pediatr Adolesc Gynecol. 2003;16(6):337–47.
26. Donnez J, Dolmans MM, Fellah L. What if deep endometriotic nodules and uterine adenomyosis were actually two forms of the same disease? Fertil Steril. 2019;111:454–6.
27. Scott RB, Te Linde RW. Clinical external endometriosis. Obstet Gynecol. 1954;4:502–10.
28. Boretto M, Cox B, Noben M, Hendriks N, Fassbender A, Roose H, Amant F, Timmerman D, Tomassetti C, Vanhie A, Meuleman C, Ferrante M, Vankelecom H. Development of organoids from mouse and human endometrium showing endometrial epithelium physiology and long-term expandability. Development. 2017;144:1775–86.
29. Boretto M, Maenhoudt N, Luo X, Hennes A, Boeckx B, Bui B, Heremans R, Perneel L, Kobayashi H, Van Zundert I, Brems H, Cox B, Ferrante M, Uji IH, Koh KP, D'Hooghe T, Vanhie A, Vergote I, Meuleman C, Tomassetti C, Lambrechts D, Vriens J, Timmerman D, Vankelecom H. Patient-derived organoids from endometrial disease capture clinical heterogeneity and are amenable to drug screening. Nat Cell Biol. 2019;21:1041–51.
30. Koninckx PR, Ussia A, Martin DC. How organoids from endometrium and endometriosis could help to understand the pathogenesis of endometriosis. Fertil Steril. 2021;115:78–9.
31. Lagana AS, Garzon S, Gotte M, Vigano P, Franchi M, Ghezzi F, Martin DC. The pathogenesis of endometriosis: molecular and cell biology insights. Int J Mol Sci. 2019;20(22):5615.
32. Cullen TS. Adenomyoma of the round ligament. Johns Hopkins Hosp Bull. 1896;62-63:112–4.
33. Kossmann R. I. Zur Pathologie der Urnierenreste des Weibes. Gynecol Obstet Investig. 1895;1:97–131.
34. Zamecnik M, Hostakova D. Endometriosis in a mesothelial cyst of tunica vaginalis of the testis. Report of a case. Cesk Patol. 2013;49:134–6.
35. Redwine DB. Cartoon science vs evidence-based science. New York: Endometriosis Foundation of America; 2019.
36. Redwine DB. Cartoon science and the origin of endometriosis. In: Redwine D, editor. Mea culpa nunca. 12: 52; 2021.

37. Santamaria X, Mas A, Cervello I, Taylor H, Simon C. Uterine stem cells: from basic research to advanced cell therapies. Hum Reprod Update. 2018;24:673–93.
38. Evers JH. Is adolescent endometriosis a progressive disease that needs to be diagnosed and treated? Hum Reprod. 2013;28:2023.
39. Martin DC. Laparoscopic appearance of endometriosis (35-mm slide set), revised 2020, http://www.danmartinmd.com/files/lae1988.pdf. Memphis: Resurge Press; 1988.
40. Koninckx PR, Ussia A, Adamyan L, Wattiez A, Gomel V, Martin DC. Pathogenesis of endometriosis: the genetic/epigenetic theory. Fertil Steril. 2019;111:327–40.
41. Nagel W. Ueber die Entwickelung des Urogenitalsystems des Menschen. Arch Mikrosk Anat. 1889;34:269–384.
42. Marchand FJ. Beiträge zur Kenntniss der Ovarialtumoren. Abbandl der Naturf Gesellsch: Habittationsschrift, Halle; 1879. p. xiv.
43. Acien P, Bataller A, Fernandez F, Acien MI, Rodriguez JM, Mayol MJ. New cases of accessory and cavitated uterine masses (ACUM): a significant cause of severe dysmenorrhea and recurrent pelvic pain in young women. Hum Reprod. 2012;27:683–94.
44. Clement PB. The pathology of endometriosis: a survey of the many faces of a common disease emphasizing diagnostic pitfalls and unusual and newly appreciated aspects. Adv Anat Pathol. 2007;14(4):241–60. https://doi.org/10.1097/PAP.0b013e3180ca7d7b. PMID: 17592255
45. Gonzalez RS, Vnencak-Jones CL, Shi C, Fadare O. Endomyometriosis ("uterus-like mass") in an XY male: case report with molecular confirmation and literature review. Int J Surg Pathol. 2014;22(5):421–6. https://doi.org/10.1177/1066896913501385. PMID: 24651910.
46. La Greca G, Colarossi C, Di Mattia P, Gozzo C, De Zuanni M, Piombino E, Memeo L. Endomyometriosis of the rectum with disseminated peritoneal leiomyomatosis 8 years after laparoscopic myomectomy: a case report. Front Surg. 2021;8:666147. https://doi.org/10.3389/fsurg.2021.666147.
47. Kiyak H, Seckin KD, Karakis L, Karacan T, Ozyurek ES, Resit Asoglu M. Decidualized juvenile cystic adenomyoma mimicking a cornual pregnancy. Fertil Steril. 2020;113:463–5.
48. Takeuchi H, Kitade M, Kikuchi I, Kumakiri J, Kuroda K, Jinushi M. Diagnosis, laparoscopic management, and histopathologic findings of juvenile cystic adenomyoma: a review of nine cases. Fertil Steril. 2010;94:862–8.
49. Redwine DB. Mulleriosis. The single best-fit model of the origin of endometriosis. J Reprod Med. 1988;33:915–20.
50. Sampson JA. Perforating hemorrhagic (chocolate) cysts of the ovary. Their importance and especially their relation to pelvic adenomas of the endometrial type ("adenomyoma" of the uterus, rectovaginal septum, sigmoid, etc.). Trans Am Gynecol Soc. 1921b;46:162–241.
51. Marras S, Pluchino N, Petignat P, Wenger JM, Ris F, Buchs NC, Dubuisson J. Abdominal wall endometriosis: an 11-year retrospective observational cohort study. Eur J Obstet Gynecol Reprod Biol X. 2019;4:100096.
52. von Recklinghausen F. Die Adenomyome und Cystadenome der Uterus- und Tubenwandung ihre Abkunft von Resten des Wolff 'schen Korpers. In: Freund WA, editor. Klinische Notizen zu den voluminosen Adenomyomen des Uterus. Berlin: Verlag von August Hirschwald; 1896.
53. Stevens T. Adenomyoma of the rectovaginal septum. Proceedings Royal Soc Med. 1916;9:1–17.
54. Lockyer C. Fibroids and allied tumours (myoma and adenomyoma) their pathology, clinical features and surgical treatment London. Macmillan; 1918.
55. Novak E, Novak ER. Textbook of gynecology. The Williams & Wilkins Company: Baltmore; 1952.
56. Javert CT. Pathogenesis of endometriosis based on endometrial homeoplasia, direct extension, exfoliation and implantation, lymphatic and hematogenous metastasis, including five case reports of endometrial tissue in pelvic lymph nodes. Cancer. 1949;2:399–410.
57. Sampson JA. Peritoneal endometriosis due to menstrual dissemination of endometrial tissue into the peritoneal cavity. Am J Obstet Gynecol. 1927a;14:422–69.
58. Sampson JA. Metastatic or embolic endometriosis, due to the menstrual dissemination of endometrial tissue into the venous circulation. Am J Pathol. 1927b;3:93–109.

59. Chen P, Mamillapalli R, Habata S, Taylor HS. Endometriosis cell proliferation induced by bone marrow mesenchymal stem cells. Reprod Sci. 2020;28(2):426–34.
60. Sampson JA. Perforating hemorrhagic (chocolate) cysts of the ovary. Their importance and especially their relation to pelvic adenomas of the endometrial type ("adenomyoma" of the uterus, rectovaginal septum, sigmoid, etc.). Arch Surg. 1921a;3:245–323.
61. Sampson JA. Endometriosis of the sac of a right inguinal hernia, associated with a pelvic peritoneal endometriosis and an endometrial cyst of the ovary. Am J Obstet Gynecol. 1926;12:459–83.
62. Sampson JA. The development of the implantation theory for the origin of peritoneal endometriosis. Am J Obstet Gynecol. 1940;40:549–57.
63. Jacobson VC. Certain clinical and experimental aspects of ectopic endometriosis. Bull N Y Acad Med. 1925;1:385.
64. Sampson JA. The escape of foreign material from the uterine cavity into the uterine veins. Am J Obstet Gynecol. 1918;78:161–75.
65. Alifano M, Trisolini R, Cancellieri A, Regnard JF. Thoracic endometriosis: current knowledge. Ann Thorac Surg. 2006;81:761–9.
66. Lenz J, Chvatal R, Fiala L, Konecna P, Lenz D. Comparative immunohistochemical study of deep infiltrating endometriosis, lymph node endometriosis and atypical ovarian endometriosis including description of a perineural invasion. Biomed Pap Med Fac Univ Palacky Olomouc Czech Repub. 2020;165(1):69–79.
67. Signorile PG, Baldi F, Bussani R, D'armiento M, De Falco M, Baldi A. Ectopic endometrium in human foetuses is a common event and sustains the theory of mullerianosis in the pathogenesis of endometriosis, a disease that predisposes to cancer. J Exp Clin Cancer Res. 2009;28:49.
68. Signorile PG, Baldi F, Bussani R, D'Armiento M, De Falco M, Boccellino M, Quagliuolo L, Baldi A. New evidence of the presence of endometriosis in the human fetus. Reprod Biomed Online. 2010;21:142–7.
69. Koninckx PR, Martin DC. Deep endometriosis: a consequence of infiltration or retraction or possibly adenomyosis externa? Fertil Steril. 1992;58:924–8.
70. Koninckx PR, Cornillie FJ. Infiltrating endometriosis: infiltration, retraction or adenomyosis externa? In: Martin DC, editor. Atlas of endometriosis. London: Gower Med Publ; 1993.

Pathogenesis of Endometriosis: Role of Platelets in Endometriosis

4

Sun-Wei Guo

Contents

4.1 Introduction

It is often said that endometriosis shares several similarities with cancer, such as invasion and recurrence. At the cellular level, endometriotic lesions are also similar to cancer cells, as manifested in increased proliferation [1], resistance to apoptosis [2], inflammation [3, 4], angiogenesis [5], epigenetic aberration [6], and even cancer-driver mutations [7, 8]. Despite all these similarities with cancer, it is evident that endometriotic lesions differ drastically from malignant tumors in many ways. Aside from the lack of fatality, the most notable is the fact that, unlike cancer,

S.-W. Guo (✉)
Shanghai Obstetrics and Gynecology Hospital, Fudan University, Shanghai, China

Shanghai Key Laboratory of Female Reproductive Endocrine-Related Diseases, Fudan University, Shanghai, China

E. Oral (ed.), *Endometriosis and Adenomyosis*,
https://doi.org/10.1007/978-3-030-97236-3_4

endometriotic lesions do not grow unbridled. In fact, the most glaring feature of endometriotic lesions is cyclic bleeding [9], so much so that one salient commonality seemingly shared by all hormonal drugs for treating endometriosis is that they stop cyclic bleeding [9]. Yet bleeding is a quintessential hallmark of vascular injury and thus tissue injury. Once there is a tissue injury, the evolutionarily conserved program in all organisms would initiate tissue repair. In other words, endometriotic lesions thus resemble wounds. As such, they would experience the well-known four, somewhat overlapping, phases in tissue repair: hemostasis, inflammation, proliferation, and remodeling. Among all these phases, platelets are the first responder [10]. Thus, it is pertinent to review the roles of platelets in endometriosis, especially in its progression.

4.2 A Primer on Platelets

Platelets are anucleated cells originating from cytoplasmic fragmentation of megakaryocytes mostly in the bone marrow and contain a plethora of pre-synthesized bioactive molecules, stored in at least three major types of granules: α-granules, dense granules, and lysosomes. Their roles are best known in hemostasis in tissue repair and thrombosis [11]. In many ways, platelets are at pivotal nexus of tissue injury/damage and inflammatory response, destined to initiate the repair of injured tissues. If, however, platelet activation is erratic or uncontrolled, it leads to chronic inflammation associated with numeric pathological conditions, including cancer [12], fibrosis [13], and atherothrombosis [14].

4.3 Role of Platelets in Endometriosis Progression

Traditionally, endometriosis is viewed as an estrogen-dependent disease, characterized by the increased local production of estrogens due to molecular aberrations in steroidogenesis [15] and estrogen-dependent growth of endometriotic lesions. Increasingly, it also has been recognized as a pelvic inflammatory condition [16], characterized by the overexpression of inflammatory genes, the release of proinflammatory cytokines (especially tumor necrosis factor-α (TNF-α) and interleukin-1β (IL-1β)) [17, 18], NF-κB activation [4, 19, 20], and the infiltration of macrophages and lymphocytes [21–23]. Yet extensive research in the last two decades clearly indicates that inflammation and coagulation are intimately intertwined. In fact, emerging evidence indicates that inflammation also activates the coagulation cascade and coagulation modulates the inflammatory activity [24, 25]. Platelets are now increasingly viewed as inflammatory effector cells involved in the activities across the spectrum from acute inflammation to adaptive immunity [26, 27]. In fact, activated platelets are found to play a critical role in initiating inflammation [28].

In the last 5–6 years, the role of platelets in the development of endometriosis has been gradually revealed and recognized. This starts with the realization that endometriotic lesions are practically and fundamentally wounds undergoing repeated tissue injury and repair.

4.3.1 Platelet Activation by Thrombin/Thromboxane

Cyclic bleeding [9] would inevitably lead to platelet aggregation, but there is evidence also for extravasated platelets in endometriosis [29]. This raises a question as whether endometriotic lesions themselves secrete any inducers of platelet activation. In fact, it has been reported that increased production of thromboxane (TX) B2 (TXB_2), a metabolite of TXA_2, by endometriotic stromal cells stimulated with IL-1β, increases tissue factor (TF) expression as well as thrombin concentration in peritoneal fluid (PF) from women with endometriosis [29], suggesting that endometriotic lesion and its microenvironment are conducive to platelet activation and aggregation.

Indeed, it has been reported that endometriotic stromal cells secrete thrombin and TXA_2 and induce platelet activation and aggregation in a density-dependent fashion [30]. More specifically, co-culture of platelets with endometriotic stromal cells results in increased concentration of TXB_2, thrombin, and transforming growth factor β1 (TGF-β1) in a density-dependent manner [30]. Treatment of endometriotic stromal cells with hirudin (a specific thrombin inhibitor) and ozagrel (a TXA_2 synthase inhibitor), but not apyrase (an adenosine diphosphate (ADP) pathway inhibitor), resulted in significant and substantial suppression of platelet aggregation [30]. Thus, platelets and endometriotic cells mutually affect the functions of the other, collectively promoting the progression of endometriotic lesions.

4.3.2 Platelets-Mediated Suppression of Cytotoxicity in NK Cells in Endometriosis

It has long been suspected that a deficient immune system may be involved in the pathogenesis and pathophysiology of endometriosis [31, 32]. In women with endometriosis, the decreased NK cell cytotoxicity is reported as early as the 1990s [33–36]. The reduced cytotoxicity may play an essential role in the formation of lesions by permitting the survival, implantation, and proliferation of endometrial cells [37, 38]. Later research indicates the increased expression of some killer cell immunoglobulin-like receptors (KIRs), such as KIR two Ig domains and long cytoplasmic tail 1 (KIR2DL1) [39–41], KIR2DL4 [42], KIR3DL1 [39], and NKG2A [43], and the reduced expression of natural killer cell p46-related protein (NKp46), an activating receptor on NK cells [44], which may be responsible for decreased NK cell cytotoxicity in women with endometriosis.

As a key component of the innate immune system, NK cells are a subset of lymphocytes that provide the first-line defense against pathogens or transformed cells by exerting cytotoxicity and the regulation of cytokine producing effector functions

[45, 46]. The function of NK cells is tightly regulated by a plethora of functionally opposing surface receptors (inhibitory) that bind major histocompatibility complex (MHC) class I molecules and protect "self" and activating receptors that bind ligands on virus-infected or tumor cells [47]. Activating and inhibitory receptors can transduce, respectively, positive and negative signals to regulate NK cell cytotoxicity and cytokine release [48]. NK cells may play an important role in peritoneal immune surveillance, possibly eliminating endometrial cells that have been regurgitated into the pelvic cavity through retrograde menstruation, with low or absent expression of MHC class I and stress-induced expression for activating NK receptors in women without endometriosis.

NKG2D or natural killer group 2, member D, which is encoded by killer cell lectin-like receptor subfamily K, member 1 (KLRK1) gene, provides costimulatory signals to CD8αβ T cells and potently activates NK cells, so potent that it can even override inhibitory signals by MHC class I molecules or "self" signals [49, 50]. It is one of the best characterized activating receptors expressed by NK and T cells and binds to several ligands in human and mouse [51]. NKG2D ligands (NKG2DLs) include MHC class I chain-related proteins A (MICA) and B (MICB) and UL16-binding protein (ULBP) 1–6.

In endometriosis, it has been reported that the platelet count, WBC count, MPV, platelet activation rate, and the TGF-β1 concentration in the peritoneal fluid (PF) of women with endometriosis are significantly elevated when compared to those of women without endometriosis [52]. In addition, the TGF-β1 concentration correlated positively with the platelet activation rate, suggesting that activated platelets could be accountable, at least in part, for the increased TGF-β1 concentration [52]. The cytotoxicity of freshly isolated NK cells treated with PF of women with endometriosis is significantly reduced as compared with that of women without endometriosis, consistent with previously reported data [34, 36, 53]. Consistent with the report that TGF-β1 suppresses KLRK1 expression and cytotoxicity of NK cells [54–56], it is found that the platelet activation rate and the TGF-β1 concentration in the PF correlate negatively with the NKG2D expression in NK cells isolated from the PF of women with endometriosis [52]. Moreover, it has been demonstrated that the NKG2D expression level and the cytotoxicity in NK cells freshly isolated from healthy male volunteers are found to be significantly reduced if co-cultured with PF from women with endometriosis, but the TGF-β1 blockade attenuates this effect [52]. Taken together, these data suggest that platelet-derived TGF-β1 may be responsible for reduced NKG2D expression as well as reduced cytotoxicity of NK cells in women with endometriosis.

In addition, in vivo data indicate that anti-endometriosis effect of platelet depletion is mediated, at least in part, by increased NK cell cytotoxicity against endometriotic cells [57]. In fact, platelet coating, as could happen following menstruation, provides coated cells a physical shield against NK cells as well as increased MHC-I expression, effectively providing a cloak of "pseudo-self" to coated cells to shield against NK cell lysis [57]. Co-incubation of target cells with platelets reduces the expression of NKG2D ligands MICA and MICB and reduces the NK cell cytotoxicity. In addition, co-incubation of NK cells with platelets also impairs the NK cell cytotoxicity. And this impaired NK cell cytotoxicity is not due to the increased NK cell apoptosis, but, rather, through reduced NK cell degranulation and IFN-γ production, and reduced expression of activating receptors NKG2D and NKp46 and increased expression of inhibitory receptor KIR2DL1 in NK cells [57]. On the other hand, TGF-β1 neutralization abolishes the aberrant expression of NKG2D, NKp46, and KIR2DL1 and partially restores the impaired NK cell cytotoxicity induced by activated platelets and their releasates [57]. Taken together, these data provide a strong piece of evidence that activated platelets, which are aggregated in ectopic endometrium following cyclic bleeding or simply due to the release of platelet-activating molecules by endometriotic stromal cells [30], impair NK cell cytotoxicity in endometriosis through multiple mechanisms and both soluble and membrane-bound factors are required for NK cell evasion of endometriotic cells.

These data are consistent with the previous report that platelet-derived soluble factors do not induce NK cell death [58]. They are also consistent with the report that platelet-derived TGF-β1 suppresses the expression of NKG2D on NK cells, resulting in reduced cytotoxicity in women with endometriosis, but inhibition of TGF-β1 signaling reverses the reduction [52].

4.3.3 Platelets Promote Progression of Endometriotic Lesions

Inspired by the glaring hallmark of endometriotic lesions, i.e., cyclic bleeding, it has been reported that the involvement of platelets in the development of endometriosis has been reported [29, 59, 60]. Incidentally or not, platelets release copious amount of TGF-β1 upon activation [61]. In fact, platelets release far more TGF-β1 than most cell types [62]. Yet TGF-β1 is a prototypical factor in epithelial-mesenchymal transition (EMT) [63], fibroblast-to-myofibroblast transdifferentiation (FMT) [64, 65], and subsequent fibrogenesis [66]. Platelet-derived TGF-β and direct platelet-tumor cell contacts also have been shown to synergistically activate the TGF-β/Smad and NF-κB pathways in cancer cells, resulting in EMT and enhanced metastasis [67]. More importantly, as endometriotic lesions undergo cyclic and repeated bleeding (and thus injury) and repair reminiscent of fibrogenesis in other organs, it also ultimately leads to fibrosis in endometriotic lesions [29]. As such, the core pathways underlying fibrogenesis in endometriosis are likely to be similar to other organ types [68]. That is, endometriotic lesions are fundamentally wounds that undergo cyclic or *re*peated *t*issue *i*njury *a*nd *r*epair (ReTIAR), prompting EMT and FMT and resulting in smooth muscle metaplasia (SMM) and ultimately fibrosis.

Activated platelets, through the release of TGF-β1 and the induction of TGF-β/Smad signaling pathway, promote EMT, FMT, and differentiation to smooth muscle cells (SMCs) in endometriosis, resulting in increased cell contractility, collagen production, and ultimately to fibrosis. TGF-β blockade, however, reverses these processes. Prolonged exposure to activated platelets further turned endometriotic stromal cells into differentiated SMCs, giving rise to SMM as seen in endometriosis, especially deep endometriosis and adenomyosis. These data, taken together, provide a strong piece of evidence that endometriotic lesions and their microenvironment have all the necessary molecular machinery that gives rise to SMM and promotes fibrogenesis [69–71].

Traditionally, different subtypes of endometriosis, such as ovarian endometriomas (OE) and deep endometriosis (DE), are thought to have different pathogenesis and even pathophysiology [72]. Viewed with the ReTIAR prism, both OE and DE lesions are found to exhibit cellular changes consistent with EMT, FMT, SMM, and fibrosis [73]. Compared with OE, DE lesions appeared to have undergone more thorough and extensive EMT, FMT, and SMM and, consequently, displayed significantly higher fibrotic content but less vascularity and more aberrant expression of hormonal receptors [73]. In addition, DE lesions seem to have more epigenetic aberrations [73]. These findings would provide an explanation as why DE is more likely to defy medical treatment, simply because drug delivery to the target tissues becomes more difficult and because DE lesions would be less likely to respond to hormonal treatment and less likely to change at the transcriptional level due to epigenetic aberrations.

Remarkably, EMT, FMT, SMM, and fibrogenesis appear to constitute major molecular events underpinning the progression of endometriosis. In fact, alternatively activated macrophages [74] and other immune cells [75] and even sensory nerve fibers within lesions [76, 77] all participate in the promotion of lesional progression ostensibly through these molecular events. More remarkably, activated platelets also turn endothelial and mesothelial cells into collagen-producing myofibroblasts through endothelial-mesenchymal transition (EndoMT) and mesothelial-mesenchymal transition (MMT) [78, 79].

4.3.4 Platelets, Estrogen Production, and Ovarian Steroid Receptor

In endometriosis, a well-known and perhaps also a widely accepted model that encompasses various mechanisms underlying both elevated 17β-estradiol (E_2) production and increased of proinflammatory cytokines and chemokines is the feed-forward model proposed by Bulun et al. [15], in which proinflammatory cytokines activate cyclooxygenase-*2 (COX-2), resulting in* increased production of prostaglandin E_2 (PGE_2), which, in turn, stimulates some key genes involved in the production of E_2, such as steroidogenic acute regulatory protein (StAR), aromatase, and 17β-hydroxysteroid dehydrogenase type-1 (HSD17B1), resulting in elevated production of E_2, the most potent estrogen. The increased E_2 further induces estrogen receptor β (ERβ), yielding further induction of COX-2. This positive feedback process, once initiated, supposedly perpetuates if untamed, resulting in increased inflammation due to elevated PGE_2 levels and increased growth because of potent mitogenic effect of E_2 [15].

PGE_2 can activate the protein kinase A (PKA) signaling pathway via raising the intracellular levels of cyclic adenosine 3′,5′-monophosphate (cAMP) [80–82], which could enhance the binding of steroidogenic factor-1 (SF-1) to promoters of these steroidogenic genes [83], and induce phosphorylation of the transcriptional activator cAMP-response element-binding protein (CREB) [84]. The binding of SF-1 and CREB to the promoters of steroidogenic genes is responsible for inducing the expression levels and activity of these enzymes, thus promoting the estrogen biosynthesis in endometriotic stromal cells [15, 85, 86].

In wound healing, estrogen has been well documented to be actively involved [87, 88]. Numerous studies have shown that estrogen is important to wound healing and its deficiency delays or impairs wound healing [89–93]. In fact, estrogen is found to be involved in all phases of wound healing [87]. One gene expression profiling study of wound tissues from young and elder men found that among genes that were differentially expressed, 78% of them were estrogen-regulated and only 3% were age-related [94], suggesting that estrogen is more important than intrinsic aging in wound healing. Remarkably, in striking similarity to endometriotic lesions in which ERβ is shown to be overexpressed [95, 96], ERβ has been shown to play a critical role in wound healing [97, 98]. It turns out that the co-culture of endometriotic stromal cells with activated platelets can upregulate ERβ [60].

It also has been reported that activated platelets increase the E_2 production in endometriotic stromal cells through upregulation of StAR, HSD3B2, aromatase, and HSD17B1 [99]. In addition, platelets activate these genes critically involved in estrogen biosynthesis through the activation of NF-κB and/or TGF-β1, and antagonism of either signaling pathway can abolish the induction of the four genes and thus the estrogen production [99]. Platelets also induce HIF-1α, SF-1, and p-CREB, suggesting that the platelet-induced estrogen overproduction can be achieved in multiple pathways [99]. Remarkably, the product of the fold increase of the four proteins after platelet stimulation is nearly equal to the fold increase in E_2 production in endometriotic stromal cells, suggesting that the activated platelets are indeed responsible for the increased E_2 production through activation of these four genes [99].

Taken together, platelets appear to be a new yet unappreciated player in Bulun's feed-forward model, and this underscores the fact that endometriotic lesions are indeed fundamentally wounds undergoing ReTIAR.

4.3.5 Endometriosis and Hypercoagulability

While elevated platelet counts and increased plasma fibrinogen levels have been reported previously, but somewhat inconsistently [100–103], Wu et al. reported in 2015 that women with endometriosis are in a hypercoagulant state, featuring shortened thrombin time (TT) and activated partial thromboplastin time (aPTT) values, as well as elevated platelet activation rate and plasma fibrinogen levels [104]. These findings are in line with growing evidence demonstrating the important role of platelets in the progression of endometriosis [29, 30, 52, 59].

Nonetheless, the notion of hypercoagulability is subsequently questioned by another study, which only found shortened aPTT but failed to find shortened TT [105]. However, an expanded study further confirmed the shortened TT values in women with OE, along with elevated values of other coagulation measurements, such as fibrinogen, D-dimer, and fibrinogen-degradation products [106]. More remarkably, 3 months after the surgical removal of OE lesions, the hypercoagulable state was nearly resolved and addressed to homeostasis [106]. The different results found by other authors [105] may depend, at least in part, by the different choice of controls [106].

The finding of shortened TT values, along with elevated fibrinogen levels, is consistent with previous reports by our group [104, 106] and others [107]. The discrepancy found in other studies [105, 108] is mostly likely due to the selection of patients, as controls, with a diagnosis of gynecologic diseases other than endometriosis but nonetheless required surgery. This may have caused a potential bias, since these non-endometriosis gynecologic diseases may also be in a hypercoagulable state more or less, and this could be responsible for the somewhat conflicting results.

Indeed, even in healthy subjects, acute mental stress has been reported to elevate the levels of factor VIII, fibrinogen, von Willebrand factor [109], and also platelet aggregability [110], potentially forming a hypercoagulable state – even if transiently. It is conceivable that anxiety, nervousness, or even worry over the uncertainty of surgical outcome, finance, etc. can arise to a woman who is about to receive a major operation. This, coupled with other discomfort or even pain that is associated with her gynecologic condition, could heighten the tendency of hypercoagulability and may obscure the genuine difference with women with OE or endometriosis in general. It should be noted that in all studies that reported shortened TT values [104, 106, 107], the bulk of the control group were healthy women without any gynecologic conditions.

4.3.6 Therapeutic Implications

Given the promotional role of platelets in endometriosis, it is only natural to speculate that antiplatelet therapy may be effective in treating endometriosis. In fact, in traditional Chinese medicine (TCM), the treatment of endometriosis-related symptoms such as dysmenorrhea, pain, and infertility has always been the use of herbs, in various concoctions, that are now known to be antiplatelet or antithrombotic, even though there is no official name for endometriosis. Indeed, it has been reported that platelet depletion resulted in significantly reduced lesion size and improved hyperalgesia in mice with induced endometriosis [29]. The treatment with a recombinant P-selectin in mouse with induced endometriosis resulted in soluble P-selectin treatment which markedly reduced the lesion size in mouse through decreased platelet aggregation and angiogenesis, improved general hyperalgesia, and reduced the extent of macrophages infiltration, resulting in reduced fibrotic tissue content [59]. In addition, treatment with ozagrel, a TXA_2 synthase inhibitor, yields significant reduction in lesion growth along with improved hyperalgesia in mice with induced endometriosis [111]. Other antiplatelet compounds, such as scutellarin [112], andrographolide [113], and sodium tanshinone IIA [114], also show therapeutic potentials in preclinical studies.

4.4 Summary and Perspective

Platelets are the first cells to go to and aggregate at the wounding site to initiate hemostasis, inaugurating the tissue repair process of inflammation, proliferation, and tissue remodeling [115]. Activated platelets secrete a plethora of bioactive molecules, including various cytokines/chemokines and growth factors, including PDGF and TGF-β1 [62]. As such, the involvement of platelets in endometriosis seems to be beyond any doubt. Yet platelets are not just passively impact on endometriotic lesions. In fact, endometriotic stromal cells also produce potent platelet-activating molecules such as thrombin and TXA_2 [30] and collagens [69], which, coupled with increased angiogenesis and thus vascular permeability, may further lead to platelet aggregation. Consequently, endometriotic lesions and platelets engage active cross-talks to maintain lesion growth and facilitate lesional progression and fibrogenesis [29, 69, 70].

Due, at least in part, to the involvement of platelets in endometriosis, women with endometriosis are in hypercoagulable state, and this may be one of the reasons for increased risk of coronary heart disease in these women [116]. Once endometriotic lesions are surgically removed, the hypercoagulable state appears to be normalized [106]. This seems to suggest that endometriotic lesions and platelet activation are mutually causative, or at least they are intimately entwined.

While the involvement of platelets in the progression of endometriosis is certain, their roles in interacting with other immune cells in the context of lesional progression are still poorly understood. For example, platelets seem to work with regulatory T (Treg) cells to form a type 2 immunity in lesional microenvironment that is conducive to lesional progression and fibrogenesis [75]. In other words, we have just scratched the surface. How platelets work with other immune cells, what their underlying molecular mechanisms are, and how to devise novel therapeutics to treat endometriosis more effectively are unresolved questions that warrant future research.

Acknowledgment This research was supported in part by grant 82071623 from the National Natural Science Foundation of China, an Excellence in Centers of Clinical Medicine grant (2017ZZ01016) from the Science and Technology Commission of Shanghai Municipality, and grant SHDC2020CR2062B from Shanghai Shenkang Center for Hospital Development.

References

1. Portelli M, et al. Endometrial seedlings. A survival instinct? Immunomodulation and its role in the pathophysiology of endometriosis. Minerva Ginecol. 2011;63(6):563–70.
2. Harada T, et al. Apoptosis and endometriosis. Front Biosci. 2007;12:3140–51.
3. Vinatier D, Dufour P, Oosterlynck D. Immunological aspects of endometriosis. Hum Reprod Update. 1996;2(5):371–84.
4. Guo SW. Nuclear factor-kappab (NF-kappaB): an unsuspected major culprit in the pathogenesis of endometriosis that is still at large? Gynecol Obstet Investig. 2007;63(2):71–97.
5. McLaren J. Vascular endothelial growth factor and endometriotic angiogenesis. Hum Reprod Update. 2000;6(1):45–55.

6. Guo SW. Epigenetics of endometriosis. Mol Hum Reprod. 2009;15(10):587–607.
7. Anglesio MS, et al. Cancer-associated mutations in endometriosis without cancer. N Engl J Med. 2017;376(19):1835–48.
8. Suda K, et al. Clonal expansion and diversification of cancer-associated mutations in endometriosis and normal endometrium. Cell Rep. 2018;24(7):1777–89.
9. Brosens IA. Endometriosis–a disease because it is characterized by bleeding. Am J Obstet Gynecol. 1997;176(2):263–7.
10. Shaw TJ, Martin P. Wound repair: a showcase for cell plasticity and migration. Curr Opin Cell Biol. 2016;42:29–37.
11. van der Meijden PEJ, Heemskerk JWM. Platelet biology and functions: new concepts and clinical perspectives. Nat Rev Cardiol. 2019;16(3):166–79.
12. Gay LJ, Felding-Habermann B. Contribution of platelets to tumour metastasis. Nat Rev Cancer. 2011;11(2):123–34.
13. Ntelis K, et al. Platelets in systemic sclerosis: the missing link connecting vasculopathy, autoimmunity, and fibrosis? Curr Rheumatol Rep. 2019;21(5):15.
14. Gawaz M, Langer H, May AE. Platelets in inflammation and atherogenesis. J Clin Invest. 2005;115(12):3378–84.
15. Bulun SE, et al. Regulation of aromatase expression in estrogen-responsive breast and uterine disease: from bench to treatment. Pharmacol Rev. 2005;57(3):359–83.
16. Burney RO, Giudice LC. Pathogenesis and pathophysiology of endometriosis. Fertil Steril. 2012;98(3):511–9.
17. Akoum A, et al. Secretion of interleukin-6 by human endometriotic cells and regulation by proinflammatory cytokines and sex steroids. Hum Reprod. 1996;11(10):2269–75.
18. Wu MY, Ho HN. The role of cytokines in endometriosis. Am J Reprod Immunol. 2003;49(5):285–96.
19. Gonzalez-Ramos R, et al. Nuclear factor-kappa B is constitutively activated in peritoneal endometriosis. Mol Hum Reprod. 2007;13(7):503–9.
20. Gonzalez-Ramos R, et al. Involvement of the nuclear factor-kappaB pathway in the pathogenesis of endometriosis. Fertil Steril. 2010;94(6):1985–94.
21. Nomiyama M, et al. Local immune response in infertile patients with minimal endometriosis. Gynecol Obstet Investig. 1997;44(1):32–7.
22. Khan KN, et al. Differential macrophage infiltration in early and advanced endometriosis and adjacent peritoneum. Fertil Steril. 2004;81(3):652–61.
23. Bacci M, et al. Macrophages are alternatively activated in patients with endometriosis and required for growth and vascularization of lesions in a mouse model of disease. Am J Pathol. 2009;175(2):547–56.
24. Petaja J. Inflammation and coagulation. An overview. Thromb Res. 2011;127(Suppl 2):S34–7.
25. Lipinski S, et al. Coagulation and inflammation. Molecular insights and diagnostic implications. Hamostaseologie. 2011;31(2):94–102, 104.
26. Semple JW, Italiano JE Jr, Freedman J. Platelets and the immune continuum. Nat Rev Immunol. 2011;11(4):264–74.
27. Vieira-de-Abreu A, et al. Platelets: versatile effector cells in hemostasis, inflammation, and the immune continuum. Semin Immunopathol. 2012;34(1):5–30.
28. Sreeramkumar V, et al. Neutrophils scan for activated platelets to initiate inflammation. Science. 2014;346(6214):1234–8.
29. Ding D, et al. Platelets are an unindicted culprit in the development of endometriosis: clinical and experimental evidence. Hum Reprod. 2015;30(4):812–32.
30. Guo SW, Du Y, Liu X. Endometriosis-derived stromal cells secrete thrombin and thromboxane A2, inducing platelet activation. Reprod Sci. 2016;23(8):1044–52.
31. Dmowski WP, Steele RW, Baker GF. Deficient cellular immunity in endometriosis. Am J Obstet Gynecol. 1981;141(4):377–83.
32. Dmowski WP, Gebel HM, Rawlins RG. Immunologic aspects of endometriosis. Obstet Gynecol Clin N Am. 1989;16(1):93–103.

33. Oosterlynck DJ, et al. Women with endometriosis show a defect in natural killer activity resulting in a decreased cytotoxicity to autologous endometrium. Fertil Steril. 1991;56(1):45–51.
34. Oosterlynck DJ, et al. The natural killer activity of peritoneal fluid lymphocytes is decreased in women with endometriosis. Fertil Steril. 1992;58(2):290–5.
35. Garzetti GG, et al. Natural killer cell activity in endometriosis: correlation between serum estradiol levels and cytotoxicity. Obstet Gynecol. 1993;81(5 Pt 1):665–8.
36. Tanaka E, et al. Decreased natural killer cell activity in women with endometriosis. Gynecol Obstet Investig. 1992;34(1):27–30.
37. Osuga Y, et al. Lymphocytes in endometriosis. Am J Reprod Immunol. 2011;65(1):1–10.
38. Sikora J, Mielczarek-Palacz A, Kondera-Anasz Z. Role of natural killer cell activity in the pathogenesis of endometriosis. Curr Med Chem. 2011;18(2):200–8.
39. Wu MY, et al. Increase in the expression of killer cell inhibitory receptors on peritoneal natural killer cells in women with endometriosis. Fertil Steril. 2000;74(6):1187–91.
40. Maeda N, et al. Aberrant expression of intercellular adhesion molecule-1 and killer inhibitory receptors induces immune tolerance in women with pelvic endometriosis. Fertil Steril. 2002;77(4):679–83.
41. Matsuoka S, et al. Expression of inhibitory-motif killer immunoglobulin-like receptor, KIR2DL1, is increased in natural killer cells from women with pelvic endometriosis. Am J Reprod Immunol. 2005;53(5):249–54.
42. Kawashima M, et al. Human leukocyte antigen-G, a ligand for the natural killer receptor KIR2DL4, is expressed by eutopic endometrium only in the menstrual phase. Fertil Steril. 2009;91(2):343–9.
43. Galandrini R, et al. Increased frequency of human leukocyte antigen-E inhibitory receptor CD94/NKG2A-expressing peritoneal natural killer cells in patients with endometriosis. Fertil Steril. 2008;89(5 Suppl):1490–6.
44. Funamizu A, et al. Expression of natural cytotoxicity receptors on peritoneal fluid natural killer cell and cytokine production by peritoneal fluid natural killer cell in women with endometriosis. Am J Reprod Immunol. 2014;71(4):359–67.
45. Caligiuri MA. Human natural killer cells. Blood. 2008;112(3):461–9.
46. Smyth MJ, et al. New aspects of natural-killer-cell surveillance and therapy of cancer. Nat Rev Cancer. 2002;2(11):850–61.
47. Lanier LL. Natural killer cell receptor signaling. Curr Opin Immunol. 2003;15(3):308–14.
48. Cheent K, Khakoo SI. Natural killer cells: integrating diversity with function. Immunology. 2009;126(4):449–57.
49. Bauer S, et al. Activation of NK cells and T cells by NKG2D, a receptor for stress-inducible MICA. Science. 1999;285(5428):727–9.
50. Groh V, et al. Costimulation of CD8alphabeta T cells by NKG2D via engagement by MIC induced on virus-infected cells. Nat Immunol. 2001;2(3):255–60.
51. Raulet DH, Guerra N. Oncogenic stress sensed by the immune system: role of natural killer cell receptors. Nat Rev Immunol. 2009;9(8):568–80.
52. Guo SW, Du Y, Liu X. Platelet-derived TGF-beta1 mediates the down-modulation of NKG2D expression and may be responsible for impaired natural killer (NK) cytotoxicity in women with endometriosis. Hum Reprod. 2016;31(7):1462–74.
53. Wu MY, et al. The suppression of peritoneal cellular immunity in women with endometriosis could be restored after gonadotropin releasing hormone agonist treatment. Am J Reprod Immunol. 1996;35(6):510–6.
54. Rook AH, et al. Effects of transforming growth factor beta on the functions of natural killer cells: depressed cytolytic activity and blunting of interferon responsiveness. J Immunol. 1986;136(10):3916–20.
55. Malygin AM, Meri S, Timonen T. Regulation of natural killer cell activity by transforming growth factor-beta and prostaglandin E2. Scand J Immunol. 1993;37(1):71–6.
56. Bellone G, et al. Regulation of NK cell functions by TGF-beta 1. J Immunol. 1995;155(3):1066–73.

57. Du Y, Liu X, Guo SW. Platelets impair natural killer cell reactivity and function in endometriosis through multiple mechanisms. Hum Reprod. 2017;32(4):794–810.
58. Kopp HG, Placke T, Salih HR. Platelet-derived transforming growth factor-beta downregulates NKG2D thereby inhibiting natural killer cell antitumor reactivity. Cancer Res. 2009;69(19):7775–83.
59. Guo SW, et al. P-selectin as a potential therapeutic target for endometriosis. Fertil Steril. 2015;103(4):990–1000 e8.
60. Zhang Q, et al. Activated platelets induce estrogen receptor beta expression in endometriotic stromal cells. Gynecol Obstet Investig. 2015;80(3):187–92.
61. Assoian RK, Sporn MB. Type beta transforming growth factor in human platelets: release during platelet degranulation and action on vascular smooth muscle cells. J Cell Biol. 1986;102(4):1217–23.
62. Assoian RK, et al. Transforming growth factor-beta in human platelets. Identification of a major storage site, purification, and characterization. J Biol Chem. 1983;258(11):7155–60.
63. Thiery JP, et al. Epithelial-mesenchymal transitions in development and disease. Cell. 2009;139(5):871–90.
64. Desmouliere A, Chaponnier C, Gabbiani G. Tissue repair, contraction, and the myofibroblast. Wound Repair Regen. 2005;13(1):7–12.
65. Gabbiani G. The myofibroblast in wound healing and fibrocontractive diseases. J Pathol. 2003;200(4):500–3.
66. Biernacka A, Dobaczewski M, Frangogiannis NG. TGF-beta signaling in fibrosis. Growth Factors. 2011;29(5):196–202.
67. Labelle M, Begum S, Hynes RO. Direct signaling between platelets and cancer cells induces an epithelial-mesenchymal-like transition and promotes metastasis. Cancer Cell. 2011;20(5):576–90.
68. Mehal WZ, Iredale J, Friedman SL. Scraping fibrosis: expressway to the core of fibrosis. Nat Med. 2011;17(5):552–3.
69. Zhang Q, et al. Platelets drive smooth muscle metaplasia and fibrogenesis in endometriosis through epithelial-mesenchymal transition and fibroblast-to-myofibroblast transdifferentiation. Mol Cell Endocrinol. 2016;428:1–16.
70. Zhang Q, et al. Cellular changes consistent with epithelial-mesenchymal transition and fibroblast-to-myofibroblast transdifferentiation in the progression of experimental endometriosis in baboons. Reprod Sci. 2016;23(10):1409–21.
71. Zhang Q, Liu X, Guo SW. Progressive development of endometriosis and its hindrance by anti-platelet treatment in mice with induced endometriosis. Reprod Biomed Online. 2016;34(2):124–36.
72. Nisolle M, Donnez J. Peritoneal endometriosis, ovarian endometriosis, and adenomyotic nodules of the rectovaginal septum are three different entities. Fertil Steril. 1997;68(4):585–96.
73. Liu X, Zhang Q, Guo SW. Histological and immunohistochemical characterization of the similarity and difference between ovarian endometriomas and deep infiltrating endometriosis. Reprod Sci. 2017;25(3):329–40.
74. Duan J, et al. The M2a macrophage subset may be critically involved in the fibrogenesis of endometriosis in mice. Reprod Biomed Online. 2018;37(3):254–68.
75. Xiao F, Liu X, Guo SW. Platelets and regulatory T cells may induce a type 2 immunity that is conducive to the progression and fibrogenesis of endometriosis. Front Immunol. 2020;11:610963.
76. Liu X, Yan D, Guo SW. Sensory nerve-derived neuropeptides accelerate the development and fibrogenesis of endometriosis. Hum Reprod. 2019;34(3):452–68.
77. Yan D, Liu X, Guo SW. Neuropeptides substance P and calcitonin gene related peptide accelerate the development and fibrogenesis of endometriosis. Sci Rep. 2019;9(1):2698.
78. Yan D, et al. Mesothelial cells participate in endometriosis fibrogenesis through platelet-induced mesothelial-mesenchymal transition. J Clin Endocrinol Metab. 2020;105(11):e4124–47.
79. Yan D, et al. Platelets induce endothelial-mesenchymal transition and subsequent fibrogenesis in endometriosis. Reprod Biomed Online. 2020;41(3):500–17.

80. Noble LS, et al. Prostaglandin E2 stimulates aromatase expression in endometriosis-derived stromal cells. J Clin Endocrinol Metab. 1997;82(2):600–6.
81. Yang S, et al. Regulation of aromatase P450 expression in endometriotic and endometrial stromal cells by CCAAT/enhancer binding proteins (C/EBPs): decreased C/EBPbeta in endometriosis is associated with overexpression of aromatase. J Clin Endocrinol Metab. 2002;87(5):2336–45.
82. Breyer RM, et al. Prostanoid receptors: subtypes and signaling. Annu Rev Pharmacol Toxicol. 2001;41:661–90.
83. Bulun SE, et al. Steroidogenic factor-1 and endometriosis. Mol Cell Endocrinol. 2009;300(1–2):104–8.
84. Hsu CC, et al. Cyclic adenosine 3′,5′-monophosphate response element-binding protein and CCAAT/enhancer-binding protein mediate prostaglandin E2-induced steroidogenic acute regulatory protein expression in endometriotic stromal cells. Am J Pathol. 2008;173(2):433–41.
85. Sun HS, et al. Transactivation of steroidogenic acute regulatory protein in human endometriotic stromal cells is mediated by the prostaglandin EP2 receptor. Endocrinology. 2003;144(9):3934–42.
86. Zeitoun KM, Bulun SE. Aromatase: a key molecule in the pathophysiology of endometriosis and a therapeutic target. Fertil Steril. 1999;72(6):961–9.
87. Horng HC, et al. Estrogen effects on wound healing. Int J Mol Sci. 2017;18(11):2325.
88. Wilkinson HN, Hardman MJ. The role of estrogen in cutaneous ageing and repair. Maturitas. 2017;103:60–4.
89. Ashcroft GS, et al. Estrogen accelerates cutaneous wound healing associated with an increase in TGF-beta1 levels. Nat Med. 1997;3(11):1209–15.
90. Ashcroft GS, et al. Estrogen modulates cutaneous wound healing by downregulating macrophage migration inhibitory factor. J Clin Invest. 2003;111(9):1309–18.
91. Hardman MJ, et al. Selective estrogen receptor modulators accelerate cutaneous wound healing in ovariectomized female mice. Endocrinology. 2008;149(2):551–7.
92. Pepe G, et al. Self-renewal and phenotypic conversion are the main physiological responses of macrophages to the endogenous estrogen surge. Sci Rep. 2017;7:44270.
93. Mukai K, et al. 17beta-Estradiol administration promotes delayed cutaneous wound healing in 40-week ovariectomised female mice. Int Wound J. 2016;13(5):636–44.
94. Hardman MJ, Ashcroft GS. Estrogen, not intrinsic aging, is the major regulator of delayed human wound healing in the elderly. Genome Biol. 2008;9(5):R80.
95. Brandenberger AW, et al. Oestrogen receptor (ER)-alpha and ER-beta isoforms in normal endometrial and endometriosis-derived stromal cells. Mol Hum Reprod. 1999;5(7):651–5.
96. Fujimoto J, et al. Expression of oestrogen receptor-alpha and -beta in ovarian endometriomata. Mol Hum Reprod. 1999;5(8):742–7.
97. Merlo S, et al. Differential involvement of estrogen receptor alpha and estrogen receptor beta in the healing promoting effect of estrogen in human keratinocytes. J Endocrinol. 2009;200(2):189–97.
98. Campbell L, et al. Estrogen promotes cutaneous wound healing via estrogen receptor beta independent of its antiinflammatory activities. J Exp Med. 2010;207(9):1825–33.
99. Qi Q, et al. Platelets induce increased estrogen production through NF-kappaB and TGF-beta1 signaling pathways in endometriotic stromal cells. Sci Rep. 2020;10(1):1281.
100. Avcioglu SN, et al. Can platelet indices be new biomarkers for severe endometriosis? ISRN Obstet Gynecol. 2014;2014:713542.
101. Yavuzcan A, et al. Evaluation of mean platelet volume, neutrophil/lymphocyte ratio and platelet/lymphocyte ratio in advanced stage endometriosis with endometrioma. J Turk Ger Gynecol Assoc. 2013;14(4):210–5.
102. Coskun B, et al. The feasibility of the platelet count and mean platelet volume as markers of endometriosis and adenomyosis: a case control study. J Gynecol Obstet Hum Reprod. 2019;2019:101626.

103. Chmaj-Wierzchowska K, et al. Novel markers in the diagnostics of endometriomas: Urocortin, ghrelin, and leptin or leukocytes, fibrinogen, and CA-125? Taiwan J Obstet Gynecol. 2015;54(2):126–30.
104. Wu Q, et al. Evidence for a hypercoagulable state in women with ovarian endometriomas. Reprod Sci. 2015;22(9):1107–14.
105. Vigano P, et al. Coagulation status in women with endometriosis. Reprod Sci. 2018;25(4):559–65.
106. Ding D, Liu X, Guo SW. Further evidence for hypercoagulability in women with ovarian endometriomas. Reprod Sci. 2018;25(11):1540–8.
107. Ding S, et al. Is there a correlation between inflammatory markers and coagulation parameters in women with advanced ovarian endometriosis? BMC Womens Health. 2019;19(1):169.
108. Ottolina J, et al. Assessment of coagulation parameters in women affected by endometriosis: validation study and systematic review of the literature. Diagnostics (Basel). 2020;10(8):567.
109. von Kanel R. Acute mental stress and hemostasis: when physiology becomes vascular harm. Thromb Res. 2015;135(Suppl 1):S52–5.
110. Larsson PT, et al. Altered platelet function during mental stress and adrenaline infusion in humans: evidence for an increased aggregability in vivo as measured by filtragometry. Clin Sci (Lond). 1989;76(4):369–76.
111. Guo SW, Ding D, Liu X. Anti-platelet therapy is efficacious in treating endometriosis induced in mouse. Reprod Biomed Online. 2016;33(4):484–99.
112. Ding D, et al. Scutellarin suppresses platelet aggregation and stalls lesional progression in mouse with induced endometriosis. Reprod Sci. 2019;26(11):1417–28.
113. Zheng Y, Liu X, Guo SW. Therapeutic potential of andrographolide for treating endometriosis. Hum Reprod. 2012;27(5):1300–13.
114. Luo M, et al. Sodium tanshinone IIA sulfonate restrains fibrogenesis through induction of senescence in mice with induced deep endometriosis. Reprod Biomed Online. 2020;41(3):373–84.
115. Nurden AT, et al. Platelets and wound healing. Front Biosci. 2008;13:3532–48.
116. Mu F, et al. Endometriosis and risk of coronary heart disease. Circ Cardiovasc Qual Outcomes. 2016;9(3):257–64.

Pathogenesis of Endometriosis: Role of Macrophages in Endometriosis

5

Khaleque N. Khan

Contents

5.1 Introduction

Endometriosis, the presence of functional endometrium outside of the uterine cavity, is a common disease, causing abdominal pain, dysmenorrhea, dyspareunia, and infertility in about 10% of the female population [1]. Even after 300 years, most of

The original version of the chapter has been revised. A correction to this chapter can be found at https://doi.org/10.1007/978-3-030-97236-3_45

K. N. Khan (✉)
Department of Obstetrics and Gynecology, The Clinical and Translational Research Center, Graduate School of Medical Science, Kyoto Prefectural University of Medicine, Kyoto, Japan
e-mail: nemokhan@koto.kpu-m.ac.jp

E. Oral (ed.), *Endometriosis and Adenomyosis*,
https://doi.org/10.1007/978-3-030-97236-3_5

the literature still claim that pathogenesis and/or pathophysiology of endometriosis is unclear [2, 3]. Besides metaplastic transformation of endometrial and peritoneal mesothelial cells, the transplantation, implantation, and growth of exfoliated menstrual debris on the peritoneal and ovarian surfaces are the widely accepted mechanisms of endometriosis [1–3]. A number of literature have already demonstrated the potential role of ovarian steroid hormones in the regeneration of endometrium after menstruation and the growth of endometriosis [4, 5]. However, as a nonself lesion in pelvic environment, the growth or persistence of endometriosis can also be regulated by innate immune system. The mitogenesis or angiogenesis of eutopic and ectopic endometrium possibly involves an extensive interplay between endometrial cells, inflammatory cells, ovarian hormones, soluble factors, and the extracellular matrix [6].

As a cell component of innate immune system, peritoneal fluid (PF) and intact tissue derived from women with endometriosis have been shown to contain higher number of activated macrophages than that found in women without endometriosis [7]. This results in the secretion of higher concentrations of growth factors including hepatocyte growth factor (HGF) and other cytokines in PF as produced by the stimulated- Macrophages (Mφ) in these patients [8, 9]. This indicates that the growth or persistence of endometriosis is a normal inflammatory response, and this was established by the accumulation of inflammatory cells in grafted endometriotic lesions in mouse endometriosis model [10].

Since mesenchymal cells retain estrogen receptor, production of different cytokines by endometrial stromal cells and its modulation by estrogen has been demonstrated [11]. Considering that infiltrated Mφ is one of the cell components of endometriotic lesion in pelvic environment, reports describing expression of steroid receptors by Mφ and the secretion of different macromolecules in response to steroid hormones are scanty. Here, we discussed the orchestrated role of Mφ, LPS, HGF, and ovarian steroid hormones in inducing pelvic inflammation and consequent development of pelvic endometriosis. We also discussed the possible effect of estrogen-suppressing agent, GnRHa, on inflammation.

5.2 Fundamentals of Macrophages

Macrophages (Mφ) are phagocytic cells of the immune system that distribute in various tissues and play a critical role in various diseases such as inflammatory disorders and growth of tumors [12]. Macrophages are critical for the growth, development, vascularization, and innervation of lesions as well as generation of pain symptoms in women suffering from endometriosis. The functional roles of Mφ include phagocytizing pathogens, apoptosis of cells and debris, antigen presentation, and modulation of other leukocyte populations [12]. Much of our knowledge regarding Mφ ontogeny is derived from studies conducted in mice. Macrophages are derived from three key populations: yolk sac of the embryo, the fetal liver, and postnatally, hematopoiesis in the bone marrow. Biologically, there are two variants of Mφ, resident tissue Mφ and bone marrow-derived Mφ. Tissue macrophages are seeded during fetal life from the fetal liver and yolk sac and undergo self-renewal. In adults, monocyte precursors extravasate from the bone marrow into the circulation, where they can undergo differentiation into macrophages and then infiltrate into the tissue [13]. Once peripheral blood monocytes are recruited to local tissue environment in response to ovarian steroid and chemokines, they undergo differentiation into Mφ by initial inflammatory mediator derived from bacterial ligands such as lipopolysaccharide (LPS) [7]. A small amount of LPS persists in pelvis as a source of gut microbiota and as a result of gut wall transmigration [14]. In tissues, Mφ modulate their phenotype dependent on local cytokines and growth factors to specific tissue or disease-associated phenotypes. LPS activates local tissue Mφ for the production of different secondary inflammatory mediators such as cytokines, growth factors, and chemokines. These chemokines together with estrogen recruit more monocytes from the peripheral blood, and a vicious cycle of tissue accumulation and subsequent differentiation into Mφ continues with the production of different macromolecules in pelvic environment (Fig. 5.1).

Based on functional roles, Mφ are broadly classified into M1 macrophages (known as classically activated Mφ) and M2 macrophages (known as alternatively activated Mφ) [15]. M1 macrophages that express specific proinflammatory biomarkers (CD40, CD68, CD80, and CD86) are potent effector cells to eliminate invading microorganisms and secrete proinflammatory cytokines (IL-1β, IL-6, IL-12, and TNFα). In contrast, M2 macrophages that express specific markers, CD163 and CD206, ameliorate inflammation and produce anti-inflammatory factors such as IL-10, TGF-β, and IL-1 receptor antagonist, but very low levels of proinflammatory cytokines. In addition, M2 macrophages are involved in tissue remodeling, angiogenesis, and tumor progression. Macrophages are a group of heterogeneous and plastic cells that switch from M1 to M2 phenotype, and vice versa, upon the induction of specific signals. M1 macrophages can be directly driven to the M2 phenotype by canonical exposure to IL-4 and IL-10 [5, 16]. Moreover, several pathways have been implicated in the M1/M2 polarization of macrophages [17].

Despite the importance of uterine Mφ, little is known about the influence of uterine Mφ and their distribution in pelvis in order to maintain uterine endometrial function and development of chronic inflammatory disorder such as endometriosis. Only a few studies have described polarization of the Mφ phenotypes M1 and M2 in the human endometrium and endometriosis. While Jansen et al. [18] demonstrated that human endometrial Mφ are predominantly M2 macrophages, other reports described contradictory results. A subsequent study indicated a significantly higher number of M1 macrophages in the endometria of women with endometriosis across the phases of menstrual cycle. The ratios of M2 macrophages in pan-macrophages (CD68+ Mφ) were significantly lower in all menstrual phases in the endometriosis group [19]. The distribution of pan-macrophages in early and advanced endometriosis and in different color appearances of peritoneal endometriosis and their pattern of change after hormonal treatment is not well described.

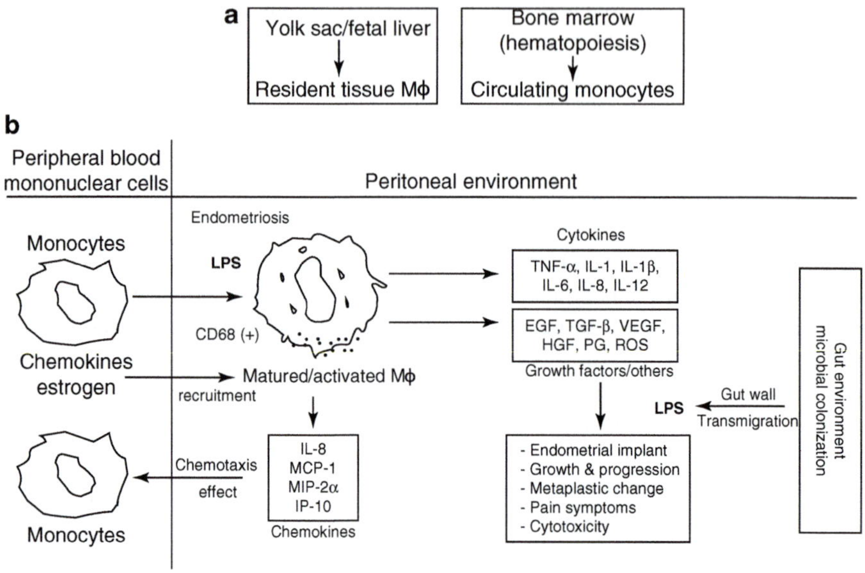

Fig. 5.1 (**a**) Shows source of two different variants of macrophages (Mφ), resident tissue Mφ derived from yolk sac/fetal liver and bone marrow-derived circulating monocytes. These monocytes can infiltrate into tissues and differentiate into activated Mφ. (**b**) The fate of peripheral blood mononuclear cell (monocytes) after their recruitment into tissues and peritoneal environment in response to the secretion of chemokines by LPS-stimulated Mφ. Estrogen itself also acts as a chemokine. The gut origin of LPS and its persistence in pelvis stimulates activated Mφ for the secretion of different cytokines, growth factors, chemokines, and other macromolecules. A vicious cycle of this cascade is involved in the growth, persistence, and progression of endometriosis. The details of this cascade are described in the text. LPS, lipopolyssachoride; TNF-α, tumor necrosis factor-alpha; IL, interleukin; EGF, epidermal growth factors; TGF-β, transforming growth factor-beta; VEGF, vascular endothelial cell growth factor; HGF, hepatocyte growth factor; PG, prostaglandin, a pain mediator; ROS, reactive oxygen species, a cytotoxic molecule; MCP-1, monocyte chemoattractant protein; MIP-2α, Mφ inflammatory protein-2alpha; and IP-10, interferon gamma-induced protein-10. LPS acts as initial inflammatory mediator, and all cytokines, growth factors, and chemokines act as secondary inflammatory mediators

5.3 Macrophages and Innate Immune Cells

As a component of innate immune system, an increase in the infiltration of Mφ was found in normal endometrium and also in the endometria of women with different reproductive diseases such as endometriosis, adenomyosis, and uterine leiomyoma [20–22]. Innate (natural or constitutive) immunity in our body depends on toll-like receptors. From flies to mammals, these proteins provide a first line defense and are implicated in infectious and autoimmune diseases. While scientists have been studying the adaptive (acquired) immune response for several decades, the recognition of the importance of innate immunity was established only during the past few years to understand the association between adaptive and innate immune system. Why is innate immunity necessary for our body? There was always a question of how adaptive immune system could defend us if it were alone, because adaptive immunity depends on the multiplication of host cells with a generation time of at least 12 h, whereas microbes can divide every 20 min. To cover this lag, the rapidly reactive innate immune system responds immediately to infectious agents, protecting the host until slower adaptive system kicks in and eventually makes memory cells for long-term response [23, 24].

Functional characterization of Toll-like receptors (TLRs) has established that innate immunity is a skillful system that detects invasion of microbial pathogens. Mammalian innate immune cells such as Mφ and dendritic cells can be activated by microbial components (nonself) such as endotoxin or lipopolysaccharide (LPS) from Gram-negative bacteria. TLRs are one group of pattern recognition receptors that are expressed on Mφ, dendritic cells, and as more recently shown, on neutrophils, natural killer (NK) cells, and endometrial epithelial/stromal cells [25, 26]. Treatment of Mφ and endometrial stromal cells with LPS significantly increased the production of a number of macromolecules such as HGF, VEGF, IL-6, IL-8, and TNFα in a dose-dependent fashion [27–29]. Among them, HGF plays a crucial role in the growth of both eutopic and ectopic endometrial cells. A significantly more growth-promoting effect of LPS was observed on endometrial cells derived from women with endometriosis when compared with similar cells derived from control women [28, 29]. The stimulatory effect of LPS was inhibited by the addition of neutralizing antibody for TLR4 and also by an LPS antagonist, polymyxin B [30]. These results indicate that as a component of innate immune system, macrophages are involved in TLR4-mediated production of proinflammatory cytokine as well as growth of endometriosis.

5.3.1 Role of Macrophages/NK Cells in Endometriosis

There are inconsistent reports in terms of the leukocyte population in the female reproductive tract. This discrepancy comes from the differences in the sampling phase in the menstrual cycle, the sample size, the analytical methods, and the antibodies used to determine immune cells. These immune cells in the reproductive tract are distributed in either an aggregated or a dispersed form in the epithelial layer, lamina propria, and stroma. Immune cells are differentially distributed in each organ of the reproductive tract. The predominant immune cells are T cells, macrophages, dendritic cells, NK cells, neutrophils, and mast cells. B cells are rare in the female reproductive tract [31]. PF from women with endometriosis has shown to contain higher numbers of activated Mφ than found in women without endometriosis [7]. Tissue infiltration of Mφ has a crucial role in enhancing the growth of endometriosis or in causing infertility [20]. The higher concentrations of growth factors and cytokines are released by activated Mφ in these patients. This indicates that growth and persistence of endometriosis is a normal inflammatory response. The increased levels of cytokines and growth factors in the PF may reflect increased synthesis of these macromolecules by the peritoneal Mφ, eutopic and ectopic endometrium, and/or mesothelial cells of the peritoneum, all of which have been shown to be capable of cytokine synthesis [11, 32].

Similar to Mφ, NK cells are important components of innate immune system and exhibit significant role in the growth of endometriosis. Uterine NK cells have also been called large granular lymphocytes, endometrial granulocytes, K cells, endometrial granulated lymphocytes, and decidual granulated lymphocytes [33]. The major phenotype of endometrial NK cells is $CD3^{-}CD56^{bright}CD16^{-}$, which distinguishes this cell subset from $CD3^{-}CD56^{dim}CD16^{+}$ NK cells in the peripheral blood [31, 33]. In the proliferative phase, only a few NK cells are scattered throughout the stroma of functional layer. In contrast, the NK cells show a dramatic increase in number after ovulation and continue to increase until a few days prior to menstruation [31].

Impaired natural killer (NK) activity in women with endometriosis is thought to promote implantation and progression of endometrial tissue. The expression of human leukocyte antigen (HLA)-G, a ligand of NK receptors, was identified on eutopic endometrium only in the menstrual phase but not in the proliferative or secretory phases. Furthermore, HLA-G-expressing cells were also detected in peritoneal fluid during the menstrual period. During retrograde menstruation, HLA-G expressing endometrial tissue may enter the peritoneal cavity and may be reduced by immunosurveillance system. Although peritoneal NK cells play an important role in this system, impairment of NK cytotoxicity via HLA-G may allow peritoneal endometrial cell survival and implantation [34]. It has been reported that there is increased platelet aggregation in endometriotic lesions and increased activation rate in the peripheral blood in women with endometriosis. Once these platelets are activated, they release copious amount of TGF-β, a molecule that suppresses NK cell function and NK Group 2, Member D (NKG2D) expression on NK cells [35]. The TGF-β1 concentration in PF carries a positive correlation with the platelet activation rate indicating that activated platelets are responsible, at least in part, for the increased TGF-β1 concentration. The cytotoxicity of freshly isolated NK cells treated with PF of women with endometriosis was significantly reduced when compared with that of women without endometriosis. Both the platelet activation rate and TGF-β1 concentration in the PF correlated negatively with the NKG2D expression in NK cells isolated from the PF. These results suggested a potential role of platelets and TGF-β1 in the impairment of NK cytotoxicity and consequent survival of endometrial cells in pelvis of women with endometriosis [35]. Another recent report from the same group provided further evidence that platelets impair NK reactivity and function in women with endometriosis through multiple mechanisms [36].

5.3.2 Macrophages and Fibrogenesis in Endometriosis

Biomaterial-mediated inflammation and fibrosis remain a prominent challenge in designing material to support tissue repair and regeneration. The primary cells involved in biomaterial-mediated fibrosis are macrophages, which modulate inflammation, fibrosis, and primarily lay down new extracellular matrix [37]. While macrophages and fibroblasts are implicated in driving biomaterial-mediated fibrosis, the signaling pathways and spatiotemporal crosstalk between these cell types remain poorly defined. In addition to pathogen scavenger activity and production of different macromolecules, Mφ are known to be a key regulator of tissue repair and fibrogenesis.

Recent report has shown that endometriotic lesions are essentially wounds that undergo repeated tissue injury and repair in response to cyclic bleeding. These events result in epithelial-mesenchymal transition (EMT), fibroblast-to-myofibroblast transdifferentiation (FMT), smooth muscle metaplasia (SMM), and ultimately fibrosis [38]. Macrophages may play some remarkable role in the fibrogenesis of endometriosis. While M1 macrophages mediate inflammation, M2 macrophages are involved in reparative anti-inflammation, tissue remodeling, and profibrotic activity [39]. On the basis of their activators, markers of activation and function, secreted cytokines, and chemokines, M2 macrophages can be further classified into four subtypes: M2a, M2b, M2c, and M2d [40]. M1 macrophages are found to be involved in early stages of wound healing whereas M2 macrophages are involved in middle stages. Although preemptive Mφ depletion before induction of endometriosis did not greatly affect lesion weight, Mφ depletion after induction resulted in reduced lesional growth and vascularization suggesting a possible role of M2 macrophages in the development of endometriosis [41].

In a mouse model of endometriosis, Duan et al. [42] demonstrated that lesional infiltration of M2 macrophages increased progressively as lesions progressed undisturbed, concomitant with progressive EMT, FMT, and fibrosis. In a separate experiment in mice, they found that diphtheria toxin-mediated Mφ depletion after induction of endometriosis significantly reduced lesional infiltration of pan-macrophages, M2 macrophages with significant reduction in fibrotic content and lesion weight. Furthermore, adoptive transfer of M2a but not M1 or M2c macrophages, after Mφ depletion, significantly increased the extent of fibrosis in endometriotic lesions [42]. The authors emphasized that a particular submit of M2 macrophage (M2a) may be involved in the growth and fibrogenesis of endometriosis.

5.4 Macrophages in Early and Advanced Endometriosis

The retrograde reflux of menstrual debris into the pelvic cavity can induce a normal inflammatory response and release different chemoattractant proteins, which in turn recruit peripheral blood mononuclear cells (PBMCs) into the peritoneal environment. These PBMCs time-dependently mature into macrophages (Mφ). The mature Mφ could be harbored either in the PF or in intact tissue, and they can produce proinflammatory mediators in response to any exogenous or endogenous stimuli [7]. As a component of the innate immune system, the activated Mφ with their liberated cytokines and growth factors are suitable for the growth of endometriosis [7, 43]. Although a link between the severity of endometriosis and Mφ activation has been reported in 1995 [44], several subsequent studies informed us regarding the tissue infiltration of these inflammatory cells and their relationship with the staging and morphologic appearances of endometriosis [45–47].

5.4.1 Mφ Infiltration in Eutopic and Ectopic Endometrium

In a case control study with eutopic and ectopic endometrial biopsy samples derived from women with and without endometriosis, we found that the tissue infiltration of CD68-stained pan-macrophages (Mφ) in the eutopic endometria was significantly higher in women with endometriosis than in women without endometriosis [47]. When we evaluated the distribution pattern of Mφ infiltration in the eutopic and ectopic endometria based on revised-ASRM staging of endometriosis, we found that women with stage I-II endometriosis harbored significantly more Mφ in their eutopic endometria than in women with stage III-IV endometriosis, and this was more marked in the secretory phase than in the proliferative phase of the menstrual cycle. The ectopic endometriotic lesions in the peritoneal cavity in women having stage I-II endometriosis also displayed higher Mφ accumulation, and this was predominant in the secretory phase [47]. These results indicate that activity status of endometriotic lesions is more dominant in early endometriosis than in advanced endometriosis.

5.4.2 Mφ Infiltration Based on Phases of Menstrual Cycle

The distribution of tissue infiltration of endometriosis according to the phases of the menstrual cycle is variable as reported by different studies. Braun et al. [48] reported that number of Mφ is decreased only in the early proliferative phase and was not significantly different in other phases of endometriotic patients. Another subsequent study reported that Mφ numbers increased in the whole proliferative phase of endometriotic patients. They counted cells that were positive for CD68, a marker of matured and activated pan-macrophages [49]. In a separate study, a higher distribution of these inflammatory cells was found in the secretory phase of the menstrual cycle [47]. Comparing to control women without endometriosis, tissue infiltration of Mφ was significantly higher in both proliferative and secretory phases in women with endometriosis. Although an apparent increase of Mφ infiltration was observed in the secretory phase, no significant difference was found between proliferative and secretory phases in women without endometriosis [47]. We examined the distribution of Mφ infiltration in the early, mid, and late proliferative phase and corresponding secretory phase of the menstrual cycle. We found that Mφ infiltration of the endometrium increased steadily throughout the cycle in both proliferative and secretory phases. In fact, a transitional increase in the accumulation of Mφ was noted from the early, mid, to late phases of the respective menstrual cycle [47].

5.4.3 Mφ Infiltration Based on Morphologic Appearance of Lesions

We examined the tissue infiltration of Mφ in different peritoneal lesions based on their color appearance and in their corresponding adjacent peritoneum. We found that red lesions and their adjacent peritoneum harbored more Mφ than in either black lesions or white lesions. The infiltrated Mφ number in the peritoneum collected from control women was not different from that of black lesions [47]. These results indicate that early endometriosis with red peritoneal lesions induces a higher inflammatory response in the pelvic cavity than advanced endometriosis by the increased recruitment and accumulation of Mφ in these tissues. These findings were coincided with a significant correlation between CD68-positive Mφ number and monocyte chemoattractant protein-1 (MCP-1) concentration in the PF of women with endometriosis. No positive correlation was found between isolated Mφ and MCP-1 levels in women without endometriosis [47].

5.4.4 Correlation Between Mφ Infiltration and HGF Expression/MVD

HGF was discovered as a mitogen for adult hepatocytes and is identical to scatter factor [50, 51]. Several lines of evidence have implied that HGF, produced by mesenchymal cells and macrophages, exerts mitogenic, motogenic (migration), morphogenic, and angiogenic activity after binding with its receptor, c-Met, on various epithelial cells derived from rodents and humans [50, 51]. The role of HGF on the proliferation, migration, and metaplastic transformation of endometrial tissue has been demonstrated both in vitro and in vivo [29, 52]. We examined the relationship between Mφ infiltration and immunoreaction of HGF in the eutopic endometrium of women with and without endometriosis and in different peritoneal lesions. We found a significant correlation between them in women with endometriosis and in those containing red peritoneal lesions [47]. We also found a similar significant association between tissue accumulation of Mφ and microvessel density (MVD) as measured by total microvessel number in the eutopic endometrium of women with endometriosis and in red lesions [47]. No relationship was found between them in control women or in other peritoneal lesions.

Collectively, our findings indicated that the growth of endometriosis is not only affected by the increased production of different mitogenic and angiogenic factors by the endometriotic tissues themselves but is also affected by the infiltrated Mφ, which is markedly accumulated in peritoneal endometriosis tissues and adjacent peritoneum. The peritoneum, which is adjacent to active endometriotic lesions, is also responsive to similar pelvic inflammation and harbors a substantial amount of Mφ. We previously reported from our laboratory that immunoexpression of HGF and its receptor, c-Met, was stronger in early endometriosis and was manifested by a strong immunoreaction in active red lesions and the corresponding eutopic endometrium of women with endometriosis than other peritoneal lesions or in control women [46]. These overexpressions of HGF and c-Met were associated with the tissue proliferation and angiogenesis as defined by the coexpression of proliferating cell nuclear antigen and von-Willbrand factor (VWF) in the same tissues [46].

Our findings suggest that growth of endometriosis does not depend on the fibrotic extension of disease, rather it depends on the tissue activity of endometriosis. We presume that extension of disease could be related to pelvic pain, but higher activity of endometriosis associated with abundant recruitment and infiltration of Mφ could be related to infertility. Our results agree with those of Donnez et al. [53, 54] and indicate that the increased tissue activity of endometriosis is associated with an increased pelvic inflammatory response.

5.5 Regulation of HGF by Basal and Stimulated Mφ

We already came to learn that different macromolecules as secreted by Mφ in the pelvic environment are involved in the growth of endometriosis. The possible mediator that stimulated Mφ for the production of different growth factors including HGF is not well known. We demonstrated that menstrual fluid and PF of women with endometriosis contains higher concentration of LPS (endotoxin) than that of those without endometriosis [30]. It is possible that as an initial inflammatory mediator, LPS could stimulate peritoneal Mφ for the production of HGF. HGF is a pleiotropic growth factor and is traditionally believed to be a source of mesenchymal cells. The possible production of HGF by the basal and LPS-stimulated Mφ derived from women with and without endometriosis was unknown.

A significant increase in the proliferation of peritoneal Mφ derived from women with endometriosis and particularly of those harboring red lesions was observed after treatment with LPS. A fourfold and threefold increase in the production of HGF was observed by the LPS-treated Mφ derived from women with revised-ASRM stage I-II endometriosis and stage III-IV endometriosis, respectively, when compared with non-LPS-treated Mφ [28]. At the transcriptional level, we found a fivefold increase in HGF mRNA expression in LPS-treated peritoneal Mφ versus basal (LPS-untreated) Mφ in women with endometriosis. The bromodeoxyuridine (BrdU) incorporation study indicated that 10–100 ng/mL of HGF enhanced the growth of endometrial epithelial cells, stromal cells, and Mφ (~50% increase) derived from women with endometriosis [28]. These results suggest that LPS could be an inflammatory mediator of Mφ stimulation in the pelvic microenvironment. Besides mesenchymal cells, HGF is also produced by peritoneal Mφ and is possibly involved in the growth or persistence of endometriosis. Besides ovarian steroid hormones, the role of innate immune system in the regulation of endometriosis is also important. Since peritoneal Mφ retain the receptor (TLR4) for LPS derived from Gram-negative bacteria [30], we can speculate that a subclinical concentration of endotoxin in pelvis could stimulate Mφ, produce different cytokines and growth factors, and interact with its neighboring cells in the pathogenesis of endometriosis.

5.6 ER/PR Expression in Mφ and Role of Ovarian Steroids

A number of publications have demonstrated the potential role of ovarian steroid hormones in the regeneration of endometrium after menstruation and the growth of endometriosis [4, 5, 55, 56]. However, as a nonself lesion in pelvic environment, the growth and/or persistence of endometriosis can also be regulated by the innate immune system. The mitogenesis or angiogenesis of eutopic and ectopic endometrium possibly involves an extensive interplay between endometrial cells, inflammatory cells, ovarian hormones, soluble factors, and the extracellular matrix [6, 49]. Since mesenchymal cells retain estrogen receptor, production of different cytokines by endometrial stromal cells and its modulation by estrogen has been demonstrated [11]. Considering that infiltrated Mφ are one of the cell components of endometriotic lesions in the pelvic environment, information of the expression of ovarian steroid receptors by macrophages and the secretion of different macromolecules in response to steroid hormones deserves attention.

RT-PCR and immunohistochemical analysis revealed that estrogen and progesterone receptors (ER/PR) were expressed in isolated peritoneal Mφ and intact tissue at the protein and mRNA levels. Macrophages derived from women with endometriosis produced significantly higher concentrations of HGF in conditioned media after treatment with estradiol (10^{-8} M) than that of basal Mφ or women without endometriosis. These effects were less evident after treatment with progesterone [57]. It was interesting to observe that treatment with antiestrogenic agent, tamoxifen (10^{-6} M), reversed the production of HGF and other macromolecules. Secretion of HGF in response to ovarian steroids was further enhanced after activation of Mφ with LPS. The mRNA expression of HGF and its receptor, c-Met, were also detected in Mφ and stroma in response to estrogen, suggesting an autocrine regulation. HGF mRNA expression was higher in cells of women with endometriosis than nonendometriosis women. Bromodeoxyuridine incorporation assay indicated that exogenous stimulation with HGF and estrogen, either alone or in combination, significantly increased cell proliferation of both endometrial stromal cells and peritoneal Mφ compared to that of nonendometriosis or nontreated cells [57].

These results suggest that besides other inflammatory mediators, ovarian steroids also participate in the production of HGF by peritoneal Mφ and may be involved in the growth of endometriosis either alone or in combination with LPS. These findings of a persistent inflammatory response in women with endometriosis and estrogen-regulated production of HGF by activated and nonactivated peritoneal Mφ further confirmed that the growth of endometriosis possibly depends on a mutual interaction between the innate immune system and ovarian steroid hormones in the pelvic microenvironment. The current therapeutic strategy of hypoestrogenic medication in women with endometriosis can also be explained by its effect on innate immune system, which may suppress different cytokines and growth factors and thereby improve the growth of endometriosis or other reproductive diseases.

5.7 Crosstalk Between Inflammation and Ovarian Steroids

Basically endometriosis is an estrogen-dependent disease and induces an inflammatory reaction in pelvic environment. An abundant number of literatures have already demonstrated individual effect of estrogen and effect of initial or secondary inflammatory mediators in the growth regulation of endometriosis [57–60]. An additive effect between inflammation and stress reaction on the growth of endometriosis has been demonstrated [61]. Therefore, it is important to know the combined effect of estrogen and inflammation in the growth of endometriosis.

In an attempt to explore the combined effect between inflammation and ovarian steroids, we demonstrated that Mφ-mediated production of HGF/VEGF/IL-6/TNFα in response to ovarian steroids was further enhanced after treatment with LPS [57]. An additive effect was observed between E_2 and LPS on promoting pelvic inflammation and on the proliferation of eutopic and ectopic endometrial stromal cells when compared with their single treatment. This effect of E_2+LPS on cell growth and peritoneal Mφ-mediated inflammation was markedly abrogated after pretreatment of cells with anti-TLR4 antibody and ICI 182720, an ER antagonist [3, 62, 63]. These findings suggest that E_2 exhibits proinflammatory response, and an immuno-endocrine crosstalk between estrogen and inflammation in pelvic environment may be involved in additive inflammatory response in pelvic environment and growth of endometriosis. Another published report on this issue supported our findings [64].

5.8 Effect of GnRHa on Tissue Inflammation

With the advent of isolation and synthesis of gonadotropin-releasing hormone (GnRH) by Schally in the early 1970s [65], interest in the clinical application of GnRH agonist (GnRHa) has grown. Now in clinical practice, GnRHa has been used for the medical treatment of prostate cancer, precocious puberty, endometriosis, adenomyosis, and uterine myoma. Traditionally, the effect of GnRHa is mediated by competitive downregulation of pituitary GnRH receptors (GnRHR), causing a state of hypoestrogenemia resulting in the resolution of pain symptoms and regression of disease.

Endogenous GnRH (GnRH I and GnRH II) and exogenous GnRHa have been demonstrated to exert antiproliferative and apoptotic effects on cultured endometriotic cells and some cancer cells derived from reproductive organs [66, 67]. The response of this hormonal medication to reproductive diseases is variable depending on the type of the medication, patients background, and GnRH receptor-ligand binding affinity for individual cells or tissues [68, 69]. In addition to central effect, multiple biological functions of GnRHa, such as in decreasing tissue inflammation, cell proliferation, and angiogenesis and in promoting cellular apoptosis, in intact tissues of women with different reproductive diseases have been demonstrated [22, 70].

Considering the effect of GnRHa on peripheral tissues, immunohistochemical analysis showed that tissue infiltration of CD68-positive Mφ and VWF-positive microvessel density were significantly decreased in the endometria of women with endometriosis, adenomyosis, and uterine myoma in the GnRHa-treated group (for a variable period of 3–6 months) when compared with that in the nontreated group [22]. A marked decrease in inflammatory and angiogenic responses was observed in lesions and myometria of these diseases. When compared with nontreated group, a significant increase in apoptotic index (apoptotic cells per 10 mm^2 area) and quantitative-histogram (Q-H) scores of activated caspase-3 after GnRHa therapy was observed in the eutopic endometria, pathological lesions, and myometria of these diseases [22]. These results suggest that GnRH agonist was able to markedly reduce the inflammatory reaction and angiogenesis and significantly induce apoptosis in tissues derived from women with endometriosis, adenomyosis, and uterine myoma. These multiple local biological effects of GnRHa may be involved in the regression of these reproductive diseases with consequent resolution of symptoms suffering from these hazardous diseases.

5.9 Summary and Perspective

We now know that besides steroid hormones, innate immunity plays a pivotal role in the initiation of an array of inflammatory reactions against regurgitated endometrial cells and subsequent development of peritoneal endometriosis. Currently, prevalent concepts on the genesis of endometriosis are retrograde dissemination of eutopic endometrial tissues during menstruation, coelomic metaplasia of the peritoneum, and compromised immuno-surveillance. However, none of these theories can explain the pathogenesis of endometriosis uniformly. A number of widely accepted mechanisms involved in the development or pathogenesis of endometriosis are summarized in Fig. 5.2. Based on our serial studies on the etiological role of bacterial endotoxin (LPS), we would propose a novel concept for the genesis of pelvic endometriosis via LPS/TLR4/Mφ-mediated engagement of innate immune response.

According to this concept, it would appear possible to integrate two conflicting thoughts of transplantation and metaplasia as reflecting the different phases of initiation and progression of pelvic endometriosis. Transplantation and consequent implantation of regurgitated endometrial cells during menstruation may trigger strong inflammatory reaction in early endometriosis. In addition, a variety of proinflammatory factors are also secreted from the infiltrated Mφ of innate immune system. During progression of the affected lesion, cellular changes of juxtaposed mesothelium into endometrioid cells and gland-like structures subsequently ensue and were described as metaplasia of peritoneal mesothelium [52, 71]. As a pleiotropic growth factor, HGF being produced by Mφ and stromal cells has been shown to serve this unique role. The multifunctional role of HGF can be performed with the aid of systemic or focal hormonal environment characterized by consistent estrogen

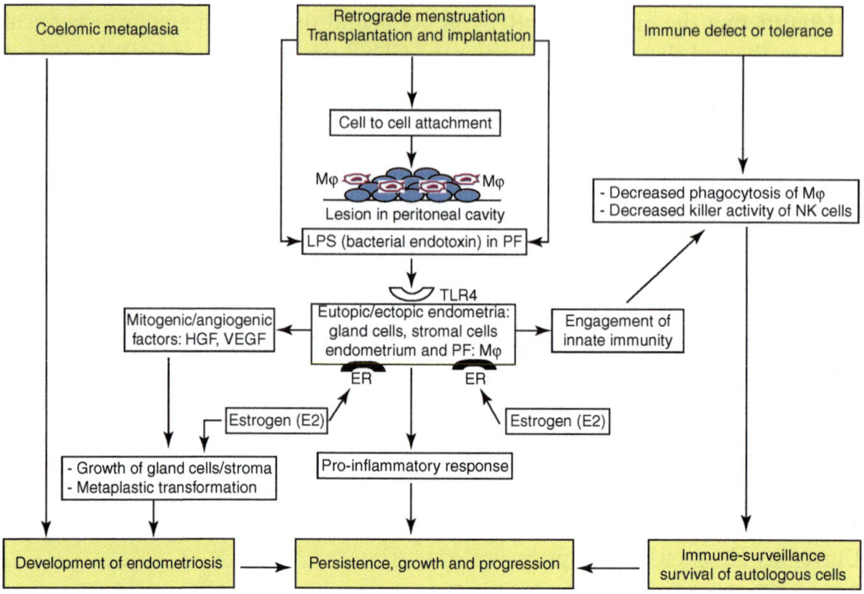

Fig. 5.2 Shows proposed concepts on the immunopathogenesis of pelvic endometriosis by hepatocyte growth factor, bacterial endotoxin (LPS) via toll-like receptor 4 (TLR4), macrophages (Mφ), and ovarian steroid hormone (estrogen, E2)) and their crosstalk in the development, persistence, and progression of endometriosis (Refs. [3, 62]). The details of the development of endometriosis, the immuno-endocrine relationship, and engagement of innate immune system in endometriosis are described in the text

synthesis. Our presenting findings demonstrate that besides other proinflammatory mediators, ovarian steroids also participate in the generation of a pelvic inflammatory response by producing different macromolecules including HGF by peritoneal Mφ. These proinflammatory mediators including HGF may be involved in the growth of endometriosis either alone or in combination with estrogen. A complete understanding of the mechanisms of endocrine-immune crosstalk in the mammalian species and the function of innate immunity via toll-like receptor system will be helpful for the future development of innovative therapies for manipulation of endometriosis.

Acknowledgments The author gratefully thanks Dr. Akira Fujishita of Saiseikai Nagasaki Hospital, Nagasaki, Japan; Prof. Tadayuki Ishimaru and Dr. Michio Kitajima of Graduate School of Biomedical Sciences, Nagasaki University, Nagasaki, Japan; and Prof. Jo Kitawaki of Kyoto Prefectural University of Medicine, Kyoto, Japan, for their constant support and scientific advice in all concerned studies as mentioned in this book chapter. The author also cordially thanks Prof. Sun-Wei Guo of Shanghai OB/GYN Hospital, Fudan Medical University, Shanghai, China, for his kind recommendation, stimulating discussion and advice during writing this chapter.

References

1. Burney RO, Giudice LC. Pathogenesis and pathophysiology of endometriosis. Fertil Steril. 2012;98(3):511–9.
2. Attar E, Bulun SE. Aromatase and other steroidogenic genes in endometriosis: translational aspects. Hum Reprod Update. 2006;12(1):49–56.
3. Khan KN, Kitajima M, Hiraki H, Fujishita A, Sekine I, Ishimaru T, Masuzaki H. Immunopathogenesis of pelvic endometriosis: role of hepatocyte growth factor, macrophages and ovarian steroids. Am J Reprod Immunol. 2008;60:383–404.
4. Sampson J. Peritoneal endometriosis due to menstrual dissemination of endometrial tissue into the peritoneal cavity. Am J Obstet Gynecol. 1927;14:422–9.
5. Thomas EJ, Prentice A. The etiology and pathogenesis of endometriosis. Reprod Med Rev. 1992;1:21–36.
6. Folkman J, Klagsbrun M. Angiogenic factors. Science. 1987;235:442–6.
7. Halme J, Becker S, Haskill S. Altered maturation and function of peritoneal macrophages: possible role in the pathogenesis of endometriosis. Am J Obstet Gynecol. 1987;156:783–9.
8. Helme J. Release of tumor necrosis factor-alpha by human peritoneal macrophages in vivo and in vitro. Am J Obstet Gynecol. 1989;161:1718–25.
9. Khan KN, Masuzaki H, Fujishita A, Hamasaki T, Kitajima M, Hasuo A, Ishimaru T. Association of interleukin 6 and estradiol with hepatocyte growth factor in peritoneal fluid of women with endometriosis. Acta Obstet Gynecol Scand. 2002;81:764–71.
10. Kitajima M, Khan KN, Fujishita A, Masuzaki H, Ishimaru T. Histomorphometric alteration and cell-type specific modulation of arylhydrocarbon receptor and estrogen receptor expression by 2,3,7,8-tetrachlorodibemzo-p-dioxin and 17b-estradiol in mouse experimental model of endometriosis. Reprod Toxicol. 2004;18:793–801.
11. Tabibzadeh SS, Santhanan V, Sehgal PB, May LT. Cytokine induced production of IFN-β2/IL-6 by freshly implanted human endometrial stromal cells: modution by estradiol 17β. J Immunol. 1989;42:3134–9.
12. Lloyd AF, Miron VE. Cellular and molecular mechanisms underpinning macrophage activation during remyelination. Front Cell Dev Biol. 2016;4:60. https://doi.org/10.3389/fcell.2016.00060.
13. Hogg C, Horne AW, Greaves E. Endometriosis-associated macrophages: origin, phenotype, and function. Front Endocrinol. 2020;11:7. https://doi.org/10.3389/fendo.2020.00007.
14. Alexander JW, Boyce ST, Babcock GF, et al. The process of microbial translocation. Ann Surg. 1990;212:496–511.
15. Nie M-F, Xie Q, Wu Y-H, He H, Zou L-J, She X-L, Wu X-Q. Serum and ectopic endometrium from women with endometriosis modulate macrophage M1/M2 polarization via the Smad2/Smad3 pathway. J Immunol Res. 2018;2018:6285813. https://doi.org/10.1155/2018/6285813.
16. Wang N, Liang H, Zen K. Molecular mechanisms that influence the macrophage m1-m2 polarization balance. Front Immunol. 2014;5:614. https://doi.org/10.3389/fimmu.2014.00614.
17. Zhang F, Wang X, Wang H, et al. TGF-beta induces M2-like macrophage polarization via SNAIL-mediated suppression of a pro-inflammatory phenotype. Oncotarget. 2016;7(32):52294–306.
18. Jansen AL, Collins J, Shipman EP, Wira CR, Guyrc PM, Piolo PA. A subset of human uterine endometrial macrophages is alternatively activated. Am J Reprod Immunol. 2012;68:374–86.
19. Takebayashi A, Kimura F, Kishi Y, Ishida M, Takahashi A, Yamanaka A, Wu D, Zheng L, Takahashi K, Suginami H, Murakami T. Subpopulations of macrophages within eutopic endometrium of endometriosis patients. Am J Reprod Immunol. 2015;73:221–31.
20. Khan KN, Fujishita A, Kitajima M, Masuzaki H, Sekine I, Ishimaru T. Infiltrated macrophage activity in intact tissue of endometriosis. Proc Endometr Res. 2002;23:137–42.
21. Miura S, Khan KN, Kitajima M, Hiraki K, Moriyama S, Masuzaki H, Samejima T, Fujishita A, Ishimaru T. Differential infiltration of macrophages and prostaglandin production by different uterine leiomyomas. Hum Reprod. 2006;21(10):2545–54.

22. Khan KN, Kitajima M, Hiraki K, Fujishita A, Sekine I, Ishimaru T, Masuzaki H. Changes in tissue inflammation, angiogenesis and apoptosis in endometriosis, adenomyosis and uterine myoma after GnRH agonist therapy. Hum Reprod. 2010;25(3):642–53.
23. Check W. Innate immunity depends on Toll-like receptors. ASM News. 2004;70:317–22.
24. Reichhart JM. TLR5 takes aim at bacterial propeller. Nat Immunol. 2003;4:1159–60.
25. Takeda K, Akira S. Toll-like receptors in innate immunity. Int Immunol. 2005;17:1–14.
26. Wira CR, Fahey JV, Sentman CL, Pioli PA, Shen L. Innate and adaptive immunity in female genital tract: cellular responses and interactions. Immunol Rev. 2005;206:306–35.
27. Fazeli A, Bruce C, Anumba DO. Characterization of Toll-like receptors in the female reproductive tract in humans. Hum Reprod. 2005;20(5):1372–8.
28. Khan KN, Masuzaki H, Fujishita A, Kitajima M, Kohno T, Sekine I, Matsuyama T, Ishimaru T. Regulation of hepatocyte growth factor by basal and stimulated-macrophages in women with endometriosis. Hum Reprod. 2005;20:49–60.
29. Khan KN, Kitajima M, Fujishita A, Sekine I, Ishimaru T, Masuzaki H. Multifunctional role of hepatocyte growth factor (HGF) in the development of pelvic endometriosis. WES e-J (review article). 2008;(July):13–20.
30. Khan KN, Kitajima M, Hiraki K, Yamaguchi N, Katamine S, Matsuyama T, Fujishita A, Nakashima M, Ishimaru T, Masuzaki H. Escherichia coli contamination of menstrual blood and effect of bacterial endotoxin on endometriosis. Fertil Steril. 2010;94(7):2860–3.
31. Lee SK, Kim CJ, Kim DJ, Kang JH. Immune cells in the female reproductive tract. Immune Netw. 2015;15(1):16–26.
32. Betjes MGH, Tuk CW, Struijik DG, Kredict RT, Arisz L, Hart M, et al. Interleukin-8 production by human peritoneal mesothelial cells in response to tumor necrosis factor-α, interleukin-1 and medium conditioned by macrophages co-cultured with Staphylococcus epidermis. J Infect Dis. 1993;168:1202–10.
33. Somerset D, Zheng AY, Kilby MD, Sansom DM, Drayson MT. Normal human pregnancy is associated with an elevation in the immune suppressive $CD25^{+}CD4^{+}$ regulatory T-cell subset. Immunology. 2004;112:38–43.
34. Maeda N, Izumiya C, Taniguchi K, Matsushima S, Fukaya T. Role of NK cells and HLA-G in endometriosis. Front Biosci (Elite Ed). 2012;S4:1568–81.
35. Guo SW, Du Y, Liu X. Platelet-derived TGF-β1 mediates the down-modulation of NKG2D expression and may be responsible for impaired natural killer (NK) cytotoxicity in women with endometriosis. Hum Reprod. 2016;31(7):1462–74.
36. Du Y, Liu X, Guo SW. Platelets impair natural killer cell cytotoxicity and function in endometriosis through multiple mechanisms. Hum Reprod. 2017;32(4):794–810.
37. Witherel CE, Abebayehu D, Barker TH, Spiller KL. Macrophage and fibroblast interactions in biomaterial-mediated fibrosis. Adv Healthc Mater. 2019;8(4):e1801451. https://doi.org/10.1002/adhm.201801451.
38. Zhang Q, Duan J, Liu X, Guo SW. Platelets drive smooth muscle metaplasia and fibrogenesis in endometriosis through epithelial-mesenchymal transition and fibroblast-to-myofibroblast transdifferentiation. Mol Cell Endocrinol. 2016;428:1–16.
39. Wynn TA, Barron L. Macrophages: master regulators of inflammation and fibrosis. Semin Liver Dis. 2010;30:245–57.
40. Hesketh M, Sahin KB, West ZE, Murray RZ. Macrophage phenotypes regulate scar formation and chronic wound healing. Int J Mol Sci. 2017;18:1545–55.
41. Bacci M, Capobianco A, Monno A, Cottone L, Di Puppo F, Camisa B, et al. Macrophages are alternatively activated in patients with endometriosis and required for growth and vascularization of lesions in a mouse model of disease. Am J Pathol. 2009;175:547–56.
42. Duan J, Liu X, Wang H, Guo SW. The M2a macrophage subset may be critically involved in the fibrogenesis of endometriosis in mice. Reprod Biomed Online. 2018;37(3):254–68.
43. Halme J, White C, Kauma S, Estes J, Haskill S. Peritoneal macrophages from patients with endometriosis release growth factor activity in vitro. J Clin Endocrinol Metab. 1988;66:1044–9.

44. Becker JL, Widen RH, Mahan CS, Yeko TR, Parsons AK, Spellacy WN. Human peritoneal macrophages and T lymphocyte populations in mild and severe endometriosis. Am J Reprod Immunol. 1995;34:179–87.
45. Khan KN, Fujishita A, Kitajima M, Masuzaki H, Sekine I, Ishimaru T. Infiltrated macrophage activity in intact tissue of endometriosis. Proc Endometr. 2002;23:137–42. (Japanese).
46. Khan KN, Masuzaki H, Fujishita A, Kitajima M, Sekine I, Ishimaru T. Immunoexpression of hepatocyte growth factor and c-Met receptor in eutopic endometrium predicts the activity of ectopic endometrium. Fertil Steril. 2003;79:173–81.
47. Khan KN, Masuzaki H, Fujishita A, Kitajima M, Sekine I, Ishimaru T. Differential macrophage infiltration in early and advanced endometriosis and adjacent peritoneum. Fertil Steril. 2004;81(3):652–61.
48. Braun DP, Ding J, Shen J, Rana N, Fernendez BB, Dmowski WP. Relationship between apoptosis and the number of macrophages in eutopic endometrium from women with and without endometriosis. Fertil Steril. 2002;78:830–5.
49. Berbic M, Schulke L, Markham R, Tokushige N, Russell P, Fraser IS. Macrophage expression in endometrium of women with and without endometriosis. Hum Reprod. 2009;24:325–32.
50. Nakamura T, Nishizawa T, Hagiya M, Seki T, Shimonishi M, Sugimura A. Molecular cloning and expression of hepatocyte growth factor. Nature. 1989;342:440–3.
51. Wiedner KM, Arakaki N, Vandekereckhove J, Weingart S, Hartmann G, Reider H. Evidence for the identity of human scatter factor and human hepatocyte growth factor. Proc Natl Acad Sci U S A. 1991;88:7001–5.
52. Sugawara J, Fukaya T, Murakami T, Yoshida H, Yajima A. Hepatocyte growth factor stimulates proliferation, migration and lumen formation of human endometrial epithelial cells in vitro. Biol Reprod. 1997;57:936–42.
53. Donnez J, Nisolle M, Smoes P, Gillet N, Beguin S, Casanas-Roux F. Peritoneal endometriosis and 'endometriotic' nodule of recto-vaginal septum are different entities. Fertil Steril. 1996;66:362–8.
54. Donnez J, Smoes P, Gillerot S, Casanas-Roux F, Nisolle M. Vascular endothelial growth factor in endometriosis. Hum Reprod. 1998;13:1686–90.
55. Fujishita A, Nakane PK, Koji T, Masuzaki H, Chavez RO, Yamabe T, Ishimaru T. Exprcssion of estrogen and progesterone receptors in endometrium and peritoneal endometriosis: an immunohistochemical and in situ hybridization study. Fertil Steril. 1997;67:856–64.
56. Nisolle M, Casana-Rouz F, Donnez J. Immunohistochemical analysis of proliferative activity and steroid receptor expression in peritoneal and ovarian endometriosis. Fertil Steril. 1997;68:912–9.
57. Khan KN, Masuzaki H, Fujishita A, Kitajima M, Sekine I, Matsuyama T, Ishimaru T. Estrogen and progesterone receptor expression in macrophages and regulation of hepatocyte growth factor by ovarian steroids in women with endometriosis. Hum Reprod. 2005;20:2004–13.
58. Khan KN, Masuzaki H, Fujishita A, Kitajima M, Hiraki K, Sekine I, Matsuyama T, Ishimaru T. Interleukin-6 and tumor necrosis factor α-mediated expression of hepatocyte growth factor by stromal cells and its involvement in the growth of endometriosis. Hum Reprod. 2005;20:2715–23.
59. Beagley KW, Gockel CM. Regulation of innate and adaptive immunity by the female sex hormones estradiol and progesterone. FEMS Immunol Med Microbiol. 2003;38:13–22.
60. Herath S, Fischer FD, Werling D, Williams EJ, Lilly ST, Dobson H, Bryant CE, Sheldon IM. Expression and function of Toll-like receptor 4 in the endometrial cells of the uterus. Endocrinology. 2006;147:562–70.
61. Khan KN, Kitajima M, Inoue T, Tateishi S, Fujishita A, Nakashima M, Masuzaki H. Additive effects of inflammation and stress reaction on Toll-like receptor 4-mediated growth of endometriotic stromal cells. Hum Reprod. 2013;28(10):2794–803.
62. Khan KN, Kitajima M, Fujishita A, Nakashima M, Masuzaki H. Toll-like receptor system and endometriosis. J Obstet Gynecol Res. 2013;39(8):1281–92.

63. Khan KN, Kitajima M, Inoue T, Fujishita A, Nakashima M, Masuzaki H. 17β-estradiol and lipopolysaccharide additively promote pelvic inflammation and growth of endometriosis. Reprod Sci. 2015;22(5):585–94.
64. Cakmak H, Guzeloglu-Kayisli O, Kayisli UA, Arici A. Immune-endocrine interactions in endometriosis. Front Biosci. 2009;E1:429–43.
65. Schally AV, Arimura A, Kastin A, Matsuo H, Baba Y, Redding TW, et al. Gonadotropin releasing hormone: one polypeptide regulates secretion of luteinizing and follicle-stimulating hormones. Science. 1971;173:1036–8.
66. Borroni R, Di Blasio AM, Gaffuri B, Santorsola R, Busacca M, Vigano P, Vignali M. Expression of GnRH receptor gene in human ectopic endometrial cells and inhibition of their proliferation by leuprolide acetate. Mol Cell Endocrinol. 2000;159:37–43.
67. Limonta P, Dondi D, Moretti RM, Maggi R, Motta M. Anti-proliferative effects of luteinizing hormone-releasing hormone agonists on the human prostatic cancer cell line LNCaP. J Clin Endocrinol Metab. 1992;75:207–12.
68. Qayum A, Gullik W, Clayton RC, Sikora K, Waxman J. The effects of gonadotropin-releasing hormone analogues in prostate cancer are mediated through specific tumor receptors. Br J Cancer. 1990;62:94–6.
69. Emons G, Schroder B, Ortaman O, Westphalen S, Schultz K, Schally AV. High affinity binding and direct antiproliferative effects of LHRH analogues in human ovarian cancer cell lines. Cancer Res. 1993;53:5439–46.
70. Khan KN, Kitajima M, Hiraki K, Fujishita A, Nakashima M, Ishimaru T, Masuzaki H. Cell proliferation effect of GnRH agonist on pathological lesions of women with endometriosis, adenomyosis and uterine myoma. Hum Reprod. 2010;25(11):2878–90.
71. Ishimaru T, Khan KN, Fujishita A, Kitajima M, Masuzaki H. Hepatocyte growth factor may be involved in cellular changes to the peritoneal mesothelium adjacent to pelvic endometriosis. Fertil Steril. 2004;81(Suppl 1):810–8.

Pathogenesis of Endometriosis: Genetics

6

Nilufer Rahmioglu and Krina T. Zondervan

Contents

6.1 Introduction

Endometriosis is a common complex condition that is caused by the interplay of multiple genetic and environmental factors. The genetic risk variants for the condition only present part of the disease risk, and environmental factors also a play an important role in disease pathogenesis either independently or through interaction with genetic factors [1]. The heritability that is the proportion of disease risk due to genetic factors for endometriosis has been estimated in two large twin studies [2, 3] that arrived at very similar estimates (49–51%). A separate study estimated 26% to be due to common genetic variation (DNA variants with a frequency >1% in the population) [4]. As the underlying pathology of endometriosis is not well understood, one way to explore underlying mechanisms is to investigate the genetic factors and their functions that are causal for the disease. For complex diseases such as

N. Rahmioglu (✉) · K. T. Zondervan
Wellcome Centre for Human Genetics, University of Oxford, Oxford, UK

Oxford Endometriosis Care Centre, Nuffield Department of Women's and Reproductive Health, John Radcliffe Hospital, University of Oxford, Oxford, UK
e-mail: nilufer@well.ox.ac.uk

E. Oral (ed.), *Endometriosis and Adenomyosis*,
https://doi.org/10.1007/978-3-030-97236-3_6

endometriosis, the most powerful and appropriate study design to detect genetic risk factors is that of a genetic association study, in which the frequencies of variants are compared between cases and controls, similar to an epidemiological case control study in which the frequency of risk-factor exposures is compared. For situations in which a disease shows a very strong pattern of familial inheritance (e.g., "monogenic" familial breast or ovarian cancer), family-based approaches are more appropriate, which we do not cover here.

6.2 Discovery of Endometriosis Genetic Susceptibility Variants

In population-based study designs, genetic variants can be investigated using hypothesis-driven or hypothesis-free association methods. The hypothesis-driven approach, candidate gene association studies, relies on prior biological understanding of the condition and testing for association in these regions that are prioritized based on previous knowledge. Similar to other complex diseases, candidate gene association studies have not generally been successful in identifying robust results for endometriosis [5]. For the results to be robust, identified associations need to be replicated in an independent study in individuals of similar ancestral background. The reason for general failure of candidate gene association studies is manyfold: (1) The prior biological knowledge on the tested regions for association may not be relevant to the disease in question; (2) the coverage of common genetic variation in candidate gene regions is often limited and does not allow the testing of all potential common genetic risk variants in these regions (either directly, or indirectly through linkage disequilibrium with other variants); (3) the number of genes included in the study are often limited to a few that make up only a small part of a potentially causal underlying pathway; (4) and the sample sizes of candidate gene studies have often been insufficient to detect common genetic variants for common complex conditions. The standard approach now to identify common genetic variants for common complex conditions is a hypothesis-free method, namely the genome-wide association study (GWAS).

6.3 Genome-Wide Association Studies

GWAS have been very successful in the identification of common genetic variants underlying complex conditions. In a GWAS, typically at least 2000 cases and 2000 controls are genotyped at a genome-wide level using an "off the shelf" microarray containing probes that capture 100,000s of single nucleotide polymorphisms (SNPs) – single base-pair DNA variants. After extensive quality control, the genotypes of SNPs nearby that are not directly genotyped can be imputed, using a reference panel that includes a comprehensive catalogue of common genetic variants in the relevant ancestry population. Subsequently, the frequency of common SNPs is tested for differences between the case and control groups. Owing to the millions of statistical tests conducted across the genome, a stringent significance threshold needs to be adopted to reduce the number of false positive findings. The standard threshold used for genome-wide significance is $p < 5 \times 10^{-8}$. A detailed overview of GWAS design is given in Zondervan and Cardon [6]. All common genome-wide significant variants identified for common complex diseases and traits through GWAS are documented in the National Human Genome Research Institute (NHGRI) GWA Catalogue (www.genome.gov/GWAStudies). This catalogue demonstrates how successful the GWAS approach has been in identifying common variants underlying complex diseases and traits: To date, the catalogue includes data on 255,015 SNP-disease associations (25 April 2021).

To date, 10 GWAS in women of European and East Asian ancestry have been published for endometriosis, varying from 171 to 58,115 included cases (Table 6.1). The largest is a meta-analysis led by the International Endogene Genomics Consortium (IEGC), for which interim results were released in 2018, comprising of 15 GWAS and a replication analysis including a total of 58,115 cases and 733,480

Table 6.1 Summary of 10 GWAS investigating associations with endometriosis

	Case and controls			Number of genome-wide significant loci	
GWAS	Ancestry	Number	Ascertainment		Reference
Adachi et al.	Japanese	696: 825	Surgically confirmed and medical records	0	Adachi et al. [7]
Uno et al.	Japanese	1423: 1318	Medical records	1	Uno et al. [8]
Painter et al.	European	3194: 7060	Surgically confirmed, medical records	1	Painter et al. [9]
Albertsen et al.	European	2019: 14,471	Surgically confirmed	3	Albertsen et al. [10]
Nyholt et al.	European and Japanese	4604: 9393	Surgically confirmed, medical records	3	Nyholt et al. [11]
Steinthorsdottir et al.	European	1840: 129,016	Surgically confirmed	3	Steinthorsdottir et al. [12]
Sapkota et al.	European and Japanese	17,045: 191,596	Surgically confirmed, medical records, and self-reported	14	Sapkota et al. [13]
Sobalska et al.	European	171: 2934	Surgically confirmed	3	Sobalska-Kwapis et al. [14]
Galarneau et al.	European	37,183: 251,258	Self-reported	14	Galarneau [15]
Rahmioglu et al.	European and Japanese	58,115: 733,480	Surgically confirmed, medical records, and self-reported	27	Rahmioglu [16]

controls [16]. An early GWAS had analyzed the effect of all SNPs combined by rASRM stage, showing a significantly higher genetic contribution to rASRM stage III/IV versus stage I/II disease (Proportion of endometriosis variation explained by common SNPs = 0.34, SD: 0.04 vs. 0.15, SD = 0.15) [9]. Therefore, subsequent GWAS meta-analyses were conducted separately for stage III/IV disease; the largest IEGC-led GWAS meta-analysis (2018) investigated association with rASRM stage III/IV disease, rASRM stage I/II disease (for the first time), and infertility-associated endometriosis subphenotypes, in addition to overall endometriosis. This study revealed 27 loci genome-wide significantly associated with endometriosis, 13 of which were novel (Table 6.2). Positionally, the lead SNPs for the identified genetic loci reside near genes that are involved in sex-steroid hormone, WNT signaling, cell adhesion/migration, cell growth/carcinogenesis, and inflammation-related pathways.

In subphenotype genome-wide association analyses, eight genome-wide significant signals were associated with stage III/IV disease and one genome-wide significant signal with infertility-associated endometriosis. Moreover, 21 of the 27 loci had larger effect sizes for stage III/IV compared to stage I/II disease (Table 6.2) suggesting that specific variants may confer risk for different subtypes of endometriosis through distinct pathways. Further studies with more detailed phenotypic data on endometriosis are needed to decipher the genetic variants that may be associated with different subtypes of the disease, and the identity of these subtypes beyond ASRM staging.

6.4 Conclusions and Future Work

The variance explained by the 27 loci together is 2.15% for overall endometriosis and 3.83% for rASRM stage III/IV disease [16], which shows that there are many more genetic susceptibility loci to be uncovered for endometriosis in larger, deeply phenotyped datasets. The most up-to-date findings show that genetic mechanisms underlying endometriosis implicate metabolic, reproductive, inflammatory, and pain-related pathways, although these are based on "nearest gene" assumptions (the notion that the gene nearest the risk variant is affected by the risk variant in terms of expression). Furthermore, the stronger associations observed with infertile endometriosis or stage III/IV endometriosis strengthen the fact that specific variants may confer risk for different subtypes of endometriosis through distinct pathways. Fine-mapping analyses are needed to identify the causal variants for each of the 27 loci. In particular, functional follow-up of identified variants is vitally important, examining their effects on transcriptomic, proteomic, metabolomic, and epigenomic data in tissues and cells relevant to endometriosis, i.e., endometrium and its cellular components.

As an example, *WNT4*/1p36.12 is a well-established locus associated with endometriosis, and the gene that sits nearest to the identified genome-wide significant variant is the *WNT4* gene. However, this positional evidence is not enough to determine whether this is the gene that involved functionally in endometriosis pathology.

Table 6.2 Twenty-seven genome-wide significant loci from the GWAS meta-analysis for endometriosis, stage III/IV, stage I/II, and infertile endometriosis [16]

Chr	Lead SNP	Position (hg19)	RA (RAF)	Overall endometriosis OR (95% CI)	Overall endometriosis p value	Stage III/IV endometriosis OR (95% CI)	Stage III/IV endometriosis p value	Stage I/II endometriosis OR (95% CI)	Stage I/II endometriosis p value	Infertile endometriosis OR (95% CI)	Infertile endometriosis p value	Nearest gene/cytoband
Previously reported loci												
1	rs12037376	22462111	A (0.19)	1.16 (1.13–1.19)	2.85×10^{-22}	1.23 (1.15–1.32)	1.33×10^{-9}	1.17 (1.08–1.26)	7.43×10^{-5}	1.21 (1.11–1.31)	4.24×10^{-6}	*WNT4/1p36.12*
2	rs11674184	11721535	T (0.61)	1.11 (1.09–1.14)	1.47×10^{-18}	1.17 (1.11–1.23)	1.13×10^{-8}	1.09 (1.02–1.16)	6.82×10^{-3}	1.05 (0.99–1.12)	0.11	*GREB1/2p25.1*
2	rs4141819	67864675	C (0.30)	1.05 (1.03–1.06)	3.08×10^{-10}	1.09 (1.03–1.15)	1.53×10^{-3}	1.07 (1.00–1.14)	0.03	1.06 (1.00–1.14)	0.05	*ETAA1/2p14*
2	rs10167914	113529183	C (0.32)	1.08 (1.05–1.11)	5.37×10^{-10}	1.13 (1.07–1.20)	1.05×10^{-5}	1.06 (1.00–1.13)	0.05	1.13 (1.05–1.19)	5.61×10^{-4}	*IL1A/2q13*
2	rs1250247	216299629	C (0.28)	1.07 (1.05–1.10)	3.88×10^{-8}	1.12 (1.06–1.18)	6.82×10^{-5}	1.09 (1.02–1.16)	9.67×10^{-3}	1.09 (1.02–1.16)	0.01	*FN1/2q35*
4	rs10012589	56002689	A (0.72)	1.10 (1.07–1.13)	5.69×10^{-13}	1.21 (1.14–1.28)	1.86×10^{-10}	1.08 (1.01–1.15)	0.02	1.11 (1.04–1.19)	2.07×10^{-3}	*KDR/4q12*
6	rs6938760	19802104	A (0.39)	1.09 (1.06–1.11)	2.89×10^{-12}	1.13 (1.08–1.19)	1.88×10^{-6}	1.06 (1.00–1.13)	0.05	1.10 (1.04–1.17)	1.16×10^{-3}	*ID4/6p22.3*
6	rs7759516	151838245	C (0.18)	1.14 (1.11–1.17)	1.35×10^{-18}	1.27 (1.19–1.35)	6.58×10^{-13}	1.03 (0.96–1.12)	0.41	1.08 (1.00–1.17)	0.04	*CCDC170/6q25.1*
6	rs71575922	152554014	G (0.16)	1.15 (1.12–1.19)	1.71×10^{-18}	1.30 (1.22–1.39)	3.63×10^{-14}	1.10 (1.02–1.19)	0.02	1.14 (1.05–1.23)	2.36×10^{-3}	*SYNE1/6q25.1*
7	rs12700667	25901639	A (0.72)	1.08 (1.05–1.11)	8.63×10^{-10}	1.20 (1.13–1.27)	3.15×10^{-9}	1.06 (0.99–1.13)	0.08	1.12 (1.05–1.20)	5.75×10^{-4}	*7p15.2/7p15.2*
7	rs55909142	46673774	C (0.6)	1.08 (1.05–1.10)	8.76×10^{-11}	1.14 (1.08–1.20)	1.61×10^{-6}	1.06 (1.00–1.13)	0.05	1.11 (1.05–1.17)	6.23×10^{-4}	*7p12.3/7p12.3*
9	rs9987548	22173075	A (0.4)	1.09 (1.06–1.12)	2.29×10^{-13}	1.19 (1.13–1.25)	6.90×10^{-11}	1.05 (0.99–1.12)	0.11	1.16 (1.09–1.24)	7.14×10^{-7}	*CDKN2-BAS1/9p21.3*

(continued)

Table 6.2 (continued)

Chr	Lead SNP	Position (hg19)	RA (RAF)	Overall endometriosis OR (95% CI)	Overall endometriosis *p* value	Stage III/IV endometriosis OR (95% CI)	Stage III/IV endometriosis *p* value	Stage I/II endometriosis OR (95% CI)	Stage I/II endometriosis *p* value	Infertile endometriosis OR (95% CI)	Infertile endometriosis *p* value	Nearest gene/cytoband
11	rs74485684	30242287	T (0.84)	1.15 (1.12–1.19)	1.32×10^{-18}	1.22 (1.14–1.31)	3.54×10^{-8}	1.10 (1.02–1.20)	0.01	1.17 (1.08–1.27)	2.34×10^{-4}	*FSHB/11p14.1*
12	rs12320196	95712695	C (0.3)	1.08 (1.05–1.10)	3.38×10^{-9}	1.14 (1.08–1.20)	2.66×10^{-6}	1.09 (1.02–1.16)	0.01	1.10 (1.03–1.17)	4.15×10^{-3}	*VEZT/12q22*
Novel loci												
1	rs1894692	169467654	A (0.98)	1.18 (1.13–1.24)	2.88×10^{-13}	1.63 (1.28–2.07)	5.99×10^{-5}	1.12 (0.88–1.43)	0.34	1.34 (1.06–1.71)	0.02	*SLC19A2/1q24.2*
1	rs495590	172152202	G (0.52)	1.07 (1.05–1.10)	6.73×10^{-10}	1.11 (1.06–1.17)	3.22×10^{-5}	1.06 (1.00–1.12)	0.05	1.07 (1.01–1.14)	0.02	*DNM3/1q24.3*
4	rs2510770	95479372	A (0.33)	1.05 (1.03–1.06)	8.25×10^{-10}	1.06 (1.01–1.12)	0.03	1.06 (0.99–1.13)	0.08	1.08 (1.01–1.15)	0.02	*PDLIM5/4q22.3*
5	rs13177597	82052282	G (0.13)	1.06 (1.04–1.08)	1.30×10^{-8}	1.15 (1.06–1.24)	6.81×10^{-4}	1.07 (0.97–1.17)	0.16	1.11 (1.01–1.22)	0.04	*ATP6AP1L/5q14.2*
7	rs62468795	23530051	G (0.85)	1.10 (1.07–1.14)	8.05×10^{-09}	1.14 (1.06–1.22)	5.2×10^{-4}	1.15 (1.06–1.26)	1.24×10^{-3}	1.08 (0.99–1.18)	0.08	*IGF2BP3/7p15.3*
8	rs10090060	75257608	A (0.58)	1.08 (1.06–1.11)	5.72×10^{-11}	1.08 (1.02–1.14)	3.85×10^{-3}	1.09 (1.02–1.15)	6.80×10^{-3}	1.11 (1.05–1.18)	4.83×10^{-4}	*GDAP1/8q21.11*
10	rs1802669	21827796	A (0.34)	1.07 (1.05–1.10)	5.52×10^{-9}	1.09 (1.03–1.15)	2.14×10^{-3}	1.09 (1.03–1.16)	6.08×10^{-3}	1.09 (1.02–1.16)	6.41×10^{-3}	*MLLT10/10p12.31*
10	rs796945	90150837	C (0.37)	1.07 (1.05–1.10)	1.78×10^{-9}	1.08 (1.03–1.14)	2.83×10^{-3}	1.05 (0.99–1.12)	0.10	1.11 (1.05–1.18)	5.80×10^{-4}	*RNLS/10q23.31*
12	rs17727841	102809630	G (0.81)	1.06 (1.04–1.08)	5.33×10^{-11}	1.17 (1.09–1.25)	4.95×10^{-6}	1.06 (0.98–1.14)	0.16	1.03 (0.95–1.11)	0.46	*IGF1/12q23.2*
14	rs7151531	93113547	C (0.29)	1.07 (1.04–1.10)	3.80×10^{-8}	1.10 (1.04–1.16)	8.37×10^{-4}	1.01 (0.95–1.08)	0.76	1.11 (1.04–1.18)	1.82×10^{-3}	*RIN3/14q32.12*

15	rs4923850	40352278	A (0.47)	1.05 (1.04–1.06)	3.07×10^{-13}	1.10 (1.04–1.15)	4.42×10^{-4}	1.03 (0.97–1.09)	0.40	1.07 (1.01–1.13)	0.03	*BMF/15q15.1*
17	rs66683298	46277748	C (0.61)	1.08 (1.06–1.11)	1.73×10^{-10}	1.10 (1.04–1.16)	3.71×10^{-4}	1.10 (1.04–1.17)	1.93×10^{-3}	1.06 (1.00–1.13)	0.04	*SKAP1/17q21.32*
17	rs76731691	63960269	G (0.94)	1.08 (1.05–1.11)	9.27×10^{-9}	1.20 (1.08–1.34)	9.77×10^{-4}	1.25 (1.10–1.42)	7.29×10^{-4}	1.14 (1.01–1.29)	0.04	*CEP112/17q24.1*

Referencing Rahmioglu et al. [16]

Powell et al. investigated the gene expression profile around this 1p36.12 cytoband and identified that the endometriosis associated variant is a significant eQTL in whole blood decreasing expression of *LINC00339* and increasing expression of *CDC42*. The eQTL for *LINC00339* was also observed in endometrium tissue with same direction of effect. However, no evidence for eQTL effects of *WNT4* was identified highlighting the importance and need for these functional studies to understand the disease-relevant mechanisms of the identified genetic risk variants [17].

Tissue-based molecular phenotyping data (transcriptomics, proteomics, and metabolomics) are not available for endometrium or its relevant cellular components in sufficiently large sample sizes from publicly available databases (e.g., the Genotype-Tissue Expression (GTEx) project [18, 19]). Two recent studies investigated the whole-transcriptome profiles utilizing RNA-sequencing ($N = 206$) and microarray-based gene expression ($N = 123$) in endometrium tissue and generated expression-quantitative trait loci (eQTL) maps to determine the genetic variants that regulate gene expression in endometrium tissue [20, 21]. The microarray-based and RNAseq-based eQTL maps identified variants that regulate expression of 198 and 327 unique genes, respectively. Such studies are very important to better understand the effect genetic risk variants have on gene expression in endometrium; however, similar profiling studies need to be conducted using other "omics" data (epigenomics, proteomics, and metabolomics). There is also need for collection of these tissue and cell types utilizing standardized protocols that will allow for collaboration between study centers to reach samples size needed for these functional investigations. The Endometriosis Phenome and Biobanking Harmonisation Project of the World Endometriosis Research Foundation has provided globally standardized protocols for data and sample collection in studies of endometriosis [22–25]. At the time of writing, 47 centers are using the standards for data and/or sample collection, with many 10,000s of samples already stored for research purposes in local study repositories. More large-scale integrated omics studies in deeply phenotyped patients are needed to understand the underlying causal mechanisms for endometriosis and dissect subtypes of this complex condition, leading to the discovery of novel, better targeted treatments.

References

1. Craig J. Complex diseases: research and applications. Nat Educ. 2008;1(1):184.
2. Saha R, Pettersson HJ, Svedberg P, Olovsson M, Bergqvist A, Marions L, Tornvall P, Kuja-Halkola R. Heritability of endometriosis. Fertil Steril. 2015;104:947–52.
3. Treloar SA, O'Connor DT, O'Connor VM, Martin NG. Genetic influences on endometriosis in an Australian twin sample. sueT@qimr.edu.au. Fertil Steril. 1999;71:701–10.
4. Lee SH, Harold D, Nyholt DR, Goddard ME, Zondervan KT, Williams J; Consortium, A.N., International Endogene, C., Genetic, Environmental Risk for Alzheimer's disease, C., et al. Estimation and partitioning of polygenic variation captured by common SNPs for Alzheimer's disease, multiple sclerosis and endometriosis. Hum Mol Genet. 2013;22:832–41.
5. Rahmioglu N, Missmer SA, Montgomery GW, Zondervan KT. Insights into assessing the genetics of endometriosis. Curr Obstet Gynecol Rep. 2012;1:124–37.

6. Zondervan KT, Cardon LR. Designing candidate gene and genome-wide case-control association studies. Nat Protoc. 2007;2:2492–501.
7. Adachi S, Tajima A, Quan J, Haino K, Yoshihara K, Masuzaki H, Katabuchi H, Ikuma K, Suginami H, Nishida N, et al. Meta-analysis of genome-wide association scans for genetic susceptibility to endometriosis in Japanese population. J Hum Genet. 2010;55:816–21.
8. Uno S, Zembutsu H, Hirasawa A, Takahashi A, Kubo M, Akahane T, Aoki D, Kamatani N, Hirata K, Nakamura Y. A genome-wide association study identifies genetic variants in the CDKN2BAS locus associated with endometriosis in Japanese. Nat Genet. 2010;42:707–10.
9. Painter JN, Anderson CA, Nyholt DR, Macgregor S, Lin J, Lee SH, Lambert A, Zhao ZZ, Roseman F, Guo Q, et al. Genome-wide association study identifies a locus at 7p15.2 associated with endometriosis. Nat Genet. 2011;43:51–4.
10. Albertsen HM, Chettier R, Farrington P, Ward K. Genome-wide association study link novel loci to endometriosis. PLoS One. 2013;8:e58257.
11. Nyholt DR, Low SK, Anderson CA, Painter JN, Uno S, Morris AP, MacGregor S, Gordon SD, Henders AK, Martin NG, et al. Genome-wide association meta-analysis identifies new endometriosis risk loci. Nat Genet. 2012;44:1355–9.
12. Steinthorsdottir V, Thorleifsson G, Aradottir K, Feenstra B, Sigurdsson A, Stefansdottir L, Kristinsdottir AM, Zink F, Halldorsson GH, Munk Nielsen N, et al. Common variants upstream of KDR encoding VEGFR2 and in TTC39B associate with endometriosis. Nat Commun. 2016;7:12350.
13. Sapkota Y, Steinthorsdottir V, Morris AP, Fassbender A, Rahmioglu N, De Vivo I, Buring JE, Zhang F, Edwards TL, Jones S, et al. Meta-analysis identifies five novel loci associated with endometriosis highlighting key genes involved in hormone metabolism. Nat Commun. 2017;8:15539.
14. Sobalska-Kwapis M, Smolarz B, Slomka M, Szaflik T, Kepka E, Kulig B, Siewierska-Gorska A, Polak G, Romanowicz H, Strapagiel D, et al. New variants near RHOJ and C2, HLA-DRA region and susceptibility to endometriosis in the Polish population-The genome-wide association study. Eur J Obstet Gynecol Reprod Biol. 2017;217:106–12.
15. Galarneau G, Fontanillas P, Clementi C, Hu-Seliger T, Parfitt DE, Tung JY, Yurttas-Beim P; the Celmatix Research Team; the 23andMe Research Team. Genome-wide association studies on endometriosis and endometriosis related infertility. BioRxiv. 2018.
16. Rahmioglu N, Banasik K, Christofidou P, Danning R, Galarneau G, Giri A, MacGregor S, Mortlock S, Sapkota Y, Schork JA, et al. Large-scale genome-wide association meta-analysis of endometriosis reveals 13 novel loci and genetically-associated comorbidity with other pain conditions. BioRxiv. 2018.
17. Powell JE, Fung JN, Shakhbazov K, Sapkota Y, Cloonan N, Hemani G, Hillman KM, Kaufmann S, Luong HT, Bowdler L, et al. Endometriosis risk alleles at 1p36.12 act through inverse regulation of CDC42 and LINC00339. Hum Mol Genet. 2016;25:5046–58.
18. Consortium, G.T. Human genomics. The Genotype-Tissue Expression (GTEx) pilot analysis: multitissue gene regulation in humans. Science. 2015;348:648–60.
19. Consortium, G.T., Laboratory, D.A., Coordinating Center-Analysis Working, G., Statistical Methods Groups-Analysis Working, G., Enhancing, G.g., Fund, N.I.H.C., NIH/NCI, NIH/NHGRI, NIH/NIMH, NIH/NIDA, et al. Genetic effects on gene expression across human tissues. Nature. 2017;550:204–13.
20. Fung JN, Mortlock S, Girling JE, Holdsworth-Carson SJ, Teh WT, Zhu Z, Lukowski SW, McKinnon BD, McRae A, Yang J, et al. Genetic regulation of disease risk and endometrial gene expression highlights potential target genes for endometriosis and polycystic ovarian syndrome. Sci Rep. 2018;8:11424.
21. Mortlock S, Kendarsari RI, Fung JN, Gibson G, Yang F, Restuadi R, Girling JE, Holdsworth-Carson SJ, Teh WT, Lukowski SW, et al. Tissue specific regulation of transcription in endometrium and association with disease. Hum Reprod. 2020;35:377–93.
22. Becker CM, Laufer MR, Stratton P, Hummelshoj L, Missmer SA, Zondervan KT, Adamson GD, Group, W.E.W. World Endometriosis Research Foundation Endometriosis Phenome and

Biobanking Harmonisation Project: I. Surgical phenotype data collection in endometriosis research. Fertil Steril. 2014;102:1213–22.
23. Fassbender A, Rahmioglu N, Vitonis AF, Vigano P, Giudice LC, D'Hooghe TM, Hummelshoj L, Adamson GD, Becker CM, Missmer SA, et al. World Endometriosis Research Foundation Endometriosis Phenome and Biobanking Harmonisation Project: IV. Tissue collection, processing, and storage in endometriosis research. Fertil Steril. 2014;102:1244–53.
24. Rahmioglu N, Fassbender A, Vitonis AF, Tworoger SS, Hummelshoj L, D'Hooghe TM, Adamson GD, Giudice LC, Becker CM, Zondervan KT, et al. World Endometriosis Research Foundation Endometriosis Phenome and Biobanking Harmonization Project: III. Fluid biospecimen collection, processing, and storage in endometriosis research. Fertil Steril. 2014;102:1233–43.
25. Vitonis AF, Vincent K, Rahmioglu N, Fassbender A, Buck Louis GM, Hummelshoj L, Giudice LC, Stratton P, Adamson GD, Becker CM, et al. World Endometriosis Research Foundation Endometriosis Phenome and Biobanking Harmonization Project: II. Clinical and covariate phenotype data collection in endometriosis research. Fertil Steril. 2014;102:1223–32.

Pathogenesis of Endometriosis: Progesterone Resistance in Women with Endometriosis

7

Ludwig Kiesel, Marie Vogel, Quang Khoi Le, and Sebastian Daniel Schäfer

Contents

7.1 Introduction

Endometriosis has been demonstrated to be an estrogen-dependent disease, and dysregulation of steroid action appears to be one of the key pathogenetic factors in altered cellular function in the endometrium as well as in lesions in women suffering from endometriosis. The high recurrence rate in women following surgery and medical therapies provides evidence for the need to develop new modalities with long-term efficacy. In addition to various other mechanisms, resistance to progesterone plays a major role not only in the pathogenesis of this enigmatic disease but also in regard to failure of long-term treatment for pain and infertility. In order to develop novel approaches to overcome resistance to therapy, detailed understanding of the

L. Kiesel (✉) · M. Vogel · Q. K. Le · S. D. Schäfer
Department of Gynecology and Obstetrics, University Hospital Münster (UKM), Münster, Germany
e-mail: ludwig.kiesel@ukmuenster.de

E. Oral (ed.), *Endometriosis and Adenomyosis*,
https://doi.org/10.1007/978-3-030-97236-3_7

mechanisms of dysregulation in the endometrium and in endometriotic lesions in women diagnosed with endometriosis is required.

7.2 Mechanisms of Progesterone Resistance in Endometriosis

In normal endometrium, steroid action is highly regulated and balanced during proliferative and secretory phase [1]. In endometriosis, however, this balance and homeostasis are disturbed with increased estrogen activity and progesterone resistance [2]. In endometriosis, there is an increased activity of the enzyme aromatase and a decreased expression of 17β-hydroxysteroid-dehydrogenase (17β-HSD-2) (Fig. 7.1). This results in an enhanced bioavailability of estradiol and further stimulation of aromatase [2]. Estrogen plays an important role in endometriotic tissue survival, inflammatory response, and cell proliferation. Progesterone induces endometrial differentiation and transition from the proliferative to the secretory phase. It stimulates the expression of the enzyme 17ß-HSD-2 which converts estradiol to its inactive form estrone [2].

In addition to hormonal imbalance, signaling factors are dysregulated in endometriosis, affecting progesterone and estrogen pathways likewise: While estradiol signaling factors are increased, progesterone signaling factors are decreased [3] (Fig. 7.2). This results in a lack of downregulation of genes that are required for

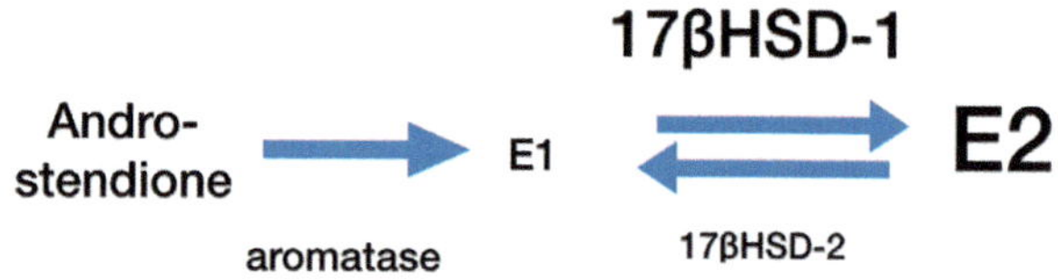

Fig. 7.1 The downregulation of 17-ßHSD-2 leads to an excess of estradiol

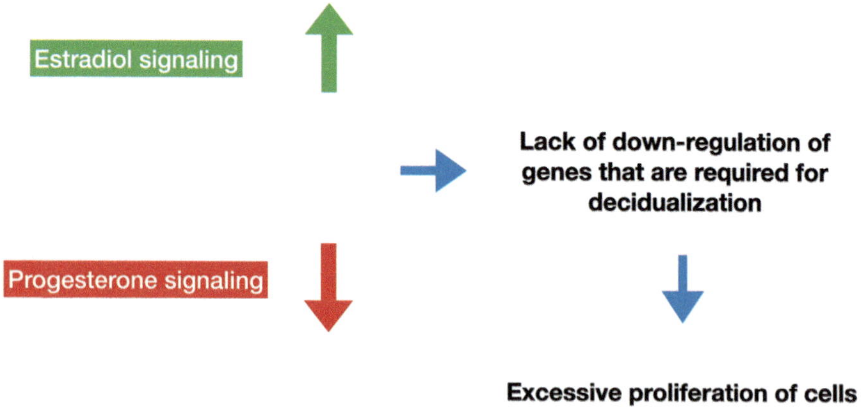

Fig. 7.2 The upregulation of E2 and downregulation of progesterone signaling lead to excessive proliferation of the cells in endometriotic lesions

decidualization, resulting in the excessive proliferation of cells. Besides, it has been reported that the loss of responsiveness to progesterone is closely linked to low numbers of progesterone receptors PR-A and PR-B. A reduced number of progesterone receptors, increased cellular estradiol levels, and altered signaling pathways cause relative progesterone resistance [3].

7.2.1 Altered Steroid Receptor Levels in Endometriosis

Endometriotic cells express estrogen receptors (ER-alpha, ER-beta, and GPER) and progesterone receptors (PR-A and PR-B) [4]. Estrogen levels can be modulated through the ER-alpha and ER-beta receptors, whereby estradiol targets the ER-alpha expression in the endometrium. Both receptors are encoded by the genes ESR1 and ESR2. It has been reported that the ratio of these two receptors is altered in endometriotic tissue with elevated ER-beta receptor levels as compared to those in normal tissue [5]. Since ER beta suppresses ER-alpha in endometriosis, the low number of ER-alpha receptors in endometriosis may result in lower progesterone receptor levels due to the failure of estradiol to induce progesterone receptor expression. In addition, the elevated ER-beta receptor levels are linked to inflammation, hyperalgesia, apoptosis inhibition, and proliferation in endometriotic tissue [5].

In normal endometrium, PR-A and PR-B levels are usually increased during the proliferative phase and reach a maximum just before ovulation (Fig. 7.3). Some studies have shown that levels of PR in endometriotic lesions are reduced in comparison to those in endometrial tissue. Other investigators demonstrated that in endometriosis, PR-A expression is greatly reduced while PR-B receptors are absent in endometriosis [3]. This results in a reduction of the expression of 17ß-HSD-2 and estradiol conversion to estrone, with an excess of estradiol [4].

In endometriosis, progesterone signaling pathways in mesenchymal stem cells (MSCs) are altered [6]. This affects not only the nuclear-, but also membrane-bound progesterone receptors and G-protein-coupled estrogen receptors [7] (Fig. 7.4). Both progesterone synthesis and the expression of the PR-A and -B are regulated by DNA methylation and the posttranscriptional silencing by miRNA [8]. In a primate model, it has been shown that progesterone resistance in endometriosis occurs due to the expression of miRNA-29c and by alteration of its targets [9]. Furthermore, the excision of endometriotic lesions decreased the expression of miRNA-29c in MSCs

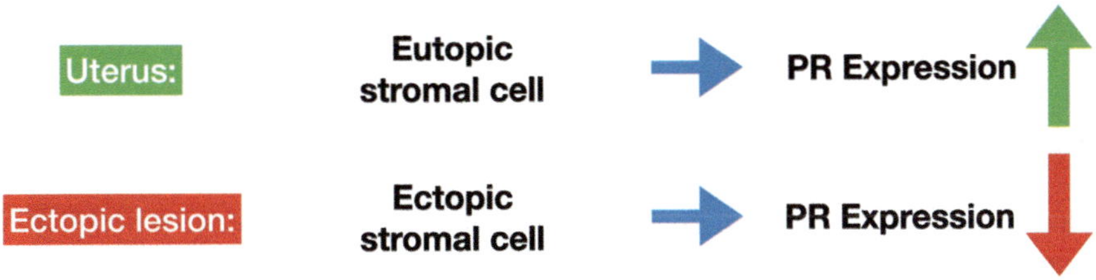

Fig. 7.3 The expression of progesterone receptors is suppressed in ectopic lesions

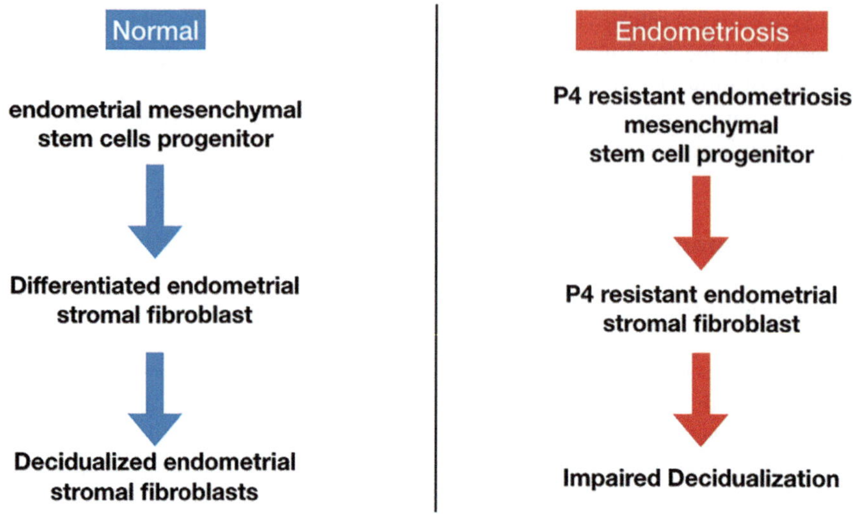

Fig. 7.4 Differences in mesenchymal stem cell progenitors lead to an impaired decidualization in endometriosis

and endometrial stem cells (EnSCs) [9]. Additional studies have revealed that low levels of PR-B might induce an increase in proliferation and apoptosis-related resistance [10].

Altered gene expression in endometriosis has been shown to be related to methylation of homeobox protein A10 (HOXA10) and A11 (HOXA11) [11]. The development of an altered response to progesterone in some endometriosis patients is also due to the lack of suppression of estrogen-responsive genes in the endometrial stromal cells during the secretory phase [3, 8]. Various mechanisms involved in progesterone resistance are summarized in Fig. 7.5.

7.3 Clinical Relevance of Progesterone Resistance

Progesterone resistance is a major factor not only in regard of the pathogenesis of endometriosis but is also relevant for the response to therapy in patients. Patients treated with progestins relapse or develop resistance to therapy in approximately 30% of the cases [6]. This includes either partial improvement while on medication or the lack of remission of endometriotic lesions (Table 7.1).

7.3.1 Prediction of Resistance to Progestin Therapy

Flores and coworkers conducted a study analyzing the histopathology in relation to response to therapy [19]. The group demonstrated that the progesterone receptor levels were significantly reduced in nonresponsive patients compared to responsive

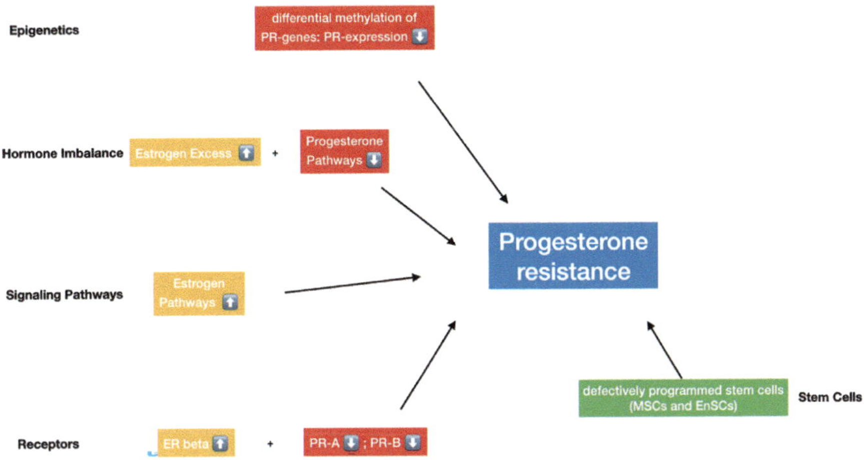

Fig. 7.5 Various mechanisms lead to the onset of progesterone resistance in endometriosis

patients. This further supports the earlier hypothesis that insufficient PR-B transcription and activity are clinically relevant for the patients' low response to progestins. The authors suggest that the use of H(Histo)-Score could help to predict progesterone resistance in patients [19].

7.3.2 Treatment Options in Patients with Progesterone Resistance

Since progesterone resistance plays a major role in affected patients, drugs that overcome resistance are needed to be taken under consideration. In resistant patients, the use of progestins may have additional effects on targets. The progestin dienogest, for example, downregulates proinflammatory cytokines, downregulates ER-beta, and increases the PR-B:PR-A RNA ratio in endometriotic tissue. This reestablishment of progesterone sensitivity may result in improved therapy outcomes in patients suffering from progesterone resistance [20]. This notion has been supported by others suggesting changing the type of drug itself, since different progestins target different mechanisms of action and therefore help reduce symptoms [21]. In addition, avoiding estrogens could be helpful for lowering symptoms in the same way that inhibiting estrogen synthesis might be beneficial. Another novel treatment option for patients who are resistant to therapy are selective progesterone receptor modulators (SPRMs). They have a strong affinity to the progesterone receptors and act as isolated agonists or antagonists. They thereby inhibit endometrial proliferation while at the same time not presenting many side effects [21]. By directly affecting downstream effects of the progesterone receptors, proliferation and prostaglandin production are altered. Mifepristone has been shown to effectively improve the patients' pain and reduce the lesion size in different trials [3].

Table 7.1 Rate of recurrence and nonresponders following progestin therapy in patients with endometriosis

Route of administration	Drug	Characteristics	Nonresponders (%)	Recurrence rate (%)	Literature
Oral progestins	NETA (Norethisterone acetate)	Rectovaginal endometriosis, low cost, and long-term treatment possible	28.9	11.9	Morotti et al. [12]
	MPA (Medroxyprogesterone acetate)	Low cost, androgenic activity	55		Harrison et al. [13]
	CPA (Cyproterone acetate)	Antiandrogenic, low progestational activity	8.9		Vercellini et al. [14]
	DNG (Dienogest)	Antiandrogenic activity, weak antigonadotropic effect, good tolerability, improves progesterone resistance, and negative effect on bone mineral density	31–34		Lang et al. [15]; Yu et al. [16]
Depot injections	MPA	150 mg i.m. or 104 mg s.c. every 3 months, almost no side-effects, and good pain relief	13.7–26.2		Carr et al. [17]
Intrauterine systems	LNG (Levonorgestrel)	Antiestrogenic and androgenic effect, good pain relief		4.8–25	Chen et al. [5, 18]

Other alternatives are changing the route of administration by considering high potency progestins, depot formulations, or levonorgestrel intrauterine systems (LNG-IUS) [20]. Brown et al. proposed to combine NSAIDs and progestins to further reduce the inflammatory response and avoid the progression of progesterone resistance [22].

Future treatment options could include novel hormonal and nonhormonal agents with tissue selective potential in endometriosis patients. Antioxidants containing N-acetyl cysteine may also have the potential to reduce symptoms [23]. Further therapeutic perspectives seem to be offered in regard to MSCs and EnSCs [24]. The use of tyrosinkinase inhibitors has been investigated to prevent further proliferative and invasive traits of endometrial MSCs in difficult courses of the disease [25]. Targeting PTEN and MiR-92a or epigenetic drivers are presently under consideration in the search for novel approaches for treatment options.

References

1. Zondervan KT, Becker CM, Koga K, Missmer SA, Taylor RN, Viganò P. Endometriosis. Nat Rev Dis Primers. 2018;4(1) https://doi.org/10.1038/s41572-018-0008-5.
2. Karim AK, Shafiee MN, Abd Aziz NH, Omar MH, Abdul Ghani NA, Lim PS, Md Zin RR, Mokhtar N. Reviewing the role of progesterone therapy in endometriosis. Gynecol Endocrinol. 2019;35(1):10–6. https://doi.org/10.1080/09513590.2018.1490404.
3. Marquardt RM, Kim TH, Shin JH, Jeong JW. Progesterone and estrogen signaling in the endometrium: what goes wrong in endometriosis? Int J Mol Sci. 2019;20(15) https://doi.org/10.3390/ijms20153822.
4. Bulun SE, Cheng YH, Pavone ME, Xue Q, Attar E, Trukhacheva E, Tokunaga H, Utsunomiya H, Yin P, Luo X, others. Estrogen receptor-beta, estrogen receptor-alpha, and progesterone resistance in endometriosis. Semin Reprod Med. 2010;28(1):36–43. https://doi.org/10.1055/s-0029-1242991.Estrogen.
5. Chen H, Malentacchi F, Fambrini M, Harrath AH, Huang H, Petraglia F. Epigenetics of estrogen and progesterone receptors in endometriosis. Reprod Sci. 2020;27(11):1967–74. https://doi.org/10.1007/s43032-020-00226-2.
6. Yotova I, Hsu E, Do C, Gaba A, Szabolcs M, Dekan S, Kenner L, Wenzl R, Tycko B. Epigenetic alterations affecting transcription factors and signaling pathways in stromal cells of endometriosis. PLoS ONE. 2017;12(1) https://doi.org/10.1371/journal.pone.0170859.
7. Houshdaran S, Oke AB, Fung JC, Vo KC, Nezhat C, Giudice LC. Steroid hormones regulate genome-wide epigenetic programming and gene transcription in human endometrial cells with marked aberrancies in endometriosis. PLoS Genet. 2020;16(6) https://doi.org/10.1371/journal.pgen.1008601.
8. Szukiewicz D, Stangret A, Ruiz-Ruiz C, Olivares EG, Soriţău O, Suşman S, Szewczyk G. Estrogen- and progesterone (P4)-mediated epigenetic modifications of endometrial stromal cells (EnSCs) and/or mesenchymal stem/stromal cells (MSCs) in the etiopathogenesis of endometriosis. Stem Cell Rev Rep. 2021; https://doi.org/10.1007/s12015-020-10115-5.
9. Joshi NR, Miyadahira EH, Afshar Y, Jeong JW, Young SL, Lessey BA, Serafini PC, Fazleabas AT. Progesterone resistance in endometriosis is modulated by the altered expression of MicroRNA-29c and FKBP4. J Clin Endocrinol Metab. 2017;102(1):141–9. https://doi.org/10.1210/jc.2016-2076.
10. Krikun G, Mor G, Alvero A, Guller S, Schatz F, Sapi E, Rahman M, Caze R, Qumsiyeh M, Lockwood CJ. A novel immortalized human endometrial stromal cell line with normal progestational response. Endocrinology. 2004;145(5):2291–6. https://doi.org/10.1210/en.2003-1606.

11. Bulun SE, Monsivais D, Kakinuma T, Furukawa Y, Bernardi L, Pavone ME, Dyson M. Molecular biology of endometriosis: from aromatase to genomic abnormalities. Semin Reprod Med. 2015;33(3):220–4. https://doi.org/10.1055/s-0035-1554053. Epub 2015 Jun 2.
12. Morotti M, Venturini PL, Biscaldi E, et al. Efficacy and acceptability of long-term norethindrone acetate for the treatment of rectovaginal endometriosis. Eur J Obstet Gynecol Reprod Biol. 2017;213:4–10.
13. Harrison RF, Barry-Kinsella C. Efficacy of medroxyprogesterone treatment in infertile women with endometriosis: a prospective, randomized, placebo-controlled study. Fertil Steril. 2000;74(1):24–30.
14. Vercellini P, De Giorgi O, Mosconi P, Stellato G, Vicentini S, Crosignani PG. Cyproterone acetate versus a continuous monophasic oral contraceptive in the treatment of recurrent pelvic pain after conservative surgery for symptomatic endometriosis. Fertil Steril. 2002;77(1):52–61.
15. Lang J, Yu Q, Zhang S, et al. Dienogest for treatment of endometriosis in Chinese women: a placebo-controlled, randomized, double-blind phase 3 study. J Women Health (2002). 2018;27(2):148–55.
16. Yu Q, Zhang S, Li H, et al. Dienogest for treatment of endometriosis in women: a 28-week, open-label, extension study. J Women Health (2002). 2019;28(2):170–7.
17. Carr B, Dmowski WP, O'Brien C, et al. Elagolix, an oral GnRH antagonist, versus subcutaneous depot medroxyprogesterone acetate for the treatment of endometriosis: effects on bone mineral density. Reprod Sci (Thousand Oaks, CA). 2014;21(11):1341–51.
18. Chen YJ, Hsu TF, Huang BS, Tsai HW, Chang YH, Wang PH. Postoperative maintenance levonorgestrel-releasing intrauterine system and endometrioma recurrence: a randomized controlled study. Am J Obstet Gynecol. 2017;216(6):582.e581–9.
19. Flores VA, Vanhie A, Dang T, Taylor HS. Progesterone receptor status predicts response to progestin therapy in endometriosis. J Clin Endocrinol Metab. 2018;103(12):4561–8. https://doi.org/10.1210/jc.2018-01227.
20. Patel BG, Rudnicki M, Yu J, Shu Y, Taylor RN. Progesterone resistance in endometriosis: origins, consequences and interventions. Acta Obstet Gynecol Scand. 2017;96(6):623–32. https://doi.org/10.1111/aogs.13156.
21. Reis FM, Coutinho LM, Vannuccini S, Batteux F, Chapron C, Petraglia F. Progesterone receptor ligands for the treatment of endometriosis: the mechanisms behind therapeutic success and failure. Hum Reprod Update. 2020;26(4):565–85. https://doi.org/10.1093/humupd/dmaa009.
22. Brown J, Crawford TJ, Datta S, Prentice A. Oral contraceptives for pain associated with endometriosis. Cochrane Database Syst Rev. 2018;2018(5) https://doi.org/10.1002/14651858.CD001019.pub3.
23. Lete I, Mendoza N, de la Viuda E, Carmona F. Effectiveness of an antioxidant preparation with N-acetyl cysteine, alpha lipoic acid and bromelain in the treatment of endometriosis-associated pelvic pain: LEAP study. Eur J Obstet Gynecol Reprod Biol. 2018;228:221–4. https://doi.org/10.1016/j.ejogrb.2018.07.002.
24. Forte A, Cipollaro M, Galderisi U. Genetic, epigenetic and stem cell alterations in endometriosis: new insights and potential therapeutic perspectives. Clin Sci. 2014;126(2):123–38. https://doi.org/10.1042/CS20130099.
25. Moggio A, Pittatore G, Cassoni P, Marchino GL, Revelli A, Bussolati B. Sorafenib inhibits growth, migration, and angiogenic potential of ectopic endometrial mesenchymal stem cells derived from patients with endometriosis. Fertil Steril. 2012;98(6):1521–1530.e2. https://doi.org/10.1016/j.fertnstert.2012.08.003.

Classification and Clinical Staging of Endometriosis

8

Jörg Keckstein, Peter Oppelt, and Gernot Hudelist

Contents

The original version of the chapter has been revised. A correction to this chapter can be found at https://doi.org/10.1007/978-3-030-97236-3_45

J. Keckstein (✉)
Endometriosis Clinic Dres. Keckstein, Villach, Austria

University Ulm, Ulm, Germany

Scientific Endometriosis Foundation (Stiftung Endometrioseforschung/SEF), Westerstede, Germany

Richard Wagner Strasse, Villach, Austria
e-mail: joerg@keckstein.at

P. Oppelt
Scientific Endometriosis Foundation (Stiftung Endometrioseforschung/SEF), Westerstede, Germany

Department of Gynecology, Obstetrics and Gynecological Endocrinology, Kepler University Hospital Linz, Johannes Kepler Universität Linz, Linz, Austria

G. Hudelist
Scientific Endometriosis Foundation (Stiftung Endometrioseforschung/SEF), Westerstede, Germany

Department of Gynaecology, Center for Endometriosis, Hospital St. John of God, Vienna, Austria

E. Oral (ed.), *Endometriosis and Adenomyosis*,
https://doi.org/10.1007/978-3-030-97236-3_8

8.1 Introduction

It was K. Rokitansky in 1860 [1] who was one of the first to describe endometriosis in detail. A large number of further publications showed how complex endometriosis is and that it is a disease with a wide variety of forms and localizations of manifestation. Many attempts have been made to describe the anatomical extent of the disease and also to classify it. The secondary adhesions caused by endometriosis have also been considered to some extent. The attempt was made to take into account the different regions or organs affected to be able to make a statement about the severity of the disease using a score. Until a few years ago, the disease was mainly assessed by surgical intervention. Primarily, the classification focused on the changes of the internal genital organs and peritoneum, but none of the systems includes a comprehensive representation of both peritoneal, ovarian, and deep endometriosis and adhesions in one system. Currently, the most commonly used AFS/rASRM classification is also used primarily with regard to fertility [2, 3].

Due to the inadequacy of the existing systems, especially because of the enormously improved surgical therapy and the much more differentiated diagnostics, attempts have been made in the past to redefine the assessment, description, and classification of endometriosis. Based on recommendations, several attempts were made to evaluate the advantages and disadvantages of the classifications most commonly used at present, so that they can be applied in the combined form if necessary [4–6].

Taking into account the existing literature and evidence, these are the revised American Society for Reproductive Medicine (rASRM) classification, the Enzian classification, and the Endometriosis Fertility Index (EFI) [7]. The consensus clearly showed the various advantages and disadvantages of the systems mentioned. A classification should allow an accurate comparison of the results of reproductive, medical, and surgical interventions.

It also became obvious that a correct morphological-anatomical description of endometriosis is an indispensable prerequisite for the comparison of different entities of the disease and therapeutic outcomes.

The analyses available to date show that the rASRM classification, with a relatively imprecise grading of findings into four stages, does not comprehensibly represent the complexity of the disease [7]. Thus, the validity of many studies is limited.

The need for an alternative or additional classification system, particularly regarding DE, is a matter of constant debate [8–21].

An ideal classification system should provide not only information about the general severity of the disease, but also a detailed description of the extent of the various lesions.

In addition, noninvasive, i.e., sonographic and MR tomographic, as well as invasive methods should be included in the description/classification.

Of course, it would be very helpful with these classifications to be able to predict correlations between the extent/localization of pathological findings and prognosis, symptoms, difficulties in surgery, and thus risk of complications.

The diagnosis and treatment of endometriosis are now increasingly performed by multidisciplinary teams like radiologists, sonographers, and various surgical specialties involving gynecological, colorectal, and urological surgeons. It is this multimodality approach that now requires the most uniform language possible in the use of classification systems for peritoneal and ovarian endometriosis including adhesions and/or deep endometriosis (DE) and adenomyosis. Currently, the rASRM, EFI, and ENZIAN classifications are used differently in a mixed or modular way to meet the needs of the sonographer and the radiologist of the specialist in reproductive medicine and the gynecological surgeon.

8.2 The rASRM Score

The American Fertility Society (AFS) first published the score in 1979 [3] with further revisions in 1985 (rAFS score) and 1996, and it is now used in revised form as the American Society for Reproductive Medicine (rASRM) score [3]. The extent of endometriosis is assessed primarily by diagnostic laparoscopy to evaluate, in particular, the lesions on the peritoneum, tube, ovary, and sacrouterina ligaments and Douglas(POD). Using a numerical scoring system for points corresponding to the size of the endometriotic lesion as well as the grade of the foci, a classification of four severity grades, namely minimal, mild, moderate, and severe endometriosis (Figs. 8.1 and 8.2) is made.

In rASRM classification, endometriosis is mainly classified by invasive procedures [3, 4].

It has been used worldwide for over 40 years for clinical and scientific publications to describe and compare clinical findings [5].

The application of the system is very sophisticated to then ultimately reduce the stages to only four categories. The classification primarily considers endometriosis at the peritoneum and ovary and adhesions but ignores DE and adenomyosis. Extragenital structures such as the bowel, bladder, rectovaginal septum (RVS), or ureter are not considered by the rASRM score. In a study by Wustlich and al., based on 63 patients with DE including recto-sigmoid endometriosis, 21% were found to have only stage 1 or 2 according to the r-ASRM scoring system [22].

During the last decade, important developments in the field of noninvasive diagnostics open new aspects in terms of accurate classification.

Few studies attempted to evaluate the applicability of transvaginal ultrasound (TVS) or magnetic resonance imaging (MRI) for noninvasive use of rASRM classification. Leonardi et al. [6, 23] Williams et al. [24] investigated the diagnostic accuracy of TVS for predicting surgically verified stages of rASRM endometriosis. Holland et al. [25] found good agreement between TVS findings and the surgical rASRM stage. Large prospective studies on the accuracy of TVS- or MRI-based endometriosis classification using the noninvasive rASRM score are lacking.

The severity of various pain symptoms caused by endometriosis with different stages of disease categorized by the rASRM score has been studied by

AMERICAN SOCIETY FOR REPRODUCTIVE MEDICINE
REVISED CLASSIFICATION OF ENDOMETRIOSIS

Patient's Name__________ Date__________

Stage I (Minimal) - 1.5
Stage II (Mild) - 6.15
Stage III (Moderate) - 16.40
Stage IV (Severe) - > 40
Total__________

Laparoscopy__________ Laparotomy__________ Photography__________
Recommended Treatment__________

Prognosis__________

	ENDOMETRIOSIS	< 1cm	1-3cm	> 3cm
PERITONEUM	Superficial	1	2	4
	Deep	2	4	6
OVARY	R Superficial	1	2	4
	Deep	4	16	20
	L Superficial	1	2	4
	Deep	4	16	20
	POSTERIOR CULDESAC OBLITERATION	Partial		Complete
		4		40
	ADHESIONS	< 1/3 Enclosure	1/3-2/3 Enclosure	> 2/3 Enclosure
OVARY	R Filmy	1	2	4
	Dense	4	8	16
	L Filmy	1	2	4
	Dense	4	8	16
TUBE	R Filmy	1	2	4
	Dense	4*	8*	16
	L Filmy	1	2	4
	Dense	4*	8*	16

*** If the fimbriated end of the fallopian tube is completely enclosed, change the point assignment to 16.**

Denote appearance of superficial implant types as red [(R), red, red-pink, flamelike, vesicular blobs, clear vesicles]. white [(W), opacifications, peritoneal defects, yellow-brown]. or black [(B) black, hemosiderin deposits, blue]. Denote percent of total described as R___%, W___%, and B___% Total should equal 100%.

Fig. 8.1 rASRM classification of endometriosis. The evaluation is performed through surgery. The stages result from the addition of points determined in particular according to the findings at the adnexa and cul-de-sac

Vercellini et al. [26] and Fedele et al. [27]. The association between rASRM stages and the degree and type of pelvic symptoms was inconsistent [28]. Little correlation between the r-ASRM stage and pain symptoms may be explained by the unclear pathophysiological behavior of the disease itself, but possibly also by the lack of a correct classification of the complex deep infiltrating disease. Chapron et al. [29] showed a correlation between the severity of dysmenorrhea and the presence of posterior deep infiltrating endometriosis (DE). There was no correlation between rASRM stages and pain symptoms in women with DE, and no correlations between the rASRM stage and postoperative natural pregnancy rates [10, 30].

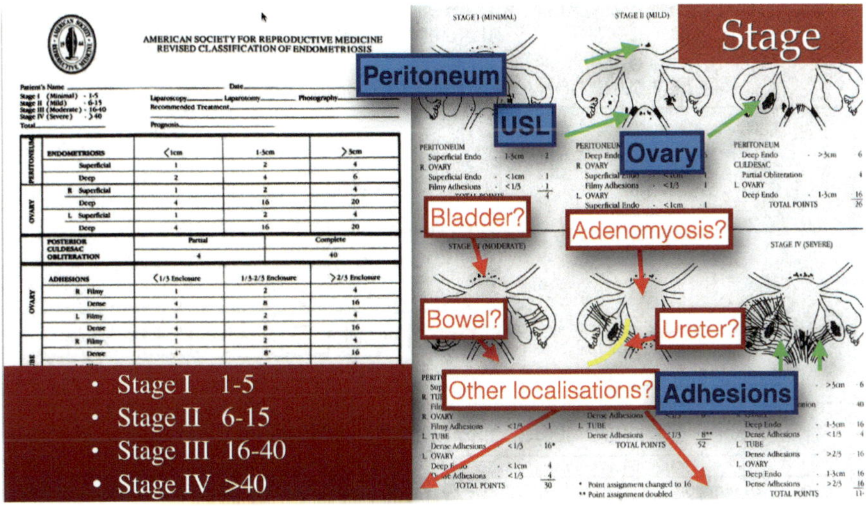

Fig. 8.2 rASRM classification. Classification into four stages by a very complex scoring system including adhesions. Mainly intraperitoneal foci are considered; the deep infiltrating foci and extragenital localizations are only minimally taken into account, if at all

Similar inconsistent results are found in the correlation of the rASRM stage and the incidence of operative difficulties and complications.

Poupon, using a nomogram, could not observe a clear correlation between rASRM stages and the occurrence of various complications [31, 32].

A problem that should not be underestimated also lies in the methodology and practical implementation of an accurate classification.

The very complex system of ASRM classification with its various exceptions is extremely error-prone and thus unreliable if not used digitally. Metzemaker [33] compared rASRM, Enzian, and EFI in paper and digital applications (EQUSUM). Not all exception rules are applied by expert endometriosis surgeons, leading to incorrect scoring.

The EQUSUM, a worldwide web-based dynamic registration and classification/scoring system for (deep) endometriosis, improves correct classification/scoring of the currently recommended rASRM, Enzian, and EFI score and is more user-friendly compared to nondigital classification.

8.3 The EFI (Endometriosis Fertility Index)

The Endometriosis Fertility Index (EFI) (Fig. 8.3) published in 2010 by Adamson et al. [17] is used to predict fertility outcomes in relation to natural conception probabilities after surgical intervention.

ENDOMETRIOSIS FERTILITY INDEX (EFI)
SURGERY FORM

LEAST FUNCTION (LF) SCORE AT CONCLUSION OF SURGERY

Score	Description		Left	Right
4	= Normal	Fallopian Tube	☐	☐
3	= Mild Dysfunction			
2	= Moderate Dysfunction	Fimbria	☐	☐
1	= Severe Dysfuction			
0	= Absent or Nonfunctional	Ovary	☐	☐

To calculate the LF score, add together the lowest score for the left side and the lowest score for the right side. If an ovary is absent on one side, the LF score is obtained by doubling the lowest score on the side with the ovary.

Lowest Score ☐ Left + ☐ Right = ☐ LF Score

ENDOMETRIOSIS FERTILITY INDEX (EFI)

Historical Factors			Surgical Factors		
Factor	**Description**	**Points**	**Factor**	**Description**	**Points**
Age			LF Score ☐		
	If age is ≤ 35 years	2		If LF Score = 7 to 8 (high score)	3
	If age is 36 to 39 years	1		If LF Score = 4 to 6 (moderate score)	2
	If age is ≥ 40 years	0		If LF Score = 1 to 3 (low score)	0
Years Infertile			AFS Endometriosis Score		
	If years infertile is ≤ 3	2		If AFS Endometriosis Lesion Score is < 16	1
	If years infertile is > 3	0		If AFS Endometriosis Lesion Score is ≥ 16	0
Prior Pregnancy			AFS Total Score		
	If there is a history of a prior pregnancy	1		If AFS total score is < 71	1
	If there is no history of prior pregnancy	0		If AFS total score is ≥ 71	0
Total Historical Factors			**Total Surgical Factors**		

EFI = TOTAL HISTORICAL FACTORS + TOTAL SURGICAL FACTORS : ☐ Historical + ☐ Surgical = ☐ EFI Score

ESTIMATED PERCENT PREGNANT BY EFI SCORE

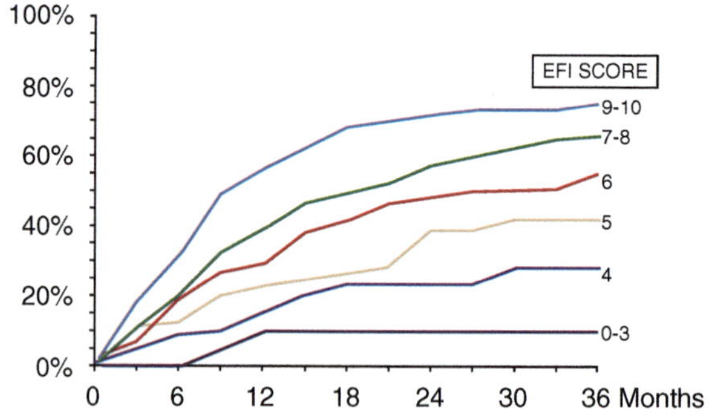

Fig. 8.3 EFI endometriosis fertility index

The EFI, a mathematical model, is based on a 10-point scoring system that includes factors such as patient age, duration of infertility and previous pregnancy, rASRM classification, and postoperative adnexal status. This is defined by a visual assessment of tubo-ovarian function by the least function (LF) score after surgery (including fallopian tubes, tubal fimbriae, and ovaries) (Fig. 8.3).

Its clinical applicability and value have been confirmed by several studies in which the validity of the external application of the EFI has been tested and positively confirmed [34, 35].

The use of the EFI has gained wide acceptance among reproductive surgeons and clinicians involved in MAR and is supported by the WES (World Endometriosis Society) for use in the classification of endometriosis [2] and an international consensus group on the recording of deep endometriosis surgery (CORDES) [21].

The following aspects should be considered:

1. EFI is a multifactorial calculation system.
2. Out of the 10 points to be calculated, only a maximum of 2 points are directly attributed to endometriosis.
3. The pathological change in the condition of the fallopian tube may also not be endometriosis-related.
4. EFI does not consider DE, extrapelvic endometriosis, or adenomyosis.

EFI is a useful model for calculating the probability of pregnancy in endometriosis or after surgical treatment of endometriosis. It cannot be described as a classification for endometriosis.

To date, only a single study has evaluated whether EFI can be used via noninvasive methods [36] Future studies will be required, possibly also using other classifications.

8.4 The Enzian Classification

Due to the problem of incomplete coverage of endometriosis using rASRM classification (deep infiltrating disease not adequately taken into account), the Scientific Endometriosis Foundation (SEF) created the ENZIAN classification in 2003 [37–39]. It accurately describes DE and can be used in combination with the r-ASRM classification. The Enzian classification, revised in 2009, classifies the various localizations of DE (vagina, uterosacral ligaments (USL), bladder, ureter, bowel, the uterus, and other extragenital locations) and the dimension of the lesions. For the complete description, a detailed code is used [40].

The Enzian classification for deep endometriosis is part of the new #Enzian classification. In Fig. 8.4, the different anatomical compartments for deep endometriosis (DE) are illustrated in red color.

The pelvis is divided into *three* compartments:

1. Compartment **A**: rectovaginal space (RVS), the vagina, and torus uterinus (craniocaudal axis).
2. Compartment **B**: USLs, the cardinal ligaments, the parametric space, and the pelvic sidewall (mediolateral axis).
3. Compartment **C**: Bowel (rectum and sigmoid) affects up to 16 cm from the anal verge, (ventrodorsal axis).

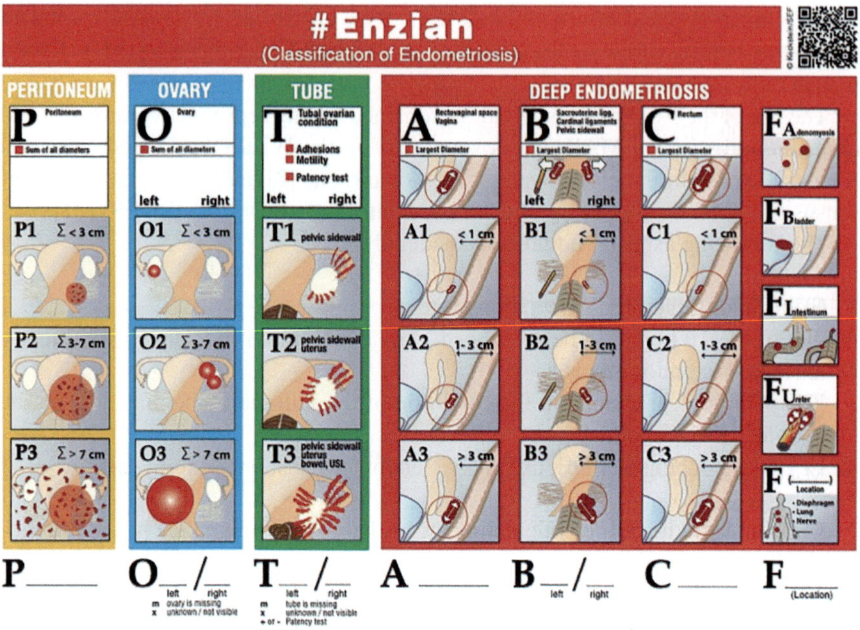

Fig. 8.4 #Enzian classification: an overview with potentially affected organs and compartments. The individual compartments are designate with the capital letters, and the various lesion sizes are numbered 1, 2, and 3 [51]

Severity is defined as follows (peritoneal lesions less than 5 mm depth of infiltration are excluded):

1. Grade 1: invasion <1 cm
2. Grade 2: invasion 1–3 cm
3. Grade 3: invasion >3 cm

Adenomyosis and other extragenital sites (**F**) are described as follows: Adenomyosis (**FA**); bladder DE (**FB**), extrinsic and/or intrinsic ureteric involvement with signs of obstruction (**FU**), bowel DE (**FI**) cranial to the rectosigmoid junction (>16 cm from anal verge; upper sigmoid, transverse colon, caecum, appendix, and small bowel), and other sites (**FO**) such as the abdominal wall, diaphragm, and involvement of nerves / sacral roots.

The description of the lesions was also primarily done by surgical procedures.

Several studies have now demonstrated the applicability of TVS or magnetic resonance imaging (MRI) for noninvasive use of the ENZIAN classification. Di Paola et al. [41] and Burla et al. [42] showed high rates of agreement between MRI-based and surgical findings. Thomassin-Naggara et al. [43] identified a significant correlation between the surgical findings and length of hospital stay using the

Enzian classification. Hudelist and Montanari et al. [28, 44] proved the high correlation between TVS findings and surgically determined DE localization and lesion size using the Enzian classification, especially for the compartments A, C, and FB described in the Enzian classification. In contrast to the rASRM score, the different DE localization correlated with the severity of the different preoperative pain symptoms [45, 46].

The Enzian classification allows a prediction of the complexity of surgical procedures: surgery duration and the risk of complications [31, 47]. A study by Roman and colleagues [48], evaluating three different surgical approaches for the treatment of intestinal endometriosis, proved that surgery times, as well as complication rates and improvement of symptoms, correlate with the classification according to the C compartment.

The nomogram developed by Poupon [32] allows prognostic calculation of the expected complications during surgery using the Enzian classification. No such correlation concerning complication rates was observed between rASRM stages I and II or between ASRM stages III and IV.

Imboden et al. [49] identified increased postoperative bladder dysfunction with radical surgery for extensive endometriosis in the Enzian B compartment.

The extent of symptoms was shown to indeed correlate with the extent of DE as classified by the Enzian score [46]. In an analysis based on 156 patients with DE and bowel involvement, Mutuku et al. [50] demonstrated a clear association between preoperative and intraoperative findings evaluated with the Enzian scoring system with a significant correlation between the extent of DE and the presence of dyspareunia. Montanari and coworkers [45] found also that disease extent depicted by the Enzian classification is associated and correlated with the presence and severity of different preoperative pain symptoms.

8.4.1 The #Enzian Classification

The Enzian classification has been objected to for various reasons and criticizations, mainly in Europe. One criticism was the necessity to use different systems at the same time, which complicates the documentation process itself.

To overcome this, the Enzian classification has recently been further developed into a comprehensive classification system, the #Enzian Classification, in the context of a consensus process of a group of experts in 2019 and 2020 [51].

The #Enzian classification is based on the known Enzian classification [40] for DE using three compartments (**A**, **B**, and **C**) as well the bladder (**FB**) the ureters (**FU**), other intestinal locations (sigmoid colon, small bowel, etc. **FI**), and other extragenital lesions (**FO**). To have comprehensive coverage of endometriosis, the involvement of the peritoneum (**P**), ovary (**O**), and adhesions is now also classified (**T**), including the tubal patency.

8.4.2 Coding of the #Enzian Classification

$$\#\textbf{Enzian}\ \textbf{P}\_,\textbf{O}\_/\_,\textbf{T}\_/\_,\textbf{A}\_,\textbf{B}\_/\_,\textbf{C}\_,\textbf{F}\_(\cdots)\ldots\ldots$$

- *Individual compartments* or organ involvement are identified with capital letters (**P, O, T, A, B, C, F**).
- The *extent of endometriosis* is represented by the numbers 1, 2, and 3 in compartment **P, O, T, A, B,** and **C**.
- *Paired organs* (ovary, tube, uterosacral ligament (USL), parametrium, and ureter). The severity is arranged separately after the letter (left / right).
- *Missing / invisible ovary or tube* is described with suffix (**m** – missing; **x**, unknown).
- *Tubal patency* (optionally) can be annotated with "**+**" (patent) or "**-**" not patent.

Example:
#Enzian summarized in the code:

• Superficial endometriosis on the peritoneum 4 cm (**P**)	= **P**2
• Ovarian endometriosis, right 4 cm(**O**)	= **O**0/2
• No adhesions on the tubo-ovarian unit (**T**) Adhesions left ovary/pelvic side wall; both tubes patent	= **T**1+/0+
• No lesion in the A compartment	= **A**0
• Deep endometriosis left USL 2 cm, right USL 3 cm (**B**)	= **B**2/2
• Deep endometriosis in the rectum 2 cm (**C**)	= **C**2
• Hydroureter right (**FU**)	= **FU**(r)
• Endometriosis in the appendix (**FI**)	= **FI** (App.)

Only affected compartments and organs should be listed:

$$\#\textbf{Enzian}\ \textbf{P}2,\textbf{O}0/2,\textbf{T}1+/0+,\textbf{B}2/2,\textbf{C}2,\textbf{FU}(\text{r}),\textbf{FI}(\text{Appendix})$$

The unique novelty of the #Enzian classification lies in the possibility of both surgical and noninvasive staging, combined with high accuracy, and serves as a common unifying language for all clinical specialties, including sonographers, radiologists, and surgeons [40, 51]. Typical sonographic features of the different phenotypes of DE, described by the IDEA [52] (International Deep Endometriosis Analysis group), are taken into account and incorporated into the #ENZIAN system.

It should be used independently of the imaging modality (TVS, MRI) and type of surgery. A prefix can be used optionally in brackets following the word #Enzian (i.e., #Enzian(**s**) P1, …) to depict the modality of evaluation of the disease when using the #Enzian:

- #Enzian(**u**) assessment by ultrasound
- #Enzian(**m**) assessment by MRI
- #Enzian(**s**) assessment by surgery

For the sonographic description, the proposal of IDEA [35] (International Deep Endometriosis Analysis Group) is taken into account and included in the # ENZIAN system. It describes the findings (localization and size) very accurately.

DiGiovanni et al. [53] recently demonstrated in a retrospective analysis of 93 women undergoing TVS and surgery for DE that preoperative evaluation of localization and size of DE lesions in different #Enzian compartments by an expert gynecological sonography is very accurate, with high sensitivity and specificity. It is the first study showing that the #Enzian classification can be applied to describe disease extent both at TVS and surgery, offering an accurate descriptive system for both noninvasive and invasive specialties. This has been confirmed by the prospective Study on 745 Patients of Montanari et al. [54].

Example:

• Superficial endometriosis on the peritoneum >7 cm (**P**)	= **P3**
• Ovarian endometriosis, left 4 cm, right normal (**O**)	= **O2/0**
• No adhesions on the tubo-ovarian unit (**T**) both tubes patent	= **T0+/0+**
• Deep endometriosis, left USL normal, right USL 2.5 cm (**B**)	= **B0/2**
• Rectum, extent not clearly visible (**C**)	= **Cx**

• #Enzian(s) P3, O2/0, T0+/0+,B0/2, Cx,

• Rectum, length of the nodule 2.4 cm(**C**)	= **C2**
• Uterus (adenomyosis)	= **FA**

Final coding with #Enzian classification, merging both, the laparoscopic and ultrasound findings (Figs. 8.5, 8.6, and 8.7):

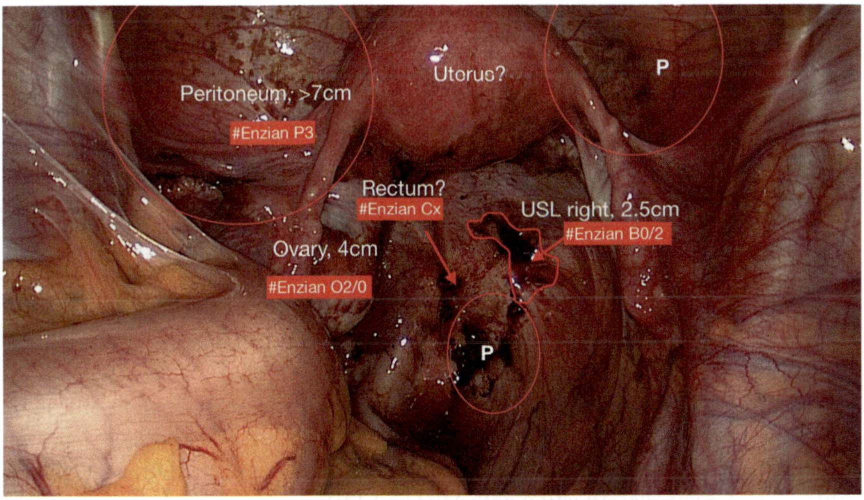

Fig. 8.5 Example of surgical classification of endometriosis; visible lesions on the peritoneum, left ovary, right USL, and rectum (#Enzian (s))

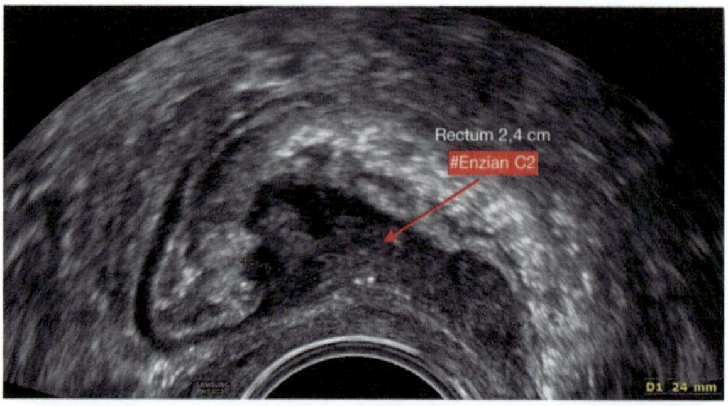

Fig. 8.6 TVS imaging of the rectal endometriosis of the same patient as in Fig. 8.5. (besides adenomyosis, ovarian and USL involvement)

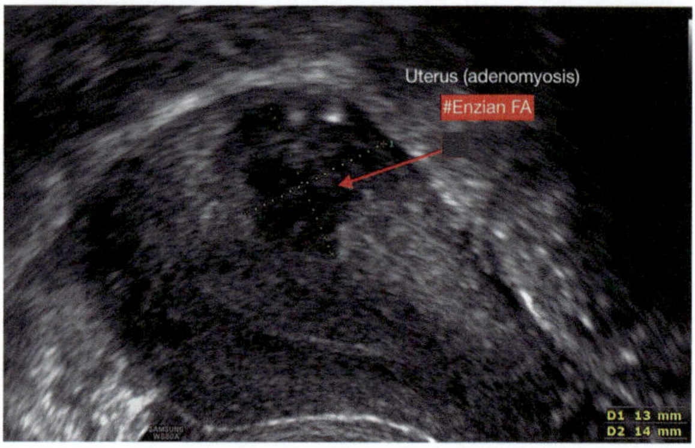

Fig. 8.7 TVS imaging of adenomyosis of the same patient as in Fig. 8.5 (besides rectal, ovarian, and USL involvement)

- #Enzian(s,u) P3, O2/0, T0+/0+, B0/2, C2$_{(u)}$, FA$_{(u)}$

8.5 Conclusion

The treatment of endometriosis has completely changed in the last years due to enormous progress in surgical therapy, but especially due to the improvement of noninvasive diagnostics. Classification of the disease has been used primarily for the postoperative staging of the disease. Unfortunately, the most commonly used rASRM classification does not correlate with symptoms, or other important parameters, and cannot be used for noninvasive diagnostics. Moreover, it does not take into account deep infiltrating endometriosis and extra pelvic endometriosis.

The EFI is better than the rASRM classification for calculating the probability of pregnancy.

It does not contain differential information on the location and extent of lesions, especially DE.

The ENZIAN classification is predominantly used to describe DE. The applicability of the Enzian classification with MRI and TVS is possible and allows to assess the difficulty of the surgical procedure and the risk of complications in surgical procedures. Whether the ENZIAN can be used to predict fertility outcomes remains to be determined.

The recently released updated version, called the #ENZIAN classification, represents a comprehensive description of peritoneal and ovarian endometriosis as well as adnexal adhesions in addition to deep endometriosis. #Enzian system is anatomically logical, easy to use, and reproducible providing clinicians with a reproducible image of the disease. The correlation between preoperative and surgical staging, namely classification of the extent of disease obtained based on the #Enzian scheme allows for consistent and clear classification of endometriosis, especially DE but also secondary adhesions. Endometriosis can be mapped completely with one single classification system applicable by preinvasive and invasive methods thereby enabling the use of one common language for describing endometriosis. In the same way as patients with cancer are described using the TNM classification, the #ENZIAN classification can be used to supplement the descriptive terms of endometriosis. The exact structural allocation of the compartments and exact description of affected organ structures may enable doctors to obtain a virtual picture of the extent of endometriosis.

References

1. Rokitansky K. Ueber Uterusdruesen-Neubildung. Zeitschrift der kaiserl königl Gesellschaft der Aerzte zu Wien. 1860;37:578–81.
2. Classification of endometriosis. The American Fertility Society. Fertil Steril. 1979;32(6):633–4.
3. Revised American Society for Reproductive Medicine classification of endometriosis: 1996. Fertil Steril. 1997;67(5):817–21.
4. Johnson NP, Hummelshoj L, Adamson GD, Keckstein J, Taylor HS, Abrao MS, et al. World Endometriosis Society consensus on the classification of endometriosis. Hum Reprod. 2017;32(2):315–24.
5. Vanhie A, Meuleman C, Tomassetti C, Timmerman D, D'Hoore A, Wolthuis A, et al. Consensus on recording deep endometriosis surgery: the CORDES statement. Hum Reprod. 2016;31(6):1219–23.
6. Keckstein J, Becker CM, Canis M, Feki A, Grimbizis GF, Hummelshoj L, et al. Recommendations for the surgical treatment of endometriosis Part 2: deep endometriosis †‡¶. Facts Views Vis Obgyn. 2019;11(4):269–97.
7. Adamson GD, Pasta DJ. Endometriosis fertility index: the new, validated endometriosis staging system. Fertil Steril. 2010;94(5):1609–15.
8. Abrao MS, Neme RM, Carvalho FM, Aldrighi JM, Pinotti JA. Histological classification of endometriosis as a predictor of response to treatment. Int J Gynaecol Obstet. 2003;82(1):31–40.
9. Abrao MS, Petraglia F, Falcone T, Keckstein J, Osuga Y, Chapron C. Deep endometriosis infiltrating the recto-sigmoid: critical factors to consider before management. Hum Reprod Update. 2015;21(3):329–39.
10. Adamson GD. Endometriosis classification: an update. Curr Opin Obstet Gynecol. 2011;23(4):213–20.
11. Koninckx PR, Ussia A, Adamyan L, Wattiez AJGS. An endometriosis classification, designed to be validated. Gynecol Surg. 2011;8(1):1–6.
12. Brosens IA, Cornillie F, Koninckx P, Vasquez G. Evolution of the revised American Fertility Society classification of endometriosis. Fertil Steril. 1985;44(5):714–6.

13. Brosens I, Donnez J, Benagiano G. Improving the classification of endometriosis. Hum Reprod. 1993;8(11):1792–5.
14. Brosens IA. Classification of endometriosis revisited. Lancet. 1993;341(8845):630.
15. Chapron C, Dubuisson JB, Chopin N, Foulot H, Jacob S, Vieira M, et al. Deep pelvic endometriosis: management and proposal for a "surgical classification". Gynecol Obstet Fertil. 2003;31(3):197–206.
16. Chapron C, Fauconnier A, Vieira M, Barakat H, Dousset B, Pansini V, et al. Anatomical distribution of deeply infiltrating endometriosis: surgical implications and proposition for a classification. Hum Reprod. 2003;18(1):157–61.
17. Exacoustos C, Malzoni M, Di Giovanni A, Lazzeri L, Tosti C, Petraglia F, et al. Ultrasound mapping system for the surgical management of deep infiltrating endometriosis. Fertil Steril. 2014;102(1):143–50 e2.
18. Redwine DB. American Fertility Society classification of endometriosis--the last word? Fertil Steril. 1990;54(1):180–1.
19. Khazali S. Endometriosis classification-The quest for the Holy Grail? J Reprod Infertil. 2016;17(2):67.
20. Van den Bosch T, de Bruijn AM, de Leeuw RA, Dueholm M, Exacoustos C, Valentin L, et al. A sonographic classification and reporting system for diagnosing adenomyosis. Ultrasound Obstet Gynecol. 2019;53(5):576–82.
21. Bouquet de Joliniere J, Major A, Ayoubi JM, Cabry R, Khomsi F, Lesec G, et al. It is necessary to purpose an add-on to the American Classification of Endometriosis? This disease can be compared to a malignant proliferation while remaining benign in most cases. EndoGram(R) is a new profile witness of its evolutionary potential. Front Surg. 2019;6:27.
22. Wustlich M. Laparoscopic assited segmental resection in endometriosis with bowel involvement (Laparoskopisch-assistierte Sigmasegmentresektionbei Endometriose mit Darmbeteiligung) [thesis]. Ulm: University Ulm; 2002.
23. Leonardi M, Espada M, Choi S, Chou D, Chang T, Smith C, et al. Transvaginal ultrasound can accurately predict the American Society of Reproductive Medicine stage of endometriosis assigned at laparoscopy. J Minim Invasive Gynecol. 2020;27(7):1581–7 e1.
24. Williams JC, Burnett TL, Jones T, Venkatesh SK, VanBuren WM. Association between kissing and retropositioned ovaries and severity of endometriosis: MR imaging evaluation. Abdom Radiol (NY). 2020;45(6):1637–44.
25. Holland TK, Yazbek J, Cutner A, Saridogan E, Hoo WL, Jurkovic D. Value of transvaginal ultrasound in assessing severity of pelvic endometriosis. Ultrasound Obstet Gynecol. 2010;36(2):241–8.
26. Vercellini P, Fedele L, Aimi G, Pietropaolo G, Consonni D, Crosignani PG. Association between endometriosis stage, lesion type, patient characteristics and severity of pelvic pain symptoms: a multivariate analysis of over 1000 patients. Hum Reprod. 2007;22(1):266–71.
27. Fedele L, Bianchi S, Bocciolone L, Di Nola G, Parazzini F. Pain symptoms associated with endometriosis. Obstet Gynecol. 1992;79(5 (Pt 1)):767–9.
28. Andres MP, Borrelli GM, Abrao MS. Endometriosis classification according to pain symptoms: can the ASRM classification be improved? Best Pract Res Clin Obstet Gynaecol. 2018;51:111–8.
29. Chapron C, Fauconnier A, Dubuisson JB, Barakat H, Vieira M, Breart G. Deep infiltrating endometriosis: relation between severity of dysmenorrhoea and extent of disease. Hum Reprod. 2003;18(4):760–6.
30. Vercellini P, Fedele L, Aimi G, De Giorgi O, Consonni D, Crosignani PG. Reproductive performance, pain recurrence and disease relapse after conservative surgical treatment for endometriosis: the predictive value of the current classification system. Hum Reprod. 2006;21(10):2679–85.
31. Nicolaus K, Zschauer S, Brauer D, Jimenez-Cruz J, Lehmann T, Rengsberger M, et al. Extensive endometriosis surgery: rASRM and Enzian score independently relate to postoperative complication grade. Arch Gynecol Obstet. 2020;301(3):699–706.

32. Poupon C, Owen C, Arfi A, Cohen J, Bendifallah S, Darai E. Nomogram predicting the likelihood of complications after surgery for deep endometriosis without bowel involvement. Eur J Obstet Gynecol Reprod Biol X. 2019;3:100028.
33. Metzemaekers J, Haazebroek P, Smeets M, English J, Blikkendaal MD, Twijnstra ARH, et al. EQUSUM: Endometriosis QUality and grading instrument for SUrgical performance: proof of concept study for automatic digital registration and classification scoring for r-ASRM, EFI and Enzian. Hum Reprod Open. 2020;2020(4):hoaa053.
34. Boujenah J, Bonneau C, Hugues JN, Sifer C, Poncelet C. External validation of the Endometriosis Fertility Index in a French population. Fertil Steril. 2015;104(1):119–23 e1.
35. Garavaglia E, Pagliardini L, Tandoi I, Sigismondi C, Vigano P, Ferrari S, et al. External validation of the Endometriosis Fertility Index (EFI) for predicting spontaneous pregnancy after surgery: further considerations on its validity. Gynecol Obstet Investig. 2015;79(2):113–8.
36. Tomassetti C, Bafort C, Vanhie A, Meuleman C, Fieuws S, Welkenhuysen M, et al. Estimation of the Endometriosis Fertility Index prior to operative laparoscopy. Hum Reprod. 2021;36(3):636–46.
37. Keckstein J, Ulrich U, Possover M, Schweppe KW. ENZIAN-Klassifikation der tief infiltrierenden Endometriose. Zentralbl Gynäkol. 2003;125:291.
38. Tuttlies F, Keckstein J, Ulrich U, Possover M, Schweppe KW, Wustlich M, et al. ENZIAN-score, a classification of deep infiltrating endometriosis. Zentralbl Gynakol. 2005;127(5):275–81.
39. Keckstein J, Wiesinger H. Deep endometriosis, including intestinal involvement--the interdisciplinary approach. Minim Invasive Ther Allied Technol. 2005;14(3):160–6.
40. Keckstein J, Hudelist G. Classification of deep endometriosis (DE) including bowel endometriosis: from r-ASRM to #Enzian-classification. Best Pract Res Clin Obstet Gynaecol. 2021;71:27–37.
41. Di Paola V, Manfredi R, Castelli F, Negrelli R, Mehrabi S, Pozzi MR. Detection and localization of deep endometriosis by means of MRI and correlation with the ENZIAN score. Eur J Radiol. 2015;84(4):568–74.
42. Burla L, Scheiner D, Samartzis EP, Seidel S, Eberhard M, Fink D, et al. The ENZIAN score as a preoperative MRI-based classification instrument for deep infiltrating endometriosis. Arch Gynecol Obstet. 2019;300(1):109–16.
43. Thomassin-Naggara I, Lamrabet S, Crestani A, Bekhouche A, Wahab CA, Kermarrec E, et al. Magnetic resonance imaging classification of deep pelvic endometriosis: description and impact on surgical management. Hum Reprod. 2020;35(7):1589–600.
44. Hudelist G, Montanari E, Salama M, Dauser B, Nemeth Z, Keckstein J. Comparison between sonography-based and surgical extent of deep endometriosis using the Enzian classification – a prospective diagnostic accuracy study. J Minim Invasive Gynecol. 2021;28(9):1643–1649.e1.
45. Montanari E, Dauser B, Keckstein J, Kirchner E, Nemeth Z, Hudelist G. Association between disease extent and pain symptoms in patients with deep infiltrating endometriosis. Reprod Biomed Online. 2019;39(5):845–51.
46. Haas D, Oppelt P, Shebl O, Shamiyeh A, Schimetta W, Mayer R. Enzian classification: does it correlate with clinical symptoms and the rASRM score? Acta Obstet Gynecol Scand. 2013;92(5):562–6.
47. Haas D, Chvatal R, Habelsberger A, Schimetta W, Wayand W, Shamiyeh A, et al. Preoperative planning of surgery for deeply infiltrating endometriosis using the ENZIAN classification. Eur J Obstet Gynecol Reprod Biol. 2013;166(1):99–103.
48. Roman H, Moatassim-Drissa S, Marty N, Milles M, Vallee A, Desnyder E, et al. Rectal shaving for deep endometriosis infiltrating the rectum: a 5-year continuous retrospective series. Fertil Steril. 2016;106(6):1438–45.e2.
49. Imboden S, Bollinger Y, Harma K, Knabben L, Fluri M, Nirgianakis K, et al. Predictive factors for voiding dysfunction after surgery for deep infiltrating endometriosis. J Minim Invasive Gynecol. 2021;28(8):1544–51.
50. Mutuku T. Prä-operative Abschätzung einer tief infiltrierenden Darmendometriose mittels Untersuchungsbefund in der ENZIAN-Klassifikation und der Symptomatik sowie Vergleich mit dem intra-operativen ENZIAN-Befund; [The assessment of deep infiltrating

endometriosis according to the preooperative investigation and symptoms in comparison to intraoperative findings with the ENZIAN-Classification] [MD Thesis]. Ulm: Universität Ulm; 2016.
51. Keckstein J, Saridogan E, Ulrich UA, Sillem M, Oppelt P, Schweppe KW, et al. The #Enzian classification: a comprehensive non-invasive and surgical description system for endometriosis. Acta Obstet Gynecol Scand. 2021;100(7):1165–75.
52. Guerriero S, Condous G, van den Bosch T, Valentin L, Leone FP, Van Schoubroeck D, et al. Systematic approach to sonographic evaluation of the pelvis in women with suspected endometriosis, including terms, definitions and measurements: a consensus opinion from the International Deep Endometriosis Analysis (IDEA) group. Ultrasound Obstet Gynecol. 2016;48(3):318–32.
53. Di Giovanni Al, Montanari E, Hudelist G, Malzoni M, Keckstein J. Comparison between sonography-based and surgical evaluation of endometriotic lesions using the #Enzian classification – a retrospective data analysis. Acta Obstet Gynecol Scand. 2021, under submission.
54. Montanari E, Bokor A, Szabó G, Kondo W, Trippia CH, Malzoni M, et al. Accuracy of sonography for non-invasive detection of ovarian and deep endometriosis using #Enzian classification: prospective multicenter diagnostic accuracy study. Ultrasound Obstet Gynecol. 2021.

Endometriosis Diagnostic Modalities: The Sonographic Diagnosis of Deep Endometriosis

9

Stefano Guerriero, Eleonora Musa, Silvia Ajossa, Angela M. Pascual, Mariachiara Pagliuca, Monica Pilloni, Manuela Neri, Luca Saba, and Luis Juan Alcazar

Contents

S. Guerriero (✉) · E. Musa · S. Ajossa · M. Pagliuca · M. Pilloni · M. Neri
Department of Obstetrics and Gynecology, University of Cagliari, Policlinico Universitario Duilio Casula, Monserrato, Cagliari, Italy
e-mail: gineca.sguerriero@tiscali.it

A. M. Pascual
Department of Obstetrics, Gynecology, and Reproduction, Hospital Universitari Dexeus, Barcelona, Spain

L. Saba
Department of Radiology, Azienda Ospedaliero Universitaria di Cagliari, Cagliari, Italy

L. J. Alcazar
Department of Obstetrics and Gynecology, Clínica Universidad de Navarra, School of Medicine, University of Navarra, Pamplona, Spain

E. Oral (ed.), *Endometriosis and Adenomyosis*,
https://doi.org/10.1007/978-3-030-97236-3_9

9.1 Introduction

Transvaginal ultrasound (TVS) is considered the primary not invasive choice in patient assessment with suspected deep endometriosis [1–3]. There are three principal types of endometriotic lesions: peritoneal or superficial endometriosis, ovarian endometriosis, and deep infiltrating endometriosis (DIE). Transvaginal ultrasound has high diagnostic accuracy for endometriomas, deep endometriotic lesions, and pelvic adhesions. However, superficial endometriotic implants are not detectable through this diagnostic tool [3]. The relevance of pelvic sonographic examination has been introduced for the first time in 2008 in the American National Guidelines (ACOG committee opinion) [4], regardless of the general pelvic examination outcomes. In fact, sonographic examination should always be performed in patient with secondary dysmenorrhea. Simultaneously, SIGO guidelines (Italian Society of Gynaecology and Obstetrics) highlighted ultrasound specific role in this diagnostic pathway [5]. Laparoscopy as the only diagnostic tool, instead, produces a sizable diagnostic delay, precisely 12 years of delay in young women [6]. For these reasons, a group of North-American experts of DIE [7] suggest to perform or order imaging to evaluate the presence of endometrioma, the presence of adenomyosis, the presence of soft markers, and the presence of nodules and masses in association with the history of patient to obtain a clinical diagnosis of endometriosis. This approach is defined as a fundamental step to reduce the delay in this chronic and invalidating disease.

The overall diagnostic performance of ultrasound for DIE lesions in rectosigmoid localization is good, as demonstrated in recent meta-analysis, with high sensitivity (91%, with 95%CI, 85–94%) and high specificity (97%, with 95%CI, 95–98%) [8], and it was significantly higher than the overall diagnostic performance of TVS for assessing DIE in USLs (Uterosacral Ligaments), RVS (Rectovaginal Septum), vaginal wall, and bladder [9]. Moreover, a recent meta-analysis has compared the diagnostic performance of TVS and MRI, respectively, concluding that it is similar to assess DIE lesions in rectosigmoid, USLs, and RVS [10]. In 2016, the IDEA (International Deep Endometriosis Analysis) group, consisting of some expert gynecological sonographers, surgeons, and radiologists, have introduced a systematic sonographic approach about the assessment in women with clinical suspicion of deep endometriosis. The purpose of IDEA consensus was the standardization of terminology, definition of anatomic localizations, and measurement lesions modality. The IDEA approach counts of four systematic steps [11]. The first step provides a routine assessment of uterus and adnexa; the principal aim is to detect adenomyosis and/or endometriomas. The second step is related to the TVS "soft markers" (site-specific tenderness and ovarian mobility). The third step provides the sliding sign used to assess the pouch of Douglas. Last, the fourth step provides a systematic evaluation of the anterior and posterior compartment for the detection of endometriosis nodules.

9.2 Uterus Assessment

During the sonographic examination, it is important to define the uterus orientation (anteverted, retroverted, or in axis), its mobility (normal, reduced, or absent, and question mark sign [12]), or other anomalies [11]. In addition, it is important to assess the adenomyosis signs and describe them with terms and definitions from the MUSA consensus (Morphological Uterus Sonographic Assessment). This is a crucial point because adenomyosis is commonly associated with deep endometriosis [13]. Adenomyosis is the presence of endometrial glands and stroma in the contest of the myometrium, and usually there are some specific sonographic signs: asymmetrical myometrial thickening (Fig. 9.1), several myometrial cysts (a typical myometrium cyst has a hyperechoic margin due to the presence of endometrial tissue), hyperechoic island with variable profile (not defined, irregular, and regular), presence of multiple fan-shaped shadows (Fig. 9.2), and subendometrial hyperechoic lines, irregular or interruption of the myometrial-endometrial junction. The myometrial endometrial junction can be studied with two-dimension views; however, the 3D assessment, particularly with the VCI (volume contrast imaging)

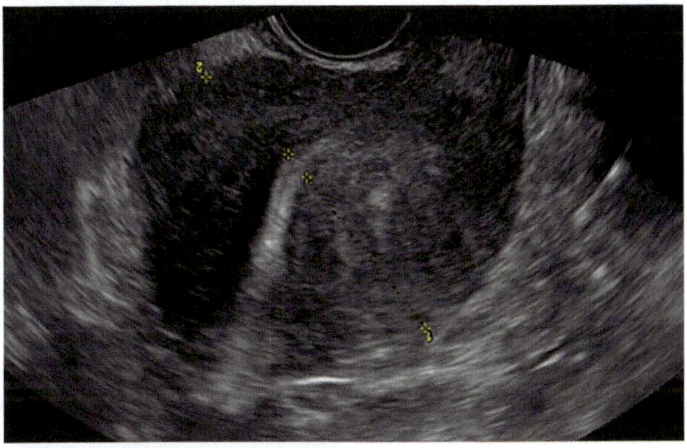

Fig. 9.1 Asymmetrical myometrium thickening

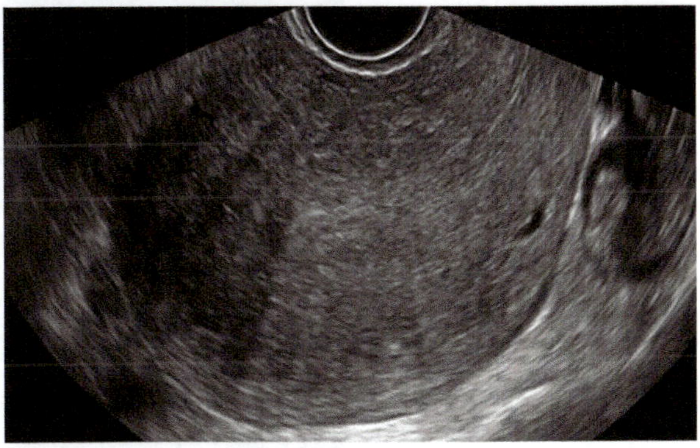

Fig. 9.2 Fan-shaped shadowing

technique set to 2 mm [14], allows a more accurate analysis. Adenomyosis might be diffuse or localized according to the myometrium involvement (respectively inferior or superior to 25%) [15].

9.3 Adnexal Assessment

Endometriomas are frequently associated with deep endometriosis [16]. A typical endometrioma (73–82% [17, 18]) is a cystic lesion with ground glass content (homogeneous hypoechoic content corresponding to the presence of blood in the cystic cavity) with a well define ovarian parenchyma, without papillary projections and solid vascularized areas [18–20] (Fig. 9.3). Less common characteristics include the following: multiple lobulations (nearly 85% <5 lobulations), hyperechoic wall foci, solid-cystic lesion (15%), and solid lesion (1%) [19–22]. The average diameter (nearly 50 mm) is almost the same in women of different age. Unilocular cysts are less common according to the increasing of age, as well as the "ground glass" content, in particular after 35 years old. Color score is similar in the different women

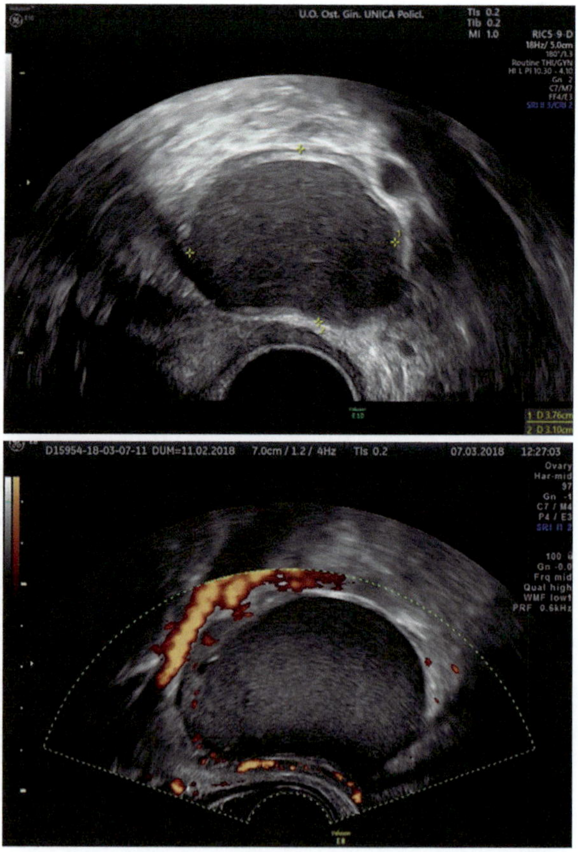

Fig. 9.3 Two examples of typical endometrioma

ages, and in most of cases color is absent or poor (color score 1–2). Sonographic accuracy is higher in younger patient with a sensibility of 90% and specificity of 97%.

9.4 Ovarian Position Assessment (Soft Markers)

The ovary visualization is followed by its position assessment. Dynamic sonographic "soft markers" are essential in this step together with the site-specific tenderness, ovarian mobility, and chiefly the ovarian adhesion to the uterus [11–21]. "Soft markers" are sonographic features suggestive of endometriosis. Using a steady and light pressure between the uterus and the ovary, the sonographer assesses possible adhesion to the uterus (Fig. 9.4), to the pelvic wall, or to the uterosacral ligaments. The kissing ovaries sign, characterized by close proximity of both ovaries, represents another sonographic feature suggestive of severe pelvic adhesions (Fig. 9.5).

9.5 Pouch of Douglas Assessment

The "sliding sign" is a new dynamic sonographic technique to appraise the pouch of Douglas. Depending on the uterus orientation, it is possible to describe two different techniques [11–24]. In case of anteverted uterus, the sliding sign can be considered positive if the rectum anterior wall slides in the posterior cervical and vaginal wall, applying a light pressure in the cervix with the TV probe. The absence of sliding between these anatomic structures can be considered as a negative sliding sign. In addition, it is possible to evaluate if the small bowel walls can freely slide to the posterior uterine wall (positive "sliding sign"). This can be evocated using the free hand throughout a gentle pelvic pressure, aiming the uterus mobilization [11–24]. The obliteration of the pouch of Douglas is due by a negative sliding sign in the posterior compartment.

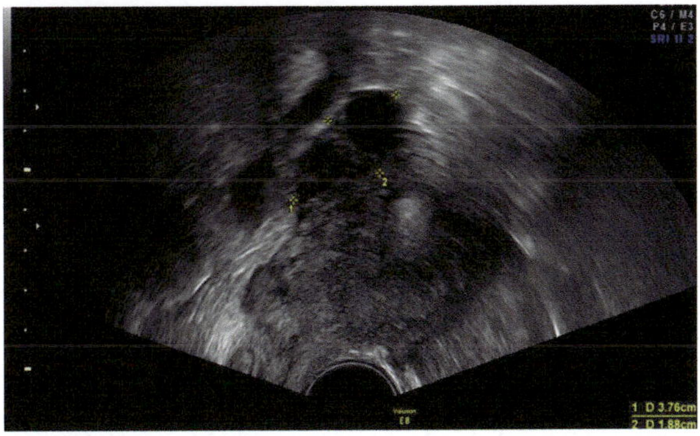

Fig. 9.4 Ovary fixed to the uterus

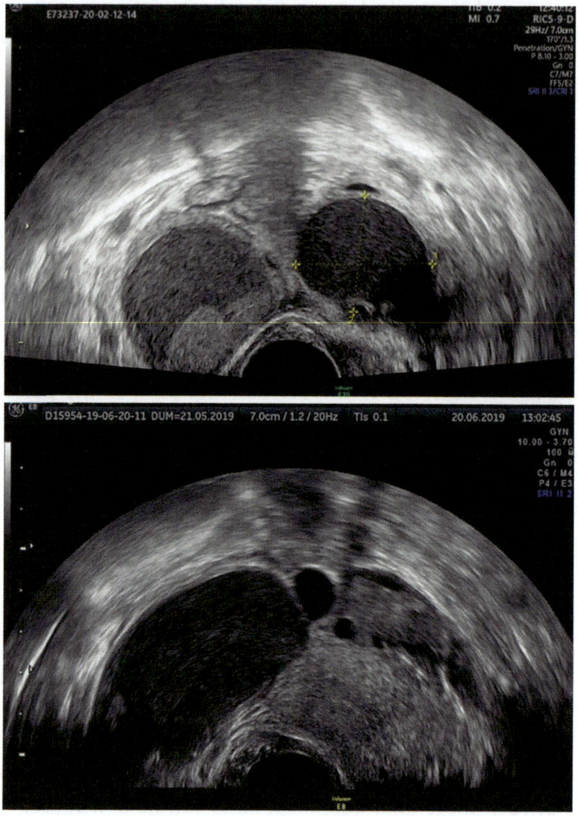

Fig. 9.5 Two examples of kissing ovaries

In case of retroverted uterus, the sliding sign is assessed throughout a gentle pressure exerted with the transvaginal probe to the posterior uterus wall. The purpose is to slide the rectum anterior wall to the uterus wall. During this maneuver, the free hand carries out a gentle pressure on the abdominal wall, thus to facilitate the sliding between these anatomic structures. If the slide happens, the sliding sign can be considered positive. The pouch of Douglas, otherwise, is considered obliterated if this sign is negative [11–24]. The presence or absence of this sign needs to be written in the report. The presurgical assessment is a simple method to assess adhesions and pelvic endometriosis in the posterior compartment, notably with the pouch of Douglas obliteration with high sensibility and specificity, respectively, of 83% and 97% [23, 24].

9.6 Deep Endometriosis Assessment

The sonographer has to look for endometriosis nodules in the anterior, posterior, and lateral compartment using the IDEA consensus model [11]. The anterior compartment is made by the uterus, the bladder, and the vesico-uterine pouch. According to the IDEA consensus [11] for the assessment of the anterior compart, the sonographer has to place the probe in the anterior fornix and a minimal vesical filling is required (100–150 ml of urine). Vesical endometriosis nodules appear as hypoechoic linear or spherical lesions [25–26] (Fig. 9.6), with or without utero-vesical adhesions assessed throughout the "sliding sign" [11].

The lateral pelvic lesions can involve the uterosacral ligaments, parameters, the pelvic lateral wall, and above all the ureters. The typical sonographic appearance of endometriotic nodules in the posterior and lateral wall is represented by hypoechoic incompressible avascular lesions (Figs. 9.7 and 9.8). The assessment of ureters juxta-vesical portion is crucial. Moreover, the view of the renal calyxes is essential to highlight possible hydronephrosis in the light of ureteral stenosis even if clinically silent.

For the posterior compartment assessment, the probe has to be placed in the posterior vaginal fornix [22–25]. The sonographer looks for hypoechoic incompressible avascular lesions in the rectovaginal septum, in the posterior fornix, in the pouch of Douglas / in the retrocervical region, in the anterior rectum wall/sigma rectum, and in the para-rectal region [22–25]. The IDEA consensus has defined the

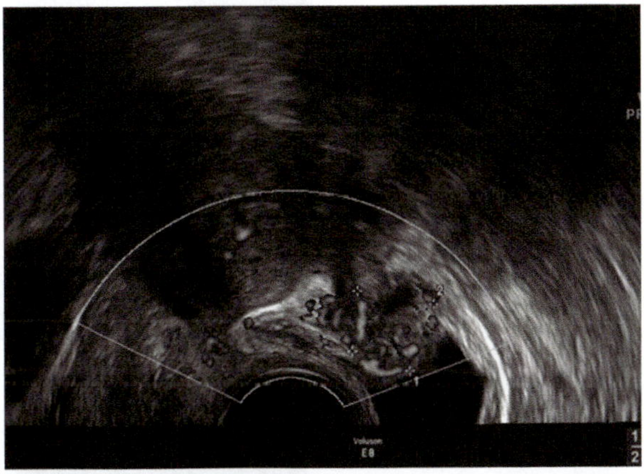

Fig. 9.6 Endometriotic vesical nodule

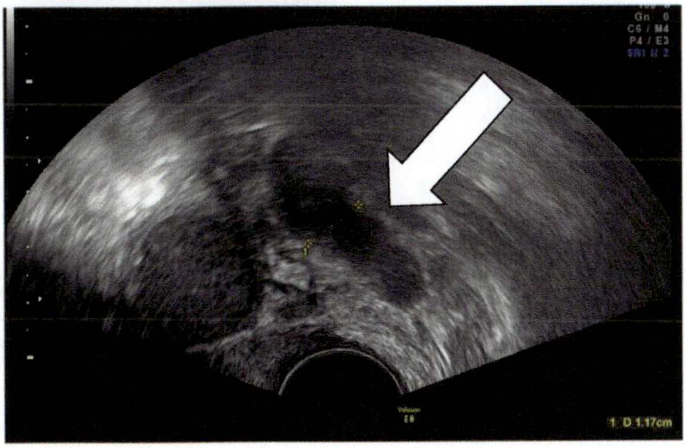

Fig. 9.7 Endometriotic nodules involving the ureter (arrow)

clinical and anatomic meaning of the rectovaginal septum. Actually, deep endometriosis seldom involves only the rectovaginal septum (which includes the vagina, the rectum, and the septum). Under those circumstances, the lesion appears as a retroperitoneal nodule in the rectovaginal area, under the posterior inferior cervical wall [7–25] (Fig. 9.9).

The endometriotic nodule involving the wall or the posterior vaginal fornix is generally a hypoechoic avascular lesion comparing to the vaginal mucosa. It can be extended to the vaginal cavity and be visible during the speculum examination [11] (Fig. 9.10a, b).

The sonographer assesses the uterosacral ligaments lesions in the retro-uterine medio-sagittal area, which are usually visualized as hypoechoic thickening with regular or irregular margins (Fig. 9.11). Commonly, lesions of the uterosacral ligaments are localized at the torus uterinus, and the typical sonographic vision is a

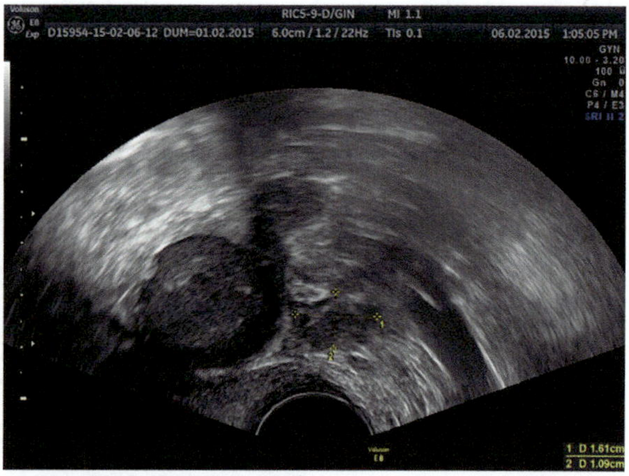

Fig. 9.8 Endometriotic nodule involving the dilated ureter (arrow)

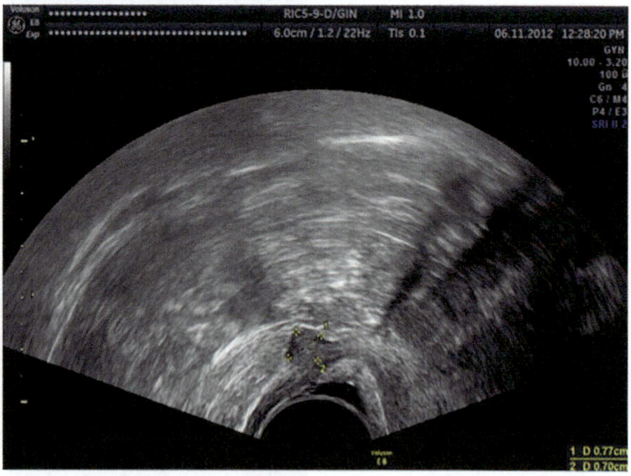

Fig. 9.9 Rectovaginal septum nodule

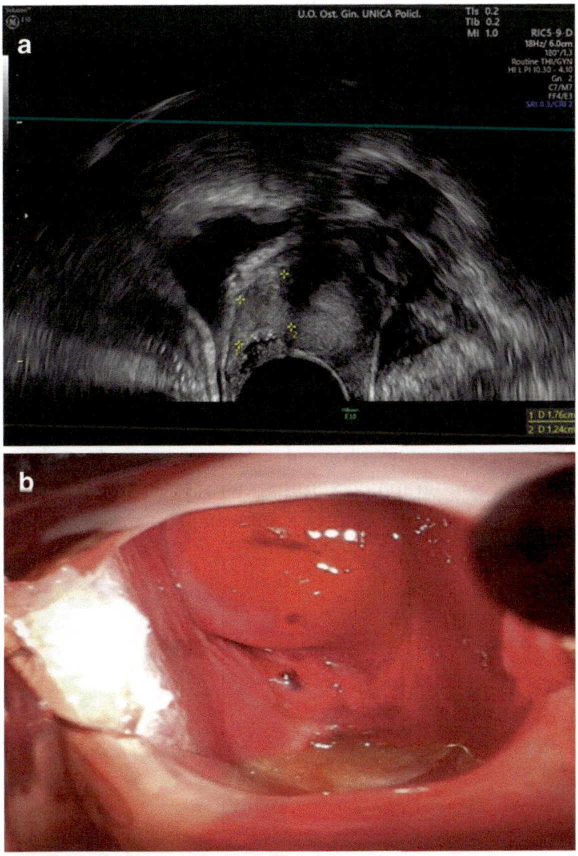

Fig. 9.10 Posterior vaginal fornix endometriotic nodule (**a**), vaginal view at speculum examination (**b**)

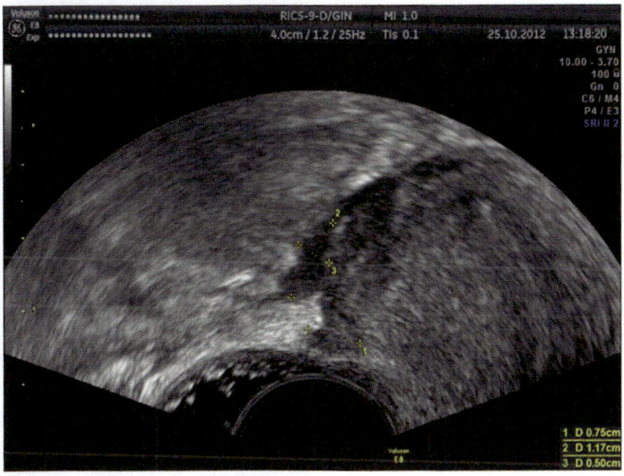

Fig. 9.11 Endometriotic nodule of uterosacral ligament

retrocervical thickening [22–25]. When endometriosis involves the rectum and/or the sigma-rectum, the sonographer has to assess the anterior rectal wall, the recto-sigmoid junction, and the sigmoid-colon for possible multifocal lesions. The typical aspect is a hypoechoic thickening of the muscular layer or a hypoechoic nodule with or without hyperechoic foci [22–25] (Fig. 9.12a, b). In some particular severe cases, it is possible to assess the "Diablo like" nodule, which is made by two closely fixed nodules: The first originates from the vaginal fornix and the second from the sigma-rectum. Regarding the necessity of a bowel preparation before TVS examination, a recent paper suggests that it can be avoided without the reduction of the accuracy but with a sure improvement of the compliance of the patient [27].

Despite the persistent idea about the learning curve difficulties for endometriosis sonographic diagnosis [28], some authors have recently pointed out that only after 40 examinations performed in 1 week of training, it is possible to reach the same diagnostic accuracy of centers of excellence [29]. Other groups [30] demonstrated that an expert gynecological sonographer can learn how to asses deep endometriosis with the sonographic examination of less than 50 patients. It has also been observed that a 2-weeks training program, based on a mix of virtual imaging navigation of

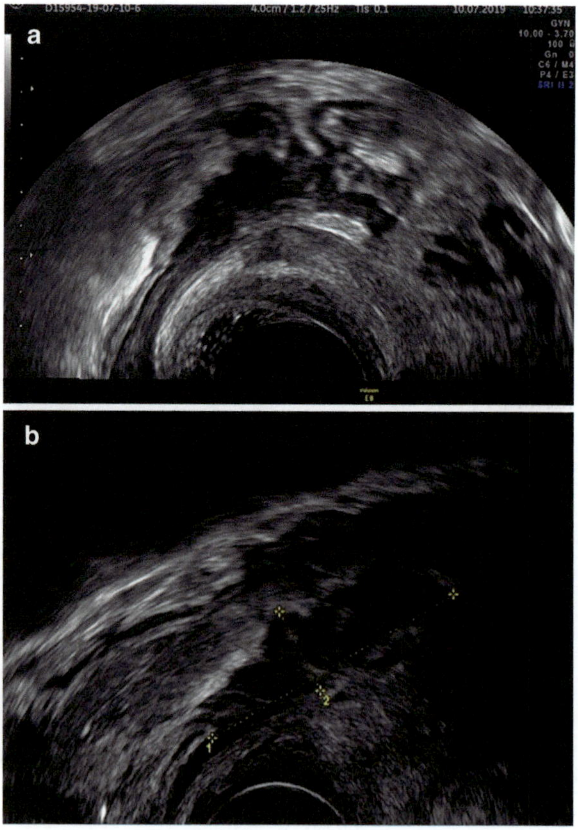

Fig. 9.12 (**a**, **b**) Bowel endometriotic nodules

patient with or without endometriosis and sonographic real session, allows a significant improvement in the diagnostic process [31].

9.7 Tenderness-Guided Transvaginal Ultrasonography

For vaginally located DIE, the use of tenderness-guided ultrasound examination is recommended [32]. In this modality, an increased amount of ultrasound gel is inserted into the transvaginal probe cover (but using only a finger glove). This "standoff" technique creates a gap between the tip of the transvaginal probe and surrounding vaginal fornices. The transvaginal probe is gently inserted into the vagina to avoid obliteration of the gel. The gradual introduction of the probe to the level of the posterior fornix may assist to visualize lesions previously not detected. During this initial ultrasound evaluation, the patient should be asked to inform the operator about the onset and the site of any tenderness experienced during the probe's placement in the posterior vaginal fornix. Particular attention must be noted to the indicated painful site which may reveal adjacent endometriosis lesions [33]. Using this modality, a better visualization of the lesion has been demonstrated [33].

9.8 Gel Sonovaginography

The sonovaginography is a sonographic transvaginal examination that allows a completion of the standard transvaginal ultrasound. Through the use of a conical tip syringe, the gel is introduced in the vagina, thus creating a better acoustic window between the transvaginal probe and the anatomic structure surrounding the vagina. This technique improves the visualization of the vaginal walls and of the anterior and posterior fornixes [34, 35]. It should be offered in circumstances of endometriosis suspicion of the posterior compartment, in particular of vaginal fornixes and rectovaginal septum involvement (Fig. 9.13).

9.9 Rectal Water-Contrast Transvaginal Ultrasonography

Similar to the vaginosonography, the introduction of water in the rectal ampule allows a distention of the rectal wall, thus improving the quality of sonographic images obtained. This technique should be offered in case of clinical suspicion of endometriotic lesions involving the rectum, the sigma-rectum, but above all to assess the local extension and possible stenosis created by the lesions. In fact, it is possible to asses with a better accuracy the bowel wall in detail: The serous layer appears thin and hyperechoic, the muscular layer is hyperechoic, and the external longitudinal smooth muscle and the internal circular smooth muscle are separated by a thin hyperechoic line (Fig. 9.14); the submucosal layer appears hyperechoic and the mucosa hypoechoic [36].

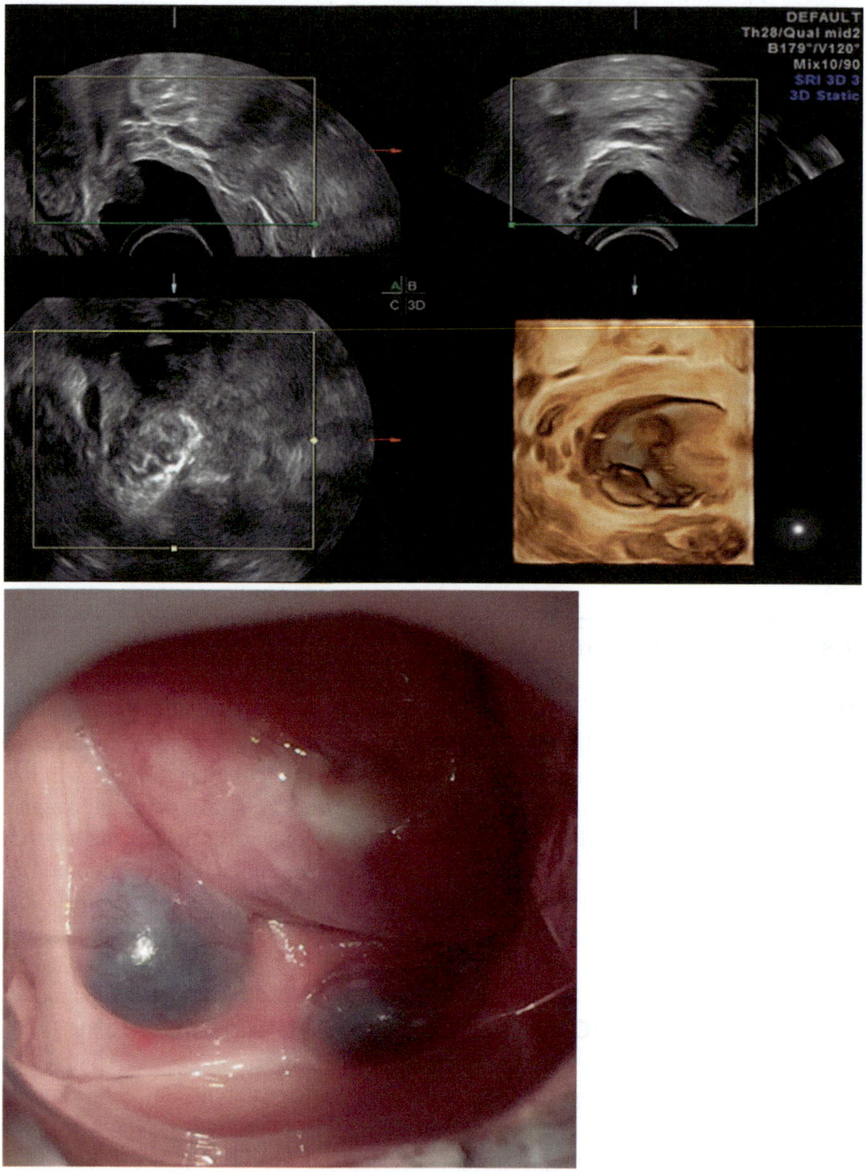

Fig. 9.13 Forniceal lesion at sonovaginography and speculum visualization of the same lesion

9.10 Three-Dimensional Ultrasonography

The use of three-dimensional (3D) image rendering has been suggested to allow a different analysis of the endometriotic nodule using new planes as coronal and lateral; this reconstruction seems to clearly show the irregular shapes and borders of the lesions [22–37]. This technique allows unrestricted access to an infinite number

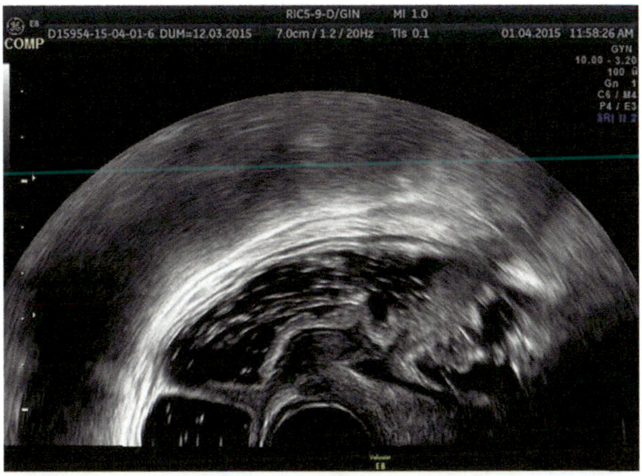

Fig. 9.14 An example of rectal water-contrast transvaginal ultrasonography

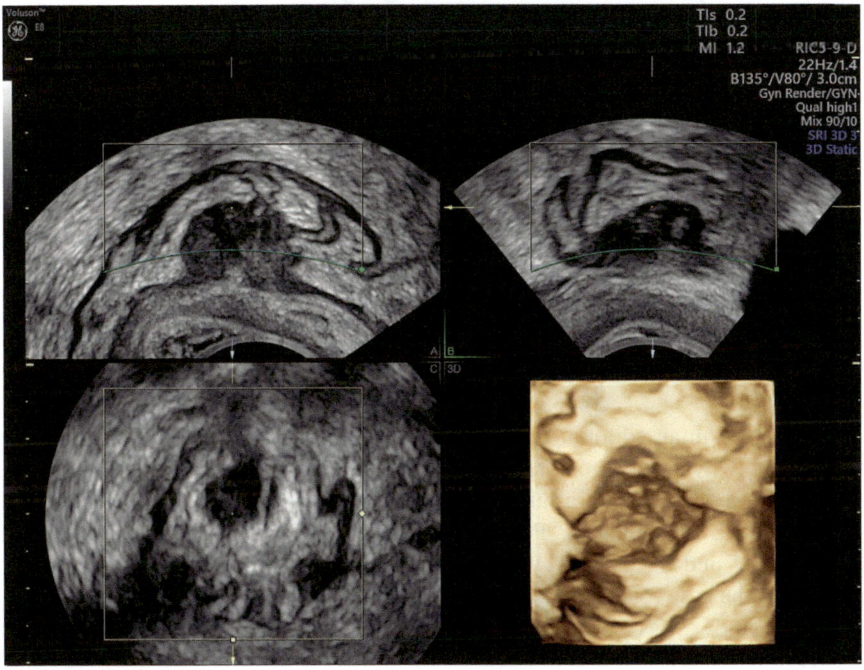

Fig. 9.15 Three-dimensional rendering of a rectosigmoid nodule

of viewing planes, which can be very useful for correctly locating lesions within the pelvis and evaluating the relationship with other organs. In addition, the stored 3D volumes can be reassessed and compared by the same or different examiners over time and also used for teaching purpose (Fig. 9.15). Guerriero et al. [26] found that the AUCs for endometriosis of intestinal location were similar for two-dimensional ultrasound and 3D. The AUCs for endometriosis of other posterior locations were significantly different (0.891, 95% CI 0.839–0.943 for 3D versus 0.789, 95% CI

0.720–0.858 for 2D; $P = 0.0193$). For the intestinal involvement, the specificity, sensitivity, positive and negative predictive value, and LR+ and LR- were 93% (89–95%), 95% (88–98%), 89% (83–92%), 97% (93–99%), 13, and 0.06, respectively, for 2D ultrasound and 97% (93–99%), 91% (84–94%), 95% (88–98%), 95% (91–96%), 25, and 0.09, respectively, for 3D ultrasound. For other posterior locations as fornix and utero-sacral ligaments, the specificity, sensitivity, positive and negative predictive value, and LR+ and LR- were 88% (82–93%), 71% (64–77%), 83% (75–90%), 79% (74–83%), 6.10, and 0.32, respectively, for 2D ultrasound and 94% (89–97%), 87% (81–91%), 92% (86–96%), 90% (85–93%), 14.0, and 0.14, respectively, for 3D ultrasound. Intraobserver agreement was substantial for both examiners (kappa 0.8754, for operator A and 0.7087, for operator B, respectively). Interobserver agreement was also substantial.

9.11 Comparison with Other Imaging Techniques

Magnetic resonance imaging (MRI) has also been used in the diagnosis of DIE. In this particular location, the diagnostic performance of TVS and MRI is similar for detecting DIE involving rectosigmoid when including only studies in which patients underwent both techniques [10]. In a recent meta-analysis of six studies (for a total 424 patients), MRI in the detection of DIE in the rectosigmoid showed a pooled sensitivity of 85% and a specificity of 95% while TVS showed a pooled sensitivity of 85% and a specificity of 96% [10]. Another meta-analysis with more cases included showed similar results [38].

9.12 Conclusion

As suggested in an editorial by Dr. Piessens [39] from Australia, it is difficult to understand why despite good test characteristics and an acceptable learning curve, even after 12 years, the ultrasound assessment of DIE is still considered a specialist assessment. Even though a "PCO assessment," a "polyp assessment," a "fibroid assessment," and an "ovarian cyst assessment" are all part of a routine examination, this is not the case for an "endometriosis assessment."

This study was partly supported by Fondazione di Sardegna grant F74I19001010007.

References

1. Exacoustos C, Manganaro L, Zupi E. Imaging for the evaluation of endometriosis and adenomyosis. Best Pract Res Clin Obstet Gynaecol. 2014;28:655–81.
2. Guerriero S, Ajossa S, Minguez JA, Jurado M, Mais V, Melis GB, Alcazar JL. Accuracy of transvaginal ultrasound for diagnosis of deep endometriosis in uterosacral ligaments, rectovaginal septum, vagina and bladder: systematic review and meta-analysis. Ultrasound Obstet Gynecol. 2015;46:534–45.

3. Reid S, Condous G. Endometriomas and pelvic endometriosis. In: Guerriero S, et al., editors. Managing ultrasonography in human reproduction. A pratical handbook. Springer; 2017.
4. ACOG Committee Opinion No. 760. American College of Obstetricians and Gynecologists. Dysmenorrhea and endometriosis in the adolescent. Obstet Gynecol. 2018;132:e249–58.
5. Linee guida per la diagnosi e il trattamento dell'endometriosi. Italian J Gynaecol Obstet. 2018;30(2). ISSN 2385–0868.
6. Arruda MS, Petta CA, Abrão MS, Benetti-Pinto CL. Time elapsed from onset of symptoms to diagnosis of endometriosis in a cohort study of Brazilian women. Hum Reprod. 2003;18:756–9.
7. Agarwal SK, Chapron C, Giudice LC, Laufer MR, Leyland N, Missmer SA, Singh SS, Taylor HS. Clinical diagnosis of endometriosis: a call to action. Am J Obstet Gynecol. 2019;220(354):e1–354.e12.
8. Guerriero S, Ajossa S, Orozco R, Perniciano M, Jurado M, Melis GB, et al. Accuracy of transvaginal ultrasound for diagnosis of deep endometriosis in the rectosigmoid: systematic review and meta-analysis. Ultrasound Obstet Gynecol. 2016;47:281–9.
9. Guerriero S, Ajossa S, Minguez JA, Jurado M, Mais V, Melis GB, et al. Accuracy of transvaginal ultrasound for diagnosis of deep endometriosis in uterosacral ligaments, rectovaginal septum, vagina and bladder: systematic review and meta-analysis. Ultrasound Obstet Gynecol. 2015;46:534–45.
10. Guerriero S, Saba L, Pascual MA, Ajossa S, Rodriguez I, Mais V, et al. Transvaginal ultrasound vs magnetic resonance imaging for diagnosing deep infiltrating endometriosis: systematic review and meta-analysis. Ultrasound Obstet Gynecol. 2018;51:586–95.
11. Guerriero S, Condous G, van den Bosch T, Valentin L, Leone FP, Van Schoubroeck D, et al. Systematic approach to sonographic evaluation of the pelvis in women with suspected endometriosis, including terms, definitions and measurements: a consensus opinion from the International Deep Endometriosis Analysis (IDEA) group. Ultrasound Obstet Gynecol. 2016;48:318–32.
12. Di Donato N, Bertoldo V, Montanari G, Zannoni L, Caprara G, Seracchioli R. Question mark form of uterus: a simple sonographic sign associated with the presence of adenomyosis. Ultrasound Obstet Gynecol. 2015;46:126–7.
13. Kunz G, Beil D, Huppert P, Noe M, Kissler S, Leyendecker G. Adenomyosis in endometriosis—prevalence and impact on fertility. Evidence from magnetic resonance imaging. Hum Reprod. 2005;20(8):2309–16.
14. Votino A, Van den Bosch T, Installé A, Van Schoubroeck D, Kaijser J, Kacem Y, De Moor B, Van Pachterbeke C, Timmerman D. Optimizing the ultrasound visualization of the endometrial-myometrial junction (EMJ). Facts Views Vis Obgyn. 2015;7(1):60–3.
15. Van den Bosch T. Adenomyosis and fibroids. In: Guerriero S, et al., editors. Managing ultrasonography in human reproduction. A pratical handbook. Springer; 2017.
16. Reid S, Lu C, Condous G. Can we improve the prediction of pouch of Douglas obliteration in women with suspected endometriosis using ultrasound based models? A multicenter prospective observational study. Acta Obstet Gynecol Scand. 2015;94(12):1297–306.
17. Kupfer MC, Schwimer SR, Lebovic J. Transvaginal sonographic appearance of endometrioma: spectrum of findings. J Ultrasound Med. 1992;11:129–33.
18. Van Holsbeke C, Van Calster B, Guerriero S, Savelli L, Paladini D, Lissoni AA, Czekierdowski A, Fischerova D, Zhang J, Mestdagh G, Testa AC, Bourne T, Valentin L, Timmerman D. Endometriomas: their ultrasound characteristics. Ultrasound Obstet Gynecol. 2010;35:730–40.
19. Hudelist G, Fritzer N, Staettner S, Tammaa A, Tinelli A, Sparic R, et al. Uterine sliding sign: a simple sonographic predictor for presence of deep infiltrating endometriosis of the rectum. Ultrasound Obstet Gynecol. 2013;41:692–5.
20. Alcázar JL. Ovarian endometriosis. In: Guerriero S, Condous G, Alcázar JL, editors. How to perform ultrasonography in endometriosis. Berlin: Springer; 2018. p. 47–55.
21. Guerriero S, Ajossa S, Garau N, Alcazar JL, Mais V, Melis GB. Diagnosis of pelvic adhesions in patients with endometrioma: the role of transvaginal ultrasonography. Fertil Steril. 2010;94:742–6.

22. Pascual MA, Guerriero S, Hereter L, Barri-Soldevila P, Ajossa S, Graupera B, et al. Diagnosis of endometriosis of the rectovaginal septum using introital three-dimensional ultrasonography. Fertil Steril. 2010;94:2761–5.
23. Hudelist G, Fritzer N, Staettner S, Tammaa A, Tinelli A, Sparic R, et al. Uterine sliding sign: a simple sonographic predictor for presence of deep infiltrating endometriosis of the rectum. Ultrasound Obstet Gynecol. 2013;41:692–5.
24. Reid S, Lu C, Casikar I, Reid G, Abbott J, Cario G, et al. Prediction of pouch of Douglas obliteration in women with suspected endometriosis using a new real-time dynamic transvaginal ultrasound technique: the sliding sign. Ultrasound Obstet Gynecol. 2013;41:685–91.
25. Guerriero S, Ajossa S, Gerada M, D'Aquila M, Piras B, Melis GB. "Tenderness-guided" transvaginal ultrasonography: a new method for the detection of deep endometriosis in patients with chronic pelvic pain. Fertil Steril. 2007;88:1293–7.
26. Guerriero S, Saba L, Ajossa S, Peddes C, Angiolucci M, Perniciano M, et al. Three-dimensional ultrasonography in the diagnosis of deep endometriosis. Hum Reprod. 2014;29:1189–98.
27. Ferrero S, Scala C, Stabilini C, Vellone VG, Barra F, Maggiore LR, U. Transvaginal sonography with vs without bowel preparation in diagnosis of rectosigmoid endometriosis: prospective study. Ultrasound Obstet Gynecol. 2019;53:402–9.
28. Noventa M, Saccardi C, Litta P, Vitagliano A, D'Antona D, Abdulrahim B, et al. Ultrasound techniques in the diagnosis of deep pelvic endometriosis: algorithm based on a systematic review and meta-analysis. Fertil Steril. 2015;104:366–83.
29. Piessens S, Healey M, Maher P, Tsaltas J, Rombauts L. Can anyone screen for deep infiltrating endometriosis with transvaginal ultrasound? Aust N Z J Obstet Gynaecol. 2014;54:462–8.
30. Eisenberg VH, Alcazar JL, Arbib N, Schiff E, Achiron R, Goldenberg M, et al. Applying a statistical method in transvaginal ultrasound training: lessons from the learning curve cumulative summation test (LC-CUSUM) for endometriosis mapping. Gynecol Surg. 2017;14(19)
31. Guerriero S, Pascual MA, Ajossa S, Rodriguez I, Zajicek M, Rolla M, Llop Rams N, Yulzari V, Bardin R, Buonomo F, Comparetto O, Perniciano M, Saba S, Mais V, Alcazar JL. Learning curve for the ultrasonographic diagnosis of deep endometriosis using a structured off-line training program. Ultrasound Obstet Gynecol. 2018; https://doi.org/10.1002/uog.20176.
32. Kavallaris A, Kohler C, Kuhne-Heid R, Schneider A. Histopathological extent of rectal invasion by rectovaginal endometriosis. Hum Reprod. 2003;18(6):1323–7.
33. Bouaziz J, Soriano D. Complications of colorectal resection for endometriosis. Minerva Ginecol. 2017;69(5):477–87.
34. Saccardi C, Cosmi E, Borghero A, Tregnaghi A, Dessole S, Litta P. Comparison between transvaginal sonography, saline contrast sonovaginography and magnetic resonance imaging in the diagnosis of posterior deep infiltrating endometriosis. Ultrasound Obstet Gynecol. 2012;40:464–9.
35. Reid S, Lu C, Hardy N, Casikar I, Reid G, Cario G, Chou D, Almashat D, Condous G. Office gel sonovaginography for the prediction of posterior deep infiltrating endometriosis: a multicenter prospective observational study. Ultrasound Obstet Gynecol. 2014;44:710–8.
36. Ferrero S, Leone Roberti Maggiore U, Barra F, Scala C. Modified ultrasonographic techniques. In: How to perform ultrasonography in endometriosis. Berlin: Springer. p. 137–9.
37. Guerriero S, Alcázar JL, Ajossa S, Pilloni M, Melis GB. Three-dimensional sonographic characteristics of deep endometriosis. J Ultrasound Med. 2009;28:1061–6.
38. Moura APC, Ribeiro HSAA, Bernardo WM, Simões R, Torres US, D'Ippolito G, Bazot M, Ribeiro PAAG. Accuracy of transvaginal sonography versus magnetic resonance imaging in the diagnosis of rectosigmoid endometriosis: systematic review and metaanalysis. PLoS One. 2019;14:e0214842.
39. Piessens S. Is it time to include assessment of the most common gynaecological condition in the routine ultrasound evaluation of the pelvis? Australas J Ultrasound Med. 2019;22:83–5.

The Evil Quadruplets: Painful Conditions Coexisting with Endometriosis

10

Michael Hibner

Contents

M. Hibner (✉)
Arizona Center for Chronic Pelvic Pain, Scottsdale, AZ, USA
e-mail: mhibner@azccpp.com

E. Oral (ed.), *Endometriosis and Adenomyosis*,
https://doi.org/10.1007/978-3-030-97236-3_10

10.1 Introduction

Endometriosis has been called one of the evil quadruplets [1] because it often coexists with other conditions causing chronic pelvic pain. By itself, endometriosis produces pain in well-described mechanisms of local inflammation mediated through cytokines, direct pressure of implants on the surrounding organs, and scarring around nerve endings [2] (Fig. 10.1). Endometriosis through nerve-mediated mechanisms explained below may also lead to other pain conditions such as bladder pain syndrome/interstitial cystitis, irritable bowel syndrome, and pelvic floor muscle spasm [6]. When pain from endometriosis coexists with pain from those other conditions, it significantly augments the total pain that patient perceives and makes treatment even more difficult. In order to successfully treat endometriosis, it is important to recognize and address all the pain generators. In fact, in many patients treated for endometriosis either medically or surgically who continue to have pain, their pain is often due to those coexisting conditions and not because treatment of endometriosis have failed. One may perform the most complete surgery for endometriosis, but if muscles spasm or bladder pain is not addressed, patient will continue to be in pain.

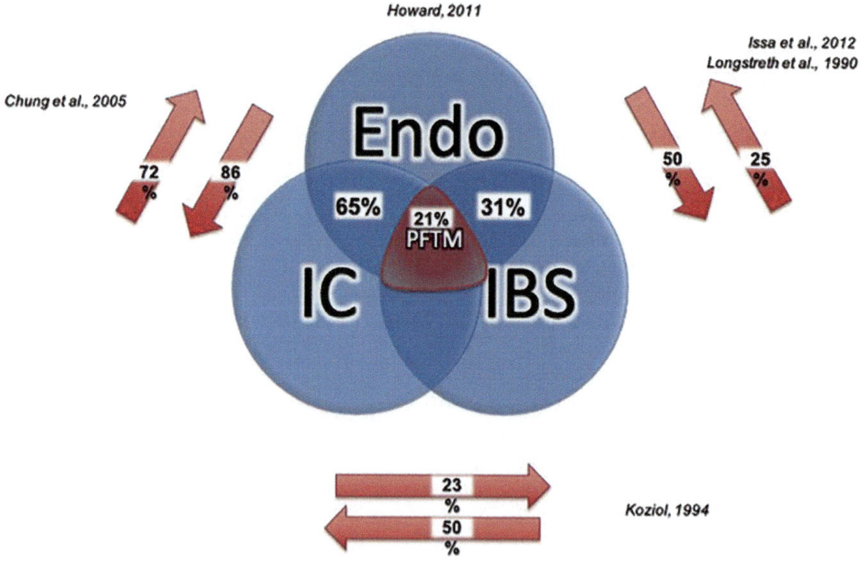

Fig. 10.1 Coexisting conditions – endometriosis, bladder pain syndrome, IBS, and spastic pelvic floor syndrome (pelvic floor tension myalgia) [3–5]

10.2 Mechanism of Coexisting Conditions

Most endometriotic implants occur on the surface of the visceral organs in the pelvis and abdomen. Pain caused by endometriosis in the peritoneal lining travels through visceral afferent fibers to the lumbosacral spinal cord. Second-order spinal neurons which receive the visceral input also receive input from other visceral nerves as well. That connection between different visceral organs at the level of spinal cord is called a viscero-visceral convergence [7] (Fig. 10.2). It explains why patients with visceral pain from endometriosis implants located on the surface of the bowel or fallopian tubes may develop pain in their bladder. This leads to so-called cross-organ sensitization between pelvic visceral organs.

The same level of spinal cord which receives visceral afferent fibers also receives convergent efferent somatic nerve fibers. This connection may lead to onset of pain in the process called viscero-somatic convergence [8] (Fig. 10.3). In this mechanism, activation of visceral fibers by endometriosis implants may lead to somatic pain located in the skin or muscle, as well as to muscle spasm mediated by efferent motor fibers. Muscle spasm in the pelvic floor may cause urinary retention and obstructive voiding [9] as well as constipation. Patients with pelvic floor muscle spasm experience pain during and after urination and bowel movement further potentiating pelvic pain. This further worsens pelvic floor muscle spasm creating a positive feedback loop of pelvic pain and spasm.

There are multiple neurotransmitters and receptors involved in the mechanisms of viscero-visceral and viscero-somatic convergence, but one with potential therapeutic implications is an N-methyl-D-aspartate (NMDA) receptor. This receptor is

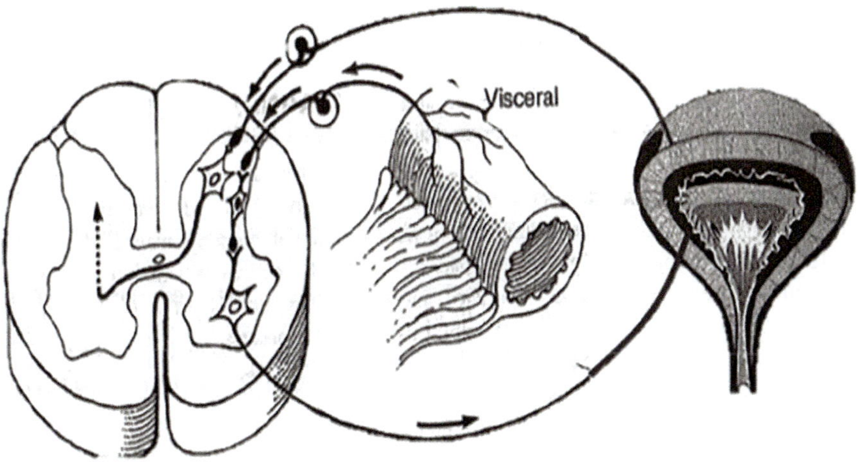

Fig. 10.2 Viscero-visceral convergence. Mechanism in which pain in one visceral organ may cause pain in another visceral organ

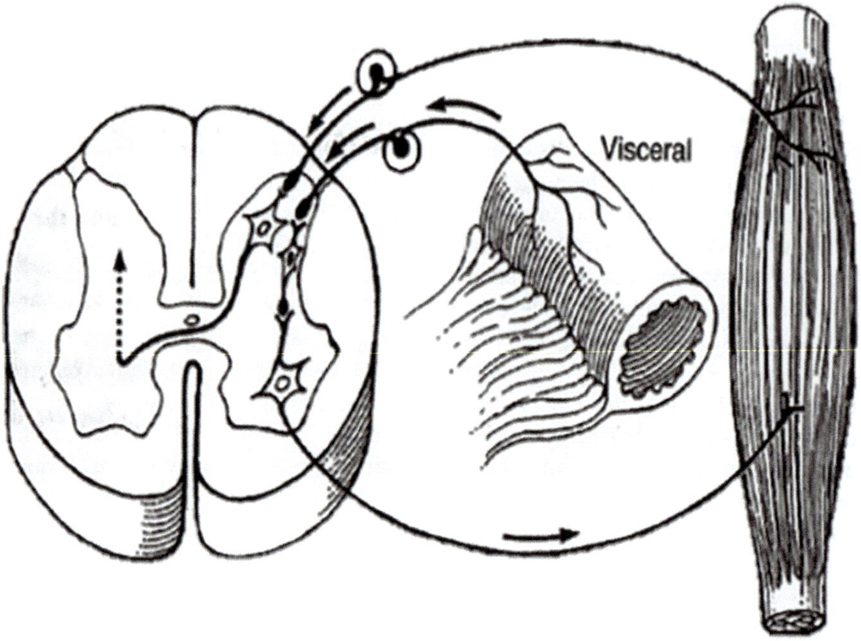

Fig. 10.3 Viscero-somatic convergence. Mechanism in which a visceral organ may cause pain in a somatic organ

expressed in primary afferents and dorsal horn neurons and is activated during transmission of visceral pain. Ketamine is one of the best-known NMDA receptor agonists, and it can be used in treatment of visceral pain and visceral convergence [10].

10.3 Bladder Pain Syndrome/Interstitial Cystitis

Interstitial cystitis/bladder pain syndrome is a condition which is characterized by the pain of the bladder during filling phase. This condition has been called by multiple different names such as interstitial cystitis (IC), bladder pain syndrome (BPS), painful bladder syndrome (PBS), and hypersensitive bladder syndrome (HBS). Even though interstitial cystitis is the most commonly used name, bladder pain syndrome was coined by NIDDK and considered the most proper name. It will be therefore used in this chapter. In 2009, Society for Urodynamics and Female Urology defined PBS as an (1) unpleasant sensation (pain, pressure, and discomfort) perceived to be related to urinary bladder (2) associated with lower urinary tract symptoms of more than 6-week duration (3) in the absence of infection or other identifiable cause [11].

10.3.1 Pathophysiology

Pathophysiology of bladder pain syndrome is not completely clear. Patients with this condition are known to have a deficiency of the glycosaminoglycan (GAG) layer of the bladder epithelium. This defect allows the irritants present in urine to penetrate bladder epithelium and cause localized inflammatory reaction in the bladder wall. This in turn leads to the release of inflammatory cytokines and nerve growth factors. Inflammation caused by this process causes mast cell activation as well as activation of capsaicin-activated nerve fibers (Fig. 10.4). This positive feedback loop causes further damage to the GAG layer allowing for more irritants to enter the bladder wall. All those inflammatory changes lead to central sensitization. In this process, NMDA receptors in the dorsal horn become activated. This leads to the decreased inhibition of dorsal horn neurons and therefore to lowering the threshold to painful stimuli not only from the bladder, but also from the surrounding organs. Researchers disagree on what is the inciting event leading to the development of bladder pain syndrome. The potential initial insult may be a bacterial infection, environmental factors, diet, stress, or autoimmune disorders [12]. Since BPS coincides with other painful conditions, it is likely that genetic factors also play a role [13]. It is thought that in patients with endometriosis it may be viscero-visceral and viscero-somatic convergence which lead to the symptoms of painful bladder syndrome.

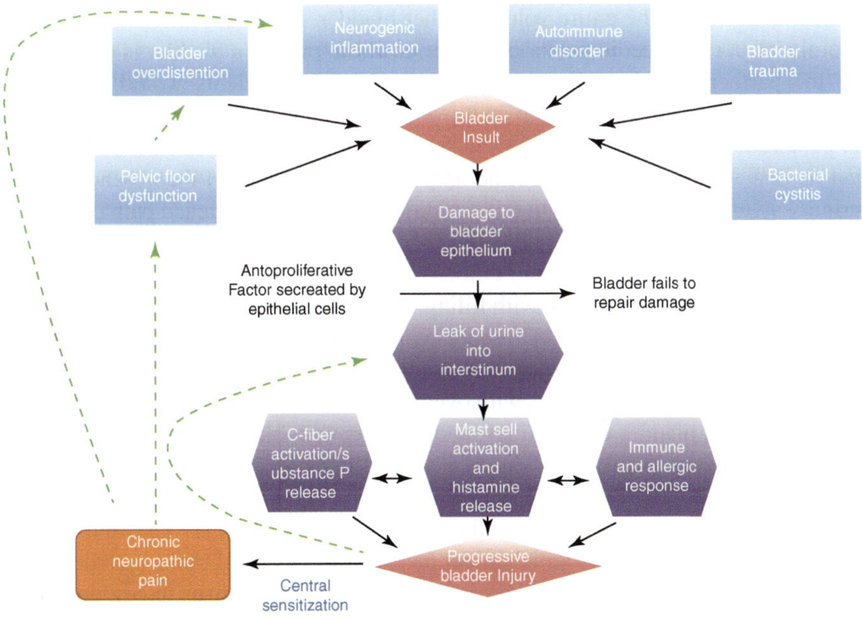

Fig. 10.4 Pathophysiology of bladder pain syndrome (BPS)

10.3.2 Epidemiology

It is difficult to estimate the prevalence of bladder pain syndrome since different practitioners use different criteria to diagnose this condition. It is estimated however that when using SUFU criteria, 2.7–6.5% of women in the United States have BPS which corresponds to 1–3% of the general population. There are therefore approximately three to eight million women in the United States suffering from bladder pain syndrome. Unfortunately, less than 50% of patients with symptoms of BPS are accurately diagnosed with this condition. Majority of patients are diagnosed in the fourth decade of life with the median age being 43. It is estimated that if the patient has chronic pelvic pain and bladder symptoms, there is 96% chance that she has BPS [14]. Patients with endometriosis are four times likely than controls to have bladder pain syndrome.

10.3.3 Symptoms

Patients with BPS typically complain of pain during filling phase of the bladder [15]. Approximately 92% of women with BPS have frequency, and 84% have urgency. Patients also frequently complain of nocturia and multiple sexual symptoms [14]. Nocturia in patients with BPS is caused by the need to avoid overfilling of the bladder. This is different from nocturia in patients with pelvic floor muscle spasm. In those patients, nocturia is caused by incomplete emptying; therefore, patient is not using the entire volume of her bladder. Pain with intercourse is most prominent in quadripedic position. In that position, patient's bladder is directly hit by the partner's penis leading to irritation and pain. Patients would frequently choose intercourse in the position on top where she controls the depth and the angle of penetration. Some patients experience lower abdominal pressure instead of pain, but in 15% of cases pain may be the only symptom of BPS in the absence of any urinary symptoms. Patients with this condition may also experience pain outside of the bladder, commonly in the vulva, lower back, and abdomen. Those may often be mistaken for other pelvic pain conditions such as vulvar vestibulitis. Symptoms of bladder pain syndrome worsen with filling of the bladder and improve with voiding which explains the symptom of frequency. It is therefore important to distinguish frequency in patients with bladder pain syndrome from frequency with pain patients with overactive bladder. Patients with overactive bladder urinate frequently because of uncontrolled bladder contractions, and patients with bladder pain syndrome urinate frequently to avoid pain. Urgency and patients with overactive bladder are generally intermittent, and in patients with BPS it is continuous. Certain foods and drinks, especially acidic, spicy, containing caffeine or alcohol, are known to trigger pain and urgency in patients with bladder pain syndrome [16]. Drinks include coffee and tea (both caffeinated and decaffeinated), soda, alcohol, citrus juices, and cranberry juice. Fruits which acidify urine are lemons, limes, oranges, grapefruit, pineapple, and kiwi fruit as well as vegetables such as chili peppers, onions, sauerkraut, tomato products, and pickles worsened BPS symptoms. Processed cheese, dark chocolate, yogurt, and sell products are also known to aggravate the bladder.

10.3.4 Diagnosis

There is a disagreement between providers and how to accurately diagnose bladder pain syndrome, and because this condition may range from mild symptoms to very severe, it is difficult to establish at which point on the spectrum of the disease the diagnoses should be made.

One of the most important aspects for diagnosing interstitial cystitis is good history consistent with symptoms outlined above [15]. Pain/urgency/frequency (PUF) questionnaire developed by Dr. Parson serves as a screening tool to aid physicians, especially those in primary care settings, to identify patients who will need to be referred to a specialist for treatment of BPS [17]. On pelvic exam, patients with bladder pain syndrome will typically have tenderness at the base of the bladder; however, lack of tenderness does not rule out bladder pain syndrome. Most of the patients with BPS exhibit spasm of the pelvic floor muscles, and it is not known if bladder pain or pelvic floor muscle spasm comes first. Another important sign appreciated on pelvic exam in patients with BPS is urethral burning elicited by light touch above urethral meatus.

Second very important step in diagnosing BPS is ruling out other conditions that are known to cause bladder pain. Patients will therefore require urine analysis and urine culture. Patients demonstrating microhematuria should be further evaluated for bladder malignancy with urine cytology. If pain begins after an encounter with the new sexual partner, patient will need vaginal culture for the presence of Mycoplasma or Ureaplasma.

Cystoscopy is required to meet the strict research criteria for diagnosing BPS, but it is not necessary in everyday clinical practice. Glomerulations seen on cystoscopy may be seen in patients without BPS, and conversely many patients with BPS may not have glomerulations. Cystoscopy is important though to rule out other causes of bladder pain and important to rule out the presence of Hunner's ulcers. Likewise, urodynamics, even though not necessary to diagnose BPS, may rule out other etiologies such as detrusor overactivity or bladder outlet obstruction. One needs to be careful though in diagnosis bladder outlet obstruction since muscle spasm in patients with BPS often causes uretheral pressures to be elevated (greater than 130 cm of H_2O).

Potassium sensitivity test, so commonly used in the past, should not be used, since in many patients without BPS test has been found to be positive [18]. The last part of the test which involves placing local anesthetic in the bladder may be helpful though. This part called bladder-anesthetic challenge test involves placing 20 mL of 2% lidocaine with 20,000 units of heparin into the bladder. Significant improvement of pain is consistent with diagnosis of BPS.

10.3.5 Treatment

When treating patients with BPS, it is particularly important to identify all the other pain generators and treat all of them appropriately. Because patients with BPS almost always demonstrate the spasm of pelvic floor muscles, which leads to obstructive voiding, the treatment of pelvic floor is an absolute must. Pain management is equally important in BPS patients since it disrupts the positive feedback between the muscles and the bladder described above. It also provides patients with overall improved quality-of-life and function.

The recommended treatment of BPS has been divided into six lines of intervention.

10.3.5.1 First-Line Interventions

Patients with bladder pain syndrome should be educated on the triggers which aggravate their bladder pain [15]. This may include information on foods and other activities (Table 10.1). It is also important to discuss with a patient that BPS is a chronic condition which may be asymptomatic with periodic flareups. Those flare-ups may be confused with urinary tract infection, and if urine analysis is not preformed, patients may be unnecessarily treated for UTI. Patients should also be educated on stress management techniques, coping mechanisms, and relaxation exercises. Reducing stress has been shown effective since reducing stress helps relax pelvic floor muscles and decrease obstructive voiding.

10.3.5.2 Second-Line Interventions

One of the most effective treatments in patients with BPS is pelvic floor physical therapy [19]. Over 80% of patients with BPS demonstrate pelvic floor muscle spasm which in addition to myofascial pain leads to voiding dysfunction. Pelvic floor physical therapy consists of myofascial release as well as other techniques such as biofeedback and dry needling. Physical therapists also educate patients on proper breathing techniques and posture. Oral medications which belong in the second-line interventions are amitriptyline, cimetidine, hydroxyzine, and pentosanpolysulfate (PPS). Some practitioners including the author of this chapter believe that PPS only has a marginal effect in treating BPS. Intravesical therapy consists of dimethyl sulfoxide instillations, and installations with heparin and/or lidocaine. The combination of heparin with alkalinized lidocaine and pH buffer is called Parsons solution and is widely used in treatment of bladder pain syndrome. This solution can be used with or without the addition of steroids such as hydrocortisone or triamcinolone. Pain management including narcotics is also a second-line intervention. Pain medications should only be used in conjunction with treatment specific to BPS, and use of narcotics should be cautious and closely monitored by a physician.

10.3.5.3 Third-Line Intervention

Cystoscopy with bladder hydrodistension may be a helpful diagnostic tool, but it is also an effective treatment in patients with BPS [15]. Hydrodistension should be performed with a pressure of 80 cm of H_2O for a period lasting from 1 to 10 min;

Table 10.1 Safe and nonsafe foods in patients with bladder pain syndrome

Food group	Safe	Not safe
Beverages	Water Juice – blueberry, pear Milk substitutes Milk shakes Tea – chamomile, peppermint Non diary creamers	Alcohol Carbonated water Juice – cranberry, orange Chocolate milk Coffee Tea – black, green Sodas Sport and energy drinks
Grains	Breads – corn, oat, whole wheat Cereals – most are safe Grains – couscous, quinoa Rice	Breads – heavily processed Cereals – heavily processes Pasta in box dishes Rice in box dishes
Fats and nuts	Nuts – almonds Oils – canola, olive, peanut, corn Margarine Lard Homemade salad dressing with safe ingredients	Nuts – hazelnuts, pecans, pistachios Salad dressing – commercially available
Eggs, meet Fish and poultry	Eggs Poultry Fish Beef Seafood – not canned Lamb Pork Protein powder	Cured meats Canned crab meat Hot dogs Sausage Smoked fish Soy products
Dairy, cheeses Frozen Desserts	Cheeses – American, mozzarella, cheddar, Feta, ricotta, string cheese Cream cheese Cottage cheese Ice cream Whipped cream	Cheeses – processed, Cheez Whiz Ice cream – citrus, chocolate Soy products
Fruits	Apples, apple sauce, blueberries, coconut, dates, pears, watermelon	Berries, citrus, dried fruit, grapes, guava, kiwi, melons, nectarines, passion fruit, papaya, pineapple, strawberries, raisins
Vegetables	Asparagus, avocado, beans, beets, broccoli, brussels sprouts, cabbage, carrots, cauliflower, celery, chives, corn, cucumber, eggplant, green beans, greens, lettuce, mushrooms, olives, parsley, pears, bell peppers, potatoes, pumpkin, radishes, squash, turnips	Chili peppers, onions, pickles, sauerkraut, soy beans, tofu
Soups	Homemade soup from safe ingredients	Bouillon, canned soups, packaged soups
Snacks	Almonds, carrots, celery, plain chips, crackers, fruit bars, vanilla milkshake, oatmeal bars, peanuts, peanut butter, popcorn, plain pretzels	Seasoned or barbecued chips Dessert cakes – in restaurant

(continued)

Table 10.1 (continued)

Food group	Safe	Not safe
Desserts and sweets	Blueberries Homemade cake Frostings Cookies – oatmeal, shortbread Muffins – carrot Cheesecake Crème brûlée Custards Pie – homemade Sweet bread Candy – licorice	Artificial sweeteners Chocolate Ice cream – chocolate Sorbets with safe fruits Pie – pecan Fruitcakes
	Maple syrup Pastries Ice cream – vanilla Pudding – tapioca, vanilla, rice Milkshake – vanilla Sweeteners – sugar, honey	
Condiments, seasonings Flavor enhancers	Allspice, almond extract, anise, basil, coriander, dill, fennel, garlic, marjoram, oregano, poppy seed, rosemary, sage, salt, thyme, tarragon, vanilla extract	Ascorbic acid, benzoates, ketchup, cayenne pepper, cloves, chili powder, horseradish, hot curry, meat tenderizes, miso, mustard, paprika. Pickles, red pepper, soy sauce, tamari, vinegar, Worcestershire sauce, MSG, sulfites
Fiber	Benefiber, plain Metamucil, bulk psyllium fiber without artificial sweetener	Metamucil with orange or berries, psyllium fiber with sugar fee sweetener, senna

however, longer protocols are used by many practitioners. In patients with Hunner's ulcers, fulguration of those ulcers has been shown to be highly effective in more than 75% of patients.

10.3.5.4 Fourth-Line Intervention

Neuromodulation such as Interstim and other nerve stimulators are not approved by FDA for treatment of BPS. Its response rate though ranges from 66% to 94%, but 28% of patients at some point demand removal due to ineffectiveness of the treatment or side effects [20].

10.3.5.5 Fifth-Line Intervention

This group consists of treatments such as botulinum toxin A injections into the detrusor muscle and cyclosporine A. This latter treatment has been found to be highly effective in patients with ulcerative form of bladder pain syndrome. Likewise, botulinum toxin A detrusor injections in some studies have been shown to be 86% effective, but they carry a significant risk of urinary retention.

10.3.5.6 Sixth-Line Intervention

Major surgery such as diversion with or without cystectomy should only be reserved for patients in whom all the other treatments have failed. The decision to have her bladder permanently removed is extremely difficult for any patient especially in light that it may not relieve the pain. Substitution cystoplasty performed to enlarge the bladder is another surgical option in patients with BPS and may be effective in patients with Hunner's ulcers.

10.3.6 Treatments That Should Not Be Offered

Several treatments used previously have been found to be ineffective for bladder pain syndrome [15]. They include prolonged antibiotic treatments, intravesical Bacillus Calmette-Guerin (BCG), high pressure/long-duration hydrodistention, and long-term systemic glucocorticoids. Some of those treatments in addition to being ineffective may also be harmful.

10.4 Spastic Pelvic Floor Syndrome

Patients with significant endometriosis will often present with spasm of the pelvic floor muscles [21]. Generally in patients with endometriosis, it takes time to develop pelvic floor muscle spasm, so patients with new onset disease may not have any symptoms of pelvic floor dysfunction. Surgical procedures and manipulation of pelvic organs in those patients may further irritate pelvic muscles and increase spasm.

10.4.1 Pathophysiology

Pelvic floor muscle spasm in patients with endometriosis occurs in the previously described mechanism of viscero-somatic convergence. In this mechanism, the painful impulse from the visceral organ or peritoneal surface travels to the dorsal horn of the spinal cord through the afferent fibers. Those neurons "converge" with the nuclei of the efferent motor fibers innervating pelvic floor. The painful visceral stimulus therefore leads to spasm of pelvic floor muscles [21].

Not all the patients with pelvic floor muscle spasm have endometriosis or other painful intraperitoneal process. There are numerous patients who have developed pelvic floor muscle spasm as a result of physical trauma to the pelvis (accidents, vaginal delivery, or pelvic surgery), psychological trauma such as sexual or domestic violence, or having spasm without any preceding event or condition [22].

10.4.2 Epidemiology

The incidence of pelvic floor muscle spasm in patients with endometriosis is not well known. The likelihood of pelvic muscles going into spasm depends on the severity of the disease, amount of pain it is causing, and age at onset of endometriosis as well as the number of previous surgical interventions. Patients with endometriosis managed by general OB/GYN practitioners may have lower incidence of pelvic floor muscle spasm than those cared for by pelvic pain specialists. In highly specialized pain practices, the incidence of pelvic floor muscle spasm in patients with endometriosis may be much higher due to the fact that patients have already failed treatments with other providers.

10.4.3 Diagnosis

Pelvic floor muscle spasm can be easily appreciated on pelvic exam. Superficial muscles which include the ischiocavernosus, bulbospongiosus, and transversus perineal muscle are palpated during single digit exam with patient in dorsal lithotomy position. Transvaginal or transrectal palpation allows to assess deeper muscles such as pubococcygeus, puborectalis, and iliococcygeus. Those muscles are collectively known as levator ani muscles. The obturator internus muscle is palpated against the posterior surface of the pubic bone while patient presses her ipsilateral knee against the nonexamining hand of the provider (Fig. 10.5).

Digital rectal exam will aid not only with assessment of the anal sphincter but also coccyx, coccygeal muscles and attachment of pubococcygeus and iliococcygeus to coccyx.

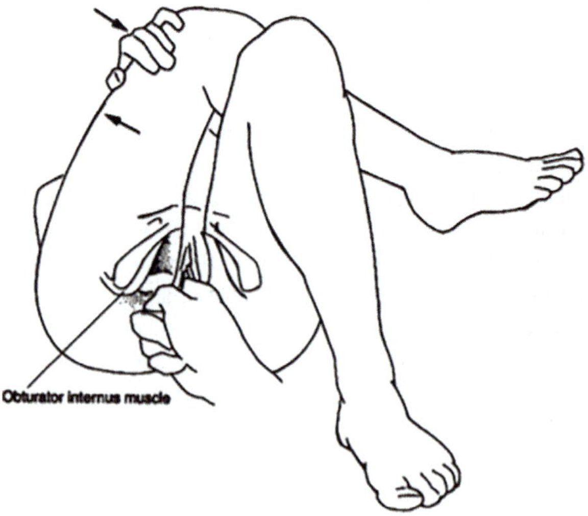

Fig. 10.5 Examination of obturator internus muscle

During the exam, patient may be asked to squeeze and relax the pelvic floor, and lack of relaxation is consistent with pelvic floor muscle spasm. This exam may be extremely uncomfortable to patient and elicit significant amounts of pain and should always be performed with one finger.

10.4.4 Treatment

The mainstay of treatment of pelvic floor spasm is pelvic floor physical therapy [22]. Pelvic floor physical therapists not only provide manual treatments, but also education important to those patients. It consists of proper breathing techniques, proper posture, sitting as well as learning the relaxation techniques. Manual therapy includes trigger point massage, trigger point release, and joint mobilization. Strengthening of the core muscles is equally important in patients with pelvic floor muscle spasm. Biofeedback in addition to manual techniques is used to teach patients to relax pelvic floor.

Medical treatments consist of various muscle relaxants. No particular oral muscle relaxant is preferred in patients with pelvic floor muscle spasm; however, vaginal or rectal suppositories containing muscle relaxants seem to work better than oral formulations. Medications such as diazepam, baclofen, gabapentin, lidocaine, and ketamine have been used in suppository formulations. Because compounded medications may be expensive, and usually not covered by insurance, an alternative may be to use valium oral tablets vaginally.

Patients who have failed muscle relaxants and pelvic floor physical therapy may benefit from injection of botulinum toxin into pelvic floor muscles [23]. Different toxins are available commercially, but onabotulinum toxin A (Botox) is the most commonly used. Doses of onabotulinum toxin A range from 100 to 400 units, and most providers use 200 units diluted in 20 ml of normal sterile saline. This injection is best done transvaginally using pudendal nerve block needle in volumes of 1 ml per injection. Some physicians choose to do those injections under CT or ultrasound guidance, but doing them transvaginally allows for palpation of spasming muscles. Regardless of the route, this injection is very painful, so it should be done with some level of sedation or anesthesia. Most commonly injected muscles are pubococcygeus, obturator internus, transversus perineal, and bulbocavernosus. In patients with endometriosis, spasm is usually bilateral, and therefore injections are done bilaterally. Immediately after the injection, pain may increase before botulinum toxin takes effect. Onabotulinum toxin A takes 5–7 days to start working, but it may take 2 weeks for patients to feel a relief of pain. When the toxin starts working, patients often notice that they have less hesitancy, and they are able to empty their bladder more completely. If patient does not report any relief of pain 2–3 weeks after the injection, she needs to be examined to assess the degree of muscle spasm. If there is still spasm, patient did not get enough onanbotulinum toxin A or it was not injected in the correct location. If there is a relaxation of the muscle, but patient still reports pain, it must be caused by something else than muscle spasm. It is important to emphasize that patient after botulinum toxin A injection needs to continue pelvic floor physical therapy since ultimately it is the therapy that will cause the muscles to stay in the relaxed stage.

10.5 Irritable Bowel Syndrome

Irritable bowel syndrome (IBS) is defined as presence of abdominal pain in association with change of bowel habits and in the absence of detecting any organic disease. IBS may present with predominance of constipation (IBS-C), diarrhea (IBS-D), or mixed symptoms with alternating constipation and diarrhea (IBS-M). It has been estimated that up to 30% of patients develop IBS symptoms after enteric infection (IBS-PI).

10.5.1 Epidemiology

Prevalence of IBS in different countries varies from 7% to 21%, and in North America it is estimated to be 12% [24]. This disease is more commonly found in younger women, and after age 50 the prevalence drops by 25%. IBS has significant impact on the economy costing over $20 billion annually.

10.5.2 Pathophysiology

Pathophysiology of IBS is very complex. Potential causes include motility of the G.I. tract, visceral hypersensitivity, inflammation, bacterial overgrowth, and food sensitivity [25]. Genetics may also play a role.

10.5.3 Diagnosis

Diagnosis of IBS is based on the symptom-based criteria. Pain in patients with IBS is generally diffuse and intermittent. It may range from mild to severe and lasting from minutes to days. In order to diagnose patients with IBS, Rome IV criteria were developed, and the hallmark of this criteria is that abdominal pain must be associated with at least two of the following: defecation, change in stool frequency, or change in stool form [26] (Table 10.2).

Table 10.2 Rome IV criteria

Rome IV criteria for diagnosing IBS
Recurrent abdominal pain, on average, at least 1 day/week in the prior 3 months, associated with two or more of the following criteria:
Related to defecation
Associated with a change in frequency of stool
Associated with a change in form (appearance) of stool

Physical exam is helpful to rule out an acute process in the abdomen such as appendicitis or diverticulitis. Patients with IBS may be diffusely tender but, generally, do not have rebound or guarding. Additional tests such as laboratory evaluation, radiological tests, and endoscopic evaluation are helpful in ruling out any other condition that would explain pain.

10.5.4 Treatment

Treatment is based on which symptom is predominant, and diet may be one of the most important factors.

10.5.4.1 Diet

In order to find the proper diet, certain foods have to be eliminated in the process. Patients with lactose intolerance have symptoms resembling IBS; therefore, this condition should be ruled out first [27]. Short chain carbohydrates are completely absorbed in the small bowel, leading to fermentation and gas production. Foods such as legumes, lactose, fructose, and sorbitol should be therefore eliminated for several weeks. This includes many different fruits and vegetables as well as ice cream and yogurt. Patients with IBS may be inclined to increase the consumption of fiber; however, fiber has not been shown to improve symptoms of this disease.

10.5.4.2 Probiotics

Probiotics may be beneficial in treatment of IBS, and single strain probiotics seem to be more effective than multistrain. No single brand has been found to be more effective than any other though [28].

10.5.4.3 Gluten

Patients without celiac disease who choose to go on gluten-free diet often experience significant improvement in GI symptoms [29].

10.5.4.4 IBS-C

Patients with IBS-C type of the disease experience infrequent and hard stools. Treatment of those patients include medications that decrease intestinal transit as well as antispasmodics to relieve intestinal cramping. The first-line treatment recommended is polyethylene glycol, an osmotic laxative. Bisacodyl and senna which are stimulant laxatives are not recommended for prolonged use due to possible dependency.

10.5.4.5 IBS-D

Patients with this form of IBS may be limited with the daily activities due to significant diarrhea. One of the most common treatments for this condition are over the counter antidiarrhea medications such as the loperamide. It works by slowing down the gut motility, allowing for greater absorption of liquid from the stool. Prescription medications such alosteron, rifaximin, and eluxadoline are also helpful in treatment of this form of IBS [30]. Antispasmodics such as dicoclymine and hyoscamine when used on as-needed basis help with relief of symptoms. Patients also benefit from psychotherapeutic interventions to help manage stress, anxiety, and depression so frequently displayed in this disease.

10.6 Suggestions from the Author

Successful treatment of pain in patients with endometriosis depends on addressing all the sources of pain. Patients with endometriosis often have multiple sources of pain including pelvic floor muscle spasm, bladder pain, and abdominal pain caused by irritable bowel syndrome. They can usually tell the difference between those pains, but if they cannot, pain from the muscles and pain from the bladder can be demonstrated to the patient during pelvic exam. Palpation of the muscles and bladder in those cases will elicit pain, and the provider can ask a question "is this the pain you are usually feeling?" Treatment of those additional sources of pain can be done prior to treatment of endometriosis, concurrently or after endometriosis has been addressed. This choice of treatment should be based on predominant symptoms and patient's wishes. Likewise, patients who underwent surgery for endometriosis and continue to be in pain may have pain originating in the pelvic floor muscles or/and bladder.

If the provider decides to proceed with treatment of pelvic floor muscle spasm, it is absolutely necessary to work in conjunction with pelvic floor physical therapist. They can be found on the website of International Pelvic Pain Society (pelvicpain.org), Women's Section of American Physical Therapy Association (aptapelvichealth.org), or Hermann and Wallace Pelvic Rehabilitation Institute (hermanwallace.com). Medical treatments of pelvic floor muscle spasm without concurrent pelvic floor physical therapy will most likely fail as muscles have to learn to stay in the relaxed state.

Bladder pain syndrome/interstitial cystitis is best managed by a pelvic pain specialist or urogynecologist. In my practice, I find that most of my patients develop bladder pain in response to pelvic floor muscle spasm; therefore, treatment of pelvic floor muscle spasm is one of the most important steps in treatment of bladder pain syndrome. In my practice, I use vaginal suppositories with muscle relaxants, onabotulinum toxin A injection to pelvic floor muscles, and pelvic floor physical therapy. I am also a big proponent of 30-minutes bladder hydrodistension in those patients.

Irritable Bowel Syndrome (IBS) is best managed by a GI specialist. Diagnosis of this conditions requires ruling out other gastrointestinal conditions which may require preforming colonoscopy or EGD. For that reason, IBS should be managed by someone who is equipped and privileged to preform those procedures.

To summarize, patients with endometriosis often have multiple sources of pain in addition to endometriosis pain. The best course of action for those patients is to identify all the sources of pain prior to surgical treatment of endometriosis. Patients who are undergoing surgical resection of endometriosis can have onabotulinum toxin A injection to pelvic floor muscles and cystoscopy with 30 min bladder hydrodistension done at the time of endometriosis surgery. Patients will then need to continue pelvic floor physical therapy to retrain the muscles to stay in the relaxed state.

References

1. Chung MK, Chung RP, Gordon D. Interstitial cystitis and endometriosis in patients with chronic pelvic pain: the "Evil Twins" syndrome. JSLS. 2005;9(1):25–9. http://www.pubmedcentral.nih.gov/articlerender.fcgi?artid=3015562&tool=pmcentrez&rendertype=abstract.
2. Morotti M, Vincent K, Becker CM. Mechanisms of pain in endometriosis. Eur J Obstet Gynecol Reprod Biol. 2017; https://doi.org/10.1016/j.ejogrb.2016.07.497.
3. Longstreth GF, Preskill DB, Youkeles L. Irritable bowel syndrome in women having diagnostic laparoscopy or hysterectomy. Relation to gynecologic features and outcome. Dig Dis Sci. 1990;35(10):1285–90. https://doi.org/10.1007/BF01536421. PMID: 2145139
4. Howard FM. Surgical treatment of endometriosis. Obstet Gynecol Clin North Am. 2011;38(4):677–86. https://doi.org/10.1016/j.ogc.2011.09.004. PMID: 22134016
5. Koziol JA. Epidemiology of interstitial cystitis. Urol Clin North Am. 1994;21(1):7–20. PMID: 8284848
6. Butrick CW. Patients with chronic pelvic pain: endometriosis or interstitial cystitis/painful bladder syndrome? J Soc Laparoendosc Surg. 2007;11(2):182–9. http://www.pubmedcentral.nih.gov/articlerender.fcgi?artid=3015726&tool=pmcentrez&rendertype=abstract.
7. Giamberardino MA, Costantini R, Affaitati G, et al. Viscero-visceral hyperalgesia: characterization in different clinical models. Pain. 2010;151(2):307–22. https://doi.org/10.1016/j.pain.2010.06.023.
8. Issa B, Onon TS, Agrawal A, et al. Visceral hypersensitivity in endometriosis: a new target for treatment? Gut. 2012;61(3):367–72. https://doi.org/10.1136/gutjnl-2011-300306.
9. Kuo TLC, Ng LG, Chapple CR. Pelvic floor spasm as a cause of voiding dysfunction. Curr Opin Urol. 2015; https://doi.org/10.1097/MOU.0000000000000174.
10. Visser E, Schug SA. The role of ketamine in pain management. Biomed Pharmacother. 2006; https://doi.org/10.1016/j.biopha.2006.06.021.
11. Hanno P, Dmochowski R. Status of international consensus on interstitial cystitis/bladder pain syndrome/painful bladder syndrome: 2008 snapshot. Neurourol Urodyn. 2009; https://doi.org/10.1002/nau.20687.
12. Butrick CW. Interstitial cystitis/bladder pain syndrome. Management of the pain disorder: a urogynecology perspective. Urol Clin North Am. 2012; https://doi.org/10.1016/j.ucl.2012.06.007.
13. Warren JW, Jackson TL, Langenberg P, Meyers DJ, Xu J. Prevalence of interstitial cystitis in first-degree relatives of patients with interstitial cystitis. Urology. 2004; https://doi.org/10.1016/j.urology.2003.08.027.
14. Berry SH, Elliott MN, Suttorp M, et al. Prevalence of symptoms of bladder pain syndrome/interstitial cystitis among adult females in the United States. J Urol. 2011; https://doi.org/10.1016/j.juro.2011.03.132.
15. Hanno PM, Burks DA, Clemens JQ, et al. AUA guideline for the diagnosis and treatment of interstitial cystitis/bladder pain syndrome. J Urol. 2011; https://doi.org/10.1016/j.juro.2011.03.064.
16. Friedlander JI, Shorter B, Moldwin RM. Diet and its role in interstitial cystitis/bladder pain syndrome (IC/BPS) and comorbid conditions. BJU Int. 2012; https://doi.org/10.1111/j.1464-410X.2011.10860.x.
17. Parsons CL, Dell J, Stanford EJ, et al. Increased prevalence of interstitial cystitis: previously unrecognized urologic and gynecologic cases identified using a new symptom

questionnaire and intravesical potassium sensitivity. Urology. 2002; https://doi.org/10.1016/S0090-4295(02)01829-0.

18. Hanno P. Is the potassium sensitivity test a valid and useful test for the diagnosis of interstitial cystitis? Int Urogynecol J. 2005;16(6):428–9. https://doi.org/10.1007/s00192-005-1306-5.
19. FitzGerald MP, Payne CK, Lukacz ES, et al. Randomized multicenter clinical trial of myofascial physical therapy in women with interstitial cystitis/painful bladder syndrome and pelvic floor tenderness. J Urol. 2012;187(6):2113–8. https://doi.org/10.1016/j.juro.2012.01.123.
20. Laviana A, Jellison F, Kim J-H. Sacral neuromodulation for refractory overactive bladder, interstitial cystitis, and painful bladder syndrome. Neurosurg Clin. 2014;25(1):33–46. https://doi.org/10.1016/j.nec.2013.08.001.
21. Aredo JV, Heyrana KJ, Karp BI, Shah JP, Stratton P. Relating chronic pelvic pain and endometriosis to signs of sensitization and myofascial pain and dysfunction. Semin Reprod Med. 2017;35(1):88–97. https://doi.org/10.1055/s-0036-1597123.
22. Hartmann D, Sarton J. Chronic pelvic floor dysfunction. Best Pract Res Clin Obstet Gynaecol. 2014; https://doi.org/10.1016/j.bpobgyn.2014.07.008.
23. Nesbitt-Hawes EM, Won H, Jarvis SK, Lyons SD, Vancaillie TG, Abbott JA. Improvement in pelvic pain with botulinum toxin type A – single vs. repeat injections. Toxicon. 2013;63:83–7. https://doi.org/10.1016/j.toxicon.2012.11.018.
24. Chey WD, Kurlander J, Eswaran S. Irritable bowel syndrome: a clinical review. JAMA. 2015;313(9):949–58. https://doi.org/10.1001/jama.2015.0954.
25. Saha L. Irritable bowel syndrome: pathogenesis, diagnosis, treatment, and evidence-based medicine. World J Gastroenterol. 2014;20(22):6759–73. https://doi.org/10.3748/wjg.v20.i22.6759.
26. Vork L, Weerts ZZRM, Mujagic Z, et al. Rome III vs Rome IV criteria for irritable bowel syndrome: a comparison of clinical characteristics in a large cohort study. Neurogastroenterol Motil. 2018;30(2):e13189. https://doi.org/10.1111/nmo.13189.
27. Yang J, Deng Y, Chu H, et al. Prevalence and presentation of lactose intolerance and effects on dairy product intake in healthy subjects and patients with irritable bowel syndrome. Clin Gastroenterol Hepatol. 2013;11(3):262–268.e1. https://doi.org/10.1016/j.cgh.2012.11.034.
28. Zhang Y, Li L, Guo C, et al. Effects of probiotic type, dose and treatment duration on irritable bowel syndrome diagnosed by Rome III criteria: a meta-analysis. BMC Gastroenterol. 2016;16(1):62. https://doi.org/10.1186/s12876-016-0470-z.
29. Vazquez–Roque MI, Camilleri M, Smyrk T, et al. A controlled trial of gluten-free diet in patients with irritable bowel syndrome-diarrhea: effects on bowel frequency and intestinal function. Gastroenterology. 2013;144(5):903–911.e3. https://doi.org/10.1053/j.gastro.2013.01.049.
30. Camilleri M. Peripheral mechanisms in irritable bowel syndrome. N Engl J Med. 2012;367(17):1626–35. https://doi.org/10.1056/NEJMra1207068.

Part II

Endometriosis: Across the Lifespan

In Utero and Early-Life

11

Marwan Habiba and Giuseppe Benagiano

Contents

11.1 Brief Historical Background

In Chaps. 1 and 25 of this volume, we provided a history of the evolution of the modern understanding of endometriosis and adenomyosis. We indicated that available literature shows that the majority of work and of cases managed in early clinical practice were encountered in reproductive age women. This is not surprising as ectopic endometrial foci are responsive to estrogens and progestogens. The theory of retrograde menstruation is widely celebrated as the best-fitting hypothesis for endometriosis; it entails that regurgitated endometrial or endosalpingeal epithelium

M. Habiba (✉)
Department of Health Sciences, University of Leicester and University Hospitals of Leicester, Leicester, UK
e-mail: mah6@Leicester.ac.uk

G. Benagiano
Department of Maternal and Child Health, Gynaecology and Urology, Sapienza University of Rome, Rome, Italy

E. Oral (ed.), *Endometriosis and Adenomyosis*,
https://doi.org/10.1007/978-3-030-97236-3_11

that flows through the fallopian tubes and onto the surface of the peritoneum triggers the development of ectopic epithelial implants. Acceptance of this theory of causation reinforces the notion that endometriosis is a disease of reproductive age women. Despite being widely accepted, retrograde menstruation does not explain all the features of the endometriosis, its occurrence at distant sites, or the presence of lesions in the absence of menstrual cycles. Brosens et al. [1] pointed to the significance of the study of endometriosis in nonreproductive-age women. This is an important area of research, but our knowledge remains fragmentary and hindered because of the infrequent need for pelvic surgery in children or prepubertal girls and because of the known limitations of noninvasive testing. However, the few cases encountered in the fetus and in the premenarche can provide valuable insight into the pathophysiology of endometriosis.

Prior to the distinction being drawn between endometriosis and adenomyosis, Von Recklinghausen advocated that adenomyosis originates from congenital remnants of the Wolffian duct [2]. Others have theorized a link to Müllerian remnants [3]. Batt and Yeh [4] proposed the theory of the existence of a new variant they named "Müllerianosis". They argued that – distinct from the more common acquired type – some endometriotic lesions develop from embryonic epithelial rests. According to this hypothesis, those lesions may contain endometrial, endosalpingeal, and endocervical tissue, singly or in combination. Instances include lesions found outside the pelvis and genital tract, or in peritoneal "defects" or pockets. The embryonic origin theory projects the root cause of endometriosis to events early in fetal life. Although rare, the finding of aberrant endometrial tissue in fetal or prepubertal girls can have an important impact on our understanding of disease pathogenesis. There are limited reports of cases of what may be considered adenomyosis or endometriosis in fetuses and children [5–7]. Baldi at al [8]. provided additional information pointing to the possible existence of endometriotic foci in human fetuses.

11.2 The Possible Fetal Origin of Ectopic Endometrium

Information on the development of ectopic endometrial foci during fetal life may be deduced from the embryogenesis of the reproductive tract. In 1759, Caspar Wolff described an embryonic structure within the *urogenital ridge*, which he named *mesonephros* (named after him as the *Wolffian body*) [9]. The *mesonephric duct* (*Wolffian duct*) stems from the mesonephros and runs caudad to join the cloaca, situated at the terminal end of the lower embryonic intestine (the hindgut). The first description of the early formation of the female internal genital organs was made by Johannes Müller [10] in 1830. He described two ducts, coined *paramesonephric ducts* (named after him the *Müllerian ducts*). These could be found running lateral to the mesonephric ducts, extending caudally and then crossing medially to terminate at a small tubercle in the primitive urogenital sinus. Within this context, a fist detailed description of the fetal endometrium was presented in 1934 by Spivack [11].

Müllerian duct epithelial cells develop adjacent to the rostral mesonephric epithelium, as antero-lateral invaginations of the coelomic epithelium from the intermediate mesoderm. The Müllerian duct opens into the coelomic cavity with a funnel-like structure that will give rise to the fimbrial end of the Fallopian tube. The Müllerian duct lining develops into the endosalpinx and the endometrium. It is possible that fragments of the Müllerian duct epithelium become displaced to adjacent sites, giving rise to ectopic foci.

During the early development stages, the uterine lumen is lined by a single layer of epithelium devoid of glands. Glands begin to appear when the fetus reaches approximately 550 grams in weight. Initially, the glands are straight, short, and simple. Robboy et al. [12] described elongated and branched glands in the uterus and cervix by 18 weeks. Barberini et al. [13] reported that between 12 and 18 weeks' gestation, the endocervix is lined by a simple columnar epithelial cell layer with short microvilli and simple primary cilia. The definitive histological features of the endometrium begin to take shape near term with invaginations or primordial glands [14]. However, elongated and branched uterine and cervical glands were noted within the stroma as early as 20 weeks' gestation [12]. Structural differentiation and the formation of a uterine cavity and its lining are complete by month 7 [15]. Basal vacuoles and stromal edema appear during month 8, and apocrine secretion, glandular glycogen, and predecidualization occur during the last month of pregnancy. Between 18 and 20 weeks, the epithelium at the utero-tubal junction exhibits tall polyhedral cells, with microvilli and fewer ciliated cells [16]. An important observation when exploring the presence of ectopic endometrium in human fetus is that the endometrium is only partly responsive to hormone action [17]. At months 7–8, there is an increase in gland number, and the epithelium becomes pseudostratified due to proliferation and comprises only two to three rows of cell nuclei. Pseudostratification, however, can appear as early as 16–20 weeks and is suggestive of an estrogenic response [18].

11.2.1 Endometrial Glands Development

Uterine gland development or adenogenesis is critical for endometrial function. Assuming that gland genesis occurs in humans in a similar way to that in experimental animals, formation begins with an invagination of the luminal epithelium and is inhibited by progestogens acting on epithelial progesterone receptors (PR) [19–21]. Nevertheless, the exact mechanisms in the human and the relation to PR remain unknown. Several relevant factors have been identified including FOXA2, a glandular epithelium-specific transcription factor found in humans and all studied animals [21], and the "Indian hedgehog" signaling pathway (regulated by the Ihh gene) [22]. Endometrial glandular development is completed after birth. Glands are definitely less developed in infancy compared to the adult [23]. Interestingly, some degree of glandular development occurs in infancy in spite of the lack of circulating steroid hormones. By 6 years of age, glands extend from one-third to one-half of the distance from the myometrium and continue to increase in depth until puberty [23].

A unique characteristic of neonatal endometrium is the possibility of shedding soon after birth. Neonatal uterine bleeding (NUB), which suggests endometrial maturation, was first documented in the early nineteenth century [24]. Many early reports followed [25, 26]. The observation that NUB occurs in only a minority of neonates points to an intrinsic, ontogenetic resistance to the action of progesterone [27]. The phenomenon of uterine bleeding in neonates is far from being universal, which contrasts with the universal postnatal sharp drop of circulating progesterone. In fact, visible vaginal bleeding is observed in 3–5% of neonates, but occult bleeding is far more common and in one study was found to be as high as 61.3% [28]. Neonatal uterine bleeding occurs through degeneration and regression and is distinct from the adult menstrual loss.

Full endometrial maturation may not be complete till after menarche, and it is possible that progesterone resistance persists beyond the early neonatal period [29, 30]. Spivack [11] observed follicle development, including cyst formation, in the majority of premature and term neonatal ovaries, but developed endometrial glands were present only in a minority of cases. Ober and Bernstein [17] also noted the lack of correlation between ovarian and endometrial features. In the majority of cases, the neonatal endometrium is in a "resting phase" (i.e., inactive or proliferative) and appears thin and lined by one layer of cuboidal or columnar surface epithelium; the glands are simple and embedded in compact or loose stroma. The poor progestogenic response occurs despite the high circulating progesterone levels near term [31], indicating that the fetal endometrium possesses an intrinsic (coined "ontogenetic") progesterone resistance [32]. An interesting, but unexplained, phenomenon is the occurrence of isolated prepubertal menstruation [33], characterized by the occurrence of vaginal bleeding in prepubertal girls with no other signs of sexual development and no detectable abnormality. Pinto and Garden [34] reported four cases with no endometrial echo on ultrasound. This casts doubt on increased endometrial thickness as a cause and the possibility that the underlying mechanism resides in increased sensitivity to estrogen. The onset of uterine growth precedes the onset of puberty and continues after menarche well into the second decade [35]. Brosens et al. [30] stressed that uterine biological immaturity, possibly compounded by sociodemographic factors, accounts for the increased incidence of obstetrical disorders in very young mothers. Around menarche, the uterine response to steroid hormones may be uncoupled from ovulatory maturation of the hypothalamic-pituitary-ovarian axis. The origin of the endometrium from the proliferation and invagination of the coelomic epithelium points to the shared origin with the pelvic peritoneum and a possible route for the development of early ectopic pelvic endometriosis through coelomic metaplasia.

11.3 Development of Ectopic Endometrial Foci During Fetal Life

Meyer [36] concluded that a mucosal invasion of the myometrium was seldom visible. Emge [37] referred to the report by Meyer in 1897 [5] of the identification of a mucosal invasion in a fetus at term and to the reports by Albrecht, Erbslöh,

Holden, Javert, and Philipp of the existence of ectopic foci of endometrium in autopsies of children between 4 and 14 years of age. Emge [37] believed that these reports supported the existence of a type of congenital adenomyosis present prior to cyclic ovarian activities. He also cited cases of persistent primary dysmenorrhea that were later found to have adenomyosis and advocated "further search of the evidence in premenarchial uteri obtainable at autopsies." Congenital endometriosis also remains a possibility. Holden reported a case of adenomyosis in a 14-year old who had severe dysmenorrhea starting 6 months after menarche. But the extensive work by Meyer which was detailed in his monogram dated 1899 [38] describes ectopic mucosa within fetal and neonatal uteri in the context of regressing rudimentary developmental structures. Meyer examined 100 specimens and identified remnants of Gartner Duct in 12 out of 12 cases (100%) at months 2–3, in 6 out of 21 cases (28.5%) at months 4–6 and in 11 cases (out of 12 cases at months 7–8 and 55 newborns, 16.4%) and in 3 out of 18 children up to 7 years (16.6%). He viewed this as evidence of the universal presence of Gartner duct tissue during early embryology. He regarded residual remnant tissue as incapable of progressing to future disease.

Signorile et al. [7] reported the identification of ectopic endometrial tissue in 4 out of 36 cases autopsied in an investigation of female human fetuses of various gestational age (16, 18, 24, and 25 weeks). Endometrial tissue was identified using CA125 together with positivity for estrogen-receptor antibodies. Sporadic ectopic staining was identified in the rectovaginal septum, in proximity to the pouch of Douglas, close to the posterior wall of the uterus, in the rectal tube and in the wall of the uterus. Although neither CA125 nor estrogen receptor is a specific marker of endometrium, Batt and Yeh [4] took this as supportive evidence for the occurrence of congenital endometriosis. Molecular events during a critical window of embryogenesis could result in aberrant development of the female genital system [8]. The high incidence of endometriosis in the presence of uterine anomalies renders the identification of any such factors, and whether they may be relevant to any particular phenotype, a priority area. Bouquet De Jolinière et al. [39] reported on the identification of ectopic foci of glandular structures surrounded by densely distributed stromal cells in their study of seven fetal autopsies between 18 and 36 weeks' gestation. Using serial sections of the uterine myometrium, two fetuses with gestational ages of 25 weeks and of 36 weeks had ectopic bodies within the myometrium, and six cases were identified with embryonic tubular ducts in the broad ligament, the ovarian ligament, and under the fallopian tube serosa. They hypothesized that aberrant migration of Müllerian ducts could cause spread of embryonic cells, which could result in the growth of ectopic foci. Aberrant Müllerian structures were described by Lauchlan [40] in terms of a "giant shadow" cast by the primary Müllerian system and derived from the peritoneum or the coelom, characterized by the lack of organization. The identification of developmental remnants is perhaps unsurprising, but their relevance to endometriosis remains speculative. Schuster and Mackeen [41] reported an unusual case of a fetus with a 7.0 × 4.5 cm pelvic mass identified using antenatal ultrasound. The mass, which was removed on day 2 of postnatal life was a hemorrhagic ovarian cyst with focal endometriosis.

11.4 Perimenarcheal Endometriosis

The most widely recognized theory of the origins of endometriosis is that by Sampson. It was developed in the 1920s based on the assumption that retrograde menstrual effluent contains viable cells from the superficial endometrium capable of implantation. More recent research has demonstrated that menstrual blood contains a mixture of endometrial mesenchymal stem cells (eMSCs) and stromal fibroblasts. In addition, epithelial and epithelial progenitor cells (eEPs) may be present [42, 43]. eMSCs isolated from ectopic lesions show greater invasiveness and capacity to stimulate neoangiogenesis, compared to those in eutopic endometrium [44]. These cells presumably first attach and then breach the peritoneum [45]. The same situation may occur at birth in neonates experiencing the phenomenon known as neonatal uterine bleeding (NUB) [46, 47]. This mechanism could therefore explain cases of premenarcheal or early postmenarcheal endometriosis.

Evidence of what may be considered the initial stages of endometriosis formation in female infants has been provided by Arcellana et al. [48]. The neonate had McKusick-Kaufman syndrome and died approximately 8 hours after birth. At autopsy, an intact transverse vaginal septum, with hydrocolpos containing 200 mL of cloudy fluid, was observed. Examination of the peritoneal cavity revealed hemorrhagic endometrial reflux and implantation of epithelial fragments on the bowel serosa, as well as adhesions around the ovaries and the upper portion of the uterus. These findings are consistent with the model of implantation of premenarcheal endometriosis.

The presence of endometriosis has been observed, although rarely, in normal young girls before menarche. This needs to be distinguished from disease associated with congenital obstructive anomalies of the lower genital tract that appears after menarche or in the presence of cryptomenorrhea. A classic form of endometriosis was documented in five premenarcheal girls aged between 8.5 and 13 years and with Tanner stage I-III breast development [49]. All these girls experienced chronic pelvic pain for >6 months. Endometriosis was diagnosed on laparoscopy, and all had lesions that were typical of peritoneal endometriosis. However, histologically the lesions comprised stromal tissue, vascular proliferation, hemosiderin deposits, and/or adhesions but no glandular tissue. Two cases required a second look laparoscopy some years later, and at this point, repeat biopsy confirmed the presence of endometrial glands. Similar cases have also been described in literature including a case of peritoneal endometriosis in a 9-year-old [50] and one with a large ovarian endometrioma in an 11-year-old premenarcheal girl [51].

When discussing perimenarcheal endometriosis, special attention should be paid to the presence of congenital obstructive anomalies of the reproductive tract, particularly those defined by the presence of a uterus didelphis with an obstructed hemivagina and ipsilateral renal agenesis or dysplasia. This condition, coined Herlyn-Werner-Wünderlich syndrome (HWWS), seems to be specifically associated to a variant of endometriosis. Tong et al. [52] described a series of 94 young girls affected by HWWS in whom endometriosis was diagnosed at laparoscopy or laparotomy in 19% of cases. All had cystic ovarian endometriosis. The median time between menarche and the onset of cyclic pelvic pain was 1 year (range 0–16 years), while the median time between menarche and the diagnosis of pelvic endometriosis was 3 years (range 1–16 years). The early presence of endometriosis in these girls supports the hypothesis that it is caused by retrograde shedding of eMSCs.

Overall, the reported incidence of endometriosis in teenagers with genital tract anomalies varies between 11% and 40% [53]. The incidence appears to be greater in anomalies associated with genital tract outflow obstruction [54, 55]. Of interest is the observation that treating the anomaly by correcting the outflow obstruction may be curative [56].

Traditionally, endometriosis was believed to be rare in adolescence, but increased awareness has helped to achieve earlier diagnosis. However, similar to the case in the adult, estimates of the prevalence of endometriosis vary widely, ranging from 19% to 73%. The high incidence in adolescent girls is supported by the observation that a large proportion of reproductive age women with endometriosis can trace their symptoms to early postmenarche.

The different appearance of peritoneal endometriosis is classified as early-active (red, glandular, or vesicular), advanced (black, puckered), and healed (white, fibrotic) implants [28, 57, 58]. In adolescence, there is a higher prevalence of active peritoneal lesions characterized by intense angiogenesis. There is also evidence that some lesions may be transient [59–61] and that it may more easily recur [62].

Thus, more research is needed to assess the significance of these lesions and their contribution to our understanding of disease etiology. The potential role of antecedents of endometriosis and whether these could be activated by factors such as the vascular endothelial growth factor, maternal steroids, or prepubertal estrogen are areas that warrant future research. The effect of Anti-Müllerian hormone and its receptors in relation to the suppression of endometrium is also an area that warrants further research. There is still considerable uncertainty about whether mechanisms such as coelomic metaplasia, embryonic Müllerian rests, or persistence of other forms of embryonic endometriosis are relevant to this variant of the disease. Mesenchymal stem cells may be the principal source of endometriosis outside the peritoneal cavity, and it is possible that they play a role also in the pathophysiology of premenarcheal and adolescent endometriosis. Progenitor cells may originate and implant into the peritoneum as a consequence of retrograde neonatal uterine bleeding.

References

1. Brosens I, Puttemans P, Benagiano G. Endometriosis: a life cycle approach? Am J Obstet Gynecol. 2013;209:307–16.
2. von Recklinghausen F. Die Adenomyomata und Cystadenomata der Uterus und Tubenwandung: Ihre Abkunft von Resten des Wolffischen Körpers [*The adenomyomas and cystadenomas of the uterus and tube wall: their origin from remnants of the Wolffian body*]. Berlin: August Hirschwald Verlag; 1896.
3. Kossman R. Die Abstammung der Drüseneinschlüsse in der Uterus und der Tuben [*The lineage of the glandular inclusions in the uterus and tubes*]. Arch Gynakol. 1897;54:359–81.
4. Batt RE, Yeh J. Müllerianosis: four developmental (embryonic) mullerian diseases. Reprod Sci. 2013;20:1030–7.

5. Meyer R. Ueber die genese der cystadenome und adenomyome des uterus, mit demonstrationene. Ztschr Geburtsh Gynäkol. 1897;37:327–35.
6. Holden FC. Adenomyoma of the uterus. Am J Obstet Gynecol. 1931;22:801.
7. Signorile PG, Baldi F, Bussani R, D'Armiento M, De Falco M, Baldi A. Ectopic endometrium in human foetuses is a common event and sustains the theory of müllerianosis in the pathogenesis of endometriosis, a disease that predisposes to cancer. J Exp Clin Cancer Res. 2009;28:49–53.
8. Baldi A, Signorile PG. New evidence in endometriosis. Int J Cell Biol Biochem. 2015;60:19–22.
9. Wolff CF. Theoria generationis [*The theory of embryology*]. Litteris Hendelianis: Halae ad Salam; 1759.
10. Müller J. Bildungsgeschichte der genitalien aus anatomischen untersuchungen an embryonen des menschen und der thiere [*History of genital development from anatomical investigations on embryos of man and animals*]. Düsseldorf: bei Arnz. 1830;
11. Spivack M. Polycystic ovaries in the newborn and early infancy and their relation to the structure of the endometrium. Am J Obstet Gynecol. 1934;27:157–73.
12. Robboy SJ, Kurita T, Baskin L, Cunha GR. New insights into human female reproductive tract development. Differentiation. 2017;97:9–22.
13. Barberini F, Makabe S, Motta PM. A three-dimensional study of human fetal endocervix with special reference to its epithelium. Histol Histopathol. 1998;13:635–45.
14. Valdés-Dapena MA. Histology of the fetus and newborn. In: Uterus and vagina. Philadelphia, London, Toronto: W.B. Saunders Company; 1979. p. 479–500.
15. Rosa P. Endocrinologie sexuelle du fœtus féminin [Sexual endocrinology of the female fetus], vol. 1. Paris, France: Paris: Masson et Cie; 1955. p. 262–72.
16. Benagiano G, Brosens I, Habiba M. Adenomyosis: a life-cycle approach. Reprod Biomed Online. 2015;30:220–32.
17. Ober WB, Bernstein J. Observations on the endometrium and ovary in the newborn. Pediatrics. 1955;16:445–60.
18. Wang T. Human fetal endometrium – light and electron microscopic study. Arch Gynecol Obstet. 1989;246:169–79.
19. Bartol FF, Wiley AA, Goodlett DR. Ovine uterine morphogenesis: histochemical aspects of endometrial development in the fetus and neonate. J Anim Sci. 1988;66:1303–13.
20. Stewart CA, Wang Y, Bonilla-Claudio M, Martin JF, Gonzalez G, Taketo MM, Behringer RR. CTNNB1 in mesenchyme regulates epithelial cell differentiation during Müllerian duct and postnatal uterine development. Mol Endocrinol. 2013;27:1442–54.
21. Kelleher AM, DeMayo FJ, Spencer TE. Uterine glands: developmental biology and functional roles in pregnancy. Endocr Rev. 2019;40:1424–45.
22. Franco HL, Rubel CA, Large MJ, Wetendorf M, Fernandez-Valdivia R, Jeong JW, Spencer TE, Behringer RR, Lydon JP, DeMayo FJ. Epithelial progesterone receptor exhibits pleiotropic roles in uterine development and function. FASEB J. 2012;26:1218–27.
23. Gray CA, Bartol FF, Tarleton BJ, Wiley AA, Johnson GA, Bazer FW, Spencer TA. Developmental biology of uterine glands. Biol Reprod. 2001;65:1311–23.
24. Carus CG. IV. Blut abgang aus den geburts heilen einen neugebornen kindes. [*IV Vaginal bleedingin a newborn child*]. Zeitschrift fürNatür und Heilkusw. 1822;2:106–7.
25. Cullingworth CJ. Haemorrhage from the genital organs in the recently born female child. Liverpool and Manchester. Med Surg Rep. 1876;4:48–57.
26. Halban J. Über Fetale Menstruation und ihre Bedeutung [On the fetal menstruation and its meaning] Proc Versammlung Deutscher Naturvorscher und Aertze in Breslau (VII.76). Berliner KlinWochenschr. 1904;48:1254–6.
27. Brosens I, Benagiano G. The endometrium from the neonate to the adolescent. J Matern Fetal Neonatal Med. 2016;29:1195–9.
28. Brosens I, Puttemans P, Benagiano G. Endometriosis: a life cycle approach? Am J Obstet Gynecol. 2013;209:307–16.
29. Zhang K, Pollack S, Ghods A, Dicken C, Isaac B, Adel G, Zeitlian G, Santoro N. Onset of ovulation after menarche in girls: a longitudinal study. J Clin Endocrinol Metab. 2008;93:1186–94.

30. Brosens I, Muter J, Gargett C, Puttemans P, Benagiano G, Brosens JJ. The impact of uterine immaturity on obstetrical syndromes during adolescence. Am J Obstet Gynecol. 2017;217:546–55.
31. Tulchinsky D, Okada DM. Hormones in human pregnancy. IV. Plasma progesterone. Am J Obstet Gynecol. 1975;121:293–9.
32. Brosens I, Ćurčić A, Vejnović T, Gargett CE, Brosens JJ, Benagiano G. The perinatal origins of major reproductive disorders in the adolescent: research avenues. Placenta. 2015b;36:341–4.
33. Heller ME, Dewhurst J, Grant DB. Premature menarche without other evidence of precocious puberty. Arch Dis Child. 1979;54:472–5.
34. Pinto SM, Garden AS. Prepubertal menarche: a defined clinical entity. Am J Obstet Gynecol. 2006;195:327–9.
35. Holm K, Laursen EM, Brocks V, Muller J. Pubertal maturation of the internal genitalia: an ultrasound evaluation of 166 healthy girls. Ultrasound Obstet Gynecol. 1995;6:175–81.
36. Meyer R. Über adenomatöse Schleimhautwucherungen in der Uterus – und Tubenwand und ihre pathologisch-anatomische Bedeutung [Article in german] On the the adenomatous mucosal growths in the uterus – and tubal wall and their pathological-anatomical features. Virchows Arch Pathol Anat Physiol Klin Med. 1903;172:394–409.
37. Emge LA. The elusive adenomyosis of the uterus. Am J Obstet Gynecol. 1962;83:1541–63.
38. Meyer R. Ueber epitheliale Gebilde im Myometrium des foetalen und kindlichen uterus einschliesslich des Gartner'schen Ganges. Berlin: Verlag von S. Karger; 1899.
39. Bouquet De Jolinière J, Ayoubi JM, Gianaroli L, Dubuisson JB, Gogusev J, Feki A. Endometriosis: a new cellular and molecular genetic approach for understanding the pathogenesis and evolutivity. Front Surg. 2014;1:16.
40. Lauchlan SC. The secondary Müllerian system. Obstet Gynecol Surv. 1972;27:133–46.
41. Schuster M, Mackeen DA. Fetal endometriosis: a case report. Fertil Steril. 2015;103:160–2.
42. Musina RA, Belyavski AV, Tarusova OV, Solovyova EV, Sukhikh GT. Endometrial mesenchymal stem cells isolated from the menstrual blood. Bull Exp Biol Med. 2008;145:539–43.
43. Gargett CE, Schwab KE, Deane JA. Endometrial stem/progenitor cells: the first 10 years. Hum Reprod Update. 2016;22:137–63.
44. Kao AP, Wang KH, Chang CC, et al. Comparative study of human eutopic and ectopic endometrial mesenchymal stem cells and the development of an in vivo endometriotic invasion model. Fertil Steril. 2011;95:1308–15.
45. Witz CA, Thomas MR, Montoya-Rodriguez IA, Nair AS, Centonze VE, Schenken RS. Short-term culture of peritoneum explants confirms attachment of endometrium to intact peritoneal mesothelium. Fertil Steril. 2001;75:385–90.
46. Brosens I, Brosens JJ, Benagiano G. Neonatal uterine bleeding as an antecedent of pelvic endometriosis. Hum Reprod. 2013;28:2893–7.
47. Gargett E, Schwab KE, Puttemans P, Brosens JJ, Benagiano G, Brosens I. Potential role of endometrial stem/progenitor cells in the pathogenesis of early-onset endometriosis. Mol Hum Reprod. 2014;20:591–8.
48. Arcellana RC, Robinson TW, Tyson RW, Joyce MR. McKusick-Kaufman syndrome with legal complications of hydrometrocolpos and congenital endometriosis. J Perinatol. 1996;16:220–3.
49. Marsh EE, Laufer MR. Endometriosis in premenarcheal girls who do not have an associated obstructive anomaly. Fertil Steril. 2005;83:758–60.
50. Ebert AD, Fuhr N, David M, Schneppel L, Papadopoulos T. Histological confirmation of endometriosis in a 9-year-old girl suffering from unexplained cyclic pelvic pain since her eighth year of life. Gynecol Obstet Investig. 2009;67:158–61.
51. Gogacz M, Sarzynski M, Napierała R, Sierocinska-Sawa J, Semczuk A. Ovarian endometrioma in an 11-year-old girl before menarche: a case study with literature review. J Pediatr Adolesc Gynecol. 2012;25:e5–7.
52. Tong J, Zhu L, Chen N, Lang J. Endometriosis in association with Herlyn-Werner-Wunderlich syndrome. Fertil Steril. 2014;102:790–4.
53. Dovey S, Sanfilippo J. Endometriosis and the adolescent. Clin Obstet Gynecol. 2010;53:420–8.

54. Olive DL, Henderson DY. Endometriosis and Müllerian anomalies. Obstet Gynecol. 1987;69:412–5.
55. Yang Y, Wang Y, Yang J, Wang S, Lang J. Adolescent endometriosis in China: a retrospective analysis of 63 cases. J Pediatr Adolesc Gynecol. 2012;25:295–9.
56. Sanfilippo JS, Wakim NG, Schikler KN, Yussman MA. Endometriosis in association with uterine anomaly. Am J Obstet Gynecol. 1986;154:39–43.
57. Vasquez G, Cornillie F, Brosens IA. Peritoneal endometriosis: scanning electron microscopy and histology of minimal pelvic endometriotic lesions. Fertil Steril. 1984;42:696–703.
58. Murphy AA, Green WR, Bobbie D. Unsuspected endometriosis documented by scanning electron microscopy in visually normal peritoneum. Fertil Steril. 1986;46:522–4.
59. Wiegerinck MA, Van Dop PA, Brosens IA. The staging of peritoneal endometriosis by the type of active lesion in addition to the revised American Fertility Society classification. Fertil Steril. 1993;60:461–4.
60. Stripling MC, Martin DC, Chatman DL, Van der Zwaag R, Poston WM. Subtle appearance of pelvic endometriosis. Fertil Steril. 1988;49:427–31.
61. Martin DC, Hubert GD, Van der Zwaag R, El-Zeky FA. Laparoscopic appearances of peritoneal endometriosis. Fertil Steril. 1989;51:63–7.
62. Kalu E, McAuley W, Richardson R. Teenagers, adolescents, endometriosis and recurrence: a retrospective analysis of recurrence following primary operative laparoscopy. Gynecol Surg. 2008;5:209–12.

Endometriosis in Adolescence

12

Jessica Y. Shim and Marc R. Laufer

Contents

J. Y. Shim (✉)
Division of Gynecology, Boston Children's Hospital, Boston, MA, USA
e-mail: Jessica.Shim@childrens.harvard.edu

M. R. Laufer
Division of Gynecology, Boston Children's Hospital, Boston, MA, USA

Center for Infertility and Reproductive Surgery, Brigham and Women's Hospital, Boston, MA, USA

Harvard Medical School, Boston, MA, USA

E. Oral (ed.), *Endometriosis and Adenomyosis*,
https://doi.org/10.1007/978-3-030-97236-3_12

12.1 Prevalence and Epidemiology

In 1948, Meigs reported the incidence of endometriosis in adolescents to be 6% [1]. Others have attempted to estimate the prevalence of endometriosis in adolescents, although these estimates vary depending on symptoms and the modality used for diagnosis. The prevalence of endometriosis in adolescents who present for investigation, however, appears to be high. The prevalence among adolescents undergoing laparoscopic investigation for pelvic pain not responsive to nonsteroidal anti-inflammatory drugs and oral contraceptive pills is 50–70% [2–4]. A 2013 systematic review by Janssen et al. [5] sought to review the prevalence of endometriosis diagnosed by laparoscopy in adolescents; based on 15 selected studies, they identified the overall prevalence of visually confirmed endometriosis was 62% in all adolescents undergoing laparoscopic investigation, 75% in girls with chronic pelvic pain resistant to treatment, and 70% in girls with dysmenorrhea. Although laparoscopy has been the gold standard for confirming endometriosis, other studies have included the use of imaging, such as magnetic resonance imaging (MRI) or ultrasound, to aid in the diagnosis or as an alternative to laparoscopy [6–8]. A 2020 systematic review by Hirsch et al. [9] included studies diagnosing endometriosis via both laparoscopy and imaging in adolescents, and the prevalence ranged from 25% to 100%, with a mean prevalence of 64%.

Prevalence estimates are unfortunately limited as some adolescents are asymptomatic or have atypical presentations leading to underdiagnosis. Delays in diagnosis from the onset of symptoms are common worldwide, ranging from 4 to 11 years [10–14]. In a registry of 4000 adult women with endometriosis, two-thirds of women responded to a survey and reported their first pelvic symptoms started before age 20, and 1 in 5 had pain before age 15 [15]. Symptomatic cases have been cited at earlier ages, including prior to menarche [16] and in others soon after menarche [17, 18]. The early manifestations of endometriosis suggest the origin of endometriosis is likely multifactorial and not simply after years of retrograde menstruation.

12.2 Risk Factors

Several predisposing factors make adolescents uniquely vulnerable to endometriosis. A family history of endometriosis may predispose young women to the disease, although the precise mechanism or mechanisms remain unclear. In a systematic genetic study of 234 cases of histologically confirmed endometriosis, endometriosis occurred at a 6.9% rate in first-degree relatives of women with the disease, compared to a 1% rate in relatives of controls [19]. Endometriosis that occurs in families tends to be more severe compared to sporadic cases, and a similar and earlier age of onset of symptoms occur in affected families [20, 21]. Due to the demonstration of familial clustering of endometriosis, the disease is considered by most investigators to be inherited in a polygenic or multifactorial mode [20].

Endometriosis has also been reported in up to 40% of adolescents with reproductive tract anomalies [22]. Obstructive anomalies that have been implicated include imperforate hymen, transverse vaginal septum, and vaginal agenesis [23, 24]. The presence of an obstructive anomaly supports the concept of retrograde flow as predisposing an adolescent to endometriosis. Although repair or relief of the obstruction has been associated with resolution of endometriosis [25], a case series demonstrated that endometriosis may not always resolve following repair of an obstructive anomaly [26]. This may be due to the obstruction seeding the peritoneal cavity or to other risk factors.

Increased exposure to menstruation and endogenous estrogen may predispose adolescents to acquiring endometriosis. Identified risk factors include earlier menarche (before age 11–13), nulliparity, shorter menstrual cycle intervals, and heavy menstrual bleeding [27–29]. In a laparoscopy cohort, women diagnosed with endometriosis were found to be a taller height and a leaner body habitus since adolescence [30]. Sociodemographic factors include ethnicity, with Caucasian/white and Asian women having higher reported rates of endometriosis in comparison to Hispanic and black women, although this underreporting may be contributed by implicit bias, potentially different presenting symptoms of endometriosis, and racial disparities in healthcare access [31, 32]. Childhood sexual and physical abuse are associated with an increased risk of endometriosis [33].

Modifiable and early life risk factors may also contribute to the development of endometriosis in adolescents. Prior studies have postulated lower birth weight, prematurity, and maternal diethylstilbestrol as increase risk factors for endometriosis; intense physical activity, passive smoke exposure, and skin sensitivity have also been raised as increased risk factors but remain understudied [34]. In an investigation of in utero and early life factors in relation to endometriosis, exposure to breastfeeding in early life was associated with lower odds of surgically diagnosed endometriosis and secondhand smoke during childhood was associated with greater odds of endometriosis in adolescents [35]. Exposures in adolescence may also further impact endometriosis risk into adulthood. Even dietary exposures seem to be implicated; in a longitudinal cohort study, lower rates of laparoscopically confirmed endometriosis were diagnosed among adult women who in adolescence consumed greater amounts of total dairy foods [36]. These findings support the need for further investigation of early life influences, and if early life interventions may reduce endometriosis burden in later life.

12.3 Pathophysiology

The pathophysiology of endometriosis remains controversial despite decades of research. The most recognized theory behind endometriosis is Sampson's theory [37] of retrograde menstruation, but it alone cannot explain the wide ranges of manifestations of endometriosis, including endometriosis in early adolescence. Retrograde menstruation is a common physiologic event in nearly all menstruating women with patent tubes, with or without endometriosis present [38]. Early-onset or adolescent endometriosis therefore appears to be distinct from adult endometriosis, or at least contributed by other mechanisms [39]. One of the theories behind adolescent endometriosis is the seeding of naive endometrial progenitor cells into the pelvic cavity at the time of neonatal uterine bleeding. Neonatal uterine bleeding is a less common phenomenon affecting only 5% of newborn girls, characterized by decidual transformation and endometrial shedding in the neonatal uterus [40, 41]. The implantation model via neonatal uterine bleeding was described in a case report by Arcellana et al. [42], of a demised female infant with McKusick-Kaufman syndrome. The infant's postmortem examination revealed an intact transverse vaginal septum, hemorrhagic endometrial reflux, and implantation of epithelial fragments on the bowel serosa and adhesions around the ovaries and upper uterus. It is postulated that the relatively longer neonatal cervix and thick cervical secretions may facilitate retrograde seeding of endometrial mesenchymal stem cells and stromal fibroblasts during the early neonatal period [38, 43]. Other theories on the origins of endometriosis include Halban's [44] theory on vascular or lymphatic spread of endometrial cells, Meyer's [45] theory of embryologically totipotent cells undergoing metaplastic transformation, innate or acquired properties of the endometrium, and defective immune clearance [46]. No unifying theory explains all cases of endometriosis, and challenging cases such as premenarcheal endometriosis supports alternative theories to Sampson's theory, such as coelomic metaplasia and Müllerian embryonic rests. [17]

As part of a pursuit to further characterize adolescent endometriosis, studies have attempted to describe its physiologic environment and distinguishing features. Increasing evidence has pointed to endometriosis being a pelvic inflammatory condition. A multicenter nested case-control study demonstrated significant differences in peritoneal fluid cytokines when comparing adolescents with endometriosis to adults with and without endometriosis [47]. A more pro-invasive cytokine profile was observed in adolescents compared to adults, despite greater use of hormones for treatment. Whether observed cytokine profiles are a source or a result of endometriosis remains to be definitively determined. But, these findings at least suggest adolescents with endometriosis have a unique inflammatory milieu that may contribute to greater and/or earlier symptomatology [47].

12.4 Clinical Presentation

Endometriosis is the leading cause of secondary dysmenorrhea in adolescents, and it is also the most common finding in young women undergoing laparoscopy for chronic pelvic pain [48]. Unlike adults, endometriosis is less likely to present as the classic symptom of dysmenorrhea, or as infertility or endometriomas. In a retrospective study by Laufer et al. [2], the classic symptom of cyclic pain was present by itself in 9.4% of adolescent subjects, whereas 28.1% of subjects had acyclic pain alone, and 62.5% had both cyclic and acyclic pain. Therefore, the majority (90.6%) of adolescents with endometriosis experienced acyclic pain. In a 2018 prospective study by DiVasta et al. [49], general acyclic pain was common for adolescents (66%) and lasted for days at a time (40%). Most participants also experienced moderate-severe menstrual pain, commonly starting at menarche.

Inquiring about general pelvic pain is crucial as it is the predominant symptom in premenarcheal endometriosis. A small case series by Marsh and Laufer [17] identified five premenarcheal girls with chronic pelvic pain who had been evaluated with a standard medical and gastrointestinal evaluation without definitive findings for an etiology for their pain. All five subjects were laparoscopically confirmed to have stage I endometriosis based on the standard American Society for Reproductive Medicine Classification of Endometriosis [50], and none of them had an obstructive anomaly of the reproductive tract. Thus, premenarcheal girls and postmenarcheal adolescents should be asked about their pelvic pain symptoms, even in the absence of menstruation. A pain diary may be helpful for the patient and/or caregiver in documenting the frequency and character of pain.

Another manifestation of pelvic pain commonly reported by women with endometriosis is dyspareunia. Adolescents and young adults with endometriosis experience dyspareunia twice as often as their peers without endometriosis; the burden of dyspareunia has an additive negative impact on physical health and mental health [51]. A thorough review of systems in adolescents with endometriosis may reveal multiple pain symptoms including non-gynecologic sources. In a case series of 25 female individuals (mean age, 17.2 years) with laparoscopically confirmed endometriosis, 52% of patients reported at least 1 genitourinary symptom, and 56% reported at least 1 gastrointestinal symptom [52]. Genitourinary symptoms reported were bladder pain, flank pain, back pain, dysuria, urinary frequency and urgency, incontinence, hematuria, and nocturia; gastrointestinal symptoms included nausea, constipation, diarrhea, and hematochezia. More adolescents with endometriosis than adults report nausea accompanying their general pelvic pain, and they experience general pelvic pain relief after a bowel movement [49]. The presence of urinary or gastrointestinal symptoms may in part be secondary to overlap with functional pain syndromes such as interstitial cystitis and irritable bowel syndrome (IBS) [53, 54]. A large prospectively enrolled cohort study showed that the odds of IBS was five-fold higher among adolescents with endometriosis than without, and the presence of acyclic pelvic pain was a strong predictor of the likelihood of IBS [55]. Another commonly reported pain disorder among adolescents with endometriosis is migraines. A cross-sectional study found a higher prevalence of migraines among adolescents with endometriosis compared to those without endometriosis [56]. The study also demonstrated a linear relationship between migraine pain severity and the odds of endometriosis, suggesting heightened pain sensitivity for adolescents with endometriosis.

Interestingly, there is a higher self-reported rate of autoimmune diagnoses in women with endometriosis compared to the general female population. Thus, adolescents may exhibit non-pain symptoms and should be screening by their provider for other comorbidities so as to receive comprehensive healthcare [57]. A 2019 systematic review and meta-analysis suggested an increased risk of autoimmune diseases including systemic lupus erythematosus, Sjögren's syndrome, rheumatoid arthritis, autoimmune thyroid disorder, celiac disease, multiple sclerosis, inflammatory bowel disease, and Addison disease [58]. However, only a few studies were of high quality and well-designed. It is unclear whether endometriosis is a risk factor or a consequence of autoimmune disease, but this adds evidence to the chronic and inflammatory nature of endometriosis.

Adolescents with endometriosis commonly report their symptoms as interfering with their functionality and quality of life. There is a high prevalence of pelvic pain that negatively impacts work, school, daily activities, exercise, and sleep to a moderate-extreme degree [49]. In a study of 250 adolescents with dysmenorrhea and symptoms suspicious for endometriosis, 12% of those age 14–20 years lost days of school or work each month due to pain [59]. A population-based study by Gallagher et al. [60] provided evidence that adolescents and young adults with endometriosis experience deficits in physical health-related and mental health-related quality of life. In addition to pain, participants had difficulty completing daily activities (e.g., "climbing several flights of stairs," "bathing or dressing yourself") and trouble engaging in social activities with family, friends, and groups. Unfortunately, diagnostic delay is common, despite the significant impact on quality of life. In the study by Gallagher et al. [60], the mean age at surgical diagnosis was 16.3 years (SD = 2.5), representing an average diagnostic delay of 2.8 years from onset of first symptoms.

Diagnostic delay is contributed by multiple factors. Firstly, many healthcare providers, including pediatricians, gynecologists, and family medicine practitioners, may not be aware of the many symptoms of endometriosis in adolescents. In addition, many women perceive their symptoms as an extreme of normality and consider themselves to be "unlucky" rather than ill. Women may not come forward with their pain symptoms partly due to embarrassment and in order to avoid stigmatization [61]. Lastly, knowledge of endometriosis is low among adolescents and those around them, including their family members and school personnel [62]. In a cross-sectional study by Zannoni et al. [59], 82% of 250 adolescents had never heard about endometriosis, and 80% expressed interest in learning more about it; these underscore the need for research on measures to create a supportive and informed social climate.

12.5 Evaluation

Evaluation of the adolescent patient first begins with a comprehensive history and review of systems. If the initial description of pain is vague or limited, a pain diary should be considered. The use of diaries recording pain, mood, menses, diet, medication, and other non-gynecologic symptoms can help discern the pattern of pain [63]. Since keeping a physical journal at all times may not be feasible, adolescents may find it easier to utilize pain diary and symptom tracker mobile applications. After the history, a physical examination should be performed. A physical exam is unlikely to reveal endometriosis but is helpful for assessing for other gynecologic sources of pain, such as a pelvic mass or a reproductive anomaly, or non-gynecologic etiologies of pain; these may include gastrointestinal, urinary, or musculoskeletal etiologies. Evaluation of the skin may reveal erythema ab igne, or "hot water bottle rash." Erythema ab igne presents as a reticulated hyperpigmented erythematous eruption at sites of prolonged heat exposure, and it is commonly seen in those who use of heat for relief of pain from chronic diseases such as Crohn's disease [64, 65]. An abdominal exam should be performed to locate any tenderness and palpable hernia or masses. A musculoskeletal exam can assess for abdominal wall tenderness (e.g., Carnett's sign), range of motion of the hips and spine, symptoms with pelvic compression, and bone tenderness [57].

A pelvic exam is not always necessary, particularly as adolescents are less likely to have uterosacral nodularity or distorted anatomy from advanced or deep infiltrating disease. If a pelvic examination is offered, this should be approached with sensitivity and with the goals of minimizing discomfort and anxiety [66]. The adolescent should be given the choice of having a parent or caregiver as a chaperone during the examination. If the patient consents and is sexually active, the smallest size speculum should be utilized, typically a pediatric speculum. A single digital exam or a Q-Tip (cotton swab) can be inserted into the vagina to assess for vaginal length and patency and exclude a reproductive tract anomaly. A rectal-abdominal examination may also be better tolerated than a vaginal-abdominal examination, particularly in the patient who has never been sexually active.

12.6 Laboratory/Imaging Studies

There is currently no specific blood test or biomarker that has been validated as a noninvasive diagnostic test for endometriosis. Many attempts have been made to identify and validate specific biomarkers, such as Cancer Antigen 125 (CA125) [67]. A recent evaluation of CA125 by Sasamoto et al. [68] demonstrated that average CA125 values were low in adolescents and young women with or without endometriosis, and CA125 did not correlate with pain type, severity, or frequency. Laboratory studies may include a complete blood count or an erythrocyte sedimentation rate to assess for an inflammatory or infectious process resulting in pain. A pregnancy test or sexually transmitted infection testing should be considered in the sexually active patient. Urinalysis or urine culture are helpful in excluding urinary causes of pain.

Adolescents with dysmenorrhea do not routinely need to be imaged, as most adolescents experience primary dysmenorrhea, or painful menstruation in the absence of pelvic pathology [48]. However, imaging may be helpful in patients who either present initially with symptoms suggesting secondary dysmenorrhea or they fail empiric treatment for primary dysmenorrhea and require further evaluation. Ultrasound imaging can exclude the presence of an ovarian cyst, tumor, adnexal torsion, or a reproductive tract anomaly. A pelvic ultrasound can be performed trans-abdominally instead of trans-vaginally to minimize discomfort. Alternatively, trans-rectal imaging may also be performed. In a retrospective observational study by Martire et al. [69], 270 women aged 12–26 years underwent trans-vaginal ultrasound if sexually active, and trans-rectal in never sexually active adolescents. At least one finding of endometriosis was identified in 36 (13.3%) of 270 cases; ovarian endometriomas were found in 22 (11%) patients, adenomyosis in 16 (5.2%), and deep infiltrating endometriosis in 10 (3.7%). In patients with dysmenorrhea, the detection rate of pelvic endometriosis with ultrasound increased to 20%. If the ultrasound or physical examination is concerning for an anomaly, magnetic resonance imaging should be ordered because of its high accuracy in detecting and accurately characterizing Müllerian duct anomalies [70].

12.7 Trial of Medical Therapy

A trial of medical therapy is reasonable after a thorough evaluation excludes non-gynecologic causes of pain and suggests a non-acute gynecologic source, such as primary dysmenorrhea or endometriosis. First-line treatment options include non-steroidal anti-inflammatory agents (NSAIDs), combined hormonal contraceptives, and progestin-only therapies. NSAIDs interrupt cyclooxygenase-mediated prostaglandin production and are significantly better than placebo in providing pain relief from primary dysmenorrhea, although there is no individual NSAID that is demonstrated to be superior [71]. Patient education of NSAIDs is critical, as adolescents often report little or no improvement with NSAIDs. As self-directed use of NSAIDs by adolescents is high, they have likely used subtherapeutic treatment with incorrect interval dosage and timing [48]. Providers should therefore instruct adolescents on the proper interval dosage and advise starting NSAIDs 1–2 days before menstruation and through the first 2–3 days of bleeding [72]. As each method has benefits and potential adverse effects, the decision to use one method should be patient-driven so as to improve adherence.

Hormonal therapies include combined hormonal contraception (pill, patch, ring), or progestin-only therapies (oral, injectable, or implantable). Hormonal methods prevent endometrial proliferation or ovulation, or both, and thus help to decrease prostaglandin and leukotriene production [72]. The choice of medication should be individualized and tailored to the patient, as the patient may have a prior treatment history, specific desires, or certain unacceptable adverse effects. A shared decision-making approach to hormonal contraception will improve adherence to the treatment. Combination estrogen-progestin oral contraceptive pills or progestin-only pills are most commonly prescribed as they are easily initiated and short-acting; however, there is no data suggesting one formulation is better than another for the management of dysmenorrhea. A continuous regimen may provide more rapid pain reduction than cyclic use of oral contraceptive pills, but both provide similar long-term success for managing primary dysmenorrhea [73]. Continuous regimen users should be cautioned about potential unscheduled bleeding or spotting, which generally decreases over longer treatment use.

Empiric gonadotropin-releasing (GnRH) agonists or antagonists are often considered in adult women with chronic pelvic pain and clinically suspected endometriosis. Empiric GnRH agonists for adolescents 18 years of age or younger should be avoided because of the potential adverse long-term effects on bone mineral density [74]. Patients and their parents may additionally feel uncomfortable with the potential side effects and risks of empiric GnRH agonist therapy without a definitive diagnosis. The American College of Obstetricians and Gynecologists does not endorse the use of empiric GnRH agonist therapy for treatment of adolescents with suspected primary dysmenorrhea but suggest it as an option for patients with diagnosed endometriosis and pain refractory to conservative surgical therapy and hormonal therapy [48].

A trial of 6 months of medical therapy is often conducted in adults with pelvic pain; however, this may not be practical for adolescents. Symptoms may cause significant impact an adolescent's quality of life and limit their social activities and learning. Therefore, if a patient does not experience clinical improvement with empiric treatment, treatment adherence should be assessed and a definitive diagnosis can be pursued after 3 months. The American College of Obstetricians and Gynecologists recommends the use of laparoscopy for diagnosis of endometriosis in adolescents [48]. A clinical diagnosis of endometriosis, however, can also be considered if the evaluation of symptoms, patient history, physical examination, and/or imaging raise suspicion. There has been a movement to increase the use of clinical diagnosis and treat endometriosis-associated pain without the need for a surgical diagnosis, to help remedy diagnostic delay and promote earlier intervention. A 2019 call to action by Agarwal et al. [14] proposes moving endometriosis from a histological to a clinical definition, and emphasizes the chronic, inflammatory, and progressive nature of endometriosis.

12.8 Diagnostic Surgery

Laparoscopy is an opportunity to diagnose endometriosis and treat any identifiable disease. If a gynecologist is going to proceed with laparoscopy, he or she must feel comfortable operating on adolescent patients and be familiar with the appearance of endometriosis implants in this age group. Endometriosis is staged using the revised American Society of Reproductive Medicine (ASRM) Classification of Endometriosis [50]. The staging is based on a point system that was developed to aid in fertility interventions and not pain management; thus, the extent of disease does not always correlate with the severity of symptoms [75]. Most adolescents are diagnosed with stage I or II endometriosis at laparoscopy, although some observational studies have described rates as high as 40% of stage III or IV disease [76].

Endometriosis lesions has historically been described as blue/black/gray "powder burns"; however, these may represent older and more advanced implants that are seen in adults. Adolescents typically have nonclassical or "atypical" and superficial implants such as white implants, clear vesicular lesions, and small hemorrhagic or petechial spots of the peritoneum [77] (Figs. 12.1 and 12.2). The clear and red lesions more commonly identified in adolescents may be more painful lesions of endometriosis in comparison to black lesions [78]. Moving the laparoscope closer to the peritoneum and adjusting the magnification, a "close tip technique," may be

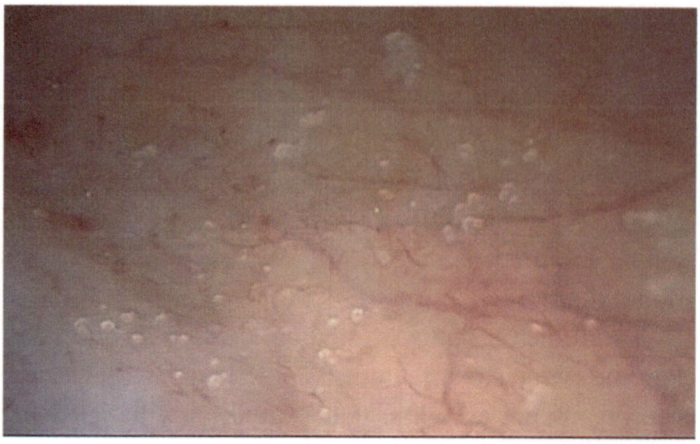

Fig. 12.1 Clear superficial lesions of endometriosis. (Reprinted from Emans [132])

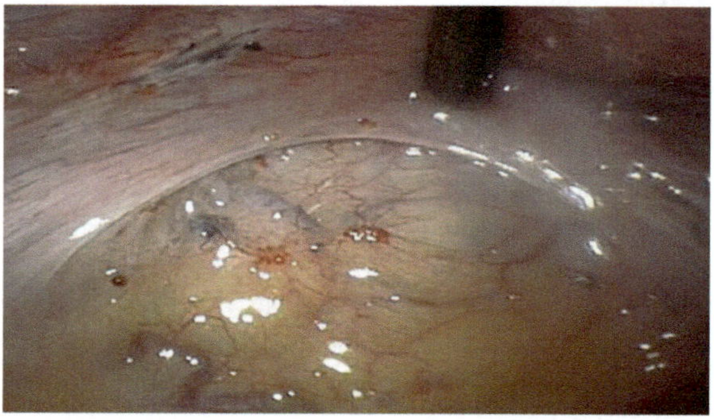

Fig. 12.2 Red peritoneal lesions of endometriosis. (Reprinted from Emans [132])

helpful in identification [79]. Another technique for visualization of lesions is by filling the pelvis with irrigation fluid (e.g., normal saline or lactated Ringer's) and submerging the laparoscope underneath the fluid; the more subtle clear lesions may be seen floating in the fluid [80]. After the lesions are identified, the fluid is removed for subsequent ablation or excision. Peritoneal windows or defects are also common in adolescents and diagnostic of endometriosis.

If no obvious or suspicious lesions are identified, a posterior cul-de-sac biopsy should be done to exclude the presence of microscopic disease. A prior retrospective study by Laufer et al. evaluated adolescents younger than 22 years of age who underwent operative laparoscopy for chronic pelvic pain unresponsive to conventional therapy; of those with a visually normal pelvis, 20% were found to have pathologically proven endometriosis from a nondirected posterior cul-de-sac biopsy [2].

12.9 Surgical Treatment

During surgery, after identification of endometriotic lesions in the pelvis, the surgeon should feel comfortable with removing or destroying as much of the disease as possible. Lysis of adhesions should also be performed if present, with the goal to restore as much of the normal anatomy as safely feasible. The gynecologist should consider surgery as one of the many tools within their "toolbox" of options for the treatment of endometriosis. Both ablation and excisional surgery have been demonstrated to be more effective than placebo at reducing pain in adult women with endometriosis [81, 82]. A retrospective cohort study by Song et al. [83] included 85 adolescents with surgically confirmed endometriosis younger than 19 years of age; pelvic pain disappeared in 41.7% of patients and improved in 38.3% of patients.

Endometriosis implants can be treated via endocoagulation, laser ablation, excision, or electrocautery [84, 85]. A combination of techniques can be utilized and tailored to the type of lesions present. In example, a surgeon may opt to use electrocautery with a monopolar L-hook electrode instrument for destroying superficial peritoneal disease, whereas he or she may excise deeper infiltrating lesions. There does not appear to be a significant difference in pain reduction between ablation and excisional treatments for stage I and II disease [86–88].

There are no data supporting the use of radical excisional surgery, or "peritoneal stripping," for superficial endometriosis. Firstly, complete excisional surgery has not been demonstrated to be curative. In a study of 17 adolescents who had complete laparoscopic excision of their endometriosis, 47% of the patients had return of pain to a level that required a subsequent laparoscopy [89, 90]. Secondly, radical excisional surgery might be overtreatment in adolescents and lead to the development of new symptoms. Laufer and Einarsson [91] published a case report on a 15-year-old young woman with ASRM-defined stage I endometriosis who underwent radical excision of the peritoneum of the anterior cul-de-sac, posterior cul-de-sac, and both pelvic sidewalls. Unfortunately, the radical excisional surgery was not curative and resulted in increased pain, extensive adhesive formation, and recurrent lesions of superficial peritoneal endometriosis. The American College of Obstetricians and Gynecologists does not recommend radical excisional surgery in adolescents due the lack of short-term and long-term outcome data about the procedure, and the potential for adhesion formation contributing to future sequelae such as bowel obstruction and infertility, and persistent pain [48].

Ovarian endometriomas are an uncommon presentation of endometriosis in adolescents that requires surgical therapy [92]. The prevalence of endometriomas in adolescents is unknown, but when present, the disease is upstaged to stage III or IV according to the ASRM classification [50]. First-line treatment of endometriomas in adolescents is cystectomy because cystectomy removes the endometriosis and leaves ovarian tissue behind versus oophorectomy. Laparoscopic cystectomy is more effective than cyst drainage or cyst wall ablation in reducing the recurrence of endometrioma or pain symptoms [93]. Attention is crucial to preserve as much of the native ovarian tissue or ovarian function.

Laparoscopy for endometriosis in adolescents should ultimately be as therapeutic as possible, with the objective of conserving as much of the normal anatomy. Unfortunately, without data-driven treatment guidelines, there is a wide variation in the use of surgical treatment for chronic pelvic pain in adolescents across the country and between types of institutions. Hung et al. [94] conducted a retrospective population-based analysis of the Nationwide Inpatient Sample in the United States from 1998 to 2016 and found the overall inpatient intervention rate was 45% for excision/ablation, 15.7% for hysterectomy, 9.5% for diagnostic laparoscopy, and 1.2% for biopsy in adolescents and young adults with chronic pelvic pain. Alarmingly, the rates of hysterectomy increased in the late 2000s while all other interventions decreased. Conservative surgical treatment should be considered first-line for adolescent women as opposed to definitive (hysterectomy with or without oophorectomy) because it is less invasive and preserves fertility and hormone production. Adolescents should be counseled that endometriosis is an extrauterine disease, therefore removal of the uterus and/or ovaries may not be curative. The reoperation rate after hysterectomy is as high as 19% [95], and women who undergo hysterectomy for endometriosis at younger than 30 years of age are more likely than older women to have residual symptoms, report a sense of loss, and to report more disruption from pain in different aspects of their lives [96].

12.10 Postoperative Medical Therapies

Because surgery is not curative, adolescents with endometriosis should be counseled on long-term medical therapy to prevent the recurrence of symptoms and the progression of disease, which could subsequently impact fertility. Medical or hormonal therapies inhibit prostaglandin production that contributes to pain, and also results in decidualization and atrophy of ectopic endometrial tissue. Long-term follow-up data in adolescents show that surgically destroyed endometriosis and postoperative medical therapy tends to retard disease progression in adolescents and young adults. In a retrospective review of adolescents with surgically destroyed endometriosis and exacerbation of pain on conventional medical therapy, no stage change was observed in 70% of patients at their subsequent laparoscopy [97]. Furthermore, this study also reported no increase in the rates of adhesion formation from the initial surgical procedure. In the absence of postoperative medical treatment, endometriosis has been demonstrated to progress to a higher stage on subsequent laparoscopy [98]. Most adolescents who remain on medical therapy do not require a subsequent surgical procedure [80]. Patients should be counseled on continuing hormonal treatment unless they are actively trying to become pregnant.

12.11 Combined Hormonal Contraception

Combined hormonal contraception is commonly utilized prior to laparoscopy and postoperatively. Combined estrogen and progestin therapy can be used long term, is generally well tolerated, inexpensive, and provides contraceptive benefits. If a pill is chosen, a monophasic regimen should be selected in the event that the pill is used continuously and withdrawal bleeds are eliminated. Oral contraceptives with ethinyl estradiol greater than 30 μg should be used in preference since there is some evidence of impaired bone accrual with lower-dose (less than 30 μg ethinyl estradiol) preparations [99]. In addition, lower ethinyl estradiol formulations are more likely to result in irregular, prolonged, frequent bleeding, or breakthrough bleeding or spotting, an undesirable symptom for those with endometriosis [100]. Alternatives to combined hormonal contraception include the transdermal patch or the vaginal ring; certain conditions may restrict use of the transdermal patch such as obesity with a body mass index greater than 30 kg/m^2 [101], and adolescents may not be willing or feel comfortable with inserting a vaginal ring. All methods are effective and safe when given in a cyclic, extended, or continues manner, but extended or continuous use is recommended for the treatment of endometriosis-associated pain.

12.12 Progestin-Only Therapies

Progestin-only therapies should be offered to those who decline estrogen-containing therapy or are not candidates to receive estrogen. Progestin-only methods include oral, injectable, and implants. While there are many formulations of combined estrogen-progestin contraceptive pills, norethindrone, desogestrel, and drospirenone are the main progestin-only oral contraceptive pills. Norethindrone is commonly available as 0.35 mg tablets daily (commercial names include Camila and Micronor). It is important to remember that the overall incidence of ovulation is 42.6% with norethindrone, in comparison to 1.1–4.6% with combined oral contraceptives [102]; therefore, norethindrone may not be an ideal choice for adolescents with recurrent functional cyst formation or ovulation pain. Drospirenone (commercial name Slynd) was approved for use in the United States in 2019 [103], and is dispensed as 24 tablets containing 4 mg drospirenone, followed by 4 placebo tablets. In contrast to norethindrone, drospirenone does consistently suppress ovulation [103]. Desogestrel (commercial names include Cerazette and Mircette) is dispensed as 75 mcg tablets daily and also inhibits ovulation [104]. Desogestrel is available in many countries excluding the United States. Norethindrone acetate (NA) is another progestin-only oral pill that is not FDA approved as a contraceptive but is indicated for the treatment of endometriosis and abnormal uterine bleeding [105]. NA can be used in a dosage from 5 to 15 mg per day and can be titrated to suppress menses and pain, although a dose greater than 10 mg per day might increase risk of hepatic adenoma formation [106]. This potential risk is likely in part by the small peripheral conversion of NA to ethinyl estradiol [107]. NA monotherapy has been demonstrated to be a well-tolerated and effective treatment for endometriosis-associated pain and bleeding in adolescents [108].

Depot medroxyprogesterone (DMPA) is another progestin-only contraceptive that is highly effective and well-received by the adolescent population [109]. DMPA is administered every 3 months in intramuscular or subcutaneous form. Adolescents should be appropriately counseled on bone health with long-term use of DMPA due to the potential loss of bone mineral density, which is temporary and reversible after discontinuation. Long-acting reversible contraceptive methods include the etonogestrel implant and the levonorgestrel intrauterine system (LNG-IUS), and both appear to improve pelvic pain, dysmenorrhea, and health-related quality of life in endometriosis [110]. While the etonogestrel implant is a very effective form of contraception, unscheduled bleeding is common and the primary reason for discontinuation [111]. As far as the LNG-IUS, there is limited but consistent evidence that it can successfully treat endometriosis-associated symptoms in adults [112]. The efficacy of the LNG-IUS for adolescent endometriosis, however, does not appear to be the same as that seen in adults. Yoost et al. [113] performed a retrospective chart review of 18 adolescents with endometriosis and LNG-IUS. Contrary to results from adult studies, the majority of patients in this adolescent cohort (67%) needed additional hormonal medications after LNG-IUS placement to achieve adequate suppression of pain or bleeding. A possible explanation is that the systemic level of hormone from the LNG-IUS may not be high enough to successfully suppress endometriosis-associated pain. A progestin-only or combination pill may therefore need to be recommended in conjunction with the LNG-IUS.

Inability to tolerate a pelvic exam should not be a limiting factor for LNG-IUS insertion. The LNG-IUS should be offered at time of diagnostic/therapeutic laparoscopy to eliminate the possible pain with insertion performed in the outpatient setting. The LNG-IUS can also be offered at a sequential date under sedation or anesthesia. While never sexually active adolescents are more likely to have an unsuccessful intrauterine device insertion in the office, insertion in this population is still successful overall with an insertion rate as high as 98.7% [114].

12.13 Androgens

Exogenous androgens are an uncommon but an accepted method of treating endometriosis. Danazol is a 17-a-ethinyltestosterone derivative that produces a high androgen/low estrogen environment, inhibiting follicular development and inducing atrophy of endometriotic implants [115]. Danazol has been demonstrated to be just as effective as GnRH agonist therapy in the treatment of endometriosis-associated symptoms [116, 117]. However, its use is limited by the occurrence of androgenic side effects, including hirsutism, acne, and weight gain. Permanent side effects are also possible, such as deepening of the voice [118]. Transgender male adolescents may therefore be more inclined than cisgender female adolescents in utilizing danazol for management of their dysmenorrhea or endometriosis symptoms.

Transmasculine adolescents may utilize testosterone for gender-affirming treatment. Testosterone should not be considered a conventional therapy for endometriosis as there may be incomplete ovulatory suppression and persistent endometrial activity [119, 120]. Shim et al. [121] reported described a cohort of 35 transmasculine adolescents who were diagnosed with dysmenorrhea. Only seven (20%) were laparoscopically evaluated for endometriosis, and it was confirmed in all seven patients. Five of the adolescents with endometriosis initiated testosterone treatment, and two continued to experience endometriosis-associated symptoms while on testosterone and concomitant progestin therapies. Transmasculine persons affected by dysmenorrhea or endometriosis should be counseled that exogenous testosterone use might not completely mitigate their symptoms, and other hormonal therapies might need to be used in conjunction with purposes including bleeding, pain, or contraception [121].

12.14 Gonadotropin-Releasing Hormone Agonists and Antagonists

If patients experience endometriosis symptoms refractory to conservative surgery and postoperative medical therapy, GnRH analogues may be advised. GnRH agonists and antagonists are both currently available for the treatment of endometriosis. Continuous GnRH by these medications downregulates the pituitary and creates a hypoestrogenic environment highly successful in suppressing endometriosis. GnRH agonists can be administered via nasal spray (nafarelin), subcutaneous or intramuscular injection (includes leuprolide), and implant (includes goserelin). The adolescent should be engaged in the decision-making process when selecting the mode of administration; the 3-month injectable agonist may be more desired as it improves patient compliance and decreases office visits. The adolescent should also be counseled on the potential "flare effect," which is when there is an initial upregulation of luteinizing hormone (LH) and follicle-stimulating hormone (FSH) prior to downregulation. The "flare effect" temporarily increase estradiol production, causing pain and withdrawal bleeding 21–28 days after initiation of therapy [80].

Adolescents who choose to initiate GnRH agonist therapy should be advised on the long-term adverse effects on bone. As adolescence is a critical time period for bone accrual, GnRH agonist therapy should be limited to patients above the age of 16 years [57]. For this reason, all adolescents who initiate GnRH agonists should receive "add-back" therapy within the first month. Add-back therapy describes the use of sex steroids to decrease the hypoestrogenic effects of the treatment such as bone demineralization, without stimulating the growth of endometriotic tissue. The most common add-back regimens include daily use of NA (5 mg), conjugated equine estrogens (CEE) (0.625 mg) plus medroxyprogesterone acetate (5 mg), or conjugated equine estrogens plus NA (2.5 or 5 mg). Combined oral contraceptives are not an appropriate add-back regimen as they negate the hypoestrogenic effects of GnRH agonists. In a randomized controlled trial of adolescents who received 12 months of GnRH agonist therapy, the combination of NA plus CEE was more effective for increasing total body bone mineral content, areal bone mineral density, and lean mass [122]. The add-back therapy of NA with CEE was also superior to NA alone for improving physical health-related QOL in the adolescent cohort [123].

Given the potential impact on bone density, patients should be counseled on adequate dietary calcium and vitamin D intake and the benefits of weight-bearing exercise. Dual energy X-ray absorptiometry screening should be considered for adolescents concluding 12 months of GnRH agonist use, and repeating testing at least every 2 years if the patient elects to stay on the therapy beyond the recommended 12 month duration. GnRH agonist therapy should be discontinued if a significant change in the bone mineral density Z-score occurs.

Adolescents should also be thoroughly counseled on the other side effects that may occur during or after GnRH agonist treatment. Hypoestrogenic symptoms are common, such as hot flashes, vaginal dryness, and decreased libido, and may result in patient dissatisfaction or discontinuation of therapy [80]. In a survey study of adolescents with endometriosis who received leuprolide depot 11.25 intramuscular injections with add-back therapy, 24 out of 25 respondents reported side effects during treatment; 80% reported side effects lasted longer than 6 months after treatment discontinuation, and 9 out of 20 reported side effects they considered irreversible, including memory loss, insomnia, and hot flashes [124].

GnRH antagonists are also an available treatment for endometriosis, although trials have not included women less than 18 years of age. One advantage of GnRH antagonists is the absence of a "flare effect" as they initiate downregulation of pituitary gonadotropins from the beginning of administration. Elagolix is an oral short-acting competitive GnRH antagonist approved in 2018 for the management of moderate to severe endometriosis-associated pain in the United States [125]. When prescribed, adolescents should be removed that elagolix does not always suppress ovulation and is not considered a contraceptive [126]. Amenorrhea may also not be realistically achieved, as the incidence varies widely from 13.9% to 65.6% in clinical trials [127]. Further long-term data are sorely needed to assess the efficacy of elagolix and other GnRH antagonists in adolescents.

12.15 Complementary Therapies

Nonhormonal therapies can be utilized to treat endometriosis-related pain, but it is important to remind the patient that nonhormonal treatments will not retard disease progression. Complementary modalities that can be offered to the adolescent include acupuncture, exercise, electrotherapy, and yoga. In a randomized, sham-controlled trial by Wayne et al., adolescents with laparoscopically confirmed endometriosis had a significant reduction in pain after Japanese-style acupuncture therapy [128].

More studies are merited to assess the efficacy and safety of complementary interventions for endometriosis in adolescents. A meta-analysis by Mira et al. identified only eight studies assessing complementary interventions for endometriosis-associated pain, and only acupuncture has demonstrated a significant improvement in outcomes [129]. There are no proven dietary treatments for the prevention or management of dysmenorrhea or endometriosis [130].

Multidisciplinary and holistic management of endometriosis can help introduce adolescents to complementary and alternative therapies, including physical therapy and biobehavioral therapy. Non-gynecology providers may include pain specialists, mental health professionals, and physical therapists. Adolescents who may find the multidisciplinary approach helpful are those with chronic pain and experience significant disability despite aggressive medical and surgical management. In these patients, a biobehavioral approach can help emphasize the patient's return to school, participation in social activities, and recognition of maladaptive behavior [131].

12.16 Support and Long-Term Follow-Up

As endometriosis is a chronic condition requiring long-term therapy, adolescents should be as much involved in the decision-making as possible to improve satisfaction and adherence to treatment. Their primary caregiver may be more involved with the initial treatment, but adolescents should be encouraged to ask questions and have their concerns addressed. Adolescents are very conscious of side effects and may become noncompliant with treatment, thus individualizing treatment is crucial [132]. In addition, as adolescents age and begin college or work, clinicians should assist in the transition of care and remind their patients to establish a relationship with a gynecologist familiar with the management of endometriosis.

Adolescents should be encouraged to identify family members or close friends who can support them when they are suffering from their endometriosis-associated symptoms. Exacerbations of pain may limit adolescents from activities such as hanging out with friends, leading to guilt or embarrassment. Education of family and friends may aid them in understanding the symptoms and treatment of endometriosis, and how to be supportive. In addition, adolescents with endometriosis find support from their peers very helpful. Adolescents can access peers through chat rooms, meetings, blogs, and phone conversations [132]. Monthly chat rooms and educational information for both patients and families are available at www.youngwomenshealth.org.

References

1. Meigs JV. Endometriosis. Ann Surg. 1948;127(5):795–808.
2. Laufer MR, Goitein L, Bush M, et al. Prevalence of endometriosis in adolescent girls with chronic pelvic pain not responding to conventional therapy. J Pediatr Adolesc Gynecol. 1997;10(4):199–202.
3. Reese KA, Reddy S, Rock JA. Endometriosis in an adolescent population: the Emory experience. J Pediatr Adolesc Gynecol. 1996;9(3):125–8.
4. Goldstein DP, De Cholnoky C, Emans SJ. Adolescent endometriosis. J Adolesc Health Care. 1980;1(1):37–41.
5. Janssen EB, Rijkers ACM, Hoppenbrouwers K, et al. Prevalence of endometriosis diagnosed by laparoscopy in adolescents with dysmenorrhea or chronic pelvic pain: a systematic review. Hum Reprod Update. 2013;19(5):570–82.
6. Ragab A, Shams M, Badawy A, et al. Prevalence of endometriosis among adolescent school girls with severe dysmenorrhea: a cross sectional prospective study. Int J Health Sci (Qassim). 2015;9(3):273–81.
7. Fong YF, Hon SK, Low LL, et al. The clinical profile of young and adolescent women with laparoscopically diagnosed endometriosis in a Singapore tertiary hospital. Taiwan J Obstet Gynecol. 2017;56(2):181–3.

8. Al-Jefout M, Alnawaiseh N, Yaghi S, et al. Prevalence of endometriosis and its symptoms among young Jordanian women with chronic pelvic pain refractory to conventional therapy. J Obstet Gynaecol Can. 2018;40(2):165–70.
9. Hirsch M, Dhillon-Smith R, Cutner AS, et al. The prevalence of endometriosis in adolescents with pelvic pain: a systematic review. J Pediatr Adolesc Gynecol. 2020;S1083–3188(2):30287–4.
10. Staal AHJ, van der Zanden M, Nap AW. Diagnostic delay of endometriosis in the Netherlands. Gynecol Obstet Investig. 2016;81(4):321–4.
11. Nnoaham KE, Hummelshoj L, Webster P, et al. Impact of endometriosis on quality of life and work productivity: a multicenter study across ten countries. Fertil Steril. 2011;96(2):366–373.e8.
12. Soliman AM, Fuldeore M, Snabes MC. Factors associated with time to endometriosis diagnosis in the United States. J Womens Health (Larchmt). 2017;26(7):788–97.
13. Hudelist G, Fritzer N, Thomas A, et al. Diagnostic delay for endometriosis in Austria and Germany: causes and possible consequences. Hum Reprod. 2012;27(12):3412–6.
14. Agarwal SK, Chapron C, Giudice LC, et al. Clinical diagnosis of endometriosis: a call to action. Am J Obstet Gynecol. 2019;220(4):354.e1–354.e12.
15. Ballweg ML. Big picture of endometriosis helps provide guidance on approach to teens: comparative historical data shows endo starting younger, is more severe. J Pediatr Adolesc Gynecol. 2003;16(3 Suppl):S21–6.
16. Marsh EE, Laufer MR. Endometriosis in premenarcheal girls who do not have an associated obstructive anomaly. Fertil Steril. 2005;83(3):758–60.
17. Goldstein DP, de Cholnoky C, Leventhal JM, Emans SJ. New insights into the old problem of chronic pelvic pain. J Pediatr Surg. 1979;14(6):675–80.
18. Yamamoto K, Mitsuhashi Y, Takaike T, et al. Tubal endometriosis diagnosed within one month after menarche: a case report. Tohoku J Exp Med. 1997;181(3):385–7.
19. Simpson JL, Elias S, Malinak LR, et al. Heritable aspects of endometriosis. I. Genetic studies. Am J Obstet Gynecol. 1980;137(3):327–31.
20. Hansen KH, Eyster KM. Genetics and genomics of endometriosis. Clin Obstet Gynecol. 2010;53(2):403–12.
21. Kennedy S, Hadfield R, Mardon H, et al. Age of onset of pain symptoms in non-twin sisters concordant for endometriosis. Hum Reprod. 1996;11(2):403–5.
22. Dovey S, Sanfilippo J. Endometriosis and the adolescent. Clin Obstet Gynecol. 2010;53(2):420–8.
23. Schifrin BS, Erez S, Moore JG. Teen-age endometriosis. Am J Obstet Gynecol. 1973;116(7):973–80.
24. Olive DL, Henderson DY. Endometriosis and Mullerian anomalies. Obstet Gynecol. 1987;69(3 Pt 1):412–5.
25. Sanfilippo JS, Wakim NG, Schikler KN, et al. Endometriosis in association with uterine anomaly. Am J Obstet Gynecol. 1986;154(1):39–43.
26. Silveira SA, Laufer MR. Persistence of endometriosis after correction of obstructive reproductive tract anomaly. J Pediatr Adolesc Gynecol. 2010;23:e89.
27. Nnoaham KE, Webster P, Kumbang J, et al. Is early age at menarche a risk factor for endometriosis? A systematic review and meta-analysis of case-control studies. Fertil Steril. 2012;98(3):702–712.e6.
28. Treloar SA, Bell TA, Nagle CM, et al. Early menstrual characteristics associated with subsequent diagnosis of endometriosis. Am J Obstet Gynecol. 2010;202(6):534.e1–6.
29. Ballard KD, Seaman HE, de Vries CS, et al. Can symptomatology help in the diagnosis of endometriosis? Findings from a national case-control study–Part 1. BJOG. 2008;115(11):1382–91.
30. Hediger ML, Hartnett HJ, Buck Louis GM. Association of endometriosis with body size and figure. Fertil Steril. 2005;84(5):1366–74.
31. Missmer SA, Hankinson SE, Spiegelman D, et al. Incidence of laparoscopically confirmed endometriosis by demographic, anthropometric, and lifestyle factors. Am J Epidemiol. 2004;160(8):784–96.

32. Bougie O, Healey J, Singh SS. Behind the times: revisiting endometriosis and race. Am J Obstet Gynecol. 2019;221(1):35.e1–5.
33. Harris HR, Wieser F, Vitonis AF, et al. Early life abuse and risk of endometriosis. Hum Reprod. 2018;33(9):1657–68.
34. Shafrir AL, Farland LV, Shah DK, et al. Risk for and consequences of endometriosis: a critical epidemiologic review. Best Pract Res Clin Obstet Gynaecol. 2018;51:1–15.
35. Sasamoto N, Farland LV, Vitonis AF, et al. In utero and early life exposures in relation to endometriosis in adolescents and young adults. Eur J Obstet Gynecol Reprod Biol. 2020;252:393–8.
36. Nodler JL, Harris HR, Chhavarro JE, et al. Dairy consumption during adolescence and endometriosis risk. Am J Obstet Gynecol. 2020;222(3):257.e1–257.e16.
37. Sampson JA. Metastatic or embolic endometriosis, due to the menstrual dissemination of endometrial tissue into the venous circulation. Am J Pathol. 1927;3(2):93–110.43.
38. Halme J, Hammond MG, Hulka JF, et al. Retrograde menstruation in healthy women and in patients with endometriosis. Obstet Gynecol. 1984;64(2):151–4.
39. Tsonis O, Barmpalia Z, Gkrozou F, et al. Endometriosis in adolescence: early manifestation of the traditional disease or a unique variant? Eur J Obstet Gynecol Reprod Biol. 2020;247:238–43.
40. Brosens I, Gargett CE, Gou SW, et al. Origins and progression of adolescent endometriosis. Reprod Sci. 2016;23(1):1282–8.
41. Ober WB, Bernstein J. Observations on the endometrium and ovary in the newborn. Pediatrics. 1955;16(4):445–60.
42. Arcellana RC, Robinson TW, Tyson RW, et al. McKusick-Kaufman syndrome with legal complications of hydrometrocolpos and congenital endometriosis. J Perinatol. 1996;16(3):220–3.
43. Brosens I, Gordts S, Benagiano G. Endometriosis in adolescents is a hidden, progressive and severe disease that deserves attention, not just compassion. Hum Reprod. 2013;28(8):2026–31.
44. Halban J. Metastatic hysteroadenosis. Wien Klin Wochenschr. 1924;37:1205–6.
45. Meyer R. Über entzundliche neterope Epithelwucherungen im weiblichen Genetalgebiet and über eine his in die Wurzel des Mesocolon ausgedehnte benigne Wucherung des Darmepithel. Virchows Arch Pathol Anat. 1909;195:487.
46. Burney RO, Giudice LC. Pathogenesis and pathophysiology of endometriosis. Fertil Steril. 2012;98(3):511–9.
47. Bailey AP, Hill AS, Beste MT, et al. Comparison of cytokines in the peritoneal fluid and conditioned medium of adolescents and adults with and without endometriosis. Am J Reprod Immunol. 2020:e13347.
48. Dysmenorrhea and endometriosis in the adolescent. ACOG Committee Opinion No. 760. American College of Obstetricians and Gynecologists. Obstet Gynecol. 2018;132:e249–58.
49. DiVasta AD, Vitonis AF, Laufer MR, Missmer SA. Spectrum of symptoms in women diagnosed with endometriosis during adolescence vs adulthood. Am J Obstet Gynecol. 2018;218(3):324.e1–324.e11.
50. American Society for Reproductive Medicine. Revised American Society for Reproductive Medicine classification of endometriosis. 1997;67(5):817–21.
51. Schneider MP, Vitonis AF, Fadayomi AB, et al. Quality of life in adolescent and young adult women with dyspareunia and endometriosis. J Adolesc Health. 2020;67(4):557–61.
52. Dun EC, Kho KA, Morozov VV, et al. Endometriosis in adolescents. JSLS. 2015;19(2):e2015.00019.
53. Butrick CW. Patients with chronic pelvic pain: endometriosis or interstitial cystitis/painful bladder syndrome? JSLS. 2007;11(2):182–9.
54. Sinaii N, Cleary SD, Ballweg ML, et al. High rates of autoimmune and endocrine disorders, fibromyalgia, chronic fatigue syndrome and atopic diseases among women with endometriosis: a survey analysis. Hum Reprod. 2002;17(1):2715–24.
55. DiVasta AD, Zimmerman LA, Vitonis AF, et al. Overlap between irritable bowel syndrome diagnosis and endometriosis in adolescents. Clin Gastroenterol Hepatol. 2020;S1542–3565(2):30324–4.

56. Miller JA, Missmer SA, Vitonis AF, et al. Prevalence of migraines in adolescents with endometriosis. Fertil Steril. 2018;109(4):685–90.
57. Shim JY, Laufer MR. Adolescent endometriosis: an update. J Pediatr Adolesc Gynecol. 2020;33(2):112–9.
58. Shigesi N, Kvaskoff M, Kirley S, et al. The association between endometriosis and autoimmune diseases: a systematic review and meta-analyses. Hum Reprod Update. 2019;25(4):486–503.
59. Zannoni L, Giorgi M, Spagnolo E, et al. Dysmenorrhea, absenteeism from school, and symptoms suspicious for endometriosis in adolescents. J Pediatr Adolesc Gynecol. 2014;27(5):258–65.
60. Gallagher JS, DiVasta AD, Vitonis AF, et al. The impact of endometriosis on quality of life in adolescents. J Adolesc Health. 2018;63(6):766–72.
61. Ballard K, Lowton K, Wright J. What's the delay? A qualitative study of women's experiences of reaching a diagnosis of endometriosis. Fertil Steril. 2006;86(5):1296–301.
62. Gupta J, Cardoso LF, Harris CS. How do adolescent girls and boys perceive symptoms suggestive of endometriosis among their peers? Findings from focus group discussions in New York City. BMJ Open. 2018;8(6):e020657.
63. Mama ST. Advances in the management of endometriosis in the adolescent. Curr Opin Obstet Gynecol. 2018;30(5):326–30.
64. Patel DP. The evolving nomenclature of erythema Ab Igne-Redness from fire. JAMA Dermatol. 2017;153(7):685.
65. Tighe MP, Morenas RA, Afzal NA, et al. Erythema ab igne and Crohn's disease. Arch Dis Child. 2008;93(5):389.
66. Gubbels A, Spivack L, Lindheim SR, et al. Adolescent endometriosis. Obstet Gynecol Surv. 2020;75(8):483–96.
67. Hirsch M, Duffy JMN, Deguara CS, et al. Diagnostic accuracy of Cancer Antigen 125 (CA125) for endometriosis in symptomatic women: a multi-center study. Eur J Obstet Gynecol Reprod Biol. 2017;210:102–7.
68. Sasamoto N, DePari M, Vitonis AF, et al. Evaluation of CA125 in relation to pain symptoms among adolescents and young adult women with and without surgically-confirmed endometriosis. PLoS One. 2020;15(8):e0238043.
69. Martire FG, Lazzeri L, Conway F, et al. Adolescence and endometriosis: symptoms, ultrasound signs and early diagnosis. Fertil Steril. 2020;114(5):1049–57.
70. Chandler TM, Maschan LS, Cooperberg PL, et al. Mullerian duct anomalies: from diagnosis to intervention. Br J Radiol. 2009;82(84):1034–42.
71. Marjoribanks J, Ayeleke RO, Farquhar C, et al. Nonsteroidal anti-inflammatory drugs for dysmenorrhoea. Cochrane Database Syst Rev. 2015;2015(7):CD001751.
72. Harel Z. Dysmenorrhea in adolescents and young adults: an update on pharmacological treatments and management strategies. Expert Opin Pharmacother. 2012;13(15):2157–70.
73. Dmitrovic R, Kunselman AR, Legro RS. Continuous compared with cyclic oral contraceptives for the treatment of primary dysmenorrhea: a randomized controlled trial. Obstet Gynecol. 2012;119(6):1143–50.
74. Propst AM, Laufer MR. Endometriosis in adolescents. Incidence, diagnosis and treatment. J Reprod Med. 1999;44(9):751–8.
75. Fedele L, Parazzini F, Bianchi S, et al. Stage and localization of pelvic endometriosis and pain. Fertil Steril. 1990;53(1):155–8.
76. Audebert A, Lecointre L, Afors K, et al. Adolescent endometriosis: report of a series of 55 cases with a focus on clinical presentation and long-term issues. J Minim Invasive Gynecol. 2015;22(5):834–40.
77. Davis GD, Thillet E, Lindemann J. Clinical characteristics of adolescent endometriosis. J Adolesc Health. 1993;14(5):362–8.
78. Demco L. Mapping the source and character of pain due to endometriosis by patient-assisted laparoscopy. J Am Assoc Gynecol Laparosc. 1998;5(3):241–5.
79. Laufer MR. Identification of clear vesicular lesions of atypical endometriosis: a new technique. Fertil Steril. 1997;68(4):739–40.

80. Laufer MR. Helping "adult gynecologists" diagnose and treat adolescent endometriosis: reflections on my 20 years of personal experience. J Pediatr Adolesc Gynecol. 2011;24(5 Suppl):S13–7.
81. Abbott J, Hawe J, Hunter D, et al. Laparoscopic excision of endometriosis: a randomized, placebo-controlled trial. Fertil Steril. 2004;82(4):878–84.
82. Sutton CJ, Ewen SP, Whitelaw N, et al. Prospective, randomized, double-blind, controlled trial of lapser laparoscopy in the treatment of pelvic pain associated with minimal, mild, and moderate endometriosis. Fertil Steril. 1993;62(4):696–700.
83. Song XC, Yu X, Luo M, et al. Clinical characteristics and postoperative symptoms of 85 adolescents with endometriosis. J Pediatr Adolesc Gynecol. 2020;33(5):519–23.
84. Practice Committee of the American Society for Reproductive Medicine. Treatment of pelvic pain associated with endometriosis. Fertil Steril. 2014;101(4):927–35.
85. Cook AS, Rock JA. The role of laparoscopy in the treatment of endometriosis. Fertil Steril. 1991;55(4):663–80.
86. Wright J, Lotfallah H, Jones K, et al. A randomized trial of excision versus ablation for mild endometriosis. Fertil Steril. 2005;83(6):1830–6.
87. Riley KA, Benton AS, Deimling TA, et al. Surgical excision versus ablation for superficial endometriosis-associated pain: a randomized controlled trial. J Minim Invasive Gynecol. 2019;26(1):71–7.
88. Healy M, Ang WC, Cheng C. Surgical treatment of endometriosis: a prospective randomized double-blinded trial comparing excision and ablation. Fertil Steril. 2010;94(7):2536–40.
89. Yeung P Jr, Sinervo K, Winer W, et al. Complete laparoscopic excision of endometriosis in teenagers: is postoperative hormonal suppression necessary? Fertil Steril. 2011;95(6):1909–12, 1912.e1.
90. Laufer MR, Missmer SA. Does complete laparoscopic excision of endometriosis in teenagers really occur? Fertil Steril. 2011;96(3):e145, author reply e146.
91. Laufer MR, Einarsson JI. Surgical management of superficial peritoneal adolescent endometriosis. J Pediatr Adolesc Gynecol. 2019;32(30):339–41.
92. Wright KN, Laufer MR. Endometriomas in adolescents. Fertil Steril. 2010;94(4):1529.e7–9.
93. Hart RJ, Hickey M, Maouris P, et al. Excisional surgery versus ablative surgery for ovarian endometriomata. Cochrane Database Syst Rev. 2008;2:CD004992.
94. Hung YC, Westfal ML, Chang DC, et al. Lack of data-driven treatment guidelines and wide variation in management of chronic pelvic pain in adolescents and young adults. J Pediatr Adolesc Gynecol. 2020;33(4):349–353.e1.
95. Shakiba K, Bena JF, McGill KM, et al. Surgical treatment of endometriosis: a 7-year follow-up on the requirement for further surgery. Obstet Gynecol. 2008;111(6):1285–92.
96. MacDonald SR, Klock SC, Milad MP. Long-term outcome of nonconservative surgery (hysterectomy) for endometriosis-associated pain in women <30 years old. Am J Obstet Gynecol. 1999;180(6 Pt 1):1360–3.
97. Doyle JO, Missmer SA, Laufer MR. The effect of combined surgical-medical intervention on the progression of endometriosis in an adolescent and young adult population. J Pediatr Adolesc Gynecol. 2009;22(4):257–63.
98. Unger CA, Laufer MR. Progression of endometriosis in non-medically managed adolescents: a case series. J Pediatr Adolesc Gynecol. 2011;24(2):e21–3.
99. Golden NH. Bones and birth control in adolescent girls. J Pediatr Adolesc Gynecol. 2020;33(3):249–54.
100. Gallo MF, Nanda K, Grimes DA, et al. 20 µg versus >20 µg estrogen combined oral contraceptives for contraception. Cochrane Database Syst Rev. 2013;2013(8):CD003989.
101. Xulane- norelgestromin and ethinyl estradiol patch. US Food and Drug Administration (FDA) approved product information. Revised 2020. US National Library of Medicine. www.dailymed.nlm.nih.gov. Accessed on 2 Oct 2020.
102. Milsom I, Korver T. Ovulation incidence with oral contraceptives: a literature review. J Fam Plann Reprod Health Care. 2008;34(4):237–46.

103. Slynd (drospirenone tablets). US FDA approved product information; Florham Park: Exeltis USA, Inc; 2019. www.accessdata.fda.gov/drugsatfda_docs/label/2019/211367s000lbl.pdf. Accessed on 2 Oct 2020.
104. Benagiano G, Primiero FM. Seventy-five microgram desogestrel minipill, a new perspective in estrogen-free contraception. Ann N Y Acad Sci. 2003;997:163–73.
105. Aygestin (norethindrone acetate). US FDA approved product information; Pomona: Duramed Pharmaceuticals, Inc; 2007. www.accessdata.fda.gov/drugsatfda_docs/label/2007/018405s023lbl.pdf. Accessed on 23 Nov 2020.
106. Brady PC, Missmer SA, Laufer MR. Hepatic adenomas in adolescents and young women with endometriosis treated with norethindrone acetate. J Pediatr Adolesc Gynecol. 2017;30(3):422–4.
107. Chu MC, Zhang X, Gentzschein E, et al. Formation of ethinyl estradiol in women during treatment with norethindrone acetate. J Clin Endocrinol Metab. 2007;92(6):2205–7.
108. Kaser DJ, Missmer SA, Berry KF, et al. Use of norethindrone acetate alone for postoperative suppression of endometriosis symptoms. J Pediatr Adolesc Gynecol. 2012;25(2):105–8.
109. Cromer BA, Smith RD, Blair JM, et al. A prospective study of adolescents who choose among levonorgestrel implant (Norplant), medroxyprogesterone acetate (Depo-Provera), or the combined oral contraceptive pill as contraception. Pediatrics. 1994;94(5):687–94.
110. Carvalho N, Margatho D, Cursino K, et al. Control of endometriosis-associated pain with etonogestrel-releasing contraceptive implant and 52-mg levonorgestrel-releasing intrauterine system: randomized clinical trial. Fertil Steril. 2018;110(6):1129–36.
111. Darney P, Patel A, Rosen K, et al. Safety and efficacy of a single-rod etonogestrel implant (Implanon): results from 11 international clinical trials. Fertil Steril. 2009;91(5):1646–53.
112. Abou-Setta AM, Al-Inany HG, Farquhar CM. Levonorgestrel-releasing intrauterine device (LNG-IUD) for symptomatic endometriosis following surgery. Cochrane Datatbase Syst Rev. 2006;4:CD005072.
113. Yoost J, LaJoie AS, Hertweck P, et al. Use of the levonorgestrel intrauterine system in adolescents with endometriosis. J Pediatr Adolesc Gynecol. 2013;26(2):120–4.
114. Kebodeaux CA, Schwartz BI. Experience with intrauterine device insertion in never sexually active adolescents: a retrospective cohort study. Am J Obstet Gynecol. 2018;219(6):600.e1–7.
115. Dmowski WP. Danazol in the treatment of endometriosis and infertility. Prog Clin Biol Res. 1982;112 Pt B:167–86.
116. Rock JA, Truglia JA, Caplan RJ. Zoladex (goserelin acetate implant) in the treatment of endometriosis: a randomized comparison with danazol. The Zoladex Endometriosis Study Group. Obstet Gynecol. 1993;82(2):198–205.
117. Selak V, Farquhar C, Prentice A, et al. Danazol for pelvic pain associated with endometriosis. Cochrane Database Syst Rev. 2001;4:CD000068.
118. Boothroyd CV, Lepre F. Permanent voice change resulting from Danazol Therapy. Aust N Z J Obstet Gynaecol. 1990;30(3):275–6.
119. Taub RL, Adriane ES, Neal-Perry G, et al. The effect of testosterone on ovulatory function in transmasculine individuals. Am J Obstet Gynecol. 2020;223(2):229.e1–8.
120. Grimstad FW, Fowler KG, New EP, et al. Uterine pathology in transmasculine persons on testosterone: a retrospective multicenter case series. Am J Obstet Gynecol. 2019;220(3):257.e1–7.
121. Shim JY, Laufer MR, Grimstad FW. Dysmenorrhea and endometriosis in transgender adolescents. J Pediatr Adolesc Gynecol. 2020;33(5):524–8.
122. DiVasta AD, Feldman HA, Gallagher JS, et al. Hormonal add-back therapy for females treated with gonadotropin-releasing hormone agonist for endometriosis: a randomized controlled trial. Obstet Gynecol. 2015;126(3):617–27.
123. Gallagher JS, Feldman HA, Stokes NA, et al. The effects of gonadotropin-releasing hormone agonist combined with add-back therapy on quality of life for adolescents with endometriosis: a randomized controlled trial. J Pediatr Adolesc Gynecol. 2017;30(2):215–22.
124. Gallagher JS, Missmer SA, Hornstein MD, et al. Long-term effects of gonadotropin-releasing hormone agonists and add-back in adolescent endometriosis. J Pediatr Adolesc Gynecol. 2018;31(4):376–81.

125. Shebley M, Polepally AR, Nader A, et al. Clinical pharmacology of Elagolix: an oral gonadotropin-releasing hormone receptor antagonist for endometriosis. Clin Pharmacokinet. 2020;59(3):297–309.
126. Ng J, Chwalisz K, Carter DC. Dose-dependent suppression of gonadotropins and ovarian hormones by Elagolix in healthy premenopausal women. J Clin Endocrinol Metab. 2017;102(5):1683–91.
127. Taylor HS, Giudice LC, Lessey BA, et al. Treatment of endometriosis-associated pain with Elagolix, an oral GnRH antagonist. N Engl J Med. 2017;377(1):28–40.
128. Wayne PM, Kerr CE, Schnyer RN, et al. Japanese-style acupuncture for endometriosis-related pelvic pain in adolescents and young women: results of a randomized sham-controlled trial. J Pediatr Adolesc Gynecol. 2008;21(5):247–57.
129. Mira TA, Buen MM, Borges MG, et al. Systematic review and meta-analysis of complementary treatments for women with symptomatic endometriosis. Int J Gynaecol Obstet. 2018;143(1):2–9.
130. Pattanittum P, Kunyanone N, Brown J, et al. Dietary supplements for dysmenorrhoea. Cochrane Database Syst Rev. 2016;3(3):CD002124.
131. Greco CD. Management of adolescent chronic pelvic pain from endometriosis: a pain center perspective. J Pediatr Adolesc Gynecol. 2003;16(3 Suppl):S17–9.
132. Emans SJ. Emans, Laufer, Goldstein's pediatric & adolescent gynecology. 7th ed. Lippincott Williams & Wilkins; 2019.

Endometriosis in Reproductive Years: Fertility

13

Omar Shebl and Carla Tomassetti

Contents

13.1 Effect of Endometriosis on Fertility

The prevalence of endometriosis was found to be over 40% in infertile women compared to up to 6% in women of reproductive age [1, 2]. This indicates a presumable association of endometriosis and infertility. The mechanisms of impact of endometriosis on fertility are still not completely answered in the literature. In severe

O. Shebl (✉)
Kepler University Hospital Linz, Department of Obstetrics, Gynaecology and Gynaecological Endocrinology, Linz, Austria
e-mail: Omar.Shebl@kepleruniklinikum.at

C. Tomassetti
University Hospitals Leuven, Department of Obstetrics and Gynaecology, Leuven University Fertility Center, Leuven, Belgium

KU Leuven, Faculty of Medicine, Department of Development and Regeneration, LEERM (Laboratory for Endometrium, Endometriosis and Reproductive Medicine), Leuven, Belgium

E. Oral (ed.), *Endometriosis and Adenomyosis*,
https://doi.org/10.1007/978-3-030-97236-3_13

endometriosis cases with pelvic adhesions and obliteration of the cul-de-sac, infertility may be caused due the occlusion of the tubal ostium [3]. Also, inflammation is accused to play a role in endometriosis linked infertility. In peritoneal fluid, inflammatory changes, such as increase of IL6, IL10, IL13, and TNF-α, have been accused to influence human reproduction [4, 5], while most endometriomas were not associated with induction of an inflammatory reaction in the nearby follicles [6]. Hormonal changes, oestrogen dominance, and progesterone resistance, which are associated with endometriosis may increase an inflammatory process and negatively affect embryo implantation [7]. Endometriosis-associated pituitary dysfunction may furthermore contribute to infertility [3, 8].

Another influencing factor applies to the oocyte development and quality. Although data are only available from ART-studies, it has been shown that endometriosis is associated with a diminished oocyte quality [9, 10], due to dysregulated mechanisms involved in steroid metabolism and biosynthesis, response to oxidative stress, and cell cycle regulation [11]. It also has been shown that the follicular fluid metabolome differs in women with endometriosis compared to a control collective [12]. Moreover, granulosa cells in the context of endometriosis undergo increased apoptosis and have an altered cell cycle that could adversely affect folliculogenesis, oocyte, and embryo quality [11]. Another potential contributing factor may be endometriosis-associated uterine hyper- and dysperistalsis, which are suspected to influence sperm ascension and disturb the transport of embryos [13]. Treatment options in women with endometriosis and infertility aim to improve these conditions to optimise reproduction.

13.2 Effect of Surgery on Infertility

As in infertile women with endometriosis, ovarian suppression treatment does not improve fertility and should therefore not be prescribed [14]; the effect of endometriosis surgery on infertility is a frequently discussed topic. Endometriosis often coexists with adenomyosis, which in itself is associated with impaired reproductive outcomes [15, 16]. Furthermore, other fertility factors such as male factor, anovulation, or others also influence fertility outcome. Therefore, the effect of surgery on a particular endometriosis type and location is difficult to analyse, mostly due to the lack of properly designed prospective randomised studies. It should also be noted that none of the studies discussed below were stratified according to the Endometriosis Fertility Index (EFI). In general, it is recommended that the decision to perform surgery should be guided by the presence or absence of pain symptoms, patient age and preferences, history of previous surgery, presence of other fertility factors, ovarian reserve, and estimated Endometriosis Fertility Index (EFI) [14]. In view of the available literature on the EFI, this tool should be used for counselling of women of their chances of becoming pregnant without ART after surgery [14].

13.3 Peritoneal Endometriosis

The only data from randomised clinical trials on the effect of surgery for endometriosis-related infertility have been performed in the population of women with rAFS stage I-II endometriosis, so presumably (predominantly) peritoneal endometriosis. In 1997, a multicentre Canadian study analysed the benefit of ablating peritoneal endometriosis implants during a laparoscopy surgery compared to diagnostic laparoscopy only. The number of recognised pregnancies in the laparoscopic surgery group was 63/172 (36.6%) compared to 37/169 (21.9%) showing a significant improvement in the pregnancy rate for laparoscopic surgery [17]. One year later a multicentre Italian trial found contradictory results for laparoscopic surgery for endometriosis lesions compared to diagnostic surgery only (12/51 (23.5%) vs. 13/45 (28.9%)) [18]; however, the interpretation of the results of this trial is hampered by the postoperative use of hormonal treatment which is contraceptive. There is moderate quality evidence that laparoscopic surgery – compared to only diagnostic laparoscopy – increases viable intrauterine pregnancy rates confirmed by ultrasound in couples with otherwise unexplained infertility, based on a Cochrane review [19]. This review, which includes three randomised studies (the aforementioned Canadian study [17], and two others [20, 21]), is unable to report on live birth, and also stresses that careful patient selection and adequate surgical experience are important in ensuring that surgery is usefully applied. A similar conclusion was made by a recent network meta-analysis [14, 22]. As peritoneal endometriosis can only reliably be diagnosed with laparoscopy, the threshold to propose diagnostic and – if endometriosis is found – simultaneous operative laparoscopy to treat peritoneal endometriosis should be guided by the presence or absence of pelvic pain symptoms and patient preferences [14, 23].

13.4 Deep Infiltrating Endometriosis

As opposed to peritoneal (or minimal/mild) endometriosis, the evaluation of the potential benefit of surgical excision of deep endometriosis on the chance of natural conception is difficult. First, there is an absolute lack of randomised studies on this subject. Second, only a minority of studies report on postoperative pregnancy rates, even in studies focused on deep lesions with colorectal involvement [24]. Interpretation of data is hampered by the unclear distinction in studied populations regarding presence or absence of bowel or urinary tract involvement, active or passive child wish (if any), the mode of conception after surgery as well as the time period for either natural evolution or ART [14, 24]. For example, a meta-analysis of Paolo Vercellini in 2012 searched the literature for spontaneous pregnancy rate after radical surgery for rectovaginal and rectosigmoid endometriosis. According to the results of the 11 selected studies, the mean postoperative conception rate in all women seeking pregnancy independently of preoperative fertility status and IVF performance was 39%, but it dropped to 24% in infertile patients who sought spontaneous conception. This illustrates that patient selection significantly influences the estimate of the effect of rectovaginal endometriosis excision on infertility [25]. On the other hand, uncontrolled single centre studies such as by Roman [26] and Meuleman [27] report high pregnancy rates in women after surgical management of even complex colorectal endometriosis, mostly spontaneously conceived [26]. As no randomised data exist, but complication rates of surgery for deep – especially for colorectal – endometriosis should be considered, the review by Darai et al. [28] has tried to evaluate pregnancy rates in those women who had been operated partially (i.e. leaving in situ the colorectal endometriosis but removing other lesions) versus completely for deep colorectal endometriosis. They conclude that there may be a potential benefit of surgery on fertility outcomes for women with colorectal endometriosis; yet, they acknowledge that further studies are required to determine whether surgical management should be first-intention or restricted to failure of MAR [28]. A systematic review from 2018 hence concluded that there may be positive aspects of deep infiltrating endometriosis surgery on the chance for a spontaneous pregnancy, but complications have to be taken into account [29].

When treatment with MAR has failed in women where endometriosis resection has not been attempted before, a retrospective study [30] found that infertile women with ≥2 IVF-ICSI failures may be referred for surgery as it appears related to reasonable postoperative pregnancy rates (43.8% in total, and 21.8% natural conceptions), particularly when endometriomas surgery is either not required or not performed. The authors also stated that surgery for DIE does not routinely delay conception, as it usually occurs during the year following surgery [30]. In conclusion, as surgical removal of deep lesions may also reduce endometriosis-associated pain and improve quality of life, those undergoing surgery should be informed on potential risks, benefits, and long-term effects on quality of life, and surgery should be performed in a centre of expertise [14]. The final decision to opt for surgery in the presence of infertility should therefore be an individualised process.

13.5 Ovarian Endometriosis

Similarly as for deep endometriosis, the scientific literature on the potential benefit of surgery for ovarian endometriosis on postoperative (natural) fertility lacks high quality evidence from randomised clinical trials. A major concern when considering surgery for ovarian endometriosis is the potential detrimental effect on ovarian reserve, which may have long-term consequences for fertility and outcome of medically assisted reproduction treatments.

For the assessment of the effect of surgery on postoperative ovarian reserve, AMH (Anti-Müllerian Hormone) assays as well as antral follicle counts (AFC) by ultrasound have been used, with conflicting results in both cohort studies (e.g. [31, 32]) as well as meta-analyses [33]. Therefore, Younis et al. have conducted a systematic review of prospective studies, to address important measured and unmeasured confounding factors, in which parallel repeat measurements of both AMH and AFC were conducted for the same women, at the same time points, and in the same setting [34]. They identified 14 prospective studies, which in total included 650 women, and concluded that endometriotic cystectomies are associated with a significant reduction in the serum AMH levels but not in the antral follicle counts, with the detrimental effects on the AMH levels consistently detectable at the early-, intermediate-, and late-postoperative time points [34]. Thus, when performing surgery for ovarian endometrioma, specific caution should be used to minimise ovarian damage [14]. Also, repeat surgery should be considered more detrimental for the ovarian reserve [35]. In search for surgical techniques that may better preserve ovarian reserve than classical cystectomy, non-cauterising techniques such as CO_2 laser vaporisation should be considered as a valuable alternative as both cystectomy and vaporisation appear to have similar long-term recurrence rates and reproductive outcomes, but AMH levels are not reduced [14, 36–38].

As mentioned before, the question whether surgical treatment of endometriomas is better than expectant management on subsequent (natural) fertility is difficult to answer, as no RCTs or high-quality prospective cohort studies were identified on this subject, nor on the indication for surgery depending on the size of the cyst [14]. Also, the potential negative effect of the presence of (an) endometrioma(s) on the rate of spontaneous ovulation – which could indirectly have an influence on fertility – remains a matter of debate. Whereas Benaglia et al. [39] in a prospective study found a reduced rate of spontaneous ovulation on the side of endometriosis-affected ovaries (31%), this could not be confirmed in a larger prospective cohort study by Leone Roberti Maggiore et al., who confirmed that even in large cysts the rate of spontaneous ovulation was not impaired on the affected side [40]. On the other hand, concerns regarding growth of the cyst while waiting for a spontaneous pregnancy should be taken into account: during a 6-month period observing spontaneous ovulation, in women with unilateral ovarian endometriosis, an increase of ovarian volume of more than 10% was observed in 24% of the women [40].

In the absence of clear-cut comparative data, and based on the added conclusions of two reviews [41, 42], the ESHRE guidelines therefore give a weak recommendation that clinicians may consider operative laparoscopy for the treatment of endometrioma-associated infertility as it may increase the chance of natural pregnancy, while informing patients on potential risks and taking specific caution to minimise ovarian damage [14]. As for deep endometriosis, the decision to perform surgery should be guided by the presence or absence of pain symptoms, patient age and preferences, history of previous surgery, presence of other infertility factors, ovarian reserve, and estimated EFI [14].

13.6 Endometriosis Fertility Index

Surgical treatment in women trying to conceive is mostly only one step in their way to get pregnant. Decision on the way women are trying to conceive after surgery frequently depends on the insight of surgery together with other factors such as age and tubal function. In 2010, Adamson and Pasta developed the Endometriosis Fertility Index (EFI): an easy-to-use score, ranged from 0 to 10 points, to estimate the chance for a non-ART conception in women after endometriosis surgery, assuming normal gamete function. Historical and surgical factors together with description of ovaries, fallopian tubes, and fimbriae are giving a score predicting the chance to conceive on a natural way within a time period up to 36 months [43]. A recent meta-analysis verified the good performance of the EFI for predicting a non-ART pregnancy, further supporting its use as a tool in postoperative fertility counselling [44]. Its clinical validity is further strengthened by a good reproducibility between different users [45], as well as its ability in reducing health-care costs by optimising fertility treatment allocation [46]. In 2021, the use of the fertility index before surgery, estimated with clinical and ultrasound findings, and after surgery, as intended, were compared. An accurate estimation of the EFI by means of presurgical clinical data was shown [47]. Especially when discussing the option of first-line surgery versus direct ART for achieving a pregnancy in women with endometriosis, this non-intended use of the fertility index score can be useful, although this is the only study so far that has evaluated this aspect of the EFI.

References

1. Meuleman C, Vandenabeele B, Fieuws S, Spiessens C, Timmerman D, D'Hooghe T. High prevalence of endometriosis in infertile women with normal ovulation and normospermic partners. Fertil Steril. 2009;92(1):68–74.
2. Abbas S, Ihle P, Köster I, Schubert I. Prevalence and incidence of diagnosed endometriosis and risk of endometriosis in patients with endometriosis-related symptoms: findings from a statutory health insurance-based cohort in Germany. Eur J Obstet Gynecol Reprod Biol. 2012;160(1):79–83.
3. Tanbo T, Fedorcsak P. Endometriosis-associated infertility: aspects of pathophysiological mechanisms and treatment options. Acta Obstet Gynecol Scand. 2017;96(6):659–67.
4. de Ziegler D, Borghese B, Chapron C. Endometriosis and infertility: pathophysiology and management. Lancet. 2010;376(9742):730–8.
5. Wang XM, Ma ZY, Song N. Inflammatory cytokines IL-6, IL-10, IL-13, TNF-α and peritoneal fluid flora were associated with infertility in patients with endometriosis. Eur Rev Med Pharmacol Sci. 2018;22(9):2513–8.
6. Opøien HK, Fedorcsak P, Polec A, Stensen MH, Åbyholm T, Tanbo T. Do endometriomas induce an inflammatory reaction in nearby follicles? Hum Reprod. 2013;28(7):1837–45.
7. Marquardt RM, Kim TH, Shin JH, Jeong JW. Progesterone and estrogen signaling in the endometrium: what goes wrong in endometriosis? Int J Mol Sci. 2019;20(15):3822.
8. Cahill DJ, Hull MG. Pituitary-ovarian dysfunction and endometriosis. Hum Reprod Update. 2000;6(1):56–66.
9. Shebl O, Sifferlinger I, Habelsberger A, Oppelt P, Mayer RB, Petek E, Ebner T. Oocyte competence in in vitro fertilization and intracytoplasmic sperm injection patients suffering from endometriosis and its possible association with subsequent treatment outcome: a matched case-control study. Acta Obstet Gynecol Scand. 2017;96(6):736–44.
10. Orazov MR, Radzinsky VY, Ivanov II, Khamoshina MB, Shustova VB. Oocyte quality in women with infertility associated endometriosis. Gynecol Endocrinol. 2019;35(sup1):24–6.
11. Corachán A, Pellicer N, Pellicer A, Ferrero H. Novel therapeutic targets to improve IVF outcomes in endometriosis patients: a review and future prospects. Hum Reprod Update. 2021;27(5):923–72.
12. Pocate-Cheriet K, Santulli P, Kateb F, Bourdon M, Maignien C, Batteux F, Chouzenoux S, Patrat C, Wolf JP, Bertho G, Chapron C. The follicular fluid metabolome differs according to the endometriosis phenotype. Reprod Biomed Online. 2020;41(6):1023–37.

13. Leyendecker G, Kunz G, Wildt L, Beil D, Deininger H. Uterine hyperperistalsis and dysperistalsis as dysfunctions of the mechanism of rapid sperm transport in patients with endometriosis and infertility. Hum Reprod. 1996;11(7):1542–51.
14. ESHRE Guideline on Endometriosis. https://www.eshre.eu/Guidelines-and-Legal/Guidelines/Endometriosis-guideline
15. Matalliotaki C, Matalliotakis M, Ieromonachou P, Goulielmos GN, Zervou MI, Laliotis A, Spandidos DA, Arici A, Matalliotakis I. Co-existence of benign gynecological tumors with endometriosis in a group of 1,000 women. Oncol Lett. 2018;15(2):1529–32.
16. Nirgianakis K, Kalaitzopoulos DR, Kohl Schwartz AS, Spaanderman M, Kramer BW, Mueller MD, Mueller M. Fertility, pregnancy and neonatal outcomes of patients with adenomyosis: a systematic review and meta-analysis. Reprod Biomed Online. 2021;42(1):185–206.
17. Marcoux S, Maheux R, Bérubé S, the Canadian Collaborative Group on Endometriosis. Laparoscopic surgery in infertile women with minimal or mild endometriosis. N Engl J Med. 1997;337:217–22.
18. Parazzini F. Ablation of lesions or no treatment in minimal-mild endometriosis in infertile women: a randomized trial. Gruppo Italiano per lo Studio dell'Endometriosi. Hum Reprod. 1999;14:1332–4.
19. Bafort C, Beebeejaun Y, Tomassetti C, Bosteels J, Duffy JMN. Laparoscopic surgery for endometriosis. Cochrane Database Syst Rev. 2020;10:CD011031.
20. Gad M, Badroui M. Evidence-based therapy for infertility associated with early stage endometriosis. Int J Gyn Obstet. 2012;2012:S548.
21. Moini A, Bahar L, Ashrafinia M, Eslami B, Hosseini R, Ashrafinia N. Fertility outcome after operative laparoscopy versus no treatment in infertile women with minimal or mild endometriosis. Int J Fert Ster. 2012;5(4):235–40.
22. Hodgson RM, Lee HL, Wang R, Mol BW, Johnson N. Interventions for endometriosis-related infertility: a systematic review and network meta-analysis. Fertil Steril. 2020;113:374–283.e372.
23. ETIC Endometriosis Treatment Italian Club. When more is not better: 10 'don'ts' in endometriosis management. An ETIC* position statement. Hum Reprod Open. 2019;2019(3):hoz009.
24. Meuleman C, Tomassetti C, Van Cleynenbreugel B, Penninckx F, Vergote I, D'Hooghe T. Surgical treatment of deeply infiltrating endometriosis with colorectal involvement. Hum Reprod Update. 2011;17:311–26.
25. Vercellini P, Barbara G, Buggio L, Frattaruolo MP, Somigliana E, Fedele L. Effect of patient selection on estimate of reproductive success after surgery for rectovaginal endometriosis: literature review. Reprod Biomed Online. 2012;24:389–95.
26. Roman H, Chanavaz-Lacheray I, Ballester M, Bendifallah S, Touleimat S, Tuech J-J, Farella M, Merlot B. High postoperative fertility rate following surgical management of colorectal endometriosis. Human Reprod. 2018;33(9):1669–76.
27. Meuleman C, Tomassetti C, Wolthuis A, Van Cleynenbreugel B, Laenen A, Penninckx F, Vergote I, D'Hoore A, D'Hooghe T. Clinical outcome after radical excision of moderate-severe endometriosis with or without bowel resection and reanastomosis: a prospective cohort study. Ann Surg. 2014;259(3):522–31.
28. Daraï E, Cohen J, Ballester M. Colorectal endometriosis and fertility. Eur J Obstet Gynecol Reprod Biol. 2017;209:86–94.
29. Iversen ML, Seyer-Hansen M, Forman A. Does surgery for deep infiltrating bowel endometriosis improve fertility? A systematic review. Acta Obstet Gynecol Scand. 2017;96:688–93.
30. Breteau P, Chanavaz-Lacheray I, Rubod C, Turck M, Sanguin S, Pop I, Resch B, Roman H. Pregnancy rates after surgical treatment of deep infiltrating endometriosis in infertile patients with at least 2 previous in vitro fertilization or intracytoplasmic sperm injection failures. J Minim Invasive Gynecol. 2020;27:1148–57.
31. Streuli I, de Ziegler D, Gayet V, Santulli P, Bijaoui G, de Mouzon J, Chapron C. In women with endometriosis anti-Muüllerian hormone levels are decreased only in those with previous endometrioma surgery. Human Reprod. 2012;27(11):3294–303.

32. Uncu G, Kasapoglu I, Ozerkan K, Seyhan A, Oral Yilmaztepe A, Ata B. Prospective assessment of the impact of endometriomas and their removal on ovarian reserve and determinants of the rate of decline in ovarian reserve. Hum Reprod. 2013;28(8):2140–5.
33. Muzii L, Di Tucci C, Di Feliciantonio M, Marchetti C, Perniola G, Panici PB. The effect of surgery for endometrioma on ovarian reserve evaluated by antral follicle count: a systematic review and meta-analysis. Hum Reprod. 2014;29(10):2190–8.
34. Younis JS, Shapso N, Ben-Sira Y, Nelson SM, Izhaki I. Endometrioma surgery-a systematic review and meta-analysis of the effect on antral follicle count and anti-Müllerian hormone. Am J Obstet Gynecol. 2022;226(1):33–51.e7.
35. Muzii L, Achilli C, Lecce F, Bianchi A, Franceschetti S, Marchetti C, Perniola G, Panici PB. Second surgery for recurrent endometriomas is more harmful to healthy ovarian tissue and ovarian reserve than first surgery. Fertil Steril. 2015;103(3):738–43.
36. Candiani M, Ottolina J, Posadzka E, Ferrari S, Castellano LM, Tandoi I, Pagliardini L, Nocun A, Jach R. Assessment of ovarian reserve after cystectomy versus 'one-step' laser vaporization in the treatment of ovarian endometrioma: a small randomized clinical trial. Human Reprod. 2018;33(12):2205–11.
37. Candiani M, Ferrari S, Bartiromo L, Schimberni M, Tandoi I, Ottolina J. Fertility outcome after CO 2 laser vaporization versus cystectomy in women with ovarian endometrioma: a comparative study. J Minim Invasive Gynecol. 2021;28(1):34–41.
38. Carmona F, Martínez-Zamora MA, Rabanal A, Martínez-Román S, Balasch J. Ovarian cystectomy versus laser vaporization in the treatment of ovarian endometriomas: a randomized clinical trial with a five-year follow-up. Fertil Steril. 2011;96:251–4.
39. Benaglia L, Somigliana E, Vercellini P, Abbiati A, Ragni G, Fedele L. Endometriotic ovarian cysts negatively affect the rate of spontaneous ovulation. Hum Reprod. 2009;24(9):2183–6.
40. Leone Roberti Maggiore U, Scala C, Venturini PL, Remorgida V, Ferrero S. Endometriotic ovarian cysts do not negatively affect the rate of spontaneous ovulation. Hum Reprod. 2015;30(2):299–307.
41. Alborzi S, Zahiri Sorouri Z, Askari E, Poordast T, Chamanara K. The success of various endometrioma treatments in infertility: a systematic review and meta-analysis of prospective studies. Reprod Med Biol. 2019;18:312–22.
42. Dan H, Limin F. Laparoscopic ovarian cystectomy versus fenestration/coagulation or laser vaporization for the treatment of endometriomas: a meta-analysis of randomized controlled trials. Gynecol Obstet Investig. 2013;76:75–82.
43. Adamson GD, Pasta DJ. Endometriosis fertility index: the new, validated endometriosis staging system. Fertil Steril. 2010;94(5):1609–15.
44. Vesali S, Razavi M, Rezaeinejad M, Maleki-Hajiagha A, Maroufizadeh S, Sepidarkish M. Endometriosis fertility index for predicting non-assisted reproductive technology pregnancy after endometriosis surgery: a systematic review and meta-analysis. BJOG. 2020;127(7):800–9.
45. Tomassetti C, Bafort C, Meuleman C, Welkenhuysen M, Fieuws S, D'Hooghe T. Reproducibility of the endometriosis fertility index: a prospective inter-/intra-rater agreement study. BJOG. 2020;127(1):107–14.
46. Ferrier C, Boujenah J, Poncelet C, Chabbert-Buffet N, Mathieu D'Argent E, Carbillon L, Grynberg M, Darai E, Bendifallah S. Use of the EFI score in endometriosis-associated infertility: a cost-effectiveness study. Eur J Obstet Gynecol Reprod Biol. 2020;253:296–303.
47. Tomassetti C, Bafort C, Vanhie A, Meuleman C, Fieuws S, Welkenhuysen M, Timmerman D, Van Schoubroeck D, D'Hooghe T. Estimation of the endometriosis fertility index prior to operative laparoscopy. Hum Reprod. 2021;36(3):636–46.

Endometriosis in Reproductive Years: ART and Endometriosis

14

Graciela Kohls and Juan Antonio Garcia-Velasco

Contents

14.1 Introduction

Endometriosis is one of the most common gynecological disorders and is an estrogen-dependant condition characterized by endometrial tissue located outside of the uterus, most commonly on the ovaries and peritoneum.

G. Kohls (✉) · J. A. Garcia-Velasco
IVI Madrid, Rey Juan Carlos University, Madrid, Spain
e-mail: Graciela.Kohls@ivirma.com

E. Oral (ed.), *Endometriosis and Adenomyosis*,
https://doi.org/10.1007/978-3-030-97236-3_14

Reduced fertility and chronic pain are the two principal clinical features of endometriosis. Endometriosis is one of the main causes of infertility, although the actual relationship between both is unclear and poorly understood.

The association between severe and advanced endometriosis and reduced fertility may be explained through the severe anatomical and functional abnormalities caused by advanced endometriosis in the female pelvis. These patients also have significantly lower ovarian reserve markers, regardless of previous ovarian surgery. The possibility that minimal or mild endometriosis may cause infertility is still a matter of debate.

14.2 Epidemiology

The true prevalence of endometriosis is uncertain because definitive diagnosis requires surgical visualization and histological confirmation, but it is estimated in around 10% in women of reproductive age [1]. In large studies the prevalence of endometriosis in fertile women appears to be lower (0.5–5%), whereas in infertile women it is higher (25–40%) [1]. Moreover, the rate of infertility has been reported to be six to eight times higher in patients with endometriosis [1].

14.3 Diagnosis Delay

Endometriosis is a chronic and, in most cases, debilitating disease associated with a significant reduction of quality of life due to pain symptoms and/or infertility. In addition, several lines of evidence indicate that a significant number of women with endometriosis do develop comorbidities, such as depressive or anxiety disorders. Delaying the diagnosis of endometriosis clearly aggravates these problems [2]. Early detection is of significant importance because many complications of this chronic disease, such as infertility, may be reversed or treated earlier and for counseling fertility preservation.

Several studies have demonstrated that the length of the time interval from onset of symptoms to diagnosis is surprisingly long and it could be around 3–11 years [2–6] (Table 14.1).

Table 14.1 Diagnosis delay

	Diagnosis delay (years)
USA [3–5]	11.7
UK [3–5]	7.9
Brazil [6]	7
China [5]	3.3
Italy [5]	10.7
Germany and Austria [2]	10.4
UK and Spain [4, 5]	6.7
Norway [4]	6.7
Ireland and Belgium [5]	4–5

Several factors cause the delay of the diagnosis like nonspecific symptoms, widespread use of oral contraceptives that attenuate the symptoms, misdiagnosis, the normalization of menstrual pain, clinical examinations that are nondiscriminatory without transvaginal sonography (TVS), lack of sensitive and specific biomarkers, etc.

14.4 Pathogenesis and Pathophysiology

The pathogenesis and pathophysiological characteristics of pelvic endometriosis are complex. Potential origins of the endometriotic lesions include transplantation of endometrial tissue through retrograde menstruation and in situ coelomic metaplasia of the peritoneal lining. Vascular or lymphatic metastasis most likely occurs only rarely, in cases of extrapelvic lesions. Superficial and deep endometriotic lesions are established and maintained through interacting molecular mechanisms that promote cellular adhesion and proliferation, systemic and localized steroidogenesis, localized inflammatory response and immune dysregulation, and vascularization and innervation [7].

Since retrograde menstruation is common, other factors must determine the ability of endometrial cells to adhere to peritoneal surfaces, proliferate, and develop into endometriotic lesions. Local natural-killer-cell activity is impaired in women with endometriosis, which may contribute to immune evasion of endometrial cells. Endometrial stem-cell and progenitor-cell populations are present in eutopic endometrium, which, if shed in retrograde menstruation, may play a role in the development of endometriotic lesions [7].

The complex endocrine and proinflammatory microenvironment in and surrounding endometriotic lesions promotes their proliferation and vascularization but also nociception. The endometrium and endometriotic lesions contain nerve fibers stimulated by inflammatory mediators. The ascending nociceptive signals received in the central nervous system can lead to heightened responsiveness of nociceptive neurons to normal or subthreshold afferent input (central sensitization) and alterations in pain processing [7].

14.5 Risk Factors

Risk factors for endometriosis include obstruction of menstrual outflow (e.g., anatomic anomalies), exposure to drugs (diethylstilbestrol) in utero, prolonged exposure to endogenous estrogen (early menarche, late menopause), short and heavy menstrual cycles, low birth weight, and exposure to endocrine-disrupting chemicals found in various materials such as pesticides, metals, additives or contaminants in food, and personal care products. Twin and family studies suggest a genetic component. Consumption of red meat and trans fats is associated with an increased risk of laparoscopically confirmed endometriosis, and eating fruits, green vegetables, and omega-3 is associated with a decreased risk. Prolonged lactation and multiple pregnancies are protective. Endometriosis is associated with increased risks of autoimmune diseases and ovarian endometrioid and clear-cell cancers, as well as other cancers, including non-Hodgkin's lymphoma, thyroid cancer, and melanoma [7, 8].

14.6 Relationship Between Endometriosis and Infertility

The monthly pregnancy rate in women in their mid-reproductive years without endometriosis is around 30%, whereas in those with endometriosis, it is between only 2% and 10% [9]. This reduced pregnancy rate may even apply to women with minimal endometriosis.

The epidemiological association between endometriosis and low fertility may indicate a causal relationship (Fig. 14.1), explained by several hypotheses:

- Disorders of ovulation and fertilization, reduced quality of the oocyte and embryo, and dysfunctional implantation.
- Immunological and inflammatory disorders of the peritoneal environment.
- Tubal occlusion.
- Disorders of endometrial receptivity, for example, due to insufficient hormonal stimulation and progesterone resistance.

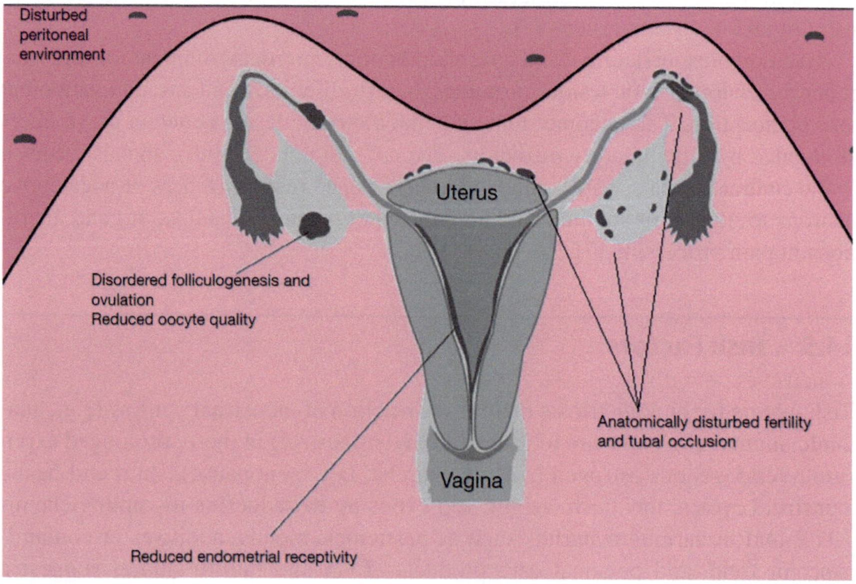

Fig. 14.1 Mechanisms that may link endometriosis with infertility

14.7 Diagnosis of Endometriosis

- *Symptoms:* Many symptoms are associated with endometriosis, ranging from pelvic and intestinal complaints to referred pain. The clinician should always suspect endometriosis when any of the following signs are reported by women of reproductive age:
  - Pelvic symptoms: Pelvic pain typically associated with endometriosis is often intramenstrual (dysmenorrhea) and progressive and of variable intensity. Painful sexual intercourse (dyspareunia), abdominal cramping, noncyclical pelvic pain, infertility, fatigue, and weariness are also symptoms of endometriosis.
  - Intestinal complaints: Periodic bloating, diarrhea/constipation, painful defecation (dyschezia), rectal bleeding.
  - Urinary symptoms: Pain (dysuria) and/or bleeding (hematuria) when urinating.
  - Referred pain to legs, back, and shoulder.

Measuring pain is not easy, but questionnaires and quality-of-life scales may be utilized to assess the impact of pain and treatment response.

- *Clinical examination:* A clinical examination may indicate endometriosis on the basis of pelvic adhesions that limit movement or cause pain during uterine or ovarian manipulation, ovarian cysts, or palpable nodules.

As an important reminder, clinical examination may be inappropriate in some patients (adolescents, sexual abuse victims, certain religious beliefs) and could be very painful in some women. Rectal examination may be of help in some of these situations.

The evidence in the medical literature is weak for diagnosing pelvic endometriosis with physical examination. Ultrasound and magnetic resonance imaging (MRI) technologies are more accurate at diagnosing ovarian and/or deep endometriosis.

- *Ultrasonography:* Transvaginal ultrasound is not useful in the early stage of endometriosis but remains the best technique for diagnosing ovarian cystic endometriosis, and it's useful for identifying and ruling out rectal endometriosis but should be performed by clinicians that are highly experienced.
- *Magnetic resonance imaging (MRI):* This is the most appropriate technique for the diagnosis of deep endometriosis, such as rectovaginal, bladder, and ureteral forms. Laparoscopy may have blind spots and this is where MRI can have a key role. MRI can help to visualize those areas that may have escaped the laparoscopic field of view. Such areas include the retroperitoneal space or lesions obscured by dense adhesions. MRI may also be helpful to assess response to treatment and the recurrence of disease.

- *Laparoscopy:* Visualization of the lesions outside the uterine cavity during the laparoscopy and histological verification of endometrial glands is the gold standard diagnostic test for endometriosis.

Controversy exists concerning whether laparoscopy should be performed in all patients when endometriosis is suspected. It could be argued that empirical treatment can be started without a definitive diagnosis, especially in young women or those who are not in need of diagnosis confirmation. Many women will not want to go through surgery if medical treatment relieves the pain [10]. Conversely, arguments to perform a laparoscopy include the patient's wish to have a definitive diagnosis or advanced disease [11].

In cases of infertility and ovarian endometriosis, laparoscopy should be approached with caution for the procedure may change from a diagnostic tool into an operative event. Surgery, especially before ART treatment, should be envisioned only in specific circumstances [12].

14.8 Biomarkers

By definition, a biomarker is a characteristic that is objectively measured and evaluated as an indicator of normal biological processes, pathogenic processes, or pharmacological responses to a therapeutic intervention. Many studies have focused on identifying biomarkers on blood or urine samples.

According to the ESHRE guideline, clinicians are recommended not to use peripheral biomarkers, including CA-125, in plasma, urine, or serum and/or biomarkers in endometrial tissue or menstrual or uterine fluids to diagnose endometriosis [13]. None of the available biomarkers consistently met the criteria for a replacement or triage diagnostic test either for detecting pelvic endometriosis or for differentiating ovarian endometrioma from other benign ovarian masses [14].

14.9 Classification of Endometriosis

Presentations of endometriosis range from superficial peritoneal lesions of varying color to cysts in the ovaries to deep endometriosis (nodules with a depth of penetration exceeding 5 mm often accompanied by fibrosis and adhesions) to extrapelvic lesions.

The most widely accepted endometriosis classification system is that of the American Society for Reproductive Medicine (ASRM). The scoring is used to determine the stages: I or minimal disease, II or mild, III or moderate, and IV or severe disease. This system is based on the location, extent, depth of invasion, and aspect of the lesions seen at the laparoscopy. The scoring assigned to each type of lesion is arbitrary and is currently not considered to be properly correlated to the symptoms, activity of the disorder, or treatment response but is useful in determining disease burden and management.

14.10 Differential Diagnosis of Endometriosis

Different conditions of the reproductive tract can cause chronic pelvic pain such as adenomyosis, pelvic adhesions, pelvic inflammatory disease, congenital anomalies of the reproductive tract, and ovarian or tubal masses. It may also be related to other non-gynecologic conditions such as irritable bowel syndrome, interstitial cystitis, fibromyalgia, and other musculoskeletal disorders. A pelvic evaluation should be carried out in order to exclude other causes of pain and specially in those women that have not responded with conventional therapy.

14.11 Treatment of Infertility Associated with Endometriosis

14.11.1 Medical Treatment

Temporary suppression of ovarian function using antigonadotropic agents is one treatment option for endometriosis-associated pain. However, none has demonstrated any efficacy in the restoration of fertility in infertile patients with endometriosis. The European Society of Human Reproduction and Embryology's *ESHRE guideline for the diagnosis and treatment of endometriosis* [13] states that the suppression of ovarian function to improve fertility in patients with minimal or mild endometriosis is not effective and should not be offered for this indication alone [13, 15]. There is no evidence of its possible efficacy in more advanced stages of the disorder either.

Regarding IVF, a Cochrane review based on a meta-analysis of 640 patients failed to find a benefit with GnRH agonist pretreatment before IVF compared with no pretreatment [16].

14.11.2 Surgical Treatment

The overall objective of surgery is to excise or coagulate the peritoneal lesions, ovarian cysts, areas of deep endometriosis, and adhesions. Laparoscopy is the safest and most effective technique. This procedure, although clearly indicated for the surgical treatment of pain caused by endometriosis, is more questionable for the treatment of infertility. Moderate and severe endometriosis may produce such distortion of the pelvis that restoration of the anatomy may be surgically impossible. Moreover, radical surgery that seeks to remove all endometriotic lesions may be detrimental to the ovarian functional reserve, which is already compromised by the endometriosis itself [13].

Contrary to the ESHRE guideline, a recent systematic review and meta-analysis concludes that operative laparoscopy may improve overall pain levels but may have little or no difference with respect to fertility-related or adverse outcomes when compared with diagnostic laparoscopy [13, 17].

There is also no consensus on the indications for surgical treatment of endometriotic cysts in infertile patients undergoing assisted reproduction because it could reduce the ovarian reserve and the effectiveness of that treatment. Large RCTs are lacking but may be now considered ethically questionable. In fact, according to the results of systematic literature reviews, surgical excision of endometriomas before IVF is associated with a need for higher amounts of gonadotrophins, lower peripheral estrogen levels, reduced number of follicles, and lower number of oocytes retrieved, but has no effect on the chances of pregnancy [18, 19]. Excision of small endometriomas before IVF is particularly discouraged in case of repetitive surgery or bilateral cysts. However, surgery remains mandatory in the presence of non-reassuring sonographic findings and can be considered in women with moderate to severe pelvic pain [14].

The diameter threshold for performing an operation before IVF should be adjusted according to the endometrioma location within the ovary. All decisions to operate a cyst beyond 3 or 4 cm are arbitrary, as there is no evidence to support one or the other. Surgeons should bear in mind that if all healthy growing follicles may be reached without damaging the endometrioma, cyst over 4 or even 5 cm do not require surgery in asymptomatic patients; however, smaller cysts that hide growing follicles, specially when the ovary is fixed, may require intervention [12].

14.11.3 Combined Medical and Surgical Treatment

It has been proposed that preoperative administration of drugs effective at controlling endometriosis could increase the beneficial effect of surgical treatment on fertility. Medical treatment could facilitate excision while reducing the surgical trauma, the duration of surgery, the formation of postoperative adhesions, and the probability of subsequent recurrence. However, there is no proof that these treatments increase fertility after surgery to a greater extent than surgery alone; therefore their use is not recommended.

Postoperative medical treatment has the advantages of encouraging the involution of residual lesions following surgery and reducing the risk of spreading the disorder associated with intraoperative rupture of endometriomas. However, studies assessing the effect of postoperative treatment on fertility have found no additional benefits to those achieved by surgery alone [20]. The ESHRE guideline therefore concludes that postoperative medical treatment offers no advantages in relation to surgical treatment.

14.11.4 Intrauterine Insemination (IUI)

The presence of endometriosis is thought to reduce the effectiveness of IUI, based on the results of studies in patients treated with artificial insemination using donor semen [21]. This negative effect persists even after the treatment of endometriosis [22]. Several randomized studies show that IUI associated with pharmacological stimulation increases fertility in patients with minimal to mild endometriosis in comparison with expectant management. IUI with ovarian stimulation is effective, but the role of unstimulated IUI is uncertain [23].

Women with stage I–II endometriosis may benefit from IUI, while those with stage III–IV endometriosis and tubal factor have the lowest IUI pregnancy rates and thus may benefit less from insemination. Overall, first-cycle chance of pregnancy with IVF is significantly higher than the cumulative pregnancy rate that can be obtained after six IUI cycles [24]. These results illustrate the significant impact of advanced endometriosis on pregnancy outcomes and suggest that providers may consider IVF over IUI for patients with advanced endometriosis [25].

14.11.5 In Vitro Fertilization (IVF)

IVF is an appropriate treatment for patients who have advanced endometriosis with reduced ovarian reserve, or if tubal function is compromised or if there is male factor infertility or advanced maternal age, and/or other treatments have failed. IVF is the only viable method in cases of severe tubal adhesion-related disease or in the presence of large endometriomas. A study concluded that patients with endometriosis-associated infertility have pregnancy rates and birth rates similar to tubal factor controls during IVF treatments. The exception is women with endometriomas, who have lower success rates compared with peritoneal endometriosis and tubal infertility [26].

Women with endometrioma have a lower mean number of oocyte retrieved and require higher FSH dosage for ovarian stimulation, suggesting that their ovarian reserve is diminished prior to IVF. Women with endometriomas should be counseled regarding their increased risk of cycle cancellation [27].

When analyzing the impact of endometriosis on uterine environment, there was no difference in pregnancy rates between women with endometriosis and tubal factor receiving donor oocytes, suggesting that endometriosis is not detrimental to embryo implantation [28, 29]. A study demonstrated that the endometrial receptivity gene signature during the window of implantation is similar in infertile women with and without endometriosis, also for different stages of endometriosis [30].

Another relevant aspect is whether patients with ovarian endometriosis who are scheduled for IVF would benefit from prior excision of the endometriomas. The chosen procedure should consider the specific condition of each patient, taking into account the likelihood of contributing to ovarian failure through intraoperative destruction of normal tissue, especially in previously operated patients [12]. While surgery did not seem to influence the live birth rate, surgical treatment of endometrioma prior to IVF could exert a further detrimental impact on ovarian reserve. There is therefore not one dogmatic recommendation as to whether women with endometrioma should or should not have surgical intervention prior to IVF and shared and informed decision with the patient is mandatory [31, 32].

In summary, there is no evidence that surgical treatment of endometriosis improves ovarian function or enhances the possibility of successful IVF. Based on current evidence, consideration should be given to individualize the care of these patients [31].

14.12 Conclusions

IVF is the most appropriate treatment for infertility, especially if there are coexisting causes for the infertility and/or other treatments have failed.

Unfortunately, IVF pregnancy rates are lower in women with endometriomas and diminished ovarian reserve. Surgical removal of ovarian endometriotic cysts prior to IVF does not offer any additional benefit in terms of fertility outcomes, and we should take into account that it could reduce even more the ovarian reserve.

References

1. Ozkan S, Murk W, Arici A. Endometriosis and infertility: epidemiology and evidence-based treatments. Ann N Y Acad Sci. 2008;1127:92–100.
2. Hudelist G, Fritzer N, Thomas A, Niehues C, Oppelt P, Haas D, et al. Diagnostic delay for endometriosis in Austria and Germany: causes and possible consequences. Hum Reprod. 2012;27:3412–6.
3. Hadfield R, Mardon H, Barlow D, Kennedy S. Delay in the diagnosis of endometriosis: a survey of women from the USA and the UK. Hum Reprod. 1996;11:878–80.
4. Ballard K, Lowton K, Wright J. What's the delay? A qualitative study of women's experiences of reaching a diagnosis of endometriosis. Fertil Steril. 2006;86:1296–301.
5. Nnoaham KE, Hummelshoj L, Webster P, D'Hooghe T, de Cicco NF, de Cicco NC, et al. Impact of endometriosis on quality of life and work productivity: a multicenter study across ten countries. Fertil Steril. 2011;96:366–73.
6. Arruda MS. Time elapsed from onset of symptoms to diagnosis of endometriosis in a cohort study of Brazilian women. Hum Reprod. 2003;18:756–9.
7. Zondervan KT, Becker CM, Missmer SA. Endometriosis. N Engl J Med. 2020;382:1244–56.
8. Giudice LC. Endometriosis. N Engl J Med. 2010;362:2389–98.
9. The Practice Committee of the American Society for Reproductive Medicine. Endometriosis and infertility. Fertil Steril. 2004;81:1441–6.
10. Kennedy S. Should a diagnosis of endometriosis be sought in all symptomatic women? Fertil Steril. 2006;86:1312–3.
11. de la Fuente JAGV G. Endometriosis and infertility, Gynaecol Forum. 2010;15:8–12.
12. Garcia-Velasco JA, Somigliana E. Management of endometriomas in women requiring IVF: to touch or not to touch. Hum Reprod. 2009;24:496–501.
13. Dunselman GAJJ, Vermeulen N, Becker C, Calhaz-Jorge C, D'Hooghe T, De Bie B, et al. ESHRE guideline: management of women with endometriosis. Hum Reprod. 2014;29:400–12.
14. When more is not better: 10 "don'ts" in endometriosis management. An ETIC position statement. ETIC Endometriosis Treatment Italian Club. Hum Reprod Open. 2019;3:1–15.
15. Hughes E, Brown J, Collins JJ, Farquhar C, Fedorkow DM, Vandekerckhove P. Ovulation suppression for endometriosis. Cochrane Database Syst Rev. 2007;3:CD000155.
16. Georgiou EX, Melo P, Baker PE, Sallam HN, Arici A, Garcia-Velasco JA, et al. Long-term GnRH agonist therapy before in vitro fertilisation (IVF) for improving fertility outcomes in women with endometriosis. Cochrane Database Syst Rev. 2019;11:CD013240.
17. Leonardi M, Gibbons T, Armour M, Wang R, Glanville E, Hodgson R, et al. When to do surgery and when not to do surgery for endometriosis: a systematic review and meta-analysis. J Minim Invasive Gynecol. 2020;27:390–407.
18. Demirol A, Guven S, Baykal C, Gurgan T. Effect of endometrioma cystectomy on IVF outcome: a prospective randomized study. Reprod Biomed Online. 2006;12:639–43.

19. Garcia-Velasco JA, Mahutte NG, Corona J, Zúñiga V, Gilés J, Arici A, et al. Removal of endometriomas before in vitro fertilization does not improve fertility outcomes: a matched, case–control study. Fertil Steril. 2004;81:1194–7.
20. Yap C, Furness S, Farquhar C. Pre and post operative medical therapy for endometriosis surgery. Cochrane Database Syst Rev. 2004;3:CD003678.
21. Jansen R. Minimal endometriosis and reduced fecundability: prospective evidence from an artificial insemination by donor program. Fertil Steril. 1986;46:141–3.
22. Toma SK, Stovall DW, Hammond MG. The effect of laparoscopic ablation or danocrine on pregnancy rates in patients with stage I or II endometriosis undergoing donor insemination. Obstet Gynecol. 1992;80:253–6.
23. Tummon IS, Asher LJ, Martin JSB, Tulandi T. Randomized controlled trial of superovulation and insemination for infertility associated with minimal or mild endometriosis. Fertil Steril. 1997;68:8–12.
24. Dmowski WP, Pry M, Ding J, Rana N. Cycle-specific and cumulative fecundity in patients with endometriosis who are undergoing controlled ovarian hyperstimulation-intrauterine insemination or in vitro fertilization-embryo transfer. Fertil Steril. 2002;78:750–6.
25. Starosta A, Gordon CE, Hornstein MD. Predictive factors for intrauterine insemination outcomes: a review. Fertil Res Pract. 2020;6:23.
26. Opøien HK, Fedorcsak P, Omland AK, Abyholm T, Bjercke S, Ertzeid G, et al. In vitro fertilization is a successful treatment in endometriosis-associated infertility. Fertil Steril. 2012;97:912–8.
27. Senapati S, Sammel MD, Morse C, Barnhart KT. Impact of endometriosis on in vitro fertilization outcomes: an evaluation of the Society for Assisted Reproductive Technologies Database. Fertil Steril. 2016;106:164–71.
28. Simón C, Gutiérrez A, Vidal A, de los Santos MJ, Tarín JJ, Remohí J, et al. Outcome of patients with endometriosis in assisted reproduction: results from in-vitro fertilization and oocyte donation. Hum Reprod. 1994;9:725–9.
29. Díaz I, Navarro J, Blasco L, Simón C, Pellicer A, Remohí J, et al. Impact of stage III–IV endometriosis on recipients of sibling oocytes: matched case-control study. Fertil Steril. 2000;74:31–4.
30. Garcia-Velasco JA, Fassbender A, Ruiz-Alonso M, Blesa D, Dhooghe T, Simon C, et al. Is endometrial receptivity transcriptomics affected in women with endometriosis? A pilot study. Reprod Biomed Online. 2015;31:647–54.
31. Hamdan M, Dunselman G, Li TCC, Cheong Y. The impact of endometrioma on IVF/ICSI outcomes: a systematic review and meta-analysis. Hum Reprod Update. 2015;21:809–25.
32. Lessey BA, Gordts S, Donnez O, Somigliana E, Chapron C, Garcia-Velasco JA, et al. Ovarian endometriosis and infertility: in vitro fertilization (IVF) or surgery as the first approach? Fertil Steril. 2018;110:1218–26.

Endometriosis in Reproductive Years: The Origin of Pain in Endometriosis and Adenomyosis

15

Sylvia Mechsner

Contents

15.1 Pathogenesis of Endometriotic Lesions

Endometriosis (EM) is a condition that is defined by endometrial-like lesions that occur outside the uterine cavity. Primarily, the disease was described as ectopic lesions on the peritoneum of the internal genital organs (endometriosis genitalis externa); lately it also comprises an emigration of endometriotic lesions into the myometrium (endometriosis genitalis interna = adenomyosis uteri (AM)). The high coincidence of these two endometriosis subtypes may arise in one common pathogenesis [1].

The "tissue injury and repair theory", by G. Leyendecker, describes the uterus as the origin of the disease. Uterine hyperperistalsis cause micro traumatization in the junctional zone (JZ), released mediators induce additional aromatase expression,

S. Mechsner (✉)
Department of Gynecology, Endometriosis Unit Charité, Charité – University Hospital Berlin, Berlin, Germany
e-mail: sylvia.mechsner@charite.de

E. Oral (ed.), *Endometriosis and Adenomyosis*,
https://doi.org/10.1007/978-3-030-97236-3_15

and the locally released oestrogen promotes proliferation and angiogenesis. This leads to changes within the JZ that can be seen sonographically as an echo-poor hem (halo phenomenon) that represents the attachment of the endometrium; in 3D ultrasound a variability of forms becomes visible [2, 3]. A new term, *archimetriosis*, describes these early changes [4]. Locally released oxytocin in turn strengthens local peristalsis and thus initiates a cycle that leads to an increasing destruction of the JZ. Presumably, within the processes of mechanical alteration and wound healing, stem cells are activated, which then leave their niche and either enter the abdominal cavity through retrograde menstruation and there cause EM or infiltrate into the myometrium and lead to AM [5, 6]. In this context of endometrial-myometrial interface disruption (EMID), an upregulation of HIF-1a (hypoxia-inducible factor 1-alpha) is likely, thereby triggering hypoxia-related molecular biological mechanisms that could also be involved in the establishment of the lesions [7]. With these ectopic lesions, extensive immunological changes occur. Extensive inflammatory reactions and multiple immunological changes are detectable in both the peritoneum and the peritoneal fluid [8]. These immunological findings are strongly associated with the occurrence of corresponding lesions, and chronic inflammation plays an increasing role within the pathophysiological theories. In line is the fact that the ectopic EML, no matter where they are located (peritoneal lesion, endometrium at the ovaries or DIE or in extragenital manifestation in the navel, the abdominal wall or the groin), consist not only of epithelial and stromal cells but also of smooth muscle cells. They all express oxytocin and vasopressin receptors as well as oestrogen and progesterone receptors [9, 10]. Therefore, these lesions not only are endometrial-like settlements but *miniature uteri*. Endometriotic lesions are always associated with surrounding fibrotic changes. It remains unclear if the surrounding tissue or the lesions themselves trigger these changes.

So a composition of uterine-like tissue (epithelial, stromal as well as smooth muscle cells) in a different variety of growth patterns (superficial or deep infiltrating), localized on different anatomical positions (intra- and extragenital) often accompanied by inflammation and fibrosis, is the root for a couple of problems.

15.2 Pathophysiologic Origin of Pain

In addition to the development of the various lesions, the effects of these are also important to understand the origin of pain. EM is a chronic disease. It recurs after surgical removal and leads to persistent treatment needs in 50% of affected cases [11]. Pain and infertility are the central problems of our patients.

15.2.1 Endometriosis-Associated Pain

The typical complaints caused by EM, such as severe dysmenorrhea, cyclic and acyclic lower abdominal pain (UBS), cyclic dysuria, dyschezia, dyspareunia as well as infertility, are well known, and yet the disease is diagnosed on average only

Table 15.1 Endometriosis related symptoms (modified from Greene et al. [12])

Typical symptoms	Unspecific symptoms
Pain	Unspecific bladder disorder
Dysmenorrhea	Unspecific bowel dysfuntion
Cyclic pelvic pain	Bloating (endobelly)
Acyclic chronic pelvic pain	Spotting, high menstrual bleeding
Dyspareunia	Vegetative concomitants: vomiting, emesis, cyclical diarrhoea, gastric disorders
Cyclic dyschezia	Headache, dizziness
Cyclic dysuria	Painful ovulation (Mittelschmerz)
Other cyclical symptoms like shoulder or umbilical pain	Irregular pelvic pain
	Lower back pain
	Pain emission in the legs
	Chronic fatique
	All symptoms together
Infertility	

10 years after the onset of the symptoms. In addition to EM-specific symptoms, non-specific complaints (Table 15.1) may lead to consultations of various medical disciplines [12]. Why are the complaints so difficult to assess and to integrate into a diagnosis of EM, and why should an early diagnosis not be feasible? After all, more than 60% of those diagnosed with EM report that the complaints started before the age of 20 [13]. There is a clear correlation between the duration and the intensity of the complaints and to the extent of the EM [13]. In this context, evolutionary aspects of endometriosis are important [4]. It is discussed that in the past young women with good uterine contractility fell pregnant easily and had a better birth outcome and thus a survival advantage. Because pregnancies and breastfeeding followed each other repeatedly in the past, there was no formation of EM/AM or at least to a lesser extent. Today, however, the primigravidas are in their 30s. Thus, women with primary dysmenorrhea and with uterine hyperperistalsis are at risk of developing archimetriosis followed by EM/AM. Therefore, the uterus has one to two decades to turn an inherently good functionality into a self-destructive force before reproduction is aspired [4].

Caused by the slow development of the disease associated with the late diagnosis, the patients develop complex complaints. Knowledge of nature and distribution of possible formations allows a better understanding of the possible effects. In general, all lesions can cause various symptoms (Fig. 15.1). Complaints usually appear in combinations; isolated symptoms are rather rare. Typical is the combination of cyclic lower abdominal pain/dysmenorrhea and dyspareunia. Depending on where the lesions are located, somatic (peritoneum, pelvic wall) or visceral (uterus, bladder or intestine) pain occurs. These two pain characteristics differ: visceral pain is dull and spasm-like, radiate, visceral organs interact with each other, so that bladder pain can be hardly distinguished to uterine-induced pain. In addition, the autonomous, visceral innervation interacts with the visceral sensory neurons that pass through the autonomous ganglia. So in severe pain also, vegetative reactions such as nausea, vomiting, collapse tendency and above all cyclic menstrual-associated

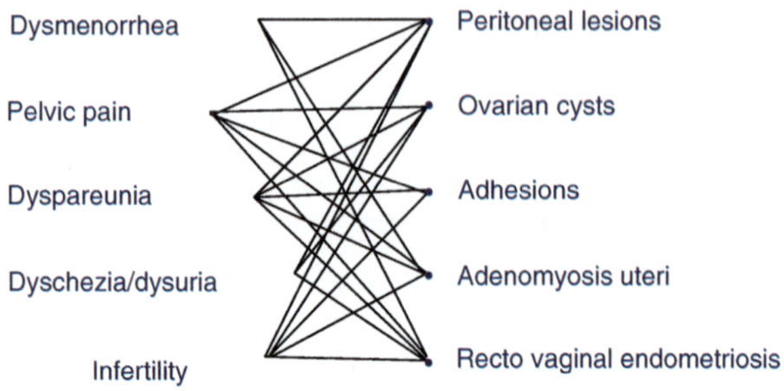

Fig. 15.1 Endometriosis-associated symptoms in correlation to the localisation of the lesions

diarrhoea are common [14]. Somatic pain, on the other hand, is rather pointed/sharp and point-shaped. Due to the high density of sensitive nerve fibres in the parietal peritoneum, they can be located more specifically.

15.3 Principles of Pain Development

A biochemical signal is needed (1), which is converted into a neural signal (2) (sensitization of pain nerve fibres via activation of the nociceptors). At the spinal level, this signal is modulated (3) and it is referred (attenuated/amplified) to the brain, where the pain perception occurs (4). Steps 1 and 2 are called peripheral and steps 3 and 4 central sensitization. Disorders of pain perception can occur at all levels.

15.3.1 Pathogenesis of Specific Forms of Pain

Dysmenorrhea and cyclic lower abdominal pain caused by peritoneal lesions can initially be understood as nociceptive inflammatory pain. There is a cyclic release of pain and inflammatory mediators. These activate visceral and peritoneal nerve fibres and lead to pain sensitivity. Inflammation and cell damage cause the pain and it disappears as the reaction subsides. This form of pain is well manageable via non-steroidal anti-inflammatory drugs (NSAIDs). Moreover, with the initiation of hormonal therapy and therapeutic amenorrhea, since then the cycle-related release of the mediators does not take place, the pain may completely disappear. Typical in AM-related dysmenorrhea is that even withdrawal bleeding under hormonal therapy with combined oral contraceptives (COC) in cyclical mode can still be painful. The mechanisms are not well understood, but it is likely that the primary disorders of the uterine layers with hyperperistalsis still result in the release of pain mediators and thus in the activation of pain fibres. Note: Persistent strong painful withdrawal bleeding under OC is to be seen as a warning! If the disease progresses, with the development of DIE (vaginal, intestinal or bladder infiltration), cyclical symptoms may also occur. In the case of rectovaginal EM, dyschezia typically occurs due to the proximity to the intestine or due to bowel infiltration. Caused by the cyclical swelling of the foci, there may also be cramp-like pain before bowel movement, stool irregularities and even cyclical subileus. Constipation followed by diarrhoea, paradoxical, or even pencil stools may occur. To look for these specific findings may help to identify a potential stenosis. A stenosis can affect the rectum, sigmoid or even the caecal pole region. If the EML infiltrates completely through the entire intestinal wall, cyclical hematochezia may occur. In addition, due to the localization of the lesion, acyclical dyspareunia is common; hence the nodes are hyperinnervated and painful when pressure is applied [15]. Bladder endometriosis typically leads to cyclical dysuria but may also cause unspecific symptoms such as pollakiuria and/or pain after voiding the bladder. Only if the bladder wall is completely infiltrated and the urothel is affected cyclical haematuria occurs.

15.3.2 Neurogenic Inflammation

Some patients develop acyclic lower abdominal pain under hormonal therapy (with and without therapeutic amenorrhea). This is an important indication that EML develops mechanisms that can be active independently of hormones. Extensive analyses have been performed regarding the innervation of these lesions [16]. Peritoneal lesions show hyperinnervation of sensitive but loss of sympathetic nerve fibres. In analogy to rheumatism research, an imbalance in the release of pro-inflammatory and anti-inflammatory sympathetic neurotransmitters seems to occur. The consequence of this imbalance may result in a neurogenic inflammation and may lead to acyclic pains. In DIE lesions, this phenomenon is known too. Therefore, especially the hormone therapy-resistant pain is important in order to adjust therapy decisions accordingly. A further complicating factor may be adhesion-related pain, which can be both somatic and visceral. The transition from initially cyclic to acyclic lower abdominal pain is characteristic.

Due to the chronic pain, patients often develop reactive depression and somatoform pain disorders, which make the clinical picture appear even more complex. Besides EM, the most important differential diagnoses of chronic lower abdominal pains are postoperative adhesions (non-EM-related), interstitial cystitis and non-specific intestinal dysfunction, the irritable colon. It is known that there is not necessarily a correlation between the extent of EM and pain intensity [14]. Therefore – and this is certainly the most difficult phenomenon for physicians to understand in the case of EM – even “inconspicuous” examination findings can cause severe pain, and conversely, patients with complex EM can be largely free of pain.

15.3.3 Development of Central Sensitization with Spinal Hyperalgesia

Physiologically, pain is a warning signal. If pain is ignored, it may increase. Moreover, pain is an individual event; the perception of pain is subjective. If severe dysmenorrhea (menstrual pain that leads to bedriddenness and incapacity to go to school or to work without the use of analgesics) remains untreated, i.e. it recurs monthly, this pain is initially perceived as nociceptive pain as described above, which also subsides as the release of the inflammatory and pain mediators decreases. If this pain occurs repeatedly, however, the body's own warning signals take effect, the pain is classified as threatening, and the modulation on the spinal level does not regulate it down, but rather increases it. At the spinal level, the release of neurotransmitters is altered and a number of modulating mechanisms are set in motion; the nociceptive field is expanded; and dysuria and/or dyschezia may occur [17]. This leads to spinal hyperalgesia with a lowered pain threshold and the perception of pain even with slight stimuli such as touch. Increasing pain frightens patients and makes pain processing more difficult. Severe cramps with pain, also accompanied by a vegetative reaction, also lead to the patient adopting a relieving posture, which is used to seek pain relief. Reactively, this leads to a reflex contraction of the pelvic floor muscles and thus to pelvic floor dysfunction, which increases the pain and can lead to dyspareunia [18]. If these tensions persist, dyspareunia develops and intensifies. Fear of pain during intercourse can strongly influence the ability to relax, and a disorder manifests itself, which takes on ever-greater proportions and no longer causes problems only cyclically, but increasingly manifests itself permanently. This phenomenon explains the often-severe pain that accompanies patients, even in the absence of pathological findings. It is essential to offer the patient pain-relief therapy. There is a correlation between the duration of pain and the occurrence of reactive depression, because patients are increasingly desperate and look for advice and help, but are often not understood [19] Fig. 15.2 illustrates the process of spinal hyperalgesia. Changes at central level develop. Functional MRI assessment demonstrates the first morphological adjustments of the brain after a pain latency of 2 years

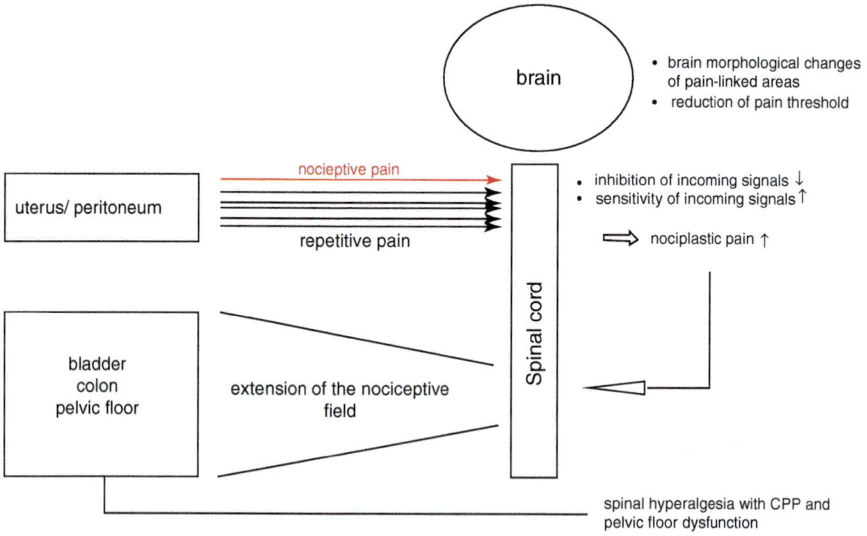

Fig. 15.2 Mechsnisms of central sensitisation and adaption on repetitve pain impulses over years. The modulation on the level of the spinal cord leads to extension of the nociceptive filed. Central changes (nociplasticity) leads to lower paintreshold and normal tough might be painful (spinal hyperalgesia)

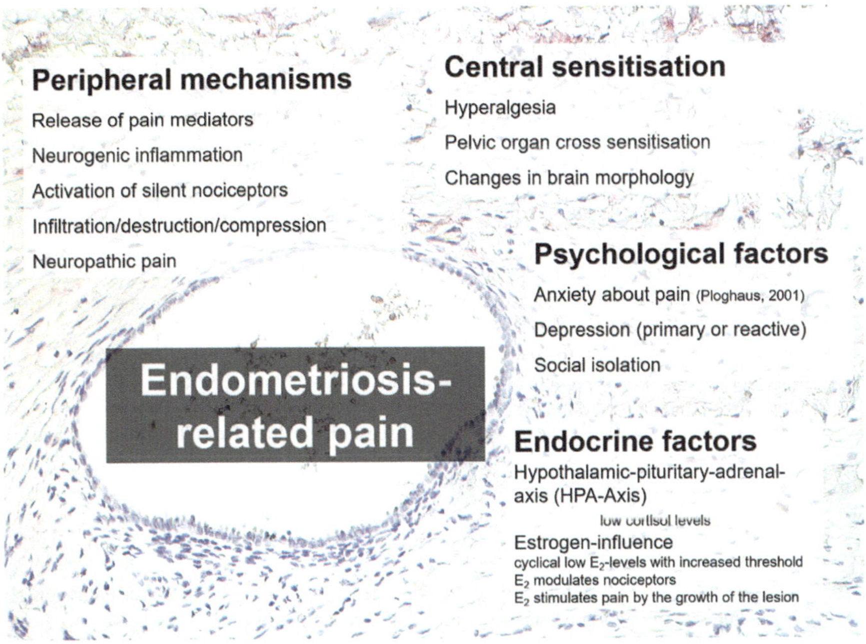

Fig. 15.3 Overview about the different pathomechanisms of pain in endometriosis

[20]. Such patients have an increased risk of developing complex chronic pain syndromes with bladder dysfunction, irritable bowel syndrome and vulvodynia [17]. Taken together, the pathogenesis of endometriosis-associated pain is very complex and certainly not yet fully understood (Fig. 15.3).

References

1. Leyendecker G, Herbertz M, Kunz G, Mall G. Endometriosis results from the dislocation of basal endometrium. Hum Reprod. 2002;17(10):2725–36.
2. Exacoustos C, Luciano D, Corbett B, De Felice G, Di Feliciantonio M, Luciano A, et al. The uterine junctional zone: a 3-dimensional ultrasound study of patients with endometriosis. Am J Obstet Gynecol. 2013;209(3):248. e1–. e7.
3. Dueholm M, Lundorf E, Hansen ES, Sørensen JS, Ledertoug S, Olesen F. Magnetic resonance imaging and transvaginal ultrasonography for the diagnosis of adenomyosis. Fertil Steril. 2001;76(3):588–94.
4. Leyendecker G, Wildt L. Evolutionäre Aspekte in der Pathogenese und Pathophysiologie von Adenomyose und Endometriose. Journal für Gynäkologische Endokrinologie/Österreich. 2019;29(4):110–21.
5. Ibrahim MG, Sillem M, Plendl J, Chiantera V, Sehouli J, Mechsner S. Myofibroblasts are evidence of chronic tissue microtrauma at the endometrial–myometrial junctional zone in uteri with adenomyosis. Reprod Sci. 2017;24(10):1410–8.
6. Cousins FL, Gargett CE. Endometrial stem/progenitor cells and their role in the pathogenesis of endometriosis. Best Pract Res Clin Obstet Gynaecol. 2018;50:27–38.

7. Guo S-W. The pathogenesis of adenomyosis Vis-à-Vis endometriosis. J Clin Med. 2020;9(2):485.
8. Symons LK, Miller JE, Kay VR, Marks RM, Liblik K, Koti M, et al. The immunopathophysiology of endometriosis. Trends Mol Med. 2018;24(9):748–62.
9. Barcena de Arellano ML, Gericke J, Reichelt U, Okuducu AF, Ebert AD, Chiantera V, et al. Immunohistochemical characterization of endometriosis-associated smooth muscle cells in human peritoneal endometriotic lesions. Hum Reprod. 2011;26(10):2721–30.
10. Mechsner S, Bartley J, Infanger M, Loddenkemper C, Herbel J, Ebert AD. Clinical management and immunohistochemical analysis of umbilical endometriosis. Arch Gynecol Obstet. 2009;280(2):235–42.
11. De Graaff A, D'hooghe T, Dunselman G, Dirksen C, Hummelshoj L, Consortium WE, et al. The significant effect of endometriosis on physical, mental and social wellbeing: results from an international cross-sectional survey. Hum Reprod. 2013;28(10):2677–85.
12. Greene R, Stratton P, Cleary SD, Ballweg ML, Sinaii N. Diagnostic experience among 4,334 women reporting surgically diagnosed endometriosis. Fertil Steril. 2009;91(1):32–9.
13. Ballweg ML. Impact of endometriosis on women's health: comparative historical data show that the earlier the onset, the more severe the disease. Best Pract Res Clin Obstet Gynaecol. 2004;18(2):201–18.
14. Mechsner S. Endometriose. Schmerz. 2016;30(5):477–90.
15. Anaf V, Simon P, El Nakadi I, Fayt I, Buxant F, Simonart T, et al. Relationship between endometriotic foci and nerves in rectovaginal endometriotic nodules. Hum Reprod. 2000;15(8):1744–50.
16. Barcena de Arellano ML, Mechsner S. The peritoneum–an important factor for pathogenesis and pain generation in endometriosis. J Mol Med (Berl). 2014;92(6):595–602.
17. Hoffman D. Central and peripheral pain generators in women with chronic pelvic pain: patient centered assessment and treatment. Curr Rheumatol Rev. 2015;11(2):146–66.
18. Aredo JV, Heyrana KJ, Karp BI, Shah JP, Stratton P. Relating chronic pelvic pain and endometriosis to signs of sensitization and myofascial pain and dysfunction. Semin Reprod Med. 2017;35(1):88–97.
19. Ng N, Wahl K, Orr NL, Noga H, Williams C, Allaire C, et al. Endometriosis and negative perception of the medical profession. J Obstet Gynaecol Can. 2020;42(3):248–55.
20. As-Sanie S, Harris RE, Napadow V, Kim J, Neshewat G, Kairys A, et al. Changes in regional gray matter volume in women with chronic pelvic pain: a voxel-based morphometry study. PAIN®. 2012;153(5):1006–14.

Endometriosis in Reproductive Years: Surgical Management of Colorectal Endometriosis

16

Horace Roman, Hanan Alsalem, Tudor Birsan, and Gernot Hudelist

Contents

16.1 Introduction

Endometriosis is a benign gynecological disorder with various variants including peritoneal, uterine, ovarian, and deep endometriosis (DE), which is characterized by subperitoneal invasion of endometriotic tissues exceeding 5 mm [1, 2]. Intestinal DE has been shown to affect between 3.8% and 37% of the patients diagnosed with endometriosis [3, 4]. Although a certain percentage of patients with bowel DE may lack

The original version of this chapter was revised to reflect a correction to Dr Hanan Alsalem's name which was misspelled in the initial publication as Hanan Amsalem. An erratum to this chapter can be found at https://doi.org/10.1007/978-3-030-97236-3_45

H. Roman (✉) · H. Alsalem
Franco-European Multidisciplinary Endometriosis Institute (IFEMEndo), Clinique Tivoli-Ducos, Bordeaux, France

T. Birsan
Center for Endometriosis, Hospital St. John of God, Vienna, Austria

G. Hudelist
Scientific Endometriosis Foundation (Stiftung Endometrioseforschung/SEF), Westerstede, Germany

Department of Gynaecology, Center for Endometriosis, Hospital St. John of God, Vienna, Austria

E. Oral (ed.), *Endometriosis and Adenomyosis*,
https://doi.org/10.1007/978-3-030-97236-3_16

relevant signs such as dyschezia, dysmenorrhea, and dyspareunia, a significant number of women with colorectal DE will face quality of life (QoL)-reducing impairment and/or additional infertility, especially due to concomitant ovarian or uterine disease and secondary adhesions involving the tuboovarian unit. Symptoms of bowel endometriosis may vary and include pain sensations such as dysmenorrhea, deep dyspareunia, and dyschezia but may also present as nonspecific alterations of bowel function including diarrhea, constipation, bloating, and rarely bowel obstruction. These digestive complaints have been related to anterior and lateral fixation and thereby impaired mobility of the rectosigmoid, partial luminal stenosis, and an inflammatory state induced and caused by DE [5, 6]. Furthermore, the extent of colorectal DE appears to correlate with the intensity of pain [7]. Nevertheless, DE-related stenosis leading to occlusion and complete bowel obstruction is a rare complication in women with this disease and has been shown to occur only in 1–2% [5]. Colorectal endometriosis usually presents with nodular enlargement and infiltration of the anterior rectal wall, either as unifocal or multifocal disease typically involving the rectum and/or sigmoid colon in over 90% of all intestinal DE cases [4, 8]. Since these anatomical changes lead to a typical tissue reaction causing nodular fibrosis, rectosigmoidal DE can be diagnosed with imaging methods such as transvaginal sonography (TVS) or magnetic resonance imaging (MRI) with high accuracy [9].

Treatment of colorectal endometriosis in symptomatic patients can be very challenging. Medical treatment options include NSAIDs and hormonal preparations and aim for reduction of DE-related symptoms. Within this, a conservative treatment approach has been demonstrated as a feasible long-term option in over 80% of these patients [10]. However, a significant number of affected women will neither respond to medical therapies nor benefit from medically assisted reproduction (MAR). As a consequence, surgical resection of DE remains the logical therapy and has been proven to effectively reduce pain symptoms and enhance fertility issues [11–13]. However, surgery for colorectal DE is complex and requires a sufficient knowledge of the extent of the disease and a multidisciplinary team setting involving gynecological and colorectal surgical expertise in the light of the fact that severe complications such as anastomotic leakage and rectovaginal fistula may arise. In the ideal scenario, resection of all deep endometriotic lesions as well as preservation and restoration of reproductive function should be accomplished. There is an ongoing debate about the risks and benefits of the ideal surgical approach to colorectal DE including rectal shaving, discoid resection, and segmental bowel resection. There are no universal and clear guidelines as to which excision technique is optimal.

16.2 Rectal Shaving

The shaving technique for the treatment of rectovaginal endometriosis was first described in 1991 [14]. The first large series was published in 1995 and was followed by another larger series from the same group that covered the period between 1997 and 2013, being the largest series so far that described about 3298 cases [15].

To present the uterus, vagina, and the rectum, a uterine manipulator is inserted the use of surgical sponge in the vagina as well as a rectal probe. The principal steps

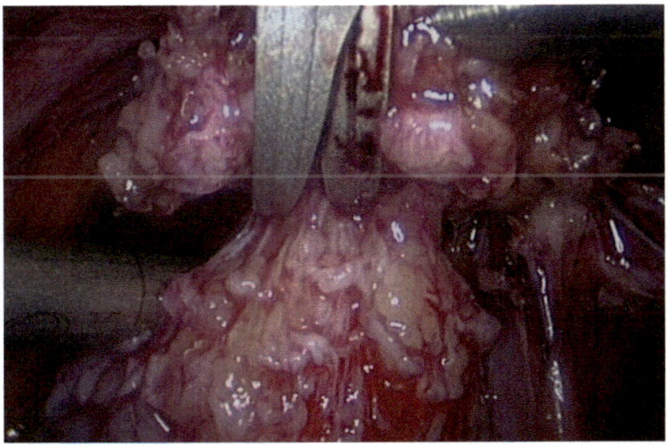

Fig. 16.1 Rectal shaving using cold scissors

of the shaving technique involve the lateral identification of the ureter and potential previously inserted ureteral stents since the rate of ureteral involvement of nodules of >3 cm is approximately 10%. When the lateral pelvic spaces are carefully dis sected, the uterosacral ligaments are transacted when involved, to leave the bowel attached to the nodule. Then, the surgeon progressively detaches the nodule from the anterior part of the rectum down to the healthy cleavage plane of rectovaginal septum.

Shaving consists of excision of the endometriotic nodule, through the thickness of rectal wall, without opening the bowel lumen (Fig. 16.1). Unfortunately, during this procedure the bowel lumen could inadvertently be breached. In such case, a bowel suture must be performed in one or two layers. Studies have reported bowel perforation during surgery to be 1.74% [16]. In all cases, the bowel was sutured during surgery and no unfavorable outcomes occurred during follow-up.

Major complications included late bowel perforation and rectovaginal fistulas. Late bowel perforation was reported in three studies. Koninckx et al. and Roman et al., respectively, described 1.7% and 2.2% of late bowel perforation requiring colostomy, while Donnez et al. reported 0.03% in a series of 3298 cases [16]. Bowel complications were reported in 0.13% of the cases (n 1/4 6/4706) operated on by the shaving technique. Rectovaginal fistulas were recorded in 0.24% of the cases (n 1/4 13/5297).

Postoperative digestive function after shaving was thoroughly assessed by our team [17–20]. In two retrospective series, better digestive functional managed outcomes for postoperative constipation and anal continence were observed in patients by shaving when compared with those undergoing bowel resection [17, 18]. However, in a recent randomized trial comparing conservative to radical rectal surgery in large deep endometriosis nodules infiltrating the rectum, no significant differences were observed in terms of gastrointestinal quality of life scores and SF36 score [21]. In conclusion, the main advantage of the shaving is the very low rate of postoperative complications and the lack of the postoperative impairment of digestive function; however the improvement of constipation is not always observed.

In 2013, a new technique was introduced, using plasma energy for rectal shaving (PlasmaJet device, Plasma Surgical, Inc., Roswell, GA) (Fig. 16.2). Rectal shaving

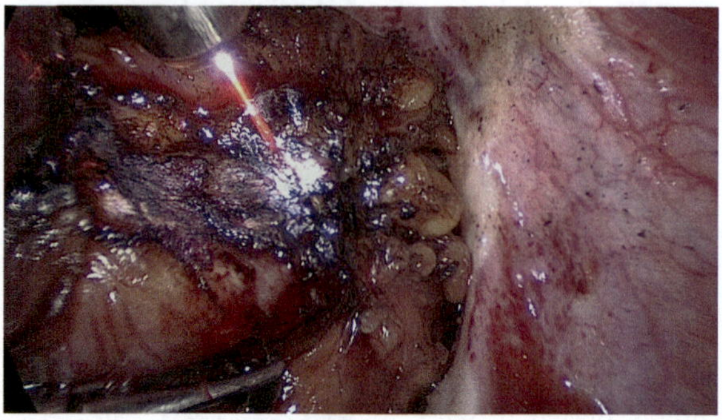

Fig. 16.2 Rectal shaving using plasma energy

using plasma energy has some particularities which are based on the specific properties of this energy: absence of lateral thermal spread around the plasma jet, ensuring safe dissection close to the rectal wall; precise ablative properties, allowing in situ ablation of rectal endometriosis implants; and kinetic energy, enhancing the dissection of subperitoneal spaces [19].

16.3 Disc Excision/The Rouen Technique

Disc excision was initially described more than 20 years ago by surgeons who reported on excision of lesions of rectovaginal endometriosis which breached the bowel lumen, requiring suturing of the bowel [22]. Other surgeons introduced the use of the transanal end-to-end anastomosis (EEA) stapler (Ethicon Endo-Surgery) to achieve suturing of the bowel concomitantly with the excision of the involved anterior rectal wall, and the procedure progressively spread worldwide [23]. Using the EEA stapler, the surgeon thus excises a full-thickness disc of the involved bowel wall which bears the endometriosis nodule and closes the resulting defect with a transverse staple line. When the low rectum is infiltrated by huge endometriotic nodules, it may be awkward to perform rectal shaving and laparoscopic or open disc excision. In response to these challenges, a new technique was introduced (the Rouen technique) using the Contour Transtar stapler (Ethicon Endo-Surgery) in combined laparoscopic and transanal full-thickness disc excision of large rectovaginal endometriosis infiltrating the low and mid rectum [24].

In a recent survey enrolling 1135 patients managed for colorectal rectovaginal endometriosis in France in 2015, disc excision was employed in only 7.3% of cases and in only 16 facilities out of 56 participating in the study [25].

The technique for full-thickness rectovaginal endometriosis excision involves at least two different steps and may be combined with both laparoscopic and transanal approaches. The first step is to perform a laparoscopy, where the goal is to achieve rectal shaving. Preliminary rectal shaving determines the size of rectal patch: the thinner and softer the shaved rectal wall, the larger the diameter of the rectal patch that can be removed using the transanal stapler [24]. The nodule is dissected away from the rectal wall and removed. In cases where the vaginal fornices are involved, a combined vaginal-laparoscopic approach may be useful. In cases where the shaved area of the rectal wall is still infiltrated by implants of endometriosis, a more complete treatment may be achieved by full-thickness disc excision of the shaved area, followed by either direct suture using several stitches or the use of transanal staplers. The first procedure does not avoid bowel opening into the pelvis, which may increase the risk of postoperative pelvic abscess. Conversely, during the disc excision procedure using transanal staplers, the bowel is never opened as resection and wall closure occur simultaneously. The surgeon may use the Contour® Transtar™ stapler when the shaved area is located between 8 and 10 cm above the anus, and the EEA circular stapler when it is located in the upper rectum. In both cases, parachute sutures placed in the middle of shaved area allow for pushing the shaved area between the opened stapler jaws; the sutures are placed laparoscopically (on the serosal aspect of the bowel wall) when the EEA stapler is used and transanally (on the mucosal aspect of the bowel wall) when the Contour Transtar stapler is employed.

When multiple nodules are revealed, they can be managed separately, in order to avoid long segmental resections. The rectal nodule can be removed using a conservative technique, while associated nodules of the colon, cecum or small bowel can be treated separately, by shaving, disc excision, or segmental resection [26].

In the FRIENDS survey, the rate of rectovaginal fistula in patients managed by disc excision was 3.6%, which was threefold higher than the rate recorded in patients managed by shaving (1.3%) and comparable to segmental resection (3.9%). This rate is similar to that reported by an Australian team in a series enrolling patients managed by disc excision using the circular transanal stapler [23].

In a more recent series of 111 patients, reported by Roman et al., the rate of rectovaginal fistula was as high as 7.2%, mainly due to the high prevalence of this event in patients with low rectovaginal endometriosis managed by the Rouen technique. When a disc excision is carried out, bowel suture is transversal and semicircular (Fig. 16.3); thus the risk of postoperative bowel stenosis is very low [19, 27].

To date, there are no large comparative studies with long-term follow-up that provide valuable answers regarding recurrence. However, various series available in the literature report low recurrence rates, with a 1.8% risk of recurrence at 2 years [24]. In the randomized trial comparing conservative surgery to colorectal resection, 5 years after the procedure, only 1 recurrence was recorded in 55 patients, and it

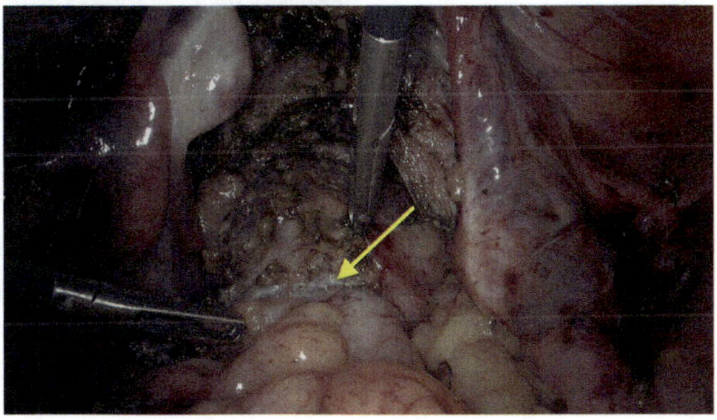

Fig. 16.3 Transanal disc excision using circular staplers

occurred after a disc excision [28]. However, the difference was neither statistically significant nor clinically relevant.

Regarding the functional outcomes, they appear to be comparable after conservative surgery and colorectal resection [20, 21]. This result is probably related to the evidence that the rectal shape is not the unique factor related to postoperative rectal function; rectal innervation plays a major role, while large rectal endometriosis nodules frequently involve parametria and rectal splanchnic nerves, leading to an impairment of rectal function independently of the volume or length of operated bowel [21]. These considerations emphasize the importance of nerve-sparing techniques, which however are not easily usable when small nerve fibers of the inferior hypogastric plexus are surrounded by deep endometriosis nodules.

16.4 Segmental Bowel Resection for DE

Segmental resection (SR) for bowel endometriosis is preferred in the case of bowel stenosis, multifocal lesions, sigmoid involvement, and lesions >3 cm or involving more than 50 percent of the bowel wall circumference [29, 30]. Within this, mobilization of the rectum is performed below the infiltrated area with the proximal dissection line close above the lesion. In contrast to bowel resection for colorectal malignancies, the mobilization and dissection of the bowel can be performed in close contact with the dorsal wall of the rectosigmoid, an approach referred to as the so-called nerve vessel-sparing technique (Fig. 16.4) [11]. However, other groups include the mesorectal tissue and blood supply in the resection specimen but aim to preserve the autonomous nerve plexus, i.e., the inferior hypogastric plexus with proven advantage of one segmental resection method, i.e., nerve vessel-sparing or non-vessel-sparing over the other so far [16]. There are several arguments for and against SR when compared to conservative approaches such as rectal shaving (RS) and discoid resection (DR). First and foremost, large rectal DE lesions exceeding

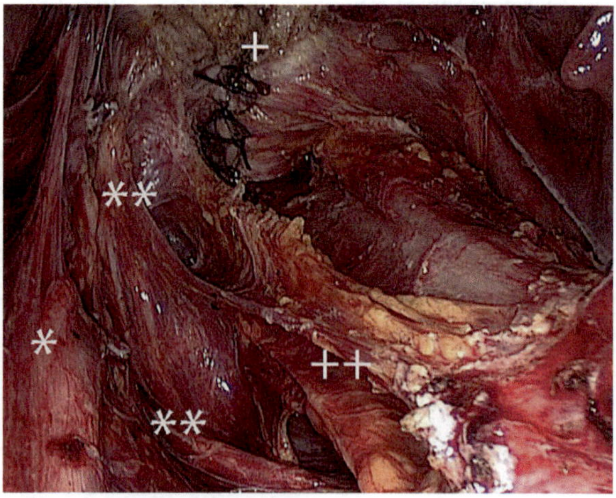

Fig. 16.4 Nerve vessel-sparing SR demonstrating the left pelvic sidewall with ureter (*), fibers of the inferior hypogastric plexus (**), mesorectal fatty tissue and vessels (++), vagina following colpectomy for DIE (+), and rectum

4–5 centimeters as well as multifocal disease may only be fully removed by SR. This is supported by the fact that recurrence rates of colorectal DE have been observed to be lower in SR patients [31]. In addition, recent evidence demonstrates that examination of the bowel segment by palpation – which should always be performed during SR and cannot be accomplished when performing DR or RS – reveals additional palpable satellite rectal DE lesions [8]. Arguments against SR primarily include possibly increased complication rates and later sequelae such as bowel stenosis or low anterior resection syndrome (LARS). Two systematic reviews have compared the published evidence regarding SR, RS, and DR including the only prospective randomized trial on SR versus DR published to date [16, 32, 33]. Within this, the mean complication rates observed for shaving, discoid excision, and SR were 2.2%, 9.7%, and 9.9%, respectively. Rectal shaving was significantly less associated with rectovaginal fistula (RVF) than DR (OR = 0.19) or SR (OR 0.26) with no significant differences between DR versus SR. No significant differences could be observed for anastomotic leakage (AL) between RS and SR or DR and SR. However, DR was observed to confer a lower risk for anastomotic stenosis compared to SR.

The problem with systematic comparisons regarding the three techniques is that pivotal risk factors influencing the risk of major complications such as distance of the stapling anastomosis from the anal verge, vaginal opening, and finally surgical experience cannot be fully taken into account. A recent work by Bokor et al. especially focused on low anterior bowel resections for DE comparing DR and nerve vessel-sparing SR in a retrospective, multicenter trial [34]. Although the results must be interpreted with caution due to the retrospective nature of the study and the differences in the use of protective ileostomies, the authors did not provide evidence for superiority of one or the other technique regarding late sequelae such as LARS but observed higher major complication rates for DR. Taking these factors into account, the risk of severe complications rising up to 9% needs to be discussed with the patients especially before embarking on full-thickness resection techniques, i.e., DR and SR. To date, there is insufficient evidence to clearly recommend one technique over the other leading to the recommendation that surgical treatment decisions should also be guided by experience and expertise.

References

1. Hudelist G, Keckstein J, Wright JT. The migrating adenomyoma: past views on the etiology of adenomyosis and endometriosis. Fertil Steril. 2009;92(5):1536–43.
2. Habib N, Centini G, Lazzeri L, Amoruso N, El Khoury L, Zupi E, et al. Bowel endometriosis: current perspectives on diagnosis and treatment. Int J Women's Health. 2020;12:35–47.
3. Remorgida V, Ferrero S, Fulcheri E, Ragni N, Martin DC. Bowel endometriosis: presentation, diagnosis, and treatment. Obstet Gynecol Surv. 2007;62(7):461–70.
4. Nezhat C, Li A, Falik R, Copeland D, Razavi G, Shakib A, et al. Bowel endometriosis: diagnosis and management. Am J Obstet Gynecol. 2018;218(6):549–62.
5. Roman H, Bridoux V, Tuech JJ, Marpeau L, da Costa C, Savoye G, et al. Bowel dysfunction before and after surgery for endometriosis. Am J Obstet Gynecol. 2013;209(6):524–30.
6. Hansen KE, Kesmodel US, Baldursson EB, Kold M, Forman A. Visceral syndrome in endometriosis patients. Eur J Obstet Gynecol Reprod Biol. 2014;179:198–203.

7. Montanari E, Dauser B, Keckstein J, Kirchner E, Nemeth Z, Hudelist G. Association between disease extent and pain symptoms in patients with deep infiltrating endometriosis. Reprod Biomed Online. 2019;39(5):845–51.
8. Roman H, Merlot B, Forestier D, Noailles M, Magne E, Carteret T, et al. Nonvisualized palpable bowel endometriotic satellites. Hum Reprod. 2021;36(3):656–65.
9. Aas-Eng MK, Montanari E, Lieng M, Keckstein J, Hudelist G. Transvaginal sonographic imaging and associated techniques for diagnosis of ovarian, deep endometriosis, and adenomyosis: a comprehensive review. Semin Reprod Med. 2020;38(2–03):216–26.
10. Egekvist AG, Marinovskij E, Forman A, Kesmodel US, Riiskjaer M, Seyer-Hansen M. Conservative approach to rectosigmoid endometriosis: a cohort study. Acta Obstet Gynecol Scand. 2017;96(6):745–50.
11. Hudelist G, Aas-Eng MK, Birsan T, Berger F, Sevelda U, Kirchner L, et al. Pain and fertility outcomes of nerve-sparing, full-thickness disk or segmental bowel resection for deep infiltrating endometriosis-a prospective cohort study. Acta Obstet Gynecol Scand. 2018;97(12):1438–46.
12. De Cicco C, Corona R, Schonman R, Mailova K, Ussia A, Koninckx P. Bowel resection for deep endometriosis: a systematic review. BJOG. 2011;118(3):285–91.
13. Bendifallah S, Roman H, Mathieu d'Argent E, Touleimat S, Cohen J, Darai E, et al. Colorectal endometriosis-associated infertility: should surgery precede ART? Fertil Steril. 2017;108(3):525–31 e4.
14. Reich H, McGlynn F, Salvat J. Laparoscopic treatment of cul-de-sac obliteration secondary to retrocervical deep fibrotic endometriosis. J Reprod Med. 1991;36(7):516.
15. Donnez J, Squifflet J. Complications, pregnancy and recurrence in a prospective series of 500 patients operated on by the shaving technique for deep rectovaginal endometriotic nodules. Hum Reprod. 2010;25:1949–58.
16. Donnez O, Roman H. Choosing the right surgical technique for deep endometriosis: shaving, disc excision, or bowel resection? Fertil Steril. 2017;108(6):931–42.
17. Roman H, Milles M, Vassilieff M, Resch B, Tuech JJ, Huet E, Darwish B, Abo C. Long-term functional outcomes following colorectal resection versus shaving for rectal endometriosis. Am J Obstet Gynecol. 2016;215(6):762.e1–9. https://doi.org/10.1016/j.ajog.2016.06.055. Epub 2016 Jul 5.
18. Roman H, Vassilieff M, Tuech JJ, et al. Postoperative digestive function after radical versus conservative surgical philosophy for deep endometriosis infiltrating the rectum. Fertil Steril. 2013;99:1695–704.
19. Marty N, Touleimat S, Moatassim-Drissa S, Millochau JC, Vallee A, Stochino Loi E, Desneyder S, Roman H. Rectal shaving using plasma energy in deep infiltrating endometriosis of the rectum: four years of experience. J Minim Invasive Gynecol. 2017;
20. Roman H, Moatassim-Drissa S, Marty N, Milles M, Vallée A, Desnyder E, Stochino Loi E, Abo C. Rectal shaving for deep endometriosis infiltrating the rectum: a 5-year continuous retrospective series. Fertil Steril. 2016;106(6):1438–45.
21. Roman H, Bubenheim M, Huet E, Bridoux V, Zacharopoulou C, Daraï E, Collinet P, Tuech JJ. Conservative surgery versus colorectal resection in deep endometriosis infiltrating the rectum: a randomized trial. Hum Reprod. 2018;33(1):47–57.
22. Nezhat C, Nezhat F, Pennington E, Nezhat CH, Ambroze W. Laparoscopic disk excision and primary repair of the anterior rectal wall for the treatment of full-thickness bowel endometriosis. Surg Endosc. 1994;8:682–5.
23. Woods RJ, Heriot AG, Chen FC. Anterior rectal wall excision for endometriosis using the circular stapler. ANZ J Surg. 2003;73(8):647–8.
24. Roman H, Darwish B, Bridoux V, Chati R, Kermiche S, Coget J, Huet E, Tuech JJ. Functional outcomes after disc excision in deep endometriosis of the rectum using transanal staplers: a series of 111 consecutive patients. Fertil Steril. 2017 Apr;107(4):977–86.
25. Roman H, FRIENDS Group. A national snapshot of the surgical management of deep infiltrating endometriosis of the rectum and the colon in France 2015: a multi-center series of 1135 cases. J Gynecol Obstet Hum Reprod. 2017;46:159–65.

26. Millochau JC, Stochino-Loi E, Darwish B, Abo C, Coget J, Chati R, Tuech JJ, Roman H. Multiple nodule removal by disc excision and segmental resection in multifocal colorectal endometriosis. J Minim Invasive Gynecol. 2018;25(1):139–46.
27. Braund S, Hennetier C, Klapczynski C, Scattarelli A, Coget J, Bridoux V, Tuech JJ, Roman H. Risk of postoperative stenosis after segmental resection versus disk excision for deep endometriosis infiltrating the rectosigmoid: a retrospective study. J Minim Invasive Gynecol. 2021;28(1):50–6.
28. Roman H, Tuech JJ, Huet E, Bridoux V, Khalil H, Hennetier C, Bubenheim M, Branduse LA. Excision versus colorectal resection in deep endometriosis infiltrating the rectum: 5-year follow-up of patients enrolled in a randomized controlled trial. Hum Reprod. 2019;34(12):2362–71.
29. Abrao MS, Petraglia F, Falcone T, Keckstein J, Osuga Y, Chapron C. Deep endometriosis infiltrating the recto-sigmoid: critical factors to consider before management. Hum Reprod Update. 2015;21(3):329–39.
30. Remorgida V, Ragni N, Ferrero S, Anserini P, Torelli P, Fulcheri E. How complete is full thickness disc resection of bowel endometriotic lesions? A prospective surgical and histological study. Hum Reprod. 2005;20(8):2317–20.
31. Bendifallah S, Vesale E, Darai E, Thomassin-Naggara I, Bazot M, Tuech JJ, et al. Recurrence after surgery for colorectal endometriosis: a systematic review and meta-analysis. J Minim Invasive Gynecol. 2020;27(2):441–51 e2.
32. Bendifallah S, Puchar A, Vesale E, Moawad G, Darai E, Roman H. Surgical outcomes after colorectal surgery for endometriosis: a systematic review and meta-analysis. J Minim Invasive Gynecol. 2020;
33. Roman H, Bubenheim M, Huet E, Bridoux V, Zacharopoulou C, Darai E, et al. Conservative surgery versus colorectal resection in deep endometriosis infiltrating the rectum: a randomized trial. Hum Reprod. 2018;33(1):47–57.
34. Bokor A, Hudelist G, Dobo N, Dauser B, Farella M, Brubel R, et al. Low anterior resection syndrome following different surgical approaches for low rectal endometriosis: a retrospective multicenter study. Acta Obstet Gynecol Scand. 2020.

Endometriosis in Peri- and Postmenopausal Year

17

Elvira Bratila, Ezgi Darici, and Engin Oral

Contents

E. Bratila
Department of Obstetrics Gynecology, "Carol Davila" University of Medicine and Pharmacy, Bucharest, Romania

Department of Obstetrics Gynecology, "Prof. Dr. Panait Sirbu" Clinical Obstetrics and Gynecology Hospital, Bucharest, Romania

E. Darici
Department of Obstetrics Gynecology, İznik State Hospital, Bursa, Turkey

E. Oral (✉)
Department of Obstetrics and Gynecology, Bezmialem Vakif University Medical Faculty, Istanbul, Turkey

E. Oral (ed.), *Endometriosis and Adenomyosis*,
https://doi.org/10.1007/978-3-030-97236-3_17

17.1 Introduction

Endometriosis is known as an estrogen-dependent disease, usually symptomatic during the fertile period of a woman's life and considered to improve after menopause. However recent analysis showed that estrogen deprivation in menopause doesn't cause the regression of all endometriosis lesions and endometriosis is not only the disease of the fertile years. Moreover, evaluation and management of endometriosis in patients over 40 requires a tailored approach since the epidemiology, clinical manifestations, and management strategies of the endometriosis disease occur differently at late reproductive years. There are many case series in the literature describing symptomatic endometriosis in menopausal patients with particular microscopic features.

As it is well known for pre-menopausal endometriosis, no existing theory can explain the appearance of all endometriosis lesions. Subsequently, it is unlikely that one single theory can explain the development of peri- and postmenopausal endometriosis. Most often peri- and postmenopausal endometriosis represents a recurrence of pre-menopausal disease [1].

The major issues which a clinician will confront during the management of patients with endometriosis over the age of 40 are fertility issues, pain, increased risk for malignancy, and the management of the menopausal symptoms. Contrary to the fertile age disease, postmenopausal endometriosis develops during an environment of ovarian estrogen deficiency and seems to have a higher predisposition to malignant transformation [2]. The disease appears to show a tendency to involve other extragenital anatomical sites and cause constrictive and obstructive implants, which is why the first choice in treatment is surgery [3].

17.2 Prevalence

Postmenopausal endometriosis was described for the first time in 1942 [4]. It is a rare disease, affecting about 2–5% of patients diagnosed with endometriosis, and the real prevalence in the general population remains unknown [5]. Punnonen et al. reported the frequency of postmenopausal endometriosis as 2.2% and the average time elapsed after menopause as 7.3 years in 11 patients with ovarian endometriosis [6]. Four years later the same group found that 19% of the patients who underwent surgery for gynecological reasons had endometriosis, and the incidence for postmenopausal endometriosis was 2.5% [7].

In a recent retrospective epidemiologic study among 42,079 women, accumulated data revealed that around 19.6% of women with surgically confirmed endometriosis were in their peri-post menopausal years [8] and, interestingly, 9 of the cases were in the upper extreme age groups: 8 were in 80–85 years and 1 case was in 90–95 years [8].

Apart from the endometriosis itself, concomitant problems as adenomyosis and uterine leiomyomas may accompany endometriosis. Oral et al. ironically named this situation as "dragon's triangle." Figure 17.1 shows the co-prevalence rates of adenomyosis (Fig. 17.1) [9, 10].

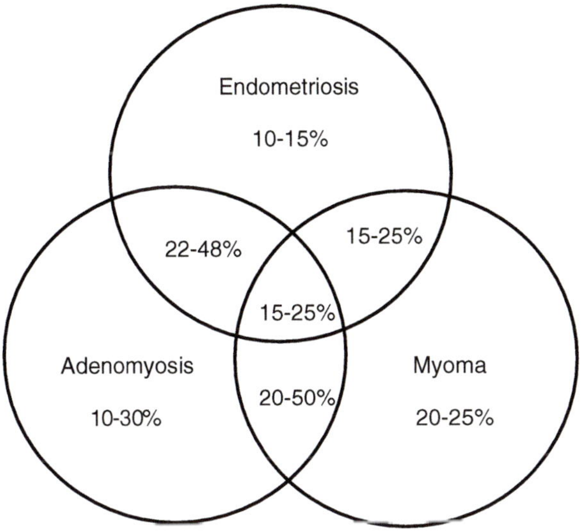

Fig. 17.1 Dragon's triangle, co-prevalence rate

17.3 Pathophysiology

Although menopause is known as an estrogen deprivation period, a small amount of estrogen may be present from both endogenous and exogenous sources [11]. Estrogen synthesis in endometriotic lesions is regulated through the presence of various enzymes present. The most studied are 17ß-hydroxysteroid dehydrogenases (17ß-HSDs) and steroidogenic acute regulatory protein (StAR), which are present in endometriosis stromal cells and promote estrogen production via aromatase [12]. That is why aromatase inhibitors have shown a good result in treating symptomatic endometriosis in menopausal patients, by inhibiting the synthesis of extra-ovarian estrogen. The synthesized estrogen through the pathways described promotes the proliferation of endometriosis lesions and the progression of the disease, and subsequently their potential malignant transformation [13].

Endometriosis lesions persist or rarely can progress even in the absence of ovarian estrogen synthesis, as they continue to be active and remain sensitive to hormonal variations after menopause. Endometriosis implants themselves can synthetize estradiol through the elevated levels of P450 aromatase activity. Cytochrome P450 is the key enzyme involved in the biosynthesis of estrogen [14]. The production of estrogen post-menopause promotes endometriosis through various pathways such as activating dorsal root ganglion neurons to produce chemokines that activate macrophages [13]. Estrogen can also activate the macrophages directly by misleading them to recognize ectopic endometriotic lesions as injuries, and stimulating neovascularization through high concentrations of VEGF, and altering the immune response [12]. Obesity, defined as a BMI over 30 kg/m^2, exogenous phytoestrogens, and hormone replacement therapies with estrogen are all risk factors for the development of menopausal endometriosis [15].

A simpler and generally accepted explanation of the presence of endometriosis in menopause is the deeply infiltrating nature of the disease, causing frequently an incomplete surgical excision at the time of surgery [16]. The remaining lesions could either evolve and become symptomatic during the perimenopausal period or be stimulated to become active by hormone replacement therapy recommended for the climacteric syndrome. Thus, it is considered that most frequently peri- and postmenopausal endometriosis represents a recurrence of the pre-menopausal disease [17]. Development of newly formed endometriosis lesions by the metaplastic transformation of peritoneal mesothelial cells into endometrial glandular cells represents a less likely possibility, but it is cited [18].

17.4 Diagnosis and Clinical Manifestations

The diagnosis of peri- and postmenopausal endometriosis is based on the same criteria as the pre-menopausal one, but the clinical presentations may show alterations. Symptoms such as infertility and dysmenorrhea present in endometriosis patients of reproductive age do not apply to this category of women, making the diagnosis more challenging.

The most frequent location of the menopausal endometriosis lesions is the ovaries, followed by the ureter, bladder, intestine, and more rarely the vagina. Extremely rare lesions have been found in the skin and liver [19].

The clinical manifestations of endometriosis occur differently at late reproductive ages. A retrospective study conducted by Ferrero et al. among 72 menopausal women showed that asymptomatic pelvic cysts were the most common clinical presentations, followed by abnormal uterine bleeding, abdominal pain, rectal bleeding, and urinary dysfunction [20]. In light of these anatomic localizations, symptoms such as abnormal vaginal bleeding, hematuria, rectal bleeding, and hemoptysis-associated pelvic pain need to be extensively investigated in postmenopausal endometriosis patients [1, 15].

A suggestive finding in ultrasound and magnetic resonance imaging, especially for patients with a history of pre-menopausal endometriosis should be sufficient for establishing the diagnosis [1, 2, 5].

Another issue to consider while evaluating a patient at her peri- and postmenopausal years is the increase in the proportion of cases of adenomyosis when compared to endometriosis. Adenomyosis appears to be more frequent in adult women in their fourth and fifth decades, and patients also need to be investigated from this aspect [21]. The presentation may be abnormal uterine bleeding, pelvic pain, or fertility problems. At the age of 40 and above, management is similar to the one at fertile ages.

17.5 Treatment

The surgical treatment is the gold standard in patients with confirmed peri- or postmenopausal endometriosis due to the higher risk of malignancy post-menopause, the capacity of the disease to invade adjacent anatomical structures, and obstructive urinary or intestinal lesions and lack of fertility desire. An aggressive excision of the uterus, fallopian tubes, ovaries and all suspected endometriosis lesions should be performed for optimization of treatment and prevention of malignant transformation [22]. For those patients for which surgical intervention is not possible, several medical therapies such as GnRH agonist and antagonists, progestins, aromatase inhibitors, combined oral contraceptives, and levonorgestrel-releasing intrauterine systems are the treatment of choice [23].

There is very little information about the medical treatment of endometriosis in menopause. The only medication that was reported as efficient in menopausal endometriosis is aromatase inhibitors. Anastrozole and letrozole have been used in patients with a history of multiple surgical interventions, and some researchers reported satisfying results in terms of pain relief and reduction in endometriosis lesions [24].

17.5.1 Management of Fertility Problems in Women with Endometriosis After the Age of 40

Since women anticipate high-level careers in contemporary lifestyle, usually fertility is postponed until the age of late 30s and early 40s. Thus, especially women with endometriosis may be obliged to face fertility problems mainly due to decreased ovarian reserve.

Endometriosis is a cause of subfertility via different suggested mechanisms such as diminished ovarian reserve, poor oocyte quality, tubal problems, fertilization and implantation problems, or even sperm problems. For women over 40 years of age, diminished ovarian reserve seems to be of utmost importance. It is known that age, previous surgery for endometrioma, and also endometrioma per se are important factors that may contribute to diminished ovarian reserve in such women. Though management should include IVF for women over 40, the first step should be ovarian reserve testing in order to decide whether to perform embryo pooling or not. After having the embryos frozen, ovarian suppression by GnRH analogs should be commenced followed by frozen-thawed embryo transfer (Fig. 17.2) [9].

17.5.2 Management of Pain Problems in Women with Endometriosis After the Age of 40

If pain is the only complaint after age 40, surgery is to be the first management option due to the risk of malignant transformation [9]. Surgical intervention should include total hysterectomy and bilateral salpingo-oophorectomy and excision/destruction of endometriotic lesions. If there are medical (e.g., cardiovascular

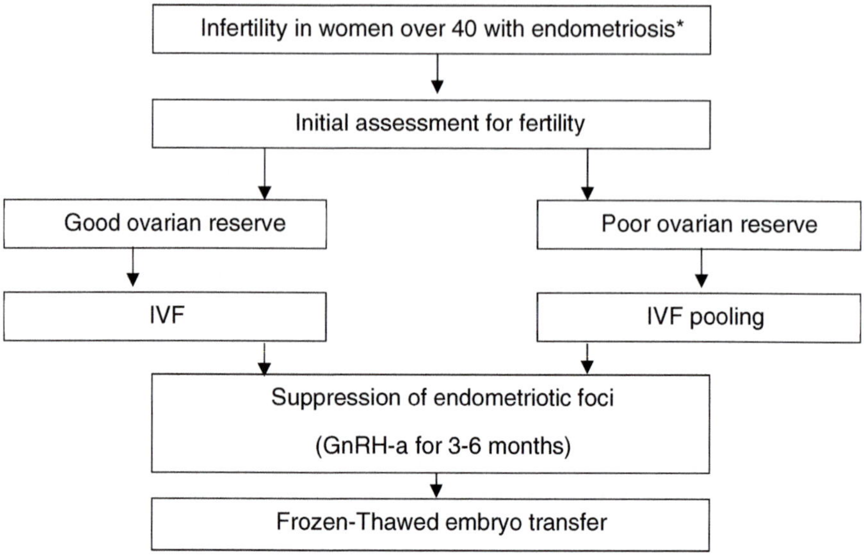

Fig. 17.2 Algorithm infertility management for women with endometriosis over the age of 40. *Surgery should be chosen in the management of women with suspicious malignancy

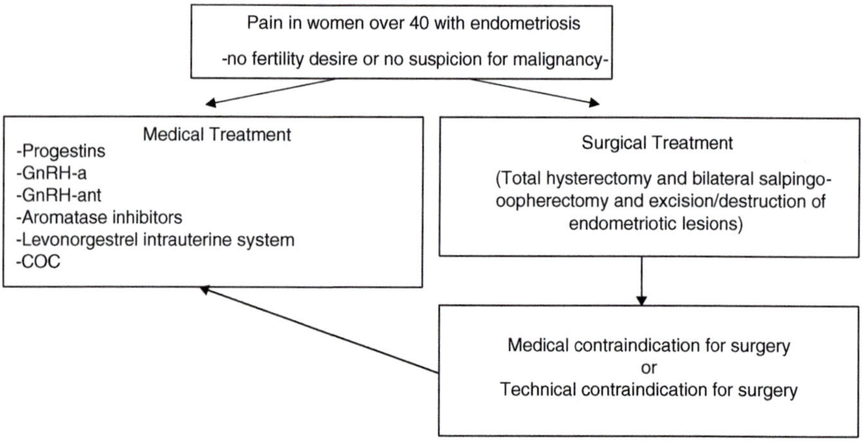

Fig. 17.3 Algorithm for pain management for women with endometriosis over 40

disease, pulmonary disease, etc.) or surgical (previous multiple operations) contraindications for a surgical approach and there is no sign for malignancy, then medical treatment is to be considered. According to data we have at the moment, there are many medical options for treatment of endometriosis, such as gonadotropin-releasing hormone agonists, progestogens, or aromatase inhibitors, gonadotropin-releasing hormone antagonists, combined oral contraceptives, and levonorgestrel intrauterine system (LNG-IUS), which also can be used in the treatment of endometriosis patients after the age 40 (Fig. 17.3) [9].

17.5.3 Hormone Replacement Therapy and Management of Menopausal Symptoms in Women with Endometriosis After the Age of 40

When the women with endometriosis do have menopausal symptoms, there may be two concerns on each pan of the scale; one is basic menopausal concerns (bones, brain, cardiovascular system, and quality of life especially in terms of vasomotor and vulvovaginal problems) and the second one is the risk of recurrence and malignancy [18, 25]. Patients undergoing menopausal hormone therapy might present a higher risk for malignant transformation, but the relationship between hormone replacement therapy and carcinomatous shift of endometriosis implants remains uncertain [26].

As recently reviewed and concluded by Zanello et al., "*women should not be denied the replacement therapy solely due to endometriosis*." Women with vasomotor symptoms, especially when they experience early or premature menopause, may use hormonal treatment [18].

Different prospective comparative studies intended to find a safe regimen to address the climacteric syndrome in this category of patients. Most studies found that the recurrence risk is low if the surgery was radical, consisting of the surgical excision of all endometriosis lesions. In these patients, the recurrence risk is similar or even lower than women who did not receive hormone replacement therapy [27]. However, when there is residual disease following surgery, the recurrence risk is significantly higher, and hormone replacement therapy should be avoided [27, 28].

The drug to be selected should be combined estrogen and progestogen unrelated to being surgically menopausal or not, since estrogen-only regimens may activate the residual endometriotic foci even in women after surgery for endometriosis and carry a higher risk of recurrence in terms of symptoms such as pelvic pain and dyspareunia but didn't report any case of malignant transformation during the follow-up period [18].

Comparison of transdermal estrogen with tibolone treatment in small groups of patients revealed that tibolone didn't cause recurrence of symptoms, unlike estrogen, which caused pelvic pain in 40% of patients and deep dyspareunia in 10%. Therefore, it is a safe option for hormone replacement therapy in operated menopausal patients [29].

The initiation time of the hormone therapy could also play a role in the recurrence risk. Women who started hormone replacement therapy immediately after the surgery for endometriosis had a significantly lower risk of disease and symptom recurrence compared to those delaying the treatment until 6 weeks after surgery [29]. Another important point is that, if the woman with endometriosis needs tamoxifen treatment, the risk of malignant transformation should be considered [15].

17.5.4 Asymptomatic Patient in Women with Endometriosis After the Age of 40

We do not know the exact prevalence of asymptomatic endometriosis at any age. The management is also quite blurred for asymptomatic patients with endometriosis. Asymptomatic endometriosis may be found by chance via imaging methods, mainly by ultrasound, or during the operations for other reasons. Although in 1996, Eric J Thomas has suggested a challenging opinion of his own by writing "*Asymptomatic endometriosis is likely to be a physiological phenomenon of very limited relevance both physician and the patient*" [30] and finished his paper by referring to an unidentified Edinburg physician's quote "*It is a very very clever doctor who can make an asymptomatic patient feel better*", there are some recent "warning" articles on asymptomatic patients with endometriosis. In their very recent retrospectively analyzed case series, Son JH et al. [31] reported 50 women with ovarian clear cell carcinoma. Of those, 11 were women with asymptomatic endometrioma and being under regular gynecological examination. The authors suggested yearly close surveillance from the age mid-30s in patients with asymptomatic endometrioma [9].

17.6 Risk of Malignant Transformation

The malignant transformation of endometriosis was first described by Sampson in 1925, which reported an incidence of about 1% [32]. Diagnosing malignant transformation of endometriosis in menopause is a clinical challenge, because of similar characteristics of both endometriosis and malignancy. Endometriosis can cause local invasion with alteration of normal anatomy as well as distant metastasis (extragenital endometriosis) similar to the oncologic disease. Distinguishing menopausal endometriosis from gynecological malignancy is very challenging in clinical practice especially in the presence of common risk factors in the etiology of both diseases: nulliparity, infertility, late pregnancy age, and short duration of contraceptive use [33].

The hypothesis behind endometriosis and cancer is a continuous source of controversy. The theories proposed are as follows:

- Endometriotic implants may directly undergo malignant transformation, perhaps through an atypical transition phase.
- Endometriosis and cancer may share common antecedent mechanisms and/or predisposing factors (genetic susceptibility, immune/angiogenic dysregulation, environmental toxin exposure).

Menopausal endometriosis seems to have a higher risk of malignant transformation, compared to endometriosis in patients of reproductive age [34]. It is now accepted that malignant transformation of endometriosis occurs most frequently in the ovaries and the lifetime risk of ovarian cancer in women with a history of endometriosis is about 1.9% compared with 1.4% in the general population [35]. This positive association is the strongest for clear cell and endometrioid carcinomas (SRR = 3.44 and SRR = 2.33, respectively) [36, 37]. Thus, patients diagnosed with ovarian endometriosis appear to have a higher risk of ovarian cancer during peri-menopause compared to the general population.

Although there is still no definite marker to confirm or exclude malignancy, for women with suspicion of malignancy, human epididymal secretory protein (HE4) is important, especially combined with CA-125 as ROMA index is accepted as the most efficient biomarker today [38].

In a retrospective analysis, Oral et al. have also drawn attention to the probable continuum of the pathological way from endometriosis to atypical endometriosis and ovarian carcinoma. Of 661 women with ovarian carcinoma or borderline ovarian tumor, 48 (4.7%) had endometriosis, and of those 48, 73% had atypical endometriosis [39]. Recently Oral et al. have also found that endometrioma-associated ovarian tumors developed in nearly 11% of women with endometriomas [40]. The risk of ovarian cancer is especially higher in women with long-standing (more than 10 years) endometriosis, or recurrent endometrioma, newly diagnosed endometrioma [35].

A higher risk of extra-ovarian cancers originating in the endometriosis lesions after the start of menopause is another problem that a peri- and postmenopausal endometriosis patient will face. The relatively positive aspect is that patients with endometriosis-related malignancies seem to bear a favorable prognosis [34, 41].

Even though there are no studies in literature describing the exact carcinogenic pathway leading from endometriosis to invasive carcinoma, several genetic mutations in PTEN, TP53, and ARIDIA genes have been identified, which may represent the molecular explanation of this malignant transformation [41].

In a very recent systematic review, Kvaskoff et al. showed that endometriosis was associated with a higher risk of ovarian and thyroid cancers, and minimally (only 4% greater risk) with breast cancer, and with a lower risk of cervical cancer [36]. In a study following a large number of 64,492 Swedish women diagnosed with endometriosis for a long period of 31 years, Melin et al. described a high risk of rare types of cancers in these women (non-Hodgkin lymphoma, endocrine and brain cancers) and ovarian cancer [42].

Bertelsen et al. studied the relationship between endometriosis and breast cancer in a large cohort of 113,427 Danish women for over 30 years. They found that the age of diagnosis is crucial. Women diagnosed with endometriosis under the age of 40 showed a reduced risk of breast cancer, while those diagnosed after the age of 40 had an increased risk [43]. The results could be interpreted according to the treatments received by the patients: the younger ones with a reduced risk received estrogen suppression therapy, while the older ones more frequently underwent hysterectomy and adnexectomy with hormone replacement therapy and had an increased prevalence of obesity.

On the other hand, the malignant transformation secondarily to hormone replacement therapy in operated menopausal patients is described. Unbalanced estrogen therapy is responsible for endometrial carcinoma, thus similarly could cause malignant transformation of endometriosis lesions. Estrogen stimulation, whether endogenous as in obese patients, or exogenous as in hormone therapy for the climacteric syndrome, could play a role in the malignancy transformation of endometriosis lesions, but the pathway is not clear. Different studies have searched a potential relationship between these aspects, and Zanetta found that hyperestrogenism, either endogenous or exogenous, is a significant risk factor for the appearance of cancer in the endometriosis lesions, especially in the ovaries [44].

The risk of malignant transformation in other anatomical sites outside the ovaries appears to be low. A review by Gücer found 20 patients with neoplasms developed in endometriosis lesions, most of them on the vagina. He didn't find any case of extra-ovarian malignant transformation in women undergoing combined hormone replacement therapy [45]. Modesitt confirmed these findings, reporting that more than half of the patients with extra-ovarian malignant transformation of endometriosis lesions in his study had been administered unbalanced estrogen therapy [46]. Other researchers have described a potential role of tamoxifen in the process of malignancy but only in a small number of cases [47]. Based on all of these observations, the general recommendation regarding hormone replacement therapy in menopausal patients operated for endometriosis is combined estrogen and progestin hormone therapy [48].

17.7 Conclusion

Although peri- and postmenopausal endometriosis is considered a rare disease, it is not uncommon and should be taken into account because of the risk of disease recurrence and malignant transformation. In these patients, hormone replacement therapy is reserved only for the severe climacteric syndrome, bone loss/osteoporosis, and genitourinary syndrome and should consist of combined estrogen-progesterone therapy.

The gold standard in treatment of a patient with confirmed peri- or postmenopausal endometriosis by anamnesis, clinical symptomatology, and imaging techniques is the surgical excision of the uterus, fallopian tubes, ovaries, and all macroscopic endometriosis lesions. For those patients for which surgical intervention is not possible, several medical therapies such as GnRH agonist and antagonists, progestins, aromatase inhibitors, combined oral contraceptives, and levonorgestrel-releasing intrauterine systems are the treatment of choice.

Peri- and postmenopausal endometriosis is still one of the least studied topics of endometriosis. Further studies are urgently needed in terms of both in epidemiology and clinical management of the disease.

References

1. Matalliotakis M, et al. Keeping an eye on perimenopausal and postmenopausal endometriosis. Diseases (Basel, Switzerland). 2019;7(1):29.
2. Morotti M, et al. Endometriosis in menopause: a single institution experience. Arch Gynecol Obstet. 2012;286
3. Secosan C, et al. Endometriosis in menopause-renewed attention on a controversial disease. Diagnostics (Basel, Switzerland). 2020;10(3):134.
4. Guy JM. Edgar Haydon (1859–1942): general practitioner and radium pioneer. J Med Biogr. 2009;17(3):127–34.
5. Oxholm D, et al. Postmenopausal endometriosis. Acta Obstet Gynecol Scand. 2007;86(10):1158–64.
6. Punnonen R, Klemi PJ, Nikkanen V. Postmenopausal endometriosis. Eur J Obstet Gynecol Reprod Biol. 1980;11(3):195–200.
7. Nikkanen V, Punnonen R. External endometriosis in 801 operated patients. Acta Obstet Gynecol Scand. 1984;63(8):699–701.
8. Haas D, et al. Endometriosis: a premenopausal disease? Age pattern in 42,079 patients with endometriosis. Arch Gynecol Obstet. 2012;286(3):667–70.
9. Oral E, Inceboz U. How can we manage patients over forty with endometriosis? Minerva Med. 2020;111(1):62–7.
10. Mueller MD. How to treat the complex patients: endometriosis, adenomyosis & uterine fibroids. In: SEUD. Italy; 2018.
11. Streuli I, et al. Endometriosis after menopause: physiopathology and management of an uncommon condition. Climacteric. 2017;20(2):138–43.
12. Ulukus M, Arici A. Immunology of endometriosis. Minerva Ginecol. 2005;57(3):237–48.
13. Bulun SE, et al. Estrogen production and metabolism in endometriosis. Ann N Y Acad Sci. 2002;955:75–85; discussion 86–8, 396–406.
14. Rylander-Rudqvist T, et al. Cytochrome P450 1B1 gene polymorphisms and postmenopausal endometrial cancer risk. Cancer Epidemiol Biomark Prev. 2004;13(9):1515–20.
15. Tan DA, Almaria MJG. Postmenopausal endometriosis: drawing a clearer clinical picture. Climacteric. 2018;21(3):249–55.
16. Gemmell LC, et al. The management of menopause in women with a history of endometriosis: a systematic review. Hum Reprod Update. 2017;23(4):481–500.
17. Haas D, et al. Endometriosis patients in the postmenopausal period: pre- and postmenopausal factors influencing postmenopausal health. Biomed Res Int. 2014;2014:746705.
18. Zanello M, et al. Hormonal replacement therapy in menopausal women with history of endometriosis: a review of literature. Medicina (Kaunas). 2019;55(8)
19. Al Kadri H, et al. Hormone therapy for endometriosis and surgical menopause. Cochrane Database Syst Rev. 2009;(1):CD005997.
20. Morotti M, et al. Endometriosis in menopause: a single institution experience. Arch Gynecol Obstet. 2012;286(6):1571–5.
21. Morassutto C, et al. Incidence and estimated prevalence of endometriosis and adenomyosis in Northeast Italy: a data linkage study. PLoS One. 2016;11(4):e0154227.
22. Rozenberg S, et al. Should we abstain from treating women with endometriosis using menopausal hormone therapy, for fear of an increased ovarian cancer risk? Climacteric. 2015;18(4):448–52.
23. Polyzos NP, et al. Aromatase inhibitors in post-menopausal endometriosis. Reprod Biol Endocrinol. 2011;9:90.
24. Fatemi HM, et al. Successful treatment of an aggressive recurrent post-menopausal endometriosis with an aromatase inhibitor. Reprod Biomed Online. 2005;11(4):455–7.

25. Alio L, et al. Endometriosis: seeking optimal management in women approaching menopause. Climacteric. 2019;22(4):329–38.
26. Moen MH, et al. EMAS position statement: managing the menopause in women with a past history of endometriosis. Maturitas. 2010;67(1):94–7.
27. Rattanachaiyanont M, et al. Hormonal replacement therapy in surgical menopause with underlying endometriosis. J Med Assoc Thail. 2003;86(8):702–7.
28. Soliman NF, Hillard TC. Hormone replacement therapy in women with past history of endometriosis. Climacteric. 2006;9(5):325–35.
29. Palep-Singh M, Gupta S. Endometriosis: associations with menopause, hormone replacement therapy and cancer. Menopause Int. 2009;15(4):169–74.
30. Thomas EJ. The relevance of asymptomatic endometriosis. Hum Reprod. 1996;11(Suppl 3):103–9.
31. Son J-H, et al. Clinicopathologic characteristics of ovarian clear cell carcinoma in the background of endometrioma: a surveillance strategy for an early detection of malignant transformation in patients with asymptomatic endometrioma. Obstet Gynecol Sci. 2019;62(1):27–34.
32. Dastur AE, Tank PD. John A Sampson and the origins of endometriosis. J Obstet Gynaecol India. 2010;60(4):299–300.
33. Fat BC, et al. Postmenopausal malignant transformation of extragenital endometriosis. A case report. Gynecol Obstet Fertil. 2008;36(1):51–5.
34. Králíčková M, Vetvicka V. Endometriosis and ovarian cancer. World J Clin Oncol. 2014;5(5):800–5.
35. Vercellini P, et al. Perimenopausal management of ovarian endometriosis and associated cancer risk: when is medical or surgical treatment indicated? Best Pract Res Clin Obstet Gynaecol. 2018;51:151–68.
36. Kvaskoff M, et al. Endometriosis and cancer: a systematic review and meta-analysis. Hum Reprod Update. 2021;27(2):393–420.
37. DePriest PD, et al. Endometrioid carcinoma of the ovary and endometriosis: the association in postmenopausal women. Gynecol Oncol. 1992;47(1):71–5.
38. Dochez V, et al. Biomarkers and algorithms for diagnosis of ovarian cancer: CA125, HE4, RMI and ROMA, a review. J Ovar Res. 2019;12(1):28.
39. Oral E, et al. Concomitant endometriosis in malignant and borderline ovarian tumours(). J Obstet Gynaecol. 2018;38(8):1104–9.
40. Oral E, et al. The prevalence of endometrioma and associated malignant transformation in women over 40 years of age. J Gynecol Obstet Human Reprod. 2020;49(5):101725.
41. Králíčková M, Losan P, Vetvicka V. Endometriosis and cancer. Womens Health (Lond). 2014;10(6):591–7.
42. Melin A, et al. Endometriosis and the risk of cancer with special emphasis on ovarian cancer. Hum Reprod. 2006;21(5):1237–42.
43. Bertelsen L, et al. Risk for breast cancer among women with endometriosis. Int J Cancer. 2007;120(6):1372–5.
44. Zanetta GM, et al. Hyperestrogenism: a relevant risk factor for the development of cancer from endometriosis. Gynecol Oncol. 2000;79(1):18–22.
45. Gücer F, Pieber D, Arikan MG. Malignancy arising in extraovarian endometriosis during estrogen stimulation. Eur J Gynaecol Oncol. 1998;19(1):39–41.
46. Modesitt SC, et al. Ovarian and extraovarian endometriosis-associated cancer. Obstet Gynecol. 2002;100(4):788–95.
47. Reimnitz C, et al. Malignancy arising in endometriosis associated with unopposed estrogen replacement. Obstet Gynecol. 1988;71(3 Pt 2):444–7.
48. Vercellini P, et al. Endometriosis: current therapies and new pharmacological developments. Drugs. 2009;69(6):649–75.

Pregnancy and Obstetric Outcomes in Endometriosis

18

Peter Oppelt and Stefan P. Renner

Contents

18.1 Introduction

Approximately 80% of patients with endometriosis are in the reproductive age group and <40 years and may face pregnancy at any time [1]. In addition to the problem of infertility, special patterns during the course of pregnancy have also been described. Toward the end of pregnancy, the question arises of which mode of delivery should be recommended.

In one study, it was shown that women without previous endometriosis treatment were more likely to give birth spontaneously and had fewer birth complications. However, if a secondary cesarean was performed during the delivery, increased rates of intraoperative and postoperative complications were observed [2]. In a study in Italy, patients with deeply infiltrating endometriosis lesions in the posterior fornix who had undergone incomplete surgery had increased rates of preterm

P. Oppelt (✉)
Department of Gynecology, Obstetrics and Gynecological Endocrinology, Kepler University Hospital Linz, Johannes Kepler Universität Linz, Linz, Austria
e-mail: Peter.Oppelt@kepleruniklinikum.at

S. P. Renner
Department of Gynecology and Obstetrics, Boeblingen Hospital, Sindelfingen–Boeblingen Clinics, Boeblingen, Germany

E. Oral (ed.), *Endometriosis and Adenomyosis*,
https://doi.org/10.1007/978-3-030-97236-3_18

delivery, placental complications (placenta previa, premature placental abruption), and pregnancy-induced hypertension [3]. The rate of cesarean procedures and also complications (hysterectomy, bladder lesions, hemoperitoneum) during cesareans were significantly increased in this group.

18.2 Pregnancy

Several studies have been published in recent years on pathological conditions occurring during pregnancy. The conditions listed below are not specific to endometriosis, but are associated with an increased incidence in connection with endometriosis.

In addition to a slightly increased rate of miscarriage, endometriosis patients also have a nearly doubled incidence of extrauterine pregnancies [4]. Premature rupture of the membranes [5] and preterm birth [6] have also been reported more frequently in pregnancy. Research is being conducted on whether the increased incidence of placenta previa and premature placental abruption [7] should be interpreted in relation to nidation or in relation to adenomyosis. Spontaneous hemoperitoneum in pregnancy (SHiP) is a very rare, although life-threatening, situation [8]. This involves sudden intra-abdominal bleeding from endometrial lesions or adenomyosis, which is still associated with a high rate of maternal morbidity and fetal morbidity and mortality. This is probably caused by de-decidualization of the ectopic endometrial tissue during the third trimester. Only a slightly higher incidence of gestational diabetes was identified in a meta-analysis [9].

Individual publications have also repeatedly reported that there is an increased incidence of preeclampsia in endometriosis. However, these data could not be confirmed in a meta-analysis [10].

18.3 Obstetrics

Although there have been several studies on potential complications of endometriosis during pregnancy, there are only a few studies on the question of which mode of birth should be recommended to endometriosis patients. The following list does not take into account general contraindications to vaginal delivery; only the mode of delivery in relation to endometriosis is considered.

High injury to the rectum in the course of spontaneous delivery is a serious complication [3, 11]. The cause is assumed to be insufficient scar tissue that does not withstand the pressure caused by intrapartum stretching and ruptures. This affects both patients who have had deeply infiltrating endometriosis removed from the rectovaginal septum or vagina and also patients who have undergone anterior rectal resections. Due to the deepening of the fetal head during delivery, maximum stretching occurs in the area of the scar tissue. Due to the limited elasticity, the tissue eventually tears. The scientific data on this issue is weak. Successful vaginal births have been described after rectal resection and in cases of untreated rectal endometriosis [12, 13], but it is not possible to draw any general treatment recommendations from this.

In a surgical study investigating cesarean section versus spontaneous childbirth after rectal resection, a better quality of life and less anterior sphincter injury were observed in the cesarean group [14].

The following four questions are frequently asked in this context and should be helpful in decision-making:

1. Should deeply infiltrating endometriosis be treated before pregnancy?
   - Patients with untreated deeply infiltrating endometriosis have a higher rate of spontaneous childbirth.
   - If a cesarean is carried out due to untreated deeply infiltrating endometriosis, intraoperative and postoperative complications are more frequent.
2. Are patients with partially treated deeply infiltrating endometriosis at greater risk in relation to childbirth? Yes, the following risks have been reported:
   - Prematurity.
   - Placenta previa.
   - Premature placental abruption.
   - Gestational hypertension.
   - Peripartum hysterectomy.
3. What advice should be given to patients with endometriosis, with or without prior treatment, in relation to childbirth?
   - Patients who have been treated for ovarian and/or peritoneal endometriosis can aim for spontaneous childbirth.
   - If previously treated or existing deeply infiltrating endometriosis is present, there are currently no contraindications against spontaneous childbirth. There have only been case reports of complications, so that a clear recommendation cannot currently be given.
   - If previously treated or existing rectal endometriosis is present, no clear recommendations can be given at present. On the basis of individual case reports, the patient should be informed about risks (including rectal injury) in the context of spontaneous delivery. It is a matter of controversy whether a primary cesarean section is indicated if the posterior fornix has been opened during the course of rectal resection. Due to a lack of data, a definite recommendation is not at present possible.
   - Surgery in the area of the sigmoid colon (without deep resection), appendix/cecum, small-bowel area, or the rest of the colon does not constitute an indication for a primary cesarean.
4. Should deeply infiltrating endometriosis be treated before pregnancy, due to the potential for complications during pregnancy or birth?
   - The data situation is poor both in relation to improvements in fertility and in relation to complications during pregnancy and birth. It is therefore not possible to make any general recommendations. Counseling should thus focus on potential infertility or pain problems, rather than on possible pregnancy-associated complications or complications during childbirth.
   - Treatment for endometriosis during pregnancy or intrapartum—e.g., during a cesarean—should be avoided. This is reserved for severe complications such as rectal rupture. Due to the vulnerability of the tissue, exploration should also be avoided during a cesarean procedure.

References

1. Haas D, Chvatal R, Reichert B, Renner S, Shebl O, Binder H, Wurm P, Oppelt P. Endometriosis: a premenopausal disease? Age pattern in 42,079 patients with endometriosis. Arch Gynecol Obstet. 2012;286(3):667–70.
2. Thomin A, Belghiti J, David C, Marty O, Bornes M, Ballester M, Roman H, Daraï E. Maternal and neonatal outcomes in women with colorectal endometriosis. BJOG. 2018;125(6):711–8.
3. Exacoustos C, Lauriola I, Lazzeri L, De Felice G, Zupi E. Complications during pregnancy and delivery in women with untreated rectovaginal deep infiltrating endometriosis. Fertil Steril. 2016;106(5):1129–1135.e1121.
4. Hjordt Hansen MV, Dalsgaard T, Hartwell D, Skovlund CW, Lidegaard O. Reproductive prognosis in endometriosis. A national cohort study. Acta Obstet Gynecol Scand. 2014;93(5):483–9.
5. Conti N, Cevenini G, Vannuccini S, Orlandini C, Valensise H, Gervasi MT, Ghezzi F, Di Tommaso M, Severi FM, Petraglia F. Women with endometriosis at first pregnancy have an increased risk of adverse obstetric outcome. J Matern Fetal Neonatal Med. 2015;28(15):1795–8.
6. Kim SG, Seo HG, Kim YS. Primiparous singleton women with endometriosis have an increased risk of preterm birth: meta-analyses. Obstet Gynecol Sci. 2017;60(3):283–8.
7. Berlac JF, Hartwell D, Skovlund CW, Langhoff-Roos J, Lidegaard Ø. Endometriosis increases the risk of obstetrical and neonatal complications. Acta Obstet Gynecol Scand. 2017;96(6):751–60.
8. Vigano P, Corti L, Berlanda N. Beyond infertility: obstetrical and postpartum complications associated with endometriosis and adenomyosis. Fertil Steril. 2015;104(4):802–12.
9. Lalani S, Choudhry AJ, Firth B, Bacal V, Walker M, Wen SW, Singh S, Amath A, Hodge M, Chen I. Endometriosis and adverse maternal, fetal and neonatal outcomes, a systematic review and meta-analysis. Human Reprod (Oxford, England). 2018;33(10):1854–65.
10. Zullo F, Spagnolo E, Saccone G, Acunzo M, Xodo S, Ceccaroni M, Berghella V. Endometriosis and obstetrics complications: a systematic review and meta-analysis. Fertil Steril. 2017;108(4):667–672.e665.
11. Menzlova E, Zahumensky J, Gürlich R, Kucera E. Rectal injury following delivery as a possible consequence of endometriosis of the rectovaginal septum. Int J Gynaecol Obstet. 2014;124(1):85–6.
12. Allerstorfer C, Oppelt P, Enzelsberger SH, Shamiyeh A, Schimetta W, Shebl OJ, Mayer RB. Delivery after operation for deeply infiltrating endometriosis. Biomed Res Int. 2016;2016:8271452.
13. Nirgianakis K, Gasparri ML, Radan AP, Villiger A, McKinnon B, Mosimann B, Papadia A, Mueller MD. Obstetric complications after laparoscopic excision of posterior deep infiltrating endometriosis: a case-control study. Fertil Steril. 2018;110(3):459–66.
14. Remzi FH, Gorgun E, Bast J, Schroeder T, Hammel J, Philipson E, Hull TL, Church JM, Fazio VW. Vaginal delivery after ileal pouch-anal anastomosis: a word of caution. Dis Colon Rectum. 2005;48(9):1691–9.

Part III

Endometriosis: Miscellaneous Clinical Presentations and Management

Recurrent Endometriosis

19

Ertan Sarıdoğan and Michael D. Mueller

Contents

Endometriosis is considered a chronic condition with a high risk of recurrence following treatment. Medical treatments are usually considered to be effective in controlling the pain symptoms of endometriosis without eliminating the lesions, and it is very common for the symptoms to recur after their discontinuation. For this reason, return of symptoms after discontinuation of medical treatment may be better described as 'relapse' instead of recurrence. Surgical treatment aims to eliminate endometriosis either as part of an organ-preserving conservative surgery or as part of a radical operation which also involves removal of the uterus with or without the ovaries. Even after surgical treatment, high recurrence rates have been reported, with estimates of 20% after 2 years and up to 50% after 5 years [1, 2]. A recent

E. Sarıdoğan (✉)
Women's Health Division, University College London Hospital, London, UK
e-mail: ertan.saridogan@nhs.net

M. D. Mueller
Department of Gynecology and Gynecological Oncology, Inselspital, Bern University Hospital, Bern, Switzerland

E. Oral (ed.), *Endometriosis and Adenomyosis*,
https://doi.org/10.1007/978-3-030-97236-3_19

population-based cohort study suggests that up to one in four who undergo minor surgery and one in five who undergo major conservative surgery with ovarian preservation require additional endometriosis surgery within 5 years following operation, whereas few endometriosis patients who undergo hysterectomy require repeat surgery. Furthermore, only 1.9% of major conservative surgery with bilateral salpingo-oophorectomy (BSO), 1.4% of hysterectomy without BSO patients and 0.4% of hysterectomy with BSO patients went on to have repeat surgery. Compared to hysterectomy with ovarian preservation, women who underwent hysterectomy and BSO are less likely to require repeat surgery (aHR0.28, 95%CI: 0.19, 0.41), although the absolutely risk of requiring repeat surgery was low after hysterectomy [3].

In this chapter we will aim to give an overview of the published data on recurrence of endometriosis following surgery, predictive factors of recurrence, preventive measures and management of recurrence.

19.1 Definition

Definition of recurrence varies in the published literature. It may be described as recurrence of pain symptoms (symptomatic recurrence) or recurrence of endometriotic lesions (anatomical recurrence). Symptomatic recurrence refers to return of one or more pain symptoms associated with endometriosis such as dysmenorrhoea, non-cyclical pelvic pain, dyspareunia or dyschezia. Many studies used this approach in defining recurrent endometriosis, as it is easier to collect data by asking the patients to report their symptoms, or complete questionnaires in person or remotely. However, grading pain is a subjective tool and may be affected by a number of factors, including the woman's personal and emotional circumstances on the day of providing the data. Furthermore, lack of data from patients who have been lost to follow up may skew the results, as they would be more likely to be unsatisfied with their outcomes.

Anatomical recurrence may be described in a number of ways: clinical examination, imaging, surgery and histology. In addition, a small number of studies used rising CA-125 levels as an indication of recurrence.

Diagnosing recurrence by clinical examination is likely to be the least reliable or accurate method of detecting anatomical recurrence. Clinical examination is subject to significant interobserver and even intraobserver variability, and co-operation of the patient during the examination, perhaps affected by how severe her pain/tenderness on the day of examination is, is likely to have an impact on its accuracy.

Both ultrasound and magnetic resonance imaging (MRI) are established modalities in diagnosing endometriomas and deep endometriosis. They would be expected to identify anatomical recurrence of these lesions as well; however, their accuracy in determining recurrence correctly and differentiating small endometriotic nodules from surgical fibrosis has not been well established. In addition, some small cystic areas containing echogenic fluid or blood products following surgical excision may resemble small endometriomas, and be diagnosed as such, although they may simply be postsurgical residues. Perhaps due to this possibility, or due to the assumption that small cysts are unlikely to be significant, many studies looking at recurrence of endometriomas after surgery use a cut-off cyst size varying between 1 and 3 cm. This cut-off is entirely arbitrary and is not based on any evidence.

Rises in CA-125 have also been used as an indication of recurrence in a couple of studies [4, 5]. An increase in the level of CA-125 by twice the level of normal was considered a sign of recurrence in women whose CA-125 had become negative after the initial surgery. CA-125 is nonspecific and is raised in a number of benign and malignant conditions; hence its usefulness is likely to be limited, similar to its use in diagnosis of endometriosis.

Histological confirmation of recurrence would be the most reliable way of demonstrating recurrence. Surgery may again have a similar accuracy in detecting anatomical recurrence. However, they are both invasive interventions. In addition, the limitations that apply to diagnostic accuracy of surgical visualisation and histopathological confirmation in diagnosing endometriosis would still apply to detecting recurrence [6]. In fact, both surgical visualisation and histopathology may have lower accuracy in detecting recurrence than diagnosing the original condition due to postsurgical fibrosis and changes in the appearance of the peritoneal surface. Furthermore, significance of anatomical recurrence without correlating it to the presence or absence of symptoms is debatable.

19.2 Mechanisms of Recurrence

Symptomatic or anatomical recurrence may be due to a number of mechanisms:

1. Incomplete removal of endometriotic lesions at surgery; this is likely to present either as persistence or early recurrence of symptoms, as discussed later.
2. Regrowth of invisible/microscopic lesions which were present at the time of surgery.
3. De novo development of new endometriotic lesions.

All three mechanisms are likely to contribute to recurrence either separately or in combination. However, the magnitude of their contribution or how they relate to the symptoms of the woman is not clearly known.

19.3 Timing of Recurrence

It has been hypothesised that rate of recurrences may have a 'U' or a 'bathtub' shape [2]. This represents an initial period when a relatively high proportion of 'recurrences' or perhaps 'persistent' symptoms is seen. This is followed by a medium-length phase where the recurrence rates are relatively low. After this phase, in the longer term, more women start experiencing recurrences. This appears a logical model based on clinical experience, although not necessarily supported by published evidence.

The initial high rates probably reflect a combination of persistent or early recurrent symptoms. This may be because the disease was not completely removed or the pain was not endometriosis related in the first place. It is also possible that patients who suffer from complex or centralised pain after long years of chronic pain may have limited benefit from surgery, although the peripheral disease may have been completely removed. It is well known that even diagnostic laparoscopy has a 'placebo effect' and women report improved pain within the first 3 months after surgery [7].

The middle part of the 'U-shaped' curve indicates that the majority of women who had successful excision of their disease have a low risk of recurrence in the 'medium term'.

The last part of the curve indicates a higher proportion of women start to experience recurrences as longer time passes, allowing regrowth or de novo development of endometriosis.

The median gap between operations has been reported to be between 30 and 36 months in a retrospective cohort in which the recurrences were confirmed surgically [8]. In this cohort the time to first recurrent endometriosis surgery was independent from the endometriosis subtype (peritoneal endometriosis, ovarian endometrioma and deep endometriosis) diagnosed at the initial surgery. Moreover, at subsequent surgery the endometriosis subtype observed was likely to be the same subtype observed previously. Interestingly, however, there was a high percentage of patients that presented with more severe lesion subtypes, particularly deep endometriosis. The trend towards more severe endometriosis subtypes in these patients implies disease progression may occur overtime irrespective of surgical removal [8].

19.4 Risk Factors for Recurrent Endometriosis

The reported risk factors for recurrence may be grouped under patient, disease and surgery related (Table 19.1) [1, 9]. There is a long list of risk factors in the published literature, and sometimes there may be conflicting reports on certain risk factors, for example, the impact of age.

19.5 Prevention of Recurrence

Postoperative medical therapies have been a subject of interest in reducing symptomatic or anatomical recurrence. In women operated on for endometriosis, it has been demonstrated that postoperative use of a levonorgestrel-intrauterine system (LNG-IUS) or a combined hormonal contraceptive for at least 18–24 months reduces the possibility of endometriosis-associated dysmenorrhoea, but not for non-menstrual pelvic pain or dyspareunia [10, 11]. A recent systematic review and meta-analysis of 17 studies using combined hormonal contraceptives, progestins, LNG-IUS or GnRH agonists showed that there was a significantly decreased risk of endometriosis recurrence in patients receiving postoperative hormonal suppression

Table 19.1 Risk factors for recurrent endometriosis

Patient related
Family history
Younger age
Higher BMI
Disease related
More advanced disease
Larger endometrioma size
Bilaterality of endometrioma
Presence of extensive adhesions
Surgery related
Incomplete surgery
Conservative or less radical surgery vs radical surgery
Coagulation/ablation vs cystectomy for endometriomas
Shaving instead of segmental or discoid resection for colorectal deep endometriosis
Positive bowel resection margins for bowel endometriosis

compared to expectant management/placebo (relative risk (RR) 0.41; 95% CI, 0.26 to 0.65) [12].

In case of endometriomas, there are more publications looking into the efficacy of postoperative medical therapies. Vercellini et al. recommended prescribing combined hormonal contraceptives for the secondary prevention of endometrioma in women not trying to become pregnant [13]. Wattanayingcharoenchai et al. [14] carried out a systematic review and network meta-analysis (NMA) on the efficacy of postoperative medical therapies in reducing endometrioma recurrence. They concluded that evidence from randomised controlled trials (RCTs) do not support the use of postoperative hormonal therapies, whereas data from cohort studies indicated a significant protective effect of LNG-IUS followed by dienogest, gonadotropin-releasing hormone agonists (GnRHa) + LNG-IUS and continuous and cyclical oral contraceptives (OC). The most effective postoperative therapy (although non-significant) was GnRHa + LNG-IUS, followed by continuous OC and GnRHa based on RCTs. Direct meta-analysis of RCTs in the Wattanayingcharoenchai et al. article indicated an approximately 40–50% reduction with OCs, but this remained statistically non-significant. There is a wide variation in the design of studies on which meta-analyses and this NMA are based on in terms of inclusion criteria, duration of treatment and definition of recurrence, and this is likely to be the reason for conflicting conclusions in different publications. It is very likely postoperative medical therapies would reduce recurrences by suppression of ovulation and reducing/eliminating menstrual flow in the long term [15].

Intraoperative measures are also expected to reduce recurrences. In women operated on for an endometrioma, performing ovarian cystectomy, instead of drainage and electrocoagulation, reduces risk of endometriosis-associated dysmenorrhoea, dyspareunia, nonmenstrual pelvic pain as well as cyst recurrence and the need for further surgery [16]. It is also very plausible to expect that completeness of surgery and performance of surgery by experienced surgeons would be expected to reduce recurrences.

19.6 Management of Recurrent Endometriosis

19.6.1 Early Recurrence

The management of early symptomatic recurrence needs to start by assessing the history of the patient and details of the previous operation as well as imaging. If it is obvious that the previous operation was incomplete based on operation records or imaging, consideration should be given to a repeat operation. It would be sensible to arrange the repeat operation at a centre with the necessary expertise to remove the residual persistent disease.

If the assessment of the previous operation details and imaging suggest that there is no residual disease, other causes of pelvic pain including the possibility of centralised chronic pain should be explored, and consideration should be given to arranging input from pain management specialists.

19.6.2 Medium-/Long-Term Recurrence

As explained earlier, the majority of patients have real anatomical recurrence in this group. Hence, thorough assessment of the patient's symptoms and their severity, extent of anatomical recurrence, age, future fertility plans, ovarian reserve in the presence of recurrent endometriomas and details of previous surgery including presence and severity of adhesions, extent of surgery, type of endometriosis and intra- and postoperative complications should be obtained. It has to be remembered that repeat surgery for recurrent endometriomas tends to be more harmful to ovarian reserve and this would be expected to have a bigger impact on a woman's future fertility or on possible future fertility treatment. Similarly, repeat operations for deep endometriosis tend to be more difficult and would carry higher risks compared to the primary operation. For these reasons, decision to reoperate in these two groups of women should be carefully considered [17]. Consideration should be given to non-organ-preserving surgery in older women who no longer plan to seek fertility or fertility treatment, if surgical treatment is chosen. The difficulty is to define the radicality of such a treatment. It has been reported that ovarian conservation is associated with a sixfold risk of recurrent pain and an eightfold risk of reoperation [18]. However, bilateral adnexectomy induces early menopause, may increase all-cause mortality and increases the risk of coronary heart disease [19]. The decision to perform bilateral adnexectomy must take into consideration the patient's age and the effect on quality of life after inducing an artificial menopause.

Medical treatment has an important role to play in the management of recurrent endometriosis for the reasons explained above. There are a number of published trials or cohorts suggesting that combined hormonal contraceptives, desogestrel, dienogest and GnRHa can be beneficial in controlling the symptoms due to recurrence after conservative surgical treatment [20–24]. Experience with past medical treatments, side effect profile and the woman's preferences should be taken into account when these options are considered.

19.7 Conclusion

Recurrence after surgical treatment of endometriosis is common; hence clinicians should be familiar with assessment of these patients. Recurrence may be due to incomplete treatment or regrowth of the condition; however persistent or recurrent symptoms after surgery have usually a more complex background. Possibilities that the symptoms may not be due to endometriosis, centralisation of pain due to prolonged exposure and side effects of previous surgery/surgeries should be considered. A multidisciplinary approach that would be able to offer surgery, medical treatment and pain management would be necessary for the management of woman with recurrent endometriosis.

References

1. Ceccaroni M, Bounous VE, Clarizia R, Mautone D, Mabrouk M. Recurrent endometriosis: a battle against an unknown enemy. Eur J Contracept Reprod Health Care. 2019;24(6):464–74. https://doi.org/10.1080/13625187.2019.1662391. Epub 2019 Sep 25.
2. Guo SW. Recurrence of endometriosis and its control. Hum Reprod Update. 2009;15(4):441–61. https://doi.org/10.1093/humupd/dmp007. Epub 2009 Mar 11.
3. Bougie O, McClintock C, Pudwell J, Brogly SB, Velez MP. Long term follow-up of endometriosis surgery in Ontario: a population-based Cohort Study. Am J Obstet Gynecol. 2021;S0002-9378(21):00467-1. https://doi.org/10.1016/j.ajog.2021.04.237. Epub ahead of print.
4. Busacca M, Chiaffarino F, Candiani M, et al. Determinants of long-term clinically detected recurrence rates of deep, ovarian, and pelvic endometriosis. Am J Obstet Gynecol. 2006;195:426–32.
5. Chen FP, Soong YK, Lee N, et al. The use of serum CA-125 as a marker for endometriosis in patients with dysmenorrhea for monitoring therapy and for recurrence of endometriosis. Acta Obstet Gynecol Scand. 1998;77:665–70.
6. Wykes CB, Clark TJ, Khan KS. Accuracy of laparoscopy in the diagnosis of endometriosis: a systematic quantitative review. BJOG. 2004;111:1204–12.
7. Sutton CJ, Ewen SP, Whitelaw N, Haines P. Prospective, randomized, double-blind, controlled trial of laser laparoscopy in the treatment of pelvic pain associated with minimal, mild, and moderate endometriosis. Fertil Steril. 1994;62:696–700.
8. Nirgianakis K, Ma L, McKinnon B, Mueller MD. Recurrence patterns after surgery in patients with different endometriosis subtypes: a long-term Hospital-Based Cohort Study. J Clin Med. 2020;9(2):496. https://doi.org/10.3390/jcm9020496. PMID: 32054117; PMCID: PMC7073694.
9. Bendifallah S, Puchar A, Vesale E, Moawad G, Daraï E, Roman H. Surgical outcomes after colorectal surgery for endometriosis: a systematic review and meta-analysis. J Minim Invasive Gynecol. 2021;28(3):453–66. https://doi.org/10.1016/j.jmig.2020.08.015. Epub 2020 Aug 22.
10. Abou-Setta AM, Houston B, Al-Inany HG, Farquhar C. Levonorgestrel-releasing intrauterine device (LNG-IUD) for symptomatic endometriosis following surgery. Cochrane Database Syst Rev. 2013;(1):CD005072. https://doi.org/10.1002/14651858.CD005072.pub3.

11. Seracchioli R, Mabrouk M, Manuzzi L, Vicenzi C, Frascà C, Elmakky A, Venturoli S. Postoperative use of oral contraceptive pills for prevention of anatomical relapse or symptom-recurrence after conservative surgery for endometriosis. Hum Reprod. 2009;24:2729–35.
12. Zakhari A, Delpero E, McKeown S, Tomlinson G, Bougie O, Murji A. Endometriosis recurrence following post-operative hormonal suppression: a systematic review and meta-analysis. Hum Reprod Update. 2021;27(1):96–107. https://doi.org/10.1093/humupd/dmaa033. PMID: 33020832; PMCID: PMC7781224.
13. Vercellini P, Somigliana E, Viganò P, De Matteis S, Barbara G, Fedele L. Post-operative endometriosis recurrence: a plea for prevention based on pathogenetic, epidemiological and clinical evidence. Reprod Biomed Online. 2010;21:259–65.
14. Wattanayingcharoenchai R, Rattanasiri S, Charakorn C, Attia J, Thakkinstian A. Postoperative hormonal treatment for prevention of endometrioma recurrence after ovarian cystectomy: a systematic review and network meta-analysis. BJOG. 2021;128(1):25–35. https://doi.org/10.1111/1471-0528.16366. Epub 2020 Jul 14. PMID: 32558987; PMCID: PMC7754428.
15. Saridogan E. Postoperative medical therapies for the prevention of endometrioma recurrence – do we now have the final answer? BJOG. 2021;128(1):36. https://doi.org/10.1111/1471-0528.16415. Epub 2020 Aug 10.
16. Hart RJ, Hickey M, Maouris P, Buckett W. Excisional surgery versus ablative surgery for ovarian endometriomata. Cochrane Database Syst Rev. 2008;2:CD004992. https://doi.org/10.1002/14651858.CD004992.pub3.
17. Working group of ESGE, ESHRE and WES, Keckstein J, Becker CM, Canis M, Feki A, Grimbizis GF, Hummelshoj L, Nisolle M, Roman H, Saridogan E, Tanos V, Tomassetti C, Ulrich UA, Vermeulen N, De Wilde RL. Recommendations for the surgical treatment of endometriosis Part 2: deep endometriosis †‡¶. Facts Views Vis Obgyn. 2020;11(4):269–97. PMID: 32322824; PMCID: PMC7162667.
18. Namnoum AB, Hickman TN, Goodman SB, Gehlbach DL, Rock JA. Incidence of symptom recurrence after hysterectomy for endometriosis. Fertil Steril. 1995;64(5):898–902. https://doi.org/10.1016/s0015-0282(16)57899-6.
19. Parker WH, Broder MS, Liu Z, Shoupe D, Farquhar C, Berek JS. Ovarian conservation at the time of hysterectomy for benign disease. Clin Obstet Gynecol. 2007;50(2):354–61. https://doi.org/10.1097/GRF.0b013e31804a838d.
20. Abdou AM, Ammar IMM, Alnemr AAA, Abdelrhman AA. Dienogest versus leuprolide acetate for recurrent pelvic pain following laparoscopic treatment of endometriosis. J Obstet Gynaecol India. 2018;68(4):306–13. https://doi.org/10.1007/s13224-018-1119-3.
21. Razzi S, Luisi S, Ferretti C, Calonaci F, Gabbanini M, Mazzini M, Petraglia F. Use of a progestogen only preparation containing desogestrel in the treatment of recurrent pelvic pain after conservative surgery for endometriosis. Eur J Obstet Gynecol Reprod Biol. 2007;135(2):188–90. https://doi.org/10.1016/j.ejogrb.2006.08.002.
22. Vercellini P, De Giorgi O, Mosconi P, Stellato G, Vicentini S, Crosignani PG. Cyproterone acetate versus a continuous monophasic oral contraceptive in the treatment of recurrent pelvic pain after conservative surgery for symptomatic endometriosis. Fertil Steril. 2002;77(1):52–61. https://doi.org/10.1016/s0015-0282(01)02951-x.
23. Koshiba A, Mori T, Okimura H, Akiyama K, Kataoka H, Takaoka O, Ito F, Matsushima H, Kusuki I, Kitawaki J. Dienogest therapy during the early stages of recurrence of endometrioma might be an alternative therapeutic option to avoid repeat surgeries. J Obstet Gynaecol Res. 2018;44(10):1970–6. https://doi.org/10.1111/jog.13725.
24. Lee JH, Song JY, Yi KW, Lee SR, Lee DY, Shin JH, Cho S, Seo SK, Kim SH. Effectiveness of dienogest for treatment of recurrent endometriosis: multicenter data. Reprod Sci. 2018;25(10):1515–22. https://doi.org/10.1177/1933719118779733.

Extrapelvic Endometriosis

20

Atilla Bokor and Nura Fitnat Topbas Selcuki

Contents

20.1 Introduction

Endometriosis is not only a disease of the pelvis, but it can also be seen in other parts of the human body. Symptoms can vary depending on the affected tissue or organ. Cyclical symptoms, which occur within the first 72 h of menstruation, are called catamenial. Catamenial symptoms are present in most of the patients, at least in early stages, and may be the only sign that leads to the final diagnosis. The prevalence is not exactly known due to the irregular clinical presentation, difficulty in diagnosis, and consultation of patients to non-gynecological specialists who are not familiar with this condition. Gold standard in diagnosis is the histopathological confirmation of endometrial glands and stroma in the excised material. A trained

A. Bokor (✉)
Department of Obstetrics and Gynecology, Semmelweis University, Budapest, Hungary

N. F. Topbas Selcuki
Department of Obstetrics and Gynecology, University of Health Sciences Turkey, Istanbul Sisli Hamidiye Etfal Training and Research Hospital, Istanbul, Turkey

E. Oral (ed.), *Endometriosis and Adenomyosis*,
https://doi.org/10.1007/978-3-030-97236-3_20

pathologist in detecting endometriosis is crucial since the excised material is not from the pelvic area. Imaging techniques and endoscopy can also be used for diagnosis depending on the affected organ system. In a systematic review conducted by Andres et al. (2020) involving 179 studies, malignancy was the most common differential diagnosis (37%) among reported visceral endometriosis cases [1]. Therefore, a clinical knowledge on the possible extrapelvic locations of endometriosis is important for an accurate diagnosis and proper treatment. Treatment depends on the localization. If complete excision is possible, this is the treatment of choice; when this is not possible, long-term medical treatment is necessary [2].

Extrapelvic endometriosis is most commonly found in the abdominal wall after surgical procedures, such as cesarean section, which is followed by inguinal and umbilical endometriosis and thoracic endometriosis syndrome. Endometriosis involving the bowel is considered intrapelvic and is discussed as a part of the deep infiltrative endometriosis. Therefore, it will not be included in this chapter. However, endometriosis involving other abdominal organs will be discussed under the visceral endometriosis section. Pelvic nerve endometriosis is discussed in a separate chapter as well. Publications addressing uncommon cases of endometriosis involving the vascular, lymphatic, and central nervous system, as well as skeletal muscle and peripheral nerves, are mostly based on case reports. These entities of limited clinical relevance will be discussed at the end.

20.2 Abdominal Wall Endometriosis: Scar, Perineal, Umbilical, and Inguinal Endometriosis

The most frequent location of the extrapelvic endometriosis is the abdominal wall [3]. Abdominal wall endometriosis (AWE) is defined by the presence of endometrial-like tissue superficial to the peritoneum, including skin, rectus abdominis muscle, and rectus sheath [4]. AWE is frequently associated with gynecologic procedures such as caesarean section, episiotomy, laparoscopic or abdominal hysterectomy [1, 5–7]. However, this definition also includes lesions that are not a result of a previous surgical procedure. In a review of 445 cases, the pooled mean time interval between index surgery and clinical presentation of AWE was reported to be 3.6 years [7]. Many cases of this entity are often misdiagnosed as hernia, hematoma, or lipoma. Therefore, patients are usually referred to general surgery clinics. Presence of intrapelvic endometriosis has been observed in 12% of AWE patients [8].

Scar endometriosis is the most common form of AWE, and the endometriotic loci are located near or at the site of the surgical incision. AWE is seen in 0.03–1.5% of women following caesarean delivery [5, 6]. Perineal endometriosis on the episiotomy scar is rarer. It is encountered in approximately 0.01–0.06% of women after vaginal birth with episiotomy [6, 9]. The etiology of scar endometriosis is thought to be iatrogenic through the transfer of endometrial cells into the surgical wound [10]. This mechanism is also called the metastatic theory. On the other hand, primary endometriotic lesions of the abdominal wall are thought to occur through the metaplastic transformation of the coelomic epithelium. Primary lesions are usually located at or around umbilicus. Therefore, these lesions are called umbilical endometriosis. Umbilical endometriosis is estimated to occur in 0.5–1.0% of all cases of endometriosis and in 0.4–4% of all extragenital endometriosis cases [5, 11]. Another form of AWE, inguinal endometriosis, is defined by the presence of endometriotic loci in the extraperitoneal portion of the round ligament, in the inguinal lymph nodes, in the subcutaneous adipose tissue, and in the wall of sacs of inguinal or femoral hernias, which occur either as primary lesions or following gynecological and/or inguinal surgeries [12–16]. The actual incidence is not known. Most of the cases are observed on the right inguinal region [16].

Symptoms include local catamenial pain, diffuse abdominal pain, palpable mass with catamenial tenderness and swelling, and rarely umbilical bleeding. AWE can be identified with transabdominal ultrasonography (TAS), computed tomography (CT), and magnetic resonance imaging (MRI) in patients who are both symptomatic or asymptomatic [5, 6, 11, 17]. The appearance of AWE at TAS, CT, and MRI depends on the phase of the patient's menstrual cycle, the chronicity of the lesion, the number of stromal and glandular elements, the amount of bleeding and associated inflammation [6, 17, 18]. TAS is usually the first-line imaging modality in evaluating focal abdominal or inguinal wall thickening identified at clinical examination. With TAS, the extent and the nature of the focal lesions can be determined and abdominal wall hernias can be excluded [18]. CT and MRI are used to exclude differential diagnoses in the anterior abdominal and pelvic wall such as hernia, abscess, hematoma, and other soft-tissue tumors [6, 17, 18]. CT can be performed with or without intravenous contrast material, although the use of contrast material improves its sensitivity and specificity. The highest reported combined sensitivity of CT imaging for the diagnosis of AWE is 0.69 (95% CI: 0.48–0.86) and specificity is 0.97 (95% CI: 0.91–1.00) [17]. MRI provides better contrast resolution than CT and TAS and is superior to CT for depicting the delineation between muscle and abdominal subcutaneous tissue and infiltration of abdominal wall structures. Furthermore, MRI is preferred in younger patients because of its improved tissue characterization and lack of ionizing radiation. Recently, for the diagnosis of umbilical endometriosis, a sensitivity of 87.1% for physical examination, 76.5% for TAS, 75.6% for CT, and 81.8% for MRI was reported [5].

Ultrasound-guided fine-needle aspiration biopsy can be performed to exclude malignancy and establish a definitive preoperative diagnosis of AWE [18]. Treatment of choice is the surgical excision of endometriotic loci. The surgical therapy of AWE is often successful following a complete excision. Use of neoadjuvant and adjuvant hormonal treatment has been reported in only a few case reports. Due to lack of data, hormonal treatment is not routinely recommended. The decision should be made according to the symptoms of the patients, extend of the disease, and the presence of pelvic endometriosis.

20.3 Visceral Endometriosis

Endometriosis is also known to affect abdominal organs. Cases of liver, kidney, pancreas, and biliary tract endometriosis have been reported in the literature [1]. Symptoms depend on the affected organ. Liver endometriosis commonly presents with abdominal pain, abdominal mass, and acute liver failure. Flank pain, hematuria, and pyelonephritis are usually associated with kidney endometriosis. Epigastric pain and acute pancreatitis can occur in patients with pancreas endometriosis. In 62% of the patients, pelvic endometriosis was reported [1]. CT is the most commonly used imaging modality. Biopsy, if possible, can lead to definitive diagnosis. Surgical excision of the endometriotic loci is the treatment of choice. However, more radical approaches such as partial nephrectomy, partial hepatectomy, and complete nephrectomy can be performed in the presence of severe disease. Hormonal treatment can be administered following surgery.

20.4 Thoracic Endometriosis Syndrome

Thoracic endometriosis syndrome (TES) encompasses a variety of symptoms and radiological findings associated with the growth of endometrial foci within the respiratory system, most commonly the lung parenchyma, pleural surfaces, and the diaphragm [19–21]. These symptoms include pneumothorax, hemothorax, hemoptysis, chest pain, pulmonary nodules, endometriosis-related diaphragmatic hernia, and endometriosis-related pleural effusion [22, 23]. Symptoms usually have a catamenial pattern [1, 20, 21]. However, non-catamenial presentation has also been reported in the literature [24]. Approximately 90% of patients with TES experience catamenial thoracic pain, which is followed by catamenial pneumothorax (80%) [25, 26]. Catamenial hemothorax is observed in 14% of the reported cases and catamenial hemoptysis in 5% [22]. In majority of the cases, a right-sided hemithorax involvement has been reported [27, 28].

Although the exact pathophysiological mechanism of TES is not yet known, a multifactorial etiology is suspected. The theories already discussed as a possible explanation for the occurrence of endometriosis such as retrograde menstruation, coelomic metaplasia, lymphatic and hematogenous dissemination, and prostaglandin F2alpha involvement are also considered in the etiology of TES [26]. The right-sided predominance can be explained by the circulation of the peritoneal fluid, which flows from the pelvis through the right paracolic gutter to the right hemidiaphragm, while deviating away from the left hemidiaphragm due to obstruction of flow by the falciform and phrenicocolic ligaments [26, 29].

Symptoms arise according to the localization of the endometriotic lesions. Pleural involvement usually presents with catamenial pneumothorax, chest and/or shoulder pain and less commonly catamenial hemothorax. Pneumothorax leads to pleuritic chest pain, cough, and shortness of breath [26]. Diaphragmatic involvement with fenestrations, which are usually present in the tendinous (central) part of the diaphragm, can cause secondary pneumothorax, serous or bloody pleural effusions, or partial thoracic herniation of abdominal organs [30, 31].

On the other hand, isolated diaphragmatic endometriosis is mostly asymptomatic, which is usually an incidental laparoscopic finding during pelvic endometriosis surgery [30]. Therefore, there is an ongoing debate on whether isolated diaphragmatic endometriosis should be considered as a part of TES or not. Endometriotic lesions of the diaphragm can cause phrenic nerve irritation. This leads to catamenial neck, shoulder, right upper quadrant, or epigastric pain [26, 32]. Parenchymal endometriotic lesions can cause mild to moderate hemoptysis and nodules can be identified with imaging.

Diagnosis of TES is challenging, as these women's symptoms may not immediately be attributed to endometriosis. Due to the respiratory related complaints, these patients usually visit thoracic clinics, which usually leads to a delay in the diagnosis. Chest X-ray (CXR), CT, and MRI are the imaging modalities of choice in diagnosis. CXR and CT are the most sensitive techniques in identifying hemothorax and pneumothorax [21, 26]. In a recent systematic review, only one study with 33 patients with diaphragmatic endometriosis evaluated the accuracy of MRI for diagnosis and reported a sensitivity of 83% with fat-suppressed T1-weighted sequences [1].

It is advisable to discuss the diagnosis and management of TES in a multidisciplinary team in a center with sufficient expertise [33]. In the case of catamenial pneumothorax, video-assisted thoracoscopic surgery (VATS) is the approach of choice for diagnosis and surgical treatment [19, 26]. Superficial lesions can be coagulated or ablated with different types of low-energy sources. The presence of larger lesions may afterwards be associated with diaphragmatic fenestrations and therefore a total excision when possible is advised [31, 34]. Small fenestrations in the diaphragm can be closed with interrupted stitches. In cases with large defects after resection, thoracoscopic suturing by a thoracic surgeon is preferable [30, 31]. Special care should be taken during the surgical interventions for the treatment of diaphragmatic endometriosis in order to preserve the phrenic nerve and vessels.

20.5 Other Sites

In a recent systematic review by Andres et al., a total of 19 case studies of nonabdominal and nonthoracic sites of endometriosis were reported [1]. These rare sites included six cases involving the central nervous system (one on brain, one on lumbar vertebra, and four on the conus medullaris). Twelve patients with endometriosis on extrapelvic muscles and peripheral nerves, and one case of nasal endometriosis. The age of this population ranged from 21 to 58 years.

In all cases involving the central nervous system, the extrapelvic muscles and the peripheral nerves, patients presented with paresthesia and catamenial pain radiating to the associated anatomical structures and dermatomes. Surgical excision was the definitive treatment in 91% of muscular and peripheral nerve endometriosis cases, with complete and partial improvement of symptoms in 90.9% and 9%, respectively. Adjuvant hormonal therapy after muscular and peripheral nerve endometriosis resection was reported in 33.3% of these cases, with GnRH-analogues and OC.

References

1. Andres MP, Arcoverde FVL, Souza CCC, Fernandes LFC, Abrão MS, Kho RM. Extrapelvic endometriosis: a systematic review. J Minim Invasive Gynecol. 2020;27(2):373–89.
2. Dunselman GA, Vermeulen N, Becker C, Calhaz-Jorge C, et al. ESHRE guideline: management of women with endometriosis. Hum Reprod. 2014;29(3):400–12.
3. Ideyi SC, Schein M, Niazi M, Gerst PH. Spontaneous endometriosis of the abdominal wall. Dig Surg. 2003;20(3):246–8.
4. Goksever Celik H, Karacan T, Kaya C, Uhri M, Savkli AO, Yalcin Bahat P, et al. Abdominal wall endometriosis: a monocentric continuous series and review of the literature. J Endometriosis Pelvic Pain Disord. 2019;11(2):95–101.
5. Hirata T, Koga K, Kitade M, Fukuda S, Neriishi K, Taniguchi F, et al. A national survey of umbilical endometriosis in Japan. J Minim Invasive Gynecol. 2020;27(1):80–7.
6. Chamié LP, Ribeiro DMFR, Tiferes DA, Macedo Neto AC, de, Serafini PC. Atypical sites of deeply infiltrative endometriosis: clinical characteristics and imaging findings. Radiographics. 2018;38(1):309–28.
7. Horton JD, Dezee KJ, Ahnfeldt EP, Wagner M. Abdominal wall endometriosis: a surgeon's perspective and review of 445 cases. Am J Surg. 2008;196(2):207–12.
8. Davis AC, Goldberg JM. Extrapelvic endometriosis. Semin Reprod Med. 2017;35(1):98–101.
9. Jubanyik KJ, Comite F. Extrapelvic endometriosis. Obstet Gynecol Clin N Am. 1997;24(2):411–40.
10. Woodward PJ, Sohaey R, Mezzetti TP. Endometriosis: radiologic-pathologic correlation. Radiographics. 2001;21(1):193–216; questionnaire 288-294.
11. Bergqvist A. Extragenital endometriosis. A review. Eur J Surg. 1992;158(1):7–12.
12. Pérez-Seoane C, Vargas J, de Agustín P. Endometriosis in an inguinal crural hernia. Diagnosis by fine needle aspiration biopsy. Acta Cytol. 1991;35(3):350–2.
13. Brzezinski A, Durst AL. Endometriosis presenting as an inguinal hernia. Am J Obstet Gynecol. 1983;146(8):982–3.
14. Quagliarello J, Coppa G, Bigelow B. Isolated endometriosis in an inguinal hernia. Am J Obstet Gynecol. 1985;152(6 Pt 1):688–9.
15. Majeski J. Scar endometriosis manifested as a recurrent inguinal hernia. South Med J. 2001;94(2):247–9.
16. Wong WSF, Lim CED, Luo X. Inguinal endometriosis: an uncommon differential diagnosis as an inguinal tumour. ISRN Obstet Gynecol. 2011;2011:272159.
17. Yarmish G, Sala E, Goldman D, Lakhman Y, Soslow R, Hricak H, et al. Abdominal wall endometriosis: differentiation from other masses using CT features. Abdom Radiol (NY). 2017;42(5):1517–23.
18. Gidwaney R, Badler RL, Yam BL, Hines JJ, Alexeeva V, Donovan V, et al. Endometriosis of abdominal and pelvic wall scars: multimodality imaging findings, pathologic correlation, and radiologic mimics. Radiographics. 2012;32(7):2031–43.
19. Alifano M, Trisolini R, Cancellieri A, Regnard JF. Thoracic endometriosis: current knowledge. Ann Thorac Surg. 2006;81(2):761–9.
20. Johnson MM. Catamenial pneumothorax and other thoracic manifestations of endometriosis. Clin Chest Med. 2004;25(2):311–9.
21. Rousset P, Rousset-Jablonski C, Alifano M, Mansuet-Lupo A, Buy J-N, Revel M-P. Thoracic endometriosis syndrome: CT and MRI features. Clin Radiol. 2014;69(3):323–30.

22. Bobbio A, Canny E, Mansuet Lupo A, Lococo F, Legras A, Magdeleinat P, et al. Thoracic endometriosis syndrome other than pneumothorax: clinical and pathological findings. Ann Thorac Surg. 2017;104(6):1865–71.
23. Kaya C, Iliman DE, Eyuboglu GM, Bahceci E. Catamenial pneumothorax: multidisciplinary minimally invasive management of a recurrent case. Kardiochir Torakochirurgia Pol. 2020;17(2):107–9.
24. Selcuki NFT, Yilmaz S, Kaya C, Usta T, Kale A, Oral E. Thoracic endometriosis; a review comparing 480 patients based on catamenial and non-catamenial symptoms. J Minim Invasive Gynecol. 2021;S1553-4650(21):00384–8.
25. Joseph J, Sahn SA. Thoracic endometriosis syndrome: new observations from an analysis of 110 cases. Am J Med. 1996;100(2):164–70.
26. Nezhat C, Lindheim SR, Backhus L, Vu M, Vang N, Nezhat A, et al. Thoracic endometriosis syndrome: a review of diagnosis and management. JSLS. 2019;23(3):e2019. Available from: https://www.ncbi.nlm.nih.gov/pmc/articles/PMC6684338/
27. Gil Y, Tulandi T. Diagnosis and treatment of catamenial pneumothorax: a systematic review. J Minim Invasive Gynecol. 2020;27(1):48–53.
28. Korom S, Canyurt H, Missbach A, Schneiter D, Kurrer MO, Haller U, et al. Catamenial pneumothorax revisited: clinical approach and systematic review of the literature. J Thorac Cardiovasc Surg. 2004;128(4):502–8.
29. Kirschner PA. Porous diaphragm syndromes. Chest Surg Clin N Am. 1998;8(2):449–72.
30. Ceccaroni M, Roviglione G, Farulla A, Bertoglio P, Clarizia R, Viti A, et al. Minimally invasive treatment of diaphragmatic endometriosis: a 15-year single referral center's experience on 215 patients. Surg Endosc. 2021;35(12):6807–17.
31. Working group of ESGE, ESHRE, and WES, Keckstein J, Becker CM, Canis M, Feki A, Grimbizis GF, et al. Recommendations for the surgical treatment of endometriosis. Part 2: deep endometriosis. Hum Reprod Open. 2020;2020(1):hoaa002.
32. Fukuda S, Hirata T, Neriishi K, Nakazawa A, Takamura M, Izumi G, et al. Thoracic endometriosis syndrome: comparison between catamenial pneumothorax or endometriosis-related pneumothorax and catamenial hemoptysis. Eur J Obstet Gynecol Reprod Biol. 2018;225:118–23.
33. Ciriaco P, Muriana P, Lembo R, Carretta A, Negri G. Treatment of thoracic endometriosis syndrome: a meta-analysis and review. Ann Thorac Surg. 2020;113(1):324–36.
34. Roman H, Darwish B, Provost D, Baste J-M. Laparoscopic management of diaphragmatic endometriosis by three different approaches. Fertil Steril. 2016;106(2):e1.

Pelvic Nerve Endometriosis (Neuropelveology)

21

Taner Usta and Shaheen Khazali

Contents

T. Usta
Acibadem Mehmet Ali Aydinlar University, Istanbul, Turkey

Endometriosis and Pelvic Pain Center, Department of Obstetrics and Gynecology, Acibadem Altunizade Hospital, Istanbul, Turkey

S. Khazali (✉)
Royal Holloway-University of London, London, UK

HCA The Lister Hospital, Centre for Endometriosis and Minimally Invasive Gynaecology (CEMIG), London, UK
e-mail: shaheen.khazali@hcaconsultant.com

E. Oral (ed.), *Endometriosis and Adenomyosis*,
https://doi.org/10.1007/978-3-030-97236-3_21

21.1 Introduction

Endometriosis is a chronic inflammatory disease affecting more than 170 million women worldwide and up to 10% of the women of reproductive age. It causes pain symptoms such as dysmenorrhea, dyspareunia, dyschezia, dysuria, and chronic pelvic pain [1, 2]. Although endometriosis affects 1 out of 10 women of reproductive age, pelvic nerve involvement is relatively rare. Endometriosis of the sciatic nerve was first described in 1946 by Schlicke, and in 1955 by Denton and Sherrill [1–3]. Since then, only a few reports on nerve endometriosis of the pelvis have been published in the literature. A review conducted by De Sousa et al. included literature on nerve endometriosis up to 2015 [4]. They reported 365 cases of endometriosis in the somatic peripheral nervous system and 13 cases (10 in the spine and 3 in the brain) of endometriosis affecting the central nervous system [4]. The most commonly affected nerves were the lumbosacral and sacral plexuses (57%, $n = 211$) and sciatic nerve (39%, $n = 140$). Other nerves were reported in significantly small numbers; five cases involved the obturator nerve and three cases reported the femoral nerve endometriosis.

Endometriotic involvement of pelvic nerves can be described in two groups; isolated group where endometriosis affects only the nerve fibers and non-isolated group where the endometriotic lesions located on or in the nerves are a continuation of the endometriotic lesions of the surrounding tissue. Somatic nerves, particularly the sciatic nerve (SN) and the sacral nerve roots are the most commonly affected nerves of the pelvis. In comparison, involvement of femoral and obturator nerves are rare. Depending on the nerve involvement, a difference in pain symptomatology can be observed. Endometriosis of the sciatic, femoral, and obturator nerves cause severe somatic pain, whereas involvement of the autonomic nerves such as inferior hypogastric and splanchnic nerves lead to visceral pelvic pain. In this chapter, we will discuss individual nerve involvement according to their frequency and then explain the appropriate diagnostic techniques and treatment modalities.

21.2 Etiology and Pathophysiology

The precise pathogenesis of endometriosis of pelvic nerves is still unknown. Multiple theories have been proposed. Nerve involvement with endometriosis generally occurs in two main ways. First, the most widely cited, yet unproven pathophysiological hypothesis is that endometrial cells are transported from the uterine cavity during menstruation and subsequently become implanted at ectopic sites. Second, the endometrial tissue in the peripheral nerves invades the epineurium and perineurium and due to monthly hormonal changes results in intraneural hemorrhage and inflammation [5]. The first and most frequent situation involves large rectovaginal or uterosacral nodules, which develop laterally through the parametrium to the lateral pelvic wall, piriformis, and levator ani muscles, where they come into contact with the sacral plexus. The second less frequent situation involves deep endometriosis nodules that occur more laterally and cranially, in contact with the pelvic wall and sciatic nerve, before exiting through the greater sciatic foramen [6]. While endometriosis is able to infiltrate and destroy sympathetic pelvic nerves, it seems unable to destroy the somatic nerves as easily. The sacral hypogastric fascia seems to be an anatomic barrier to infiltration of the pelvic wall as the Denonvilliers' fascia is an anatomic barrier to rectum infiltration in cases of endometriosis of the rectovaginal space [7].

The implantation theory can be excluded as this theory proposes that endometrial tissue passes through the fallopian tubes, then attaches and proliferates in ectopic sites in the peritoneal cavity. The theory of coelomic metaplasia or the induction theory holds that endometriosis develops from metaplasia of cells lining the pelvic peritoneum. Halban proposed the "lymphatic and vascular metastasis" theories and reported that endometriosis could arise in the retroperitoneum from lymphatic and hematogenous dissemination of endometrial cells [8].

The theory of perineural spread of endometriosis has recently been introduced as an alternative by De Sousa et al. [4, 9]. Perineural spread of endometriosis is a form of local invasion in which endometrial glands and stroma spread along the tissue of the nerve sheath. De Sousa et al. explained that the first step of the perineural spread occurs from the uterus to the lumbosacral plexus (LSP) via the visceral autonomic nerves, and the second spread is from the plexus to the spinal nerves or distally to the sciatic nerve and muscular nerve branches. Spread from the uterus to the LSP can be seen as a soft-tissue band, hyperintense on MRI T2WI and heterogeneously enhancing, extending either from the cervix or the body of the uterus toward the sciatic notch [9]. Despite all these proposed theories, data on the etiology and pathophysiology of pelvic nerve endometriosis is still very limited.

21.3 Basic Pelvic Neuroanatomy

Lumbosacral Trunk Lumbosacral trunk consists of the anterior division of S1, L5, and part of L4 (Fig. 21.1).

Femoral Nerve The femoral nerve is the largest branch of the lumbar plexus. It provides considerable sensory innervation to the anterior aspect of the thigh and knee, and motor innervation to the quadriceps muscles. In the thigh, it divides into numerous sensory and muscular branches and the saphenous nerve, its long sensory terminal branch, which continues down to the foot. It gives motor innervation to the

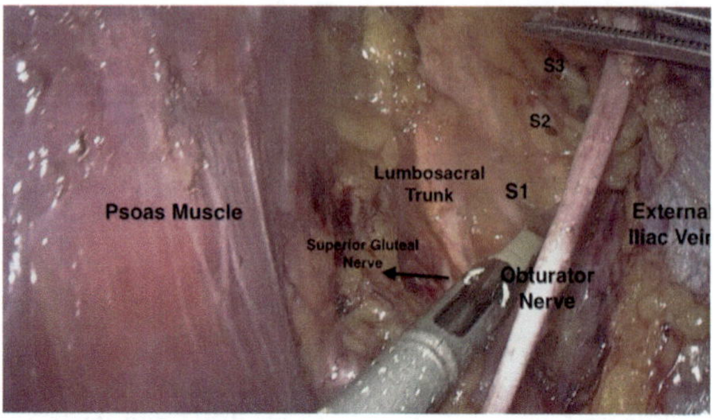

Fig. 21.1 Left lumbosacral space. (With permissions from Taner Usta)

iliopsoas, pectineus, sartorius, and quadriceps femoris (the patellar reflex is mediated by lumbar nerve L4), and sensory innervation to the anterior thigh, posterior lower leg, and hind foot.

Obturator Nerve Obturator nerve leaves the pelvic area through the obturator canal (Fig. 21.1). It sends motor branches mainly to the adductor muscles in the thigh. The anterior branch contributes a terminal sensory branch, which supplies the skin on the medial, distal part of the thigh.

Sacral Nerves The lumbosacral trunk is joined by the S2, S3, and a branch from S4 and sometimes S5 (Fig. 21.1). Together, they are called sacral plexus. The sacral plexus gives rise to five main nerves; superior gluteal nerve (SGN), inferior gluteal nerve, sciatic nerve, posterior femoral cutaneous nerve, and the pudendal nerve.

Superior Gluteal Nerve SGN feeds gluteus medius, gluteus minimus, and tensor fascia latae. If endometriosis infiltrates at this level, involving SGN, muscle atrophy may develop over time [7]. These muscles are important in maintaining the stability of the pelvis. SGN exits the pelvis above the piriformis muscle (Fig. 21.1). Superior gluteal artery and vein accompany the nerve for most of its course. During dissection, awareness of these vessels is particularly important as they can retract into the gluteal muscles if severed, making hemostasis very difficult.

Inferior Gluteal Nerve Inferior gluteal nerve supplies gluteus maximus muscle. The sciatic nerve and the inferior gluteal nerve exit the pelvis through the greater sciatic notch, caudal and inferior to the piriformis muscle.

Posterior Femoral Cutaneous Nerve This is a sensory branch of the sacral plexus. It is responsible for the sensation of the posterior thigh, buttocks, and posterior labia. It leaves the pelvis inferior to the piriformis muscle, along with the sciatic nerve.

Pudendal Nerve The pudendal nerve is a sensory and motor nerve originating from S2 to S4. It branches from the sacral plexus just proximal to the sacrospinous ligament. It exits the pelvis through the great sciatic notch and reenters the pelvis through the lesser sciatic notch. It gives off three distal branches: the perineal nerve, the inferior rectal nerve, and the dorsal nerve of the clitoris.

Sciatic Nerve The sciatic nerve (SN) is the largest somatic nerve (approximately 2 cm wide) in the human body [7, 10]. It is a major nerve of the lower limb. The roots of the SN exit the spinal cord at L4 and 5 and S1, 2, and 3. These five lumbosacral trunks (lumbosacral plexus) travel along the posterolateral aspect of the hollow of the sacrum and unite to form the sciatic nerve exiting the pelvis through the greater sciatic foramen. It innervates the posterior thigh muscles (semimembranosus, semitendinosus, and biceps femoris) as well as the hamstring portion of the abductor magnus. SN contains both sensory neurons and motor functions. It innervates (due to its terminal branches) the skin of the lateral leg, heel, and both the dorsal and plantar surfaces of the foot [10]. Damage to the SN can result in various symptoms, including lower back pain, muscle weakness, and reflex abnormalities. Symptoms are usually present in the lower leg, such as an inability to bend the knee, irradiation pain from the buttocks to the lower leg, or difficulty in rotating and bending the foot, and foot drop.

21.4 Clinical Evaluation

21.4.1 Non-discogenic Sciatica

Traditionally, sciatica, with or without lower back pain, is defined as pain along the distribution areas (lower back to the hips and buttocks and down each leg) of the sciatic nerve. The most frequent pathology of sciatica is associated with herniation of intervertebral disks [11]. Typically, sciatica is one-sided. There is a small group of patients presenting with classic sciatica misdiagnosed as having a discogenic cause. Lumbosacral imaging in such patients might show mild to moderate disc disease, which may erroneously be considered responsible for the symptoms. Sometimes, these patients undergo unnecessary surgical procedures. Non-discogenic sciatica (NDS) is uncommon and has symptoms that are similar to those of much more frequent causes of sciatica, so that it is often overlooked [12]. The neurological examination of patients with NDS usually reveals an absent Lasègue's sign (Fig. 21.2), a positive Tinel's sign with radiation into the distribution of the SN, and extremely tender deep palpation of the infragluteus region in the area of the SN between the ischial tuberosity and greater trochanter [12].

Classically, pain sets on a few days before menstruation, increases gradually and then subsides after the end of menstruation. Thus, it has also been called cyclical sciatica [13]. Major etiologies of NDS include those of traumatic, inflammatory, tumoral, vascular, and gynecological origin. The most common tumors impinging the SN are primary tumors like schwannomas, neurofibromas, and malignant peripheral nerve sheath tumors. Patients usually present with somatic, sensory (buttock and leg pain), and motor complaints (alteration of the Achillean reflex and foot

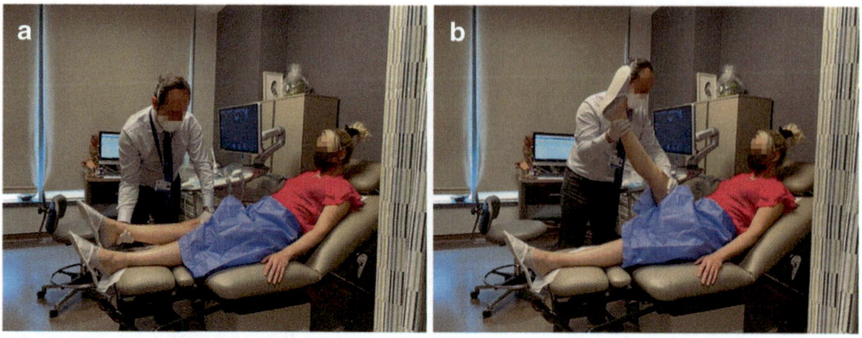

Fig. 21.2 (**a**, **b**) Straight leg raising test (Lasègue's sign). This test is used in the clinical examination of patients presenting with lower back pain. It is an important test for determining the nerve root tension. Examiner lifts the patient's leg with the knee is extended while the patient is in a supine position. If the patient experiences sciatic pain, and more specifically pain radiating down the leg (radiculopathy), when the straight leg is at an angle of between 30 and 70 degrees, then the test is positive and a herniated disk is a possible cause of the pain. (With permissions from Taner Usta)

drop owing to the involvement of S1) [6]. Sciatic pain associated with neoplasia often has an insidious onset and generally is the first symptom of disease. Other neurological symptoms, like weakness, altered gait, diminished reflexes, paresthesia, and dysesthesia, are also frequent. This symptomatology frequently mimics sciatic pain caused by disc herniation. Among gynecological pathologies, recent studies have shown extrauterine endometriosis as the principal cause. The cyclical pattern of sciatica, which coincides with menstruation, is highly suggestive of a gynecological cause.

21.4.2 Sacral Plexus Endometriosis

Endometriosis of the sacral plexus is commonly an extension and the result of invasion of deep infiltrating endometriosis involving the parametrium. Due to the anatomical proximity, deep infiltrating endometriosis affecting the sacrouterine ligament is a risky situation for S3 and S4 involvement, whereas infiltrations of cardinal ligaments and ovarian fossa correlate with S2 and S3 involvement [14]. Sacral root entrapment seems to be much more frequent than actual nerve infiltration owing to the posterior development of large rectovaginal or parametrial nodules. Conversely, intraneural endometriosis was more frequently reported in the SN and may need to require partial resection of the nerve [15] (Fig. 21.3).

SN originates from lumbar spinal nerve 5, sacral nerve root 1 and 2. Bladder has a nerve supply from sacral nerve roots 2, 3, and 4. With a detailed clinical evaluation, it is easy to exclude isolated SN and sacral nerve pathologies. Patients with endometrial nodules affecting these structures usually present with bladder, rectum, and left colon dysfunction, in addition to vaginal dryness, which is more likely due to the involvement of the inferior hypogastric plexus and the thin nerves of the

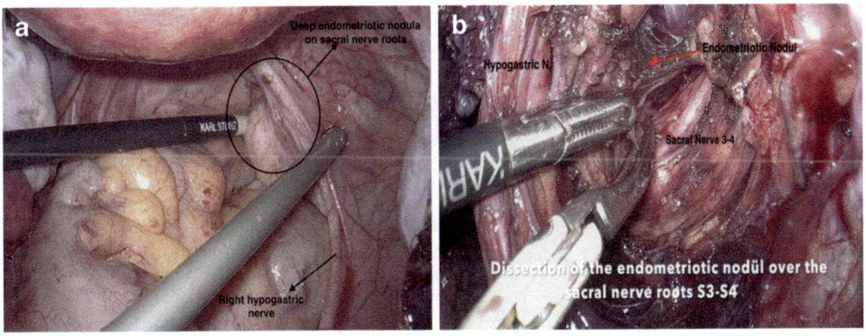

Fig. 21.3 Deep endometriotic nodule on sacral nerve roots. (**a**) Before the dissection, (**b**) after dissection. (With permissions from Taner Usta)

sacral roots [6]. Roman et al. published a retrospective case series of deep endometriosis involving the sacral roots in 49 women and the SN in 3 cases [6]. They reported that self-catheterization was required in 14 cases (27%) at 3 weeks postoperatively and in 3 women (5.8%) 12 months following surgery. Although pain reduction may be rapid after surgery, other sensory or motor complaints, including bladder dysfunction, may persists over months or years.

21.4.3 Sciatic Nerve (SN) Endometriosis

Endometriosis as the cause of sciatica by direct involvement of the SN is very rare. In 1946, Schlicke reported a case of a palpable painful nodule in the posterior part of the thigh of a woman who complained of cyclic sciatic pain, although the direct involvement of the SN was not confirmed [1, 2]. A direct association of cyclic sciatic pain and an endometriotic lesion over the SN was confirmed through surgical exploration of the SN by Denton in 1955 [1]. Although SN endometriosis was reported for the first time in 1946, few cases have been reported thus far. By far, the largest series to date was published by Possover [15]. A full clinical and neuroradiologic evaluation is mandatory in diagnosis. Pain symptoms are usually unilateral and bilateral symptoms are extremely rare. The SN endometriosis localization is of marked clinical relevance because of the important sensory and motor symptoms that may develop [16]. This condition can be very difficult to diagnose as it can present very much like a typical case of sciatica, which is commonly due to prolapsed disc compressing the adjacent nerve root as it exits the spine [17]. Although sacral endometriotic radiculopathies are usually part of parametric endometriosis, endometriosis of the SN can be isolated without any history of pelvic endometriosis [15]. Pain may begin just before menstruation and persist for several days after the end of flow. Left untreated, neuropathic pain will lose its cyclical nature, becoming constant and refractory to strong pain medications (opiates and neuroleptics). Because of nerve damage through deep infiltration of the nerve with axonal destructions, sciatic pain will be accompanied by motor deficits with gait disorder and foot drop, cramping, and/or numbness radiating down the leg [15] (Fig. 21.4).

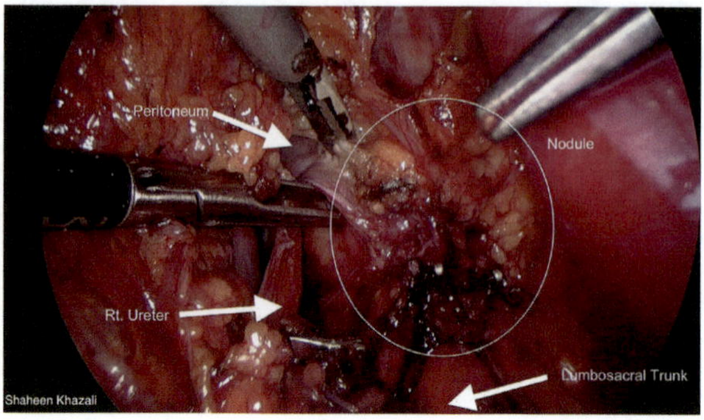

Fig. 21.4 The endometriotic nodule involving the right sciatic nerve. (With permissions from Shaheen Khazali)

The sciatica is first cyclical and occurs during menstrual periods in sciatic nerve endometriosis. It sometimes begins 1–2 days before or after the first day of the period and relieves once the menstruation ends. This is a complicated situation, as sciatica is often associated with osteomuscular etiologies and intrapelvic nerve entrapments are often neglected as a possible cause [18]. Symptoms include L5 and S1 sciatica, gluteal pain, and, sometimes, troubles of locomotion (foot drop), but never bladder dysfunctions, hyperactivity or hypersensitivity and pudendal pain is also absent [15]. Isolated sciatic endometriosis seems to develop and grow inside the SN itself and expand caudally through the greater sciatic foramen [10, 15, 17]. Therefore, a transgluteal approach for SN decompression exposes the patients to the risk of incomplete surgery by missing the endopelvic part of the lesion [14].

The most common location of endometriotic involvement of the SN is over the lateral aspect proximal to the greater sciatic foramen [15]. Isolated sciatic endometriosis is always located at the suprapiriform portion of the sciatic nerve (L5, S1, ± S2) and it is never a part of the parametric deep infiltrating endometriosis [14]. Often the lesion is located in the sciatic notch compressing other somatic nerves that share the same route when leaving the pelvis [19]. Although infiltration of the pelvic sidewall and the sacral plexus may be predominantly left-sided, SN endometriosis is predominantly right-sided. Vercellini et al. stated that the results of their systematic review demonstrated a lateral asymmetry in the location of SN endometriosis, more frequently on the right side than on the left [20].

Physical examination may reveal various neurologic deficits involving the sciatic nerve roots, with a positive straight leg raising test (Lasegue's sign), reduction/loss of the Achilles reflex, and peripheral neuropathy of the ankle. There may be localized tenderness over the sciatic notch, and transvaginal examination of the sacral plexus may induce a trigger pain with positive paresthesia of the nerve (Hoffmann–Tinel sign) [15].

21.4.4 Femoral Nerve Endometriosis

There are only few cases of femoral nerve endometriosis reported in the literature. Management requires a multidisciplinary approach between neuropelveologists (usually but not always an endometriosis surgeon), neurosurgeons, and radiologists. High-quality magnetic resonance imaging (MRI) is important to precisely identify the site of the lesion. Difficulty in treatment is the surgical approach, which may require nerve grafting and therefore long-term follow-up is necessary to confirm that nerve functions fully recover [21]. Niro et al. proposed to complete resection of the nodule and a femoral nerve transplant to the patient by laparotomic route as a treatment option.

21.4.5 Obturator Nerve Endometriosis

First reported case of obturator nerve endometriosis was operated via laparotomy in 1990 by Redwine et al., and first laparoscopic surgical treatment was performed in 2007 by Ekpo et al. [22, 23]. Reported cases of both femoral and obturator endometriosis is very limited. To the best of our knowledge, so far three cases of femoral and six cases of obturator nerve involvement have been reported [24].

21.5 Diagnosis of Nerve Endometriosis *(Neuropelveologic Diagnosis)*

Probably the main reasons for omission of pelvic nerve pathologies are that they are difficult to diagnose and treat and also there is a lack of awareness that such lesions exist [25]. The International Society of Neuropelveology (ISON) was established in 2014 by Marc Possover. One of the aims of neuropelveology is to better understand and manage the pelvic pain which is related with the pelvic nerves [26]. Neuropelveology enabled us to better understand the neural functions of the pelvic nerves and the diseases which affect these nerves. Through this better understanding, an early diagnosis became possible.

Endometriotic involvement of the pelvic nerves generate symptoms in accordance with the neural function of the affected nerve. One of the most important symptoms is pain, typically catamenial pain. The severity of the pain symptoms increases during the menstruation and alleviate once menstruation ceases. Some patients experience pain symptoms whole throughout the month although the severity varies with menstruation. The location and radiation of pain conveys important information on the localization of the lesion and involvement of the pelvic nerve. Therefore, evaluation of pain localization and radiation, bladder and intestinal function, walking, ascension and descension of stairway, ability to wear high heels, and presence of drop foot is essential in patients complaining with pelvic pain symptoms. Involvement of the autonomic nervous system (parasympathetic and sympathetic) such as the involvement of the hypogastric nerve can lead to visceral pain and vegetative symptoms. These patients usually present with urination and defecation problems. The presence of symptoms involving the bladder and the intestines can be misleading. The signs suggestive of intrapelvic nerve involvement include perineal pain or pain radiating to the lower limbs, lower urinary tract symptoms, tenesmus or dyschezia associated with gluteal pain. Its symptoms include pain, tingling, numbness, and muscle weakness on the affected nerve's dermatome. Therefore, the knowledge of dermatomes makes it possible for an accurate diagnosis, and this requires a change in the way in which pelvic surgeons are trained to think [18].

The somatic bundles of the lumbosacral plexus innervate the lower limbs, the muscle and skin of the perineum, and the pelvic floor muscles. Therefore, the symptoms suggestive of intrapelvic nerve entrapment are those such as perineal pain or pain radiating to the lower limbs, lower urinary tract symptoms, tenesmus or dyschezia associated with perineal or gluteal pain and rectal or vaginal foreign body sensation [14, 27, 28]. Any of these symptoms, in the absence of a spinal condition that could explain it, and in particular when worsening of symptoms occurs during the perimenstrual period, should alert the gynecologist to suspect sacral plexus involvement [28].

In addition to pelvic pain, in patients with sciatic involvement, gluteal pain radiating to the plantar surface of the ipsilateral foot and difficulty in walking is observed. Neurologic signs such as foot drop, weakness, and atrophy of muscles innervated by the SN, and sensory loss are also reported. Pain while straight leg test (Lasègue's sign) is frequently seen with SN involvement. Limitation of straight leg raise test is common with alteration of sensation along L5 and S1 dermatome with possible reduced power in ankle and changes to ankle reflex. Typical neurologic symptoms are pudendal and gluteal pains (S3, S4), S2 sciatica, and troubles of sensibility and functions of pelvic organs (e.g., bladder hyperactivity or sensitivity, troubles of continence, detrusor hypercontractility), but never problems with locomotion. Sphincter dysfunctions, motor or sensitive urinary urgency or voiding difficulties were explored by urodynamic testing [14].

Patient assessment should not only focus on gynecological reasons but must also include neurological disorders. Gynecologist usually focuses on the pelvic area. However, pain radiation is as important as its origin. Careful anamnesis has to be taken with detailed information of pain involving the buttocks, the pudendal area, and the lower extremities. Patients have to be evaluated by a classical neurologic workup for the lower extremities; muscle strength, evaluated and documented using the classical neurologic 0 to 5 rating scale (0, no movement; 5, normal strength); reflexes, including the patellar reflex (L3), Achilles reflex (S1), and ano-cutaneous reflex (S2) (0, absence; 1, reduced; 2, normal). Physicians have to perform toe and heel walk test. Bladder and urethral function should be evaluated by patient history, sonographic measurement of postvoiding residual volume, and urodynamic testing [15]. Possible motor deficits of hip adductors (L3–obturator nerve), knee extensors (L1-L4–femoral nerve), ankle dorsiflexion (foot drop–L5), and ankle plantar flexion (S1) should be evaluated [14]. In cases of uncertain clinical evaluation or in patients with only catamenial symptoms patients should be evaluated during menstruation. Although possible diagnostic modalities are discussed in the following sections, the gold standard in diagnosis is still the histopathological confirmation of the surgical specimen [5].

21.5.1 Electromyography

Electrophysiological studies (distal motor and sensory peripheral nerve latent period, sacral latent periods, electromyography (EMG), cortical evoked potentials, and cutaneous sympathetic potentials) provide a positive diagnosis of peripheral nerve damage and locates the disease to the nerve trunk or nerve root and is useful in establishing the prognosis for recovery [21, 29]. EMG may show denervation in muscles innervated by the SN, and nerve conduction studies may reveal slowing along the course of the nerve. In addition, EMG is useful when evaluating patients who receive medical treatment or for presurgical evaluation. It can also be applied during postsurgical follow-up to determine the efficacy of surgical intervention.

21.5.2 Urodynamic Test

Once sacral plexus involvement is suspected, careful neurologic and urodynamic evaluation should be performed [30]. Application of urodynamic tests to patients with pathologies involving the sacral 2-4 nerve plexus, which cause bladder dysfunction, can be helpful during the treatment assessment. However, a routine application of urodynamic tests during the evaluation of patients with pelvic endometriosis is not necessary.

21.6 Imaging of the Pelvic Nerves

21.6.1 Ultrasonography

Although magnetic resonance imaging (MRI) is the gold standard in the diagnosis of pelvic nerve endometriosis, ultrasonography (USG) is recommended as a feasible option for diagnostic imaging of the SN when SN endometriosis is suspected clinically [31]. It may even be used to monitor the morphological regression of the endometrial tissue in and around the nerve during pharmacological treatment. The latter may be valuable information that confirms the diagnosis and may spare the patient from undergoing invasive histological sampling or decompressive surgery. Notwithstanding the utility of MRI in the diagnosis of SN conditions, especially in assessment of intrapelvic extension of the lesion and in patients with a large body habitus, USG, in addition to its ease of access, has the advantage of higher resolution allowing better depiction of nerve structure [31]. Data on the utility of USG in the diagnosis of pelvic nerve endometriosis is limited. However, if the endometriotic lesion can be visualized with USG, USG can be used during the management and follow-up.

21.6.2 Magnetic Resonance Imaging

The diagnosis of sciatica is clinical, but MRI is a helpful tool to determinate its cause and also it can be useful in the differential diagnosis. Use of MRI in the diagnosis of SN endometriosis has been reported for the first time in 1995 [32]. MR tractography is being investigated by some authors and initial results are very promising, showing that MR tractography is superior to MR neurography for this purpose (personal communication with SK). Until a better imaging modality for diagnosis is established, MRI remains the imaging modality of choice for sciatic endometriosis. MRI is a noninvasive technique with high spatial resolution that allows a direct visualization of the spinal nerves and SN. It is the modality best suited for the study of SN involvement in extrapelvic endometriosis with a high sensitivity (90%) and specificity (98%) [33, 34]. Endometriotic cysts have a high concentration of protein and iron from recurrent and chronic hemorrhage, which reflects on MRI as a high signal on T1W sequences and low signal (shading) on T2W sequences [35–37]. On MRI, endometriotic lesion appears as solid spiculated nodules or as a focal lesion with a large cystic component and variable signal intensities due to presence of blood products [38]. Muscles denervation signs are also demonstrated, in particular in chronic disease [38]. Furthermore, it is an important investigative test to rule out other potential etiologies.

Unfortunately, not all cases of sciatic endometriosis can be identified on MRI. It has been suggested that the quality of imaging can be influenced by the phase of menstrual cycle [9]. Capek et al. described partly extraneural, partly intraneural cysts that changed in size parallel with the menstrual cycle. We believe that MRI at different phases of the menstrual cycle can be helpful in uncertain cases and can provide further insight into patients, especially those with catamenial symptoms, in whom a diagnosis often remains elusive [9].

MR neurography (MRN) is a technique that can be used to identify pelvic nerve abnormalities caused by endometriosis. However, this technique remains to be established as a potential option for the future. Contrast-enhanced short time inversion recovery (STIR) imaging sampling perfection with application-optimized contrasts using different flip angle evolution (SPACE) sequences on 3 Tesla (T) MRI, 3D STIR-SPACE imaging, is a promising technique for demonstrating sacral plexus compression and adhesion by ectopic endometrium [39].

Figure 21.5 demonstrated endometriosis infiltrating the superior gluteal nerve on the right, causing marked atrophy of the muscles innervated by this nerve (gluteus medius and gluteus minimus).

Findings may indicate a need for exploration of the lumbosacral space despite normal MRI findings. An evaluation based solely on positive MRI findings would lead to misdiagnosis of patients. Therefore, clinical evaluation is also essential. Possover et al. published three sciatic nerve endometriosis cases in 2007. They only suspected preoperative anamnestic findings such as an increase in pain during menstruation and/or a reduction in pain during a gestagen therapy [7]. They also stated that neither by preoperative examination, by CT scan, or MRI, nor by the laparoscopic inspection of the pelvis could any endometriotic lesions of the pelvic

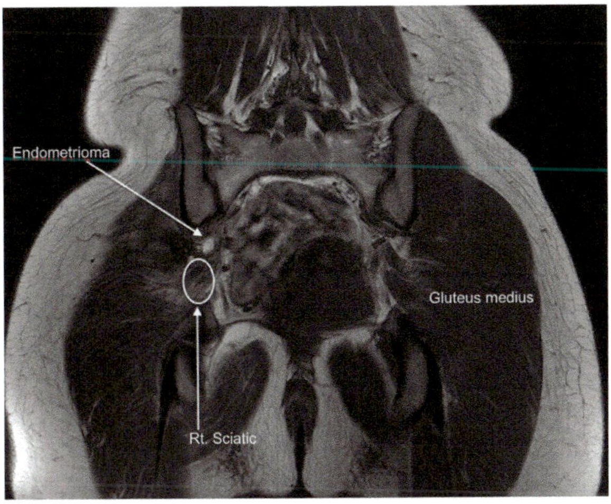

Fig. 21.5 Magnetic resonance imaging. It is showing the involvement of the right sciatic nerve and marked atrophy of the right gluteal medius and minimus muscles due to involvement of superior gluteal nerve. (With permissions from Shaheen Khazali)

retroperitoneal space be diagnosed. This is still a current issue. An experienced radiologist in both clinical aspect of the disease and interpretation of the findings is needed for accurate diagnosis. A lack in such expertise leads to late diagnosis and late onset of treatment in these patients. Therefore, clinical diagnosis carries great importance even if there are no pathologies detected with MRI.

21.7 Exclusion of Other Reasons of Sciatica

A full clinical and neuroradiologic evaluation is essentially to rule out herniation of intervertebral disks, spondylitic nerve root compression, hip-joint arthritis, arachnoiditis, primary neural tumors, metastases, gluteal artery aneurysm, and hematoma, all of which must be considered in the differential diagnosis [16]. The most frequent pathology of sciatica is associated with herniation of intervertebral disks [40]. Other possible causes of intrapelvic nerve compression include vascular entrapment, postoperative fibrosis, and muscular entrapment [41–43].

21.8 Natural Course of Nerve Endometriosis

The mechanisms of neurological pain and dysfunction in this subset of patients are from external compression of the endometriotic mass (and its surrounding fibrotic tissue) infiltrating the parametrium and pelvic wall and/or in the direct growth of endometriotic tissue into the nerve sheaths [44]. Data on the progression of intraneural nerve endometriosis over time is limited [45]. Although the involved tissue is different, nerve involvement is still considered as deep infiltrative endometriosis. Therefore, the progression of the disease is expected to be slow. Further studies are needed.

21.9 Treatment of Nerve Endometriosis

Unfortunately, due to lack of randomized prospective studies and meta-analyses, there is no agreement on what should be the gold-standard for treatment of these conditions in the international medical literature [10]. Therefore, the data presented here is based largely on case series and case studies. In the following section, first medical and then the surgical treatment is presented. Treatment is commonly based on excision of the lesion in contact with the nerve (confirming the diagnosis and giving the best chance of neurological recovery) and associated treatment of the other localizations of endometriosis (laparoscopic surgery and/or medical treatment, particularly with GnRH agonists).

21.9.1 Medical Treatment

In 1995, DeCesare and Yeko reported a case of sciatic nerve endometriosis that responded to medical management [46]. However, the data on medical treatment options is still scarce. While there have been limited reports of successful medical treatment for endometriosis of the SN, there are numerous publications of cases requiring surgical intervention due to nonresponse to medical treatment [17, 31].

Progesterone derivatives such as dienogest and norethisterone acetate (NETA) are widely used in the treatment of endometriosis related pain. Although progesterone is effective in alleviating pain, weight gain, mood changes, and abnormal uterine bleeding have been reported as side effects when used for long periods. The main problem with medical treatment is that none of the available drugs are curative and they have to be used for long periods despite of the side effects to keep the disease progression under control.

GnRH agonist was reported clinically effective on pain for SN endometriosis in a case report [16]. Motamedi et al. used hormone therapy with GnRH agonist (decapeptide) in a patient with persistent pain postsurgically, which helped improve the patient's pain [45]. The patient's pain subsided completely, but after 4 months, her neurological examinations were still unchanged. They repeated the examination at 6 months, which revealed complete foot drop on the affected side and a new EMG showed progression in the lumbosacral plexus. Endometriosis is one of the indications for GnRH agonist use and its efficacy on pain symptoms is demonstrated by the Cochrane review [45, 47]. Fedele et al. diagnosed SN endometriosis proved by clinical response to GnRH analogue treatment. However, none of the three cases included in the report by Fedele et al. had pathological MRI findings and histopathological confirmation. Authors stated that even EMG findings of marked denervation of leg and foot muscles showed good reinnervation of the muscles, after the first 12 cycles of treatment with GnRH agonist. On the other hand, all cases of claudication symptoms persisted even after GnRH agonist treatments. Carrosco et al. reported that neuropathy progression and poor pain control with medical treatments led them to decide upon surgical treatment for these patients [19]. These different treatment approaches and opinions is probably due to the extent of nerve tissue involvement. However, with this limited data, it is not possible to conclude on the effect of medical treatment on the neurological pathology along with pain. There are no data regarding the long-term efficacy of medical treatment on nerve endometriosis. In addition, it is still unknown for how long a medical treatment is appropriate, and there are no data on the recurrence rate following cease of treatment.

21.9.2 Surgical Treatment

In 2005, Volpi et al. described the first case of laparoscopic neurolysis of the SN endometriosis [48]. Possover reported that laparoscopic exploration of the SN is indicated as soon as possible before neurologic disorders appear [7]. On the other hand, Carrasco et al. recommended that if the pharmacological therapy is successful, in the absence of signs of neuropathic progression, surgery can be postponed [19]. When neuropathy progression and poor pain control occur, surgical treatment is recommended.

Although in pelvic endometriosis infiltrating the parametrial and pararectal tissues extending to the pelvic wall, the eradication of the mass with the exposure or decompression of the sacral nerve roots is usually sufficient, isolated sciatic endometriosis growing underneath the pelvic neural sheaths requires intrafascicular neurolysis of the sciatic nerve with a resection of the destroyed or involved fascial sheaths and parts of the nerve [44] (Fig. 21.3). The most frequently resected portion of the sciatic nerve was found in the cranial part corresponding to the L5 nerve root [15] (Fig. 21.4). The condition can progress and timely intervention has been recommended to prevent significant neurological injury. In a subset of 46 patients reported by Possover, who had >30% of SN destroyed by sciatic nerve with gait disturbances, recovery required at least 3 years of intensive physiotherapy [15].

When a section of tissue is removed from the body, the sensory axons within it die and degenerate, since they have been cut from their cell bodies. But we know that axons can regenerate after peripheral nerve injury [15, 49–51]. The neo-innervation which strongly supports that the complex is a potential source of sensation. The complexes became innervated like human and modeled rat endometrioma [52, 53]. In cases of deep infiltrating endometriosis of the SN, laparoscopic resection is required to obtain free margins, but this remains controversial owing to the risk of neurologic damage and irreversible gait disorders or foot drop. While some reports have claimed that microsurgical resection is the best treatment for sciatic endometriosis total recovery is not expected in advanced cases [5, 47]. However, reversal of foot drop with danazol has been reported [47]. Possover et al. reported that in patients with foot drop because of massive isolated sciatic endometriosis, surgical treatment could not result in recovery of foot flexion, but surgery is not normally the cause of the functional deterioration [14]. Furthermore, they stated that resection of endoneural endometriosis allowed axonal recovery and reconnection, with potential recovery of loss of function. This neurogenic recovery occurred in all patients, but recovery of normal gait took years [15].

Isolated sciatic endometriosis seems to develop and grow inside the sciatic nerve itself and expand caudally through the greater sciatic foramen. Isolated sciatic endometriosis requires interfascicular neurolysis of the sciatic nerve with resection of destroyed or involved parts of the nerve, whereas in sacral nerve root endometriosis, exposure or decompression of the sacral nerve roots is usually sufficient [14]. Therefore, a transgluteal approach for sciatic nerve decompression exposes the patients to the risk of incomplete surgery by missing the endopelvic part of the lesion. Only in very rare cases the extensive endometriotic infiltration of the sciatic foramen surrounding the sciatic nerve and its branches allowed just the freeing of the endopelvic part of the nerve itself, avoiding a further dissection in the gluteal region through the sciatic foramen, considering this step too dangerous [10]. If disease extends beyond the pelvis into the gluteal region, neurosurgical or orthopedic input will be required to perform a transgluteal approach [54].

Despite the high cure and improvement rate, only half of the patients experience complete remission of pain [18]. Possover reported laparoscopic exploration of isolated endometriosis of the SN in 27 patients, deep infiltrating parametric endometriosis with sacral plexus infiltration in 148 patients. A reduction in mean visual analogue scale (VAS) score of pain from 7.7 (±1.16; range 6–10) before surgery to 2.6 (±1.77; range 0–6) at 6-month after surgery was reported for sacral plexus endometriosis [14].

After surgery with nerve resection, patients usually suffer from neuropathic pain and sensorimotor disorders, possibly worse than before surgery; however, over the long term (3–5 years), most patients recover sufficient SN function and muscular compensation to achieve a normal gait [15]. Even with complete resection of endoneural endometriosis and preservation of some continuity of the SN, two additional treatments are essential: postoperative physiotherapy and medical treatment with neuroleptic agents, which must be implemented immediately after the procedure to control postoperative neuropathic pain and avoid the development of phantom pain. Postoperative physiotherapy is essential to recover function after nerve injuries. Muscles without innervation start to atrophy within the first 3 months after nerve injury, and this process reaches a critical level after 2 years [55–57]. Muscle atrophy is mainly nonreversible and hinders reinnervation when this critical time point is reached [58].

Another condition causing sciatica is pelvic peritoneal pocket also called peritoneal retraction pocket or Allen-Masterson pocket. A pelvic peritoneal pocket in association with endometriosis was first described by Sampson. Chatman and Zbella, and Redwine later demonstrated the importance of recognizing peritoneal pockets as a potential manifestation of endometriosis, as endometriosis in such structures in women with pelvic pain otherwise could remain undiagnosed and untreated [59–61]. Vilos et al. reported on 25 patients with chronic pelvic pain, cyclic pain radiating to the leg (right 15, left 9, both 1), pain over buttocks, and paresthesia of the thighs and/or knees, exacerbated during menses [40]. They found at laparoscopy pelvic peritoneal pockets in 15 patients, peritoneal endometriosis in 5, and endometriosis nodules in 5 patients. All these lesions were located in posterolateral pelvic peritoneum and they were excised [40]. After excision of the peritoneal pocket, endometriosis was confirmed histologically. Histologic evaluation of the five excised nodules showed evidence of endometriosis. Histology of peritoneal pockets included endometriosis (n = 9, 60.0%), endosalpingiosis (n = 2, 13.3%), chronic inflammation (n = 1, 6.7%), and no abnormal histology (n = 3, 20%) [40]. The patient's cyclic sciatic pain was cured. The immediate clinical outcome was complete relief of the cyclic sciatica-like pain in 19 women, marked improvement in 4, and no significant difference in 2. Since histologically at least 80% of them contain endometriosis, endosalpingiosis, or chronically inflammatory peritoneum, it is conceivable that their proximity to the lumbosacral plexus irritates areas of the sacral nerve, leading to cyclic sciatica-like pain [40]. However, it is more plausible that the pain is referred pain originating from pelvic peritoneum. Depending on the topography and deepness of infiltration, they can be the cause of some neurologic symptoms associated with endometriosis pain. Vercellini et al. showed a poor correlation between location of pain and location of superficial disease [62]. On the other hand, Hsu et al. showed a stronger correlation between location of pain and location of deep disease [63]. Carranco et al. reported on seven cases of peritoneal retraction pocket which were totally excised [64]. In all cases, endometriosis was confirmed by histopathology, and in a 6-month follow-up, all patients showed improvement of bowel, pain, and neurologic symptoms. The significance of pelvic peritoneal pockets is still unknown. Therefore, more studies are needed.

21.10 Long-Term Prognosis After Nerve Resection

Early recognition and treatment of this disorder is important to minimize the severity of nerve damage caused by the recurrent cycles of hemorrhage and fibrosis that are characteristic of endometriosis [65]. Resection of deep infiltrating endometriosis of the SN to decrease pain has been reported but neurofunctional outcomes of the SN after surgery remain unknown. Possover published 5-year follow-up on 46 sciatic nerve endometriosis patients who underwent laparoscopic neurolysis [15]. Possover reported that significant functional recovery occurred in most patients after a period of 2.5–3 years, whereas normal gait function was achieved at 4–5 years after the procedure. Evaluation of pain during the 5-year follow-up revealed the mean preoperative pain VAS score as 9.33 ± 0.65 while taking pain medication, and was reduced to 1.25 ± 1.05 at the 5-year follow-up without regular pain treatment [15]. Preoperatively, all patients reported exponential worsening of gait disorders and neuropathic pain that became refractory to medical treatments and to drug-induced amenorrhea within a short period [15]. Treating pain with drug-induced amenorrhea is legitimate, but as soon as gait disorders and foot drop appear, surgical treatment is advisable to prevent further irreversible neurogenic damage [15]. As far as we know, laparoscopic treatment can be performed with excellent results in terms of pain improvement and recurrence, as well as good functional outcome as long as part of the nerve is preserved and the patient is properly supported by intensive physiotherapy.

References

1. Denton RO, Sherrill JD. Sciatic syndrome due to endometriosis of sciatic nerve. South Med J. 1955;48(10):1027–31.
2. Schlicke CP. Ectopic endometrial tissue in the thigh. J Am Med Assoc. 1946;26(132):445.
3. Della Corte L, Di Filippo C, Gabrielli O, Reppuccia S, La Rosa VL, Ragusa R, et al. The burden of endometriosis on Women's lifespan: a narrative overview on quality of life and psychosocial wellbeing. Int J Environ Res Public Health. 2020;17(13):4683. Available from: https://www.ncbi.nlm.nih.gov/pmc/articles/PMC7370081/
4. De Sousa ACS, Capek S, Amrami KK, Spinner RJ. Neural involvement in endometriosis: review of anatomic distribution and mechanisms. Clin Anat. 2015;28(8):1029–38.
5. Mannan K, Altaf F, Maniar S, Tirabosco R, Sinisi M, Carlstedt T. Cyclical sciatica: endometriosis of the sciatic nerve. J Bone Joint Surg Br. 2008;90(1):98–101.
6. Roman H, Dehan L, Merlot B, Berby B, Forestier D, Seyer-Hansen M, et al. Postoperative outcomes after surgery for deep endometriosis of the sacral plexus and sciatic nerve: a 52-patient consecutive series. J Minim Invasive Gynecol. 2020;31:1375–83.
7. Possover M, Baekelandt J, Flaskamp C, Li D, Chiantera V. Laparoscopic neurolysis of the sacral plexus and the sciatic nerve for extensive endometriosis of the pelvic wall. Minim Invasive Neurosurg. 2007;50(1):33–6.
8. Halban J. Metastatic hysteroadenosys. Wien Klin Wochenschr. 1924;37:1205–6.
9. Capek S, Amrami KK, Howe BM, Collins MS, Sandroni P, Cheville JC, et al. Sequential imaging of intraneural sciatic nerve endometriosis provides insight into symptoms of cyclical sciatica. Acta Neurochir. 2016;158(3):507–12.
10. Ceccaroni M, Clarizia R, Alboni C, Ruffo G, Bruni F, Roviglione G, et al. Laparoscopic nerve-sparing transperitoneal approach for endometriosis infiltrating the pelvic wall and somatic nerves: anatomical considerations and surgical technique. Surg Radiol Anat. 2010;32(6):601–4.
11. Head HB, Welch JS, Mussey E, Espinosa RE. Cyclic sciatica. Report of case with introduction of a new surgical sign. JAMA. 1962;19(180):521–4.
12. Guedes F, Brown RS, Lourenço Torrão-Júnior FJ, Siquara-de-Sousa AC, Pires Amorim RM. Nondiscogenic sciatica: what clinical examination and imaging can tell us? World Neurosurg. 2020;134:e1053–61.
13. Ergun T, Lakadamyali H. CT and MRI in the evaluation of extraspinal sciatica. Br J Radiol. 2010;83(993):791–803.
14. Possover M, Schneider T, Henle K-P. Laparoscopic therapy for endometriosis and vascular entrapment of sacral plexus. Fertil Steril. 2011;95(2):756–8.
15. Possover M. Five-year follow-up after laparoscopic large nerve resection for deep infiltrating sciatic nerve endometriosis. J Minim Invasive Gynecol. 2017;24(5):822–6.
16. Fedele L, Bianchi S, Raffaelli R, Zanconato G, Zanette G. Phantom endometriosis of the sciatic nerve. Fertil Steril. 1999;72(4):727–9.
17. Saar TD, Pacquée S, Conrad DH, Sarofim M, Rosnay PD, Rosen D, et al. Endometriosis involving the sciatic nerve: a case report of isolated endometriosis of the sciatic nerve and review of the literature. Gynecol Minim Invasive Ther. 2018;7(2):81–5.
18. Lemos N, D'Amico N, Marques R, Kamergorodsky G, Schor E, Girão MJBC. Recognition and treatment of endometriosis involving the sacral nerve roots. Int Urogynecol J. 2016;27(1):147–50.
19. Carrasco AL, Gutiérrez AH, Gutiérrez PAH, González RR, Bolívar PIS, Elio RU, et al. Sciatic nerve involvement as an unusual presentation of deep endometriosis. J Endometriosis Pelvic Pain Disord. 2017;9(2):120–4.
20. Vercellini P, Chapron C, Fedele L, Frontino G, Zaina B, Crosignani PG. Evidence for asymmetric distribution of sciatic nerve endometriosis. Obstet Gynecol. 2003;102(2):383–7.
21. Niro J, Fournier M, Oberlin C, Le Tohic A, Panel P. Endometriotic lesions of the lower troncular nerves. Gynecol Obstet Fertil. 2014;42(10):702–5.

22. Redwine DB, Sharpe DR. Endometriosis of the obturator nerve. A case report. J Reprod Med. 1990;35(4):434–5.
23. Ekpo G, Senapati S, Advincula AP. Laparoscopic excision of endometriosis of the obturator nerve: a case report. J Minim Invasive Gynecol. 2007;14(6):764–6.
24. Kalkan Ü, Daniilidis A. Laparoscopic diagnosis and treatment of obturator nerve entrapment because of a deep infiltrating Endometriotic nodule: a case report. J Minim Invasive Gynecol. 2019;26(4):766–9.
25. Possover M. New surgical evolutions in management of sacral radiculopathies. Surg Technol Int. 2010;19:123–8.
26. Possover M, Forman A, Rabischong B, Lemos N, Chiantera V. Neuropelveology: new groundbreaking discipline in medicine. J Minim Invasive Gynecol. 2015;22(7):1140–1.
27. Possover M, Lemos N. Risks, symptoms, and management of pelvic nerve damage secondary to surgery for pelvic organ prolapse: a report of 95 cases. Int Urogynecol J. 2011;22(12):1485–90.
28. Lemos N, Kamergorodsky G, Ploger C, Castro R, Schor E, Girão M. Sacral nerve infiltrative endometriosis presenting as perimenstrual right-sided sciatica and bladder atonia: case report and description of surgical technique. J Minim Invasive Gynecol. 2012;19(3):396–400.
29. Lefaucheur J-P, Labat J-J, Amarenco G, Herbaut A-G, Prat-Pradal D, Benaim J, et al. What is the place of electroneuromyographic studies in the diagnosis and management of pudendal neuralgia related to entrapment syndrome? Neurophysiol Clin. 2007;37(4):223.
30. Possover M. Pathophysiologic explanation for bladder retention in patients after laparoscopic surgery for deeply infiltrating rectovaginal and/or parametric endometriosis. Fertil Steril. 2014;101(3):754–8.
31. Arányi Z, Polyák I, Tóth N, Vermes G, Göcsei Z. Ultrasonography of sciatic nerve endometriosis. Muscle Nerve. 2016;54(3):500–5.
32. Descamps P, Cottier JP, Barre I, Rosset P, Laffont J, Lansac J, et al. Endometriosis of the sciatic nerve: case report demonstrating the value of MR imaging. Eur J Obstet Gynecol Reprod Biol. 1995;58(2):199–202.
33. Roy C, Ohana M, Host P, Alemann G, Labani A, Wattiez A, et al. MR urography (MRU) of non-dilated ureter with diuretic administration: static fluid 2D FSE T2-weighted versus 3D gadolinium T1-weighted GE excretory MR. Eur J Radiol Open. 2014;6(1):6–13.
34. Gaeta M, Minutoli F, Mileto A, Racchiusa S, Donato R, Bottari A, et al. Nuck canal endometriosis: MR imaging findings and clinical features. Abdom Imaging. 2010;35(6):737–41.
35. Glastonbury CM. The shading sign. Radiology. 2002;224(1):199–201.
36. Lomoro P, Simonetti I, Nanni A, Cassone R, Di Pietto F, Vinci G, et al. Extrapelvic sciatic nerve endometriosis, the role of magnetic resonance imaging: case report and systematic review. J Comput Assist Tomogr. 2019;43(6):976–80.
37. Cimsit C, Yoldemir T, Akpinar IN. Sciatic neuroendometriosis: magnetic resonance imaging defined perineural spread of endometriosis. J Obstet Gynaecol Res. 2016;42(7):890–4.
38. Foti PV, Farina R, Palmucci S, Vizzini IAA, Libertini N, Coronella M, et al. Endometriosis: clinical features, MR imaging findings and pathologic correlation. Insights Imaging. 2018;9(2):149–72.
39. Zhang X, Li M, Guan J, Wang H, Li S, Guo Y, et al. Evaluation of the sacral nerve plexus in pelvic endometriosis by three-dimensional MR neurography. J Magn Reson Imaging. 2017;45(4):1225–31.
40. Vilos GA, Vilos AW, Haebe JJ. Laparoscopic findings, management, histopathology, and outcome of 25 women with cyclic leg pain. J Am Assoc Gynecol Laparosc. 2002;9(2):145–51.
41. Kale A, Basol G, Usta T, Cam I. Vascular entrapment of both the sciatic and pudendal nerves causing persistent sciatica and pudendal neuralgia. J Minim Invasive Gynecol. 2019;26(2):360–1. https://doi.org/10.1016/j.jmig.2018.04.014.
42. Taner U, Aysel O, Ahmet K, Gulfem B. Robot-assisted laparoscopic management of a vascular entrapment of the sacral nerve roots causing pelvic pain. J Obstet Gynaecol Res. 2019;45(8):1603–7. https://doi.org/10.1111/jog.14008.

43. Kale A, Basol G, Topcu AC, Gundogdu EC, Usta T, Demirhan R. Intrapelvic nerve entrapment syndrome caused by a variation of the Intrapelvic piriformis muscle and abnormal varicose vessels. Int Neurourol J. 2021;25(2):177. https://doi.org/10.5213/inj.2040232.116.
44. Ceccaroni M, Clarizia R, Cosma S, Pesci A, Pontrelli G, Minelli L. Cyclic sciatica in a patient with deep monolateral endometriosis infiltrating the right sciatic nerve. J Spinal Disord Tech. 2011;24(7):474–8.
45. Motamedi M, Mousavinia F, Naser Moghadasi A, Talebpoor M, Hajimirzabeigi A. Endometriosis of the lumbosacral plexus: report of a case with foot drop and chronic pelvic pain. Acta Neurol Belg. 2015;115(4):851–2.
46. DeCesare SL, Yeko TR. Sciatic nerve endometriosis treated with a gonadotropin releasing hormone agonist. A case report. J Reprod Med. 1995;40(3):226–8.
47. Streuli I, de Ziegler D, Santulli P, Marcellin L, Borghese B, Batteux F, et al. An update on the pharmacological management of endometriosis. Expert Opin Pharmacother. 2013;14(3):291–305.
48. Volpi E, Seinera P, Ferrero A, Dompè D. Laparoscopic neurolysis of the pelvic sciatic nerve in a case of catamenial footdrop. J Minim Invasive Gynecol. 2005;12(6):525–7.
49. Huebner EA, Strittmatter SM. Axon regeneration in the peripheral and central nervous systems. Results Probl Cell Differ. 2009;48:339–51.
50. Pace A, Scammell B, Dhar S. The outcome of Morton's neurectomy in the treatment of metatarsalgia. Int Orthop. 2010;34(4):511–5.
51. Ao Q, Wang Y, Cao P, Peng J. Femoral nerve regeneration and its accuracy under different injury mechanisms. Neural Regen Res. 2015;10(10):1669–73.
52. Bove GM. A model for radiating leg pain of endometriosis. J Bodyw Mov Ther. 2016;20(4):931–6.
53. Berkley KJ, Dmitrieva N, Curtis KS, Papka RE. Innervation of ectopic endometrium in a rat model of endometriosis. Proc Natl Acad Sci U S A. 2004;101(30):11094–8.
54. Jiang H, Liang Y, Li L, Gu L, Yao S. Cyclic sciatica due to endometriosis of the sciatic nerve: neurolysis with combined laparoscopic and transgluteal approaches: a case report. JBJS Case Connect. 2014;4(1 Suppl 2):1–4.
55. Kobayashi J, Mackinnon SE, Watanabe O, Ball DJ, Gu XM, Hunter DA, et al. The effect of duration of muscle denervation on functional recovery in the rat model. Muscle Nerve. 1997;20(7):858–66.
56. Aird RB, Naffziger HC. The pathology of human striated muscle following denervation. J Neurosurg. 1953;10(3):216–27.
57. Tung TH, Mackinnon SE. Nerve transfers: indications, techniques, and outcomes. J Hand Surg Am. 2010;35(2):332–41.
58. Ruijs ACJ, Jaquet J-B, Kalmijn S, Giele H, Hovius SER. Median and ulnar nerve injuries: a meta-analysis of predictors of motor and sensory recovery after modern microsurgical nerve repair. Plast Reconstr Surg. 2005;116(2):484–94; discussion 495-496.
59. Chatman DL. Pelvic peritoneal defects and endometriosis: Allen-Masters syndrome revisited. Fertil Steril. 1981;36(6):751–6.
60. Chatman DL, Zbella EA. Pelvic peritoneal defects and endometriosis: further observations. Fertil Steril. 1986;46(4):711–4.
61. Redwine DB. Peritoneal pockets and endometriosis. Confirmation of an important relationship, with further observations. J Reprod Med. 1989;34(4):270–2.
62. Vercellini P, Trespidi L, De Giorgi O, Cortesi I, Parazzini F, Crosignani PG. Endometriosis and pelvic pain: relation to disease stage and localization. Fertil Steril. 1996;65(2):299–304.
63. Hsu AL, Sinaii N, Segars J, Nieman LK, Stratton P. Relating pelvic pain location to surgical findings of endometriosis. Obstet Gynecol. 2011;118(2 Pt 1):223–30.
64. Carranco RC, Zomer MT, Berg CF, Smith AV, Koninckx P, Kondo W. Peritoneal retraction pocket defects and their important relationship with pelvic pain and endometriosis. J Minim Invasive Gynecol. 2021;28(2):168–9.
65. Zager EL, Pfeifer SM, Brown MJ, Torosian MH, Hackney DB. Catamenial mononeuropathy and radiculopathy: a treatable neuropathic disorder. J Neurosurg. 1998;88(5):827–30.

Fertility Preservation in Endometriosis

22

Henrique D'Allagnol, Ana Cobo,
and Juan Antonio Garcia-Velasco

Contents

22.1 Introduction

Endometriosis is a chronic estrogen-dependent disease with high morbidity that affects approximately 10% of women of reproductive age [1, 2]. It is strongly associated with infertility, either alone or as an adjunct to other causal factors. This disease generates a chronic systemic inflammatory process and predisposes the patient to anatomical, tubal, and ovulatory changes, being present in up to 50% of infertile couples [3].

Often, patients undergo chronic pain treatments, including long-term hormone administration (GnRH-agonists, hormonal contraceptives based on estradiol and/or progesterone), analgesics and anti-inflammatory drugs, and finally surgical treatment [2, 4]. The latter, which is being used less over time, aims to remove adhesions

H. D'Allagnol · A. Cobo · J. A. Garcia-Velasco (✉)
IVI Madrid, Rey Juan Carlos University, Madrid, Spain
e-mail: juan.garcia.velasco@ivirma.com

E. Oral (ed.), *Endometriosis and Adenomyosis*,
https://doi.org/10.1007/978-3-030-97236-3_22

and eliminate endometrial implants in the pelvic and abdominal cavities. These treatments also cause infertility, since amenorrhea is a commonly presented adverse effect [1].

Endometriotic lesions predominantly affect the ovaries, either by invagination of endometrial tissue by the ovarian cortex in situations of retrograde menstruation or by coelomic metaplasia. These lesions, called endometriomas, generate cysts that are rich in macrophages and hematic cells and can be easily detected on transvaginal ultrasound. A local deleterious impact, due to simple "mass effect" or the presence of toxic substances, could explain why these patients have less ovarian reserve (OR) and experience infertility more frequently than the healthy population [4].

Recently published studies also show an impairment of both oocyte quality and follicular quantity in this population, supporting the surgical removal of these lesions to reduce the symptoms and restore normal ovarian function when seeking pregnancy [5]. However, even more recently, it has been postulated that performing ovarian surgery to eliminate these lesions can also compromise the ovarian reserve, predisposing these women to premature ovarian failure, early menopause, and infertility [1, 6]. Experts affirm that the surgical approach should be avoided, operating only in exceptional situations, because in the effort to dry the lesions and obtain "free margins," healthy ovarian tissue with its follicular population is also eliminated [1]. This is confirmed by studies that show a sharp drop in the Anti-Mullerian Hormone (AMH) levels and antral follicle count (AFC) of postsurgical patients [7].

On the other hand, fertility preservation (FP) is increasingly used, especially in women over 35 years of age, whose decline in reproductive potential is more evident. Situations where the ovarian reserve is diminished, even when the patient's biological age is not so advanced, are also often indications for FP. These conditions include patients suffering from endometriosis, where follicular depletion occurs faster [1].

With the advent of vitrification and the high success rates in thawing (reaching 83%), the freezing of oocytes, embryos, and ovarian tissue is being increasingly used, especially oocyte preservation, given the substantial experience already acquired on the subject and the favorable results published over the years. Cryopreservation of ovarian tissue, even though it has been described for more than 20 years, is complex, expensive and little used, and then only as an alternative for emergency situations where it is impracticable to wait for controlled ovarian stimulation (COS) or where there is an indication for oophorectomy. Embryo vitrification is also less used for FP, given the ethical conflicts generated and the need for a partner at the time of oocyte extraction, in addition to controversial situations in the event of the couple separating [8].

Regardless of the technique used to preserve the fertility of these patients, especially those affected by advanced endometriosis, there is a consensus that FP can and should be proposed by the attending physician, since it increases the possibilities of future pregnancy in patients with evolutionary endometriosis or with a compromised ovarian reserve in postsurgical conditions [1, 2].

22.2 Population Characteristics

22.2.1 Endometriosis and Poor Oocyte Quality

Endometriomas can be present in up to 44% of patients with endometriosis, and their possible impact on oocyte quality has been proposed, especially in patients with advanced stages of the disease (deep endometriosis). Many studies point to a direct impact on ovarian activity due to interference with steroidogenesis [1, 9]. The reports that ovulation occurs more commonly in the contralateral ovary in the presence of endometriomas also suggest a local deleterious effect on the ovulatory mechanism or even on follicular recruitment [2, 10].

On the other hand, underlying chronic systemic inflammatory processes can also impact the quality/quantity of the follicles by increasing oxidative stress [2]. Nakahara et al. showed a higher apoptotic activity of granulosa cells and cumulus oophorus in patients with ovarian endometriomas, which may explain the poorer quality of the oocytes obtained and embryos generated after COS in these patients [11].

It is evident that in order to freeze eggs or embryos for fertility preservation, we need good quality gametes, with good rates of survival to thawing and satisfactory competence to achieve implantation and originate a live birth. A review published in 2017 reveals the scarcity of literature available on oocyte quality in patients with endometriosis. The authors cite reports of decreased expression of P450 aromatase in these oocytes, with decreased estradiol (E2) concentrations and considerable intrafollicular imbalance, resulting in increased local oxidative stress. These gametes also seem to show worse rates of in-vitro maturation, propensity to altered morphology and decreased mitochondrial cytoplasmic content [2, 9].

This increase in reactive oxygen species could promote meiotic and chromosomal abnormalities in oocytes. This could explain the lower percentages of mature oocytes found after follicular aspiration in patients with endometriosis [9].

A retrospective study published in 2019 that analyzed infertility in patients comparing endometriosis versus tubal factor showed an increase in the amount of cytoplasmic granules and vacuoles in the oocytes of patients affected by the disease. A considerably larger amount of immature oocytes was also obtained in this group ($p < 0.005$). Oocyte quality suffered a greater impact, especially when the endometriomas were more than 3 cm in diameter, suggesting a size/toxicity relationship [12].

Kitajima et al. histologically analyzed ovarian cortex samples from 13 young patients with and without endometriomas, showing a significant increase in the amount of atretic follicles in the ovaries affected by endometriotic cysts. The primordial follicle and oocyte diameters were also smaller, probably due to the ovarian inflammatory process generated by the cystic content. Immunohistochemical analysis of apoptosis confirmed increased apoptotic activity in the follicles of patients with the disease [13].

Studies in mice have also shown changes in the oocyte meiotic spindle when exposed to endometriotic content, also suggesting a possible impact on oocyte quality by the oxidative stress generated. However, studies carried out subsequently did not find clear evidence of these theories, since oocytes and embryos of women with endometriosis showed the same rates of blastulation and aneuploidy as healthy patients. The same controversy applies to reports of lower production of ATP and mitochondrial activity in these patients' oocytes, which still need confirmation [2, 14].

The impact of endometriosis on gamete quality was also analyzed in studies of women participating in oocyte donation programs. Oocytes generated by patients with this disease showed worse clinical results when transferred to healthy patients, indicating a possible qualitative impairment [15].

Following the same reasoning, another French retrospective study published in 2020 attempted to prove this impact on embryonic quality by analyzing patients with and without endometriosis and found no significant differences in the obtention of high-quality embryos between groups. The smaller number of oocytes and mature oocytes in the group with the pathology directly influenced the cumulative live birth rates, but the pregnancy rates per cycle did not differ. The results confirmed that, in this sample, the quality was equivalent between gametes obtained from patients with and without the disease [16].

In the country where this study was carried out, egg freezing in patients with advanced endometriosis has been funded by the government since 2018, which proves that public health systems are concerned about the negative impact of the disease on the reproductive capacity of endometriosis patients, which can affect up to 40% of this population [5].

The potential impairment of oocyte quality in patients with endometriosis is not yet completely clear. The studies published to date show contradictory results, and new, well-designed studies, especially including patients who have opted for fertility preservation, could elucidate the capacity of these oocytes to generate a live birth.

22.2.2 Endometriosis and Reduction of Ovarian Reserve

The impact of endometriosis on oocyte quality is a controversial topic and still needs scientific proof, but the impairment of the ovarian reserve of patients with the disease is a widespread concept. This impact on the antral follicle pool is basically explained by two factors: the evolution of the disease itself and surgical iatrogenesis. Studies comparing AMH levels and AFC show considerably lower figures in endometriosis patients, even in the absence of postsurgical cases [17, 18].

Bearing in mind that AMH and AFC are currently the most widely accepted OR markers, a study carried out in Brazil using infertile patients undergoing laparoscopy to confirm endometriosis compared AMH levels in patients with mild endometriosis and women without the disease, adjusting for the respective confounding factors. The results showed decreased levels in the group with endometriosis (1.26 vs. 2.02 ng/ml), as well as greater heterogeneity and asynchrony in the development of antral follicles [18].

Another research group carried out a prospective study to compare patients with unilateral endometriomas, bilateral endometriomas and women without the pathology in order to determine the impact of endometriomas on the ovarian reserve of nonsurgical patients [17].

There were statistically significant differences in the concentrations of AMH in patients with bilateral ovarian involvement versus those free of pathology. These data show the deleterious effect of endometriotic cysts at the ovarian level and their impact on OR, which can be explained by the effect of cytokines and the free radicals produced by them, which stimulate tissue fibrosis with vascular impairment and, consequently, interference with local perfusion. In addition, reports of proliferation of disorganized smooth muscle parallel to cysts replacing functional ovarian tissue would also account for the decrease in AMH concentration presented by these patients [17].

One of the mechanisms proposed for the local toxicity induced by endometriotic cysts is also the high concentration of free iron in their interior. This free metal can stimulate the production of free radicals, which cause damage at the cellular and vascular level [19].

The presence of iron in high concentrations alters ovarian gene expression, inducing the production and recruitment of local pro-inflammatory substances (tumor necrosis factor alpha, a proinflammatory cytokine, interleukin IL-6 and IL-8), which in the absence of homeostasis, have deleterious effects on the ovary [19, 20].

These same free radicals present within the cyst can affect the muscular layers of the vessels that supply blood to the ovaries, altering their relaxation and compliance [19].

Other studies have shown that fewer oocytes and mature oocytes are commonly aspirated in patients with endometriosis compared to patients without the pathology undergoing COS. These data, confirmed also in nonsurgical patients, can be explained by the "mass effect" exerted by endometriomas [4, 7].

Therefore, based on the currently available literature, we conclude that the presence of endometriosis, especially at the ovarian level and by different mechanisms, has a deleterious effect on follicular population. This impact can compromise the ovarian reserve of these patients and is therefore a plausible reason to propose fertility preservation to this population.

22.3 Clinical Impact of Surgical Removal of Endometriomas

One of the most controversial issues involving endometriosis is undoubtedly the indication of surgical intervention. In the past, the attitude toward the treatment of these patients was much more interventionist and active, to the point of gynecologists being "divided" into two groups of opinion, those in favor and those against early surgical management. For years, early surgical intervention was justified by the ease of removal of small lesions and by the fact that it decreased ovarian vascular involvement, in addition to facilitating the diagnosis of lesions not seen in imaging exams. Interference with ovarian functionality was considered to be minimal, and it could even increase the chances of spontaneous postsurgical pregnancy while delaying the evolution of the disease [8, 21].

One of the first studies to this effect was published in 1997, analyzing 341 women who underwent laparoscopy for endometriosis. The authors found significant differences in pregnancy rates in patients who underwent a procedure to remove endometriotic tissue, compared to those who received conservative treatment after diagnosis (30.7% vs. 17.7%). These results stimulated surgical management at the time [22].

Studies even suggested a possible capacity for ovarian self-repair after the procedure, reversing the damage caused by the surgery. These studies were based on the partial restoration of AMH in the late postoperative period, even if below the baseline [7].

Years later, surgical excision of ovarian endometriomas pre-COS was also advocated for as a way to prevent a possible increase in cyst volume during treatment. This increase was not found in other studies carried out later [23]. The greater ease of ultrasound monitoring of follicular growth during the administration of gonadotropins also justified the procedure. The overall rates of spontaneous pregnancy reported in patients affected by endometriosis were high, at approximately 73%. In addition, during oocyte extraction, the ovaries would be more accessible, thus reducing possible post-puncture complications, such as hemorrhage and formation of ovarian abscesses [2, 24–26].

However, despite the positive points mentioned above, many studies show a considerable decrease in the ovarian reserve of patients who have undergone ovarian surgery, which can have a significant impact on the ability of these women to conceive, even after assisted reproduction treatments. Studies show that after surgery, substantial falls in ovarian reserve markers are presented. Concurring with these data, fewer oocytes and embryos are generated after the surgery, thus decreasing the chances of reaching embryo transfer in assisted reproduction cycles [5, 16].

Authors concluded that after undergoing surgery to remove endometriotic foci, women undergoing COS obtain up to 1.4 fewer oocytes per stimulation than non-operated patients. This could have a direct impact on the amount of stimulations needed to vitrify a reasonable number of oocytes in cases of fertility preservation [21].

Since the infertility commonly presented by these women is due to depletion of the ovarian reserve as a consequence of the evolution of the disease or surgical iatrogenesis, the need to perform highly complex reproductive treatments has grown exponentially, currently justifying up to 25% of IVF indications [4]. These data encourage oocyte vitrification in these patients. The study by Cobo et al. in 2020 showed a significant return rate of 46.5% of patients who had their oocytes vitrified for fertility preservation in order to attempt pregnancy. This reflects the low rates of spontaneous pregnancy in patients with endometriosis who suffer from infertility, even after surgical intervention [1].

The surgical techniques for the elimination of endometriomas are laparoscopic surgical excision, electrocauterization, vaporization, and puncture of endometriotic cysts. Some of these procedures have high recurrence rates, reaching up to 66.6% [4, 21]. Regardless of the technique employed, a well-trained and experienced professional team can minimize the deleterious effects of the procedure itself, as well as avoid the use of electrocautery [5, 21]. Interestingly, in 2017, a Chinese study found no differences when comparing the retrieval of oocytes and mature oocytes in patients who had undergone ovarian surgery to remove endometriomas to the same procedure in patients who had undergone an endometriotic cyst puncture or those who had followed an expectant conduct before COS [27].

These data should be interpreted with caution, given the mechanical action exerted by surgical procedures since, in addition to removing healthy ovarian tissue, it also stimulates fibrosis at the site, occupying the space previously intended for follicular development. As described by Garcia-Velasco et al. in a study carried out in clinics in different countries, surgical removal of endometriotic cysts considerably increased the time until pregnancy, decreased the ovarian reserve (<AFC), and decreased the patient's response to COS [2].

Another study published in 2020 also reports that performing ovarian surgery before COS has a negative influence on the number of oocytes aspirated, unlike the presence of endometriomas during the process, which has not been shown to significantly interfere with the cycle [3].

Therefore, oocyte vitrification for fertility preservation before surgery seems to be the most accepted strategy today, since if the surgical procedure performed subsequently does not result in spontaneous pregnancy, the frozen oocytes will provide these women, whose ovarian reserve may be compromised post-surgery, with the opportunity to gestate [3].

The retrospective study led by Cobo et al. published in 2020 contributed significantly to our better understanding of this topic. The study aimed to evaluate the clinical results of patients with endometriosis who underwent oocyte vitrification, as well as the impact of ovarian surgery on COS. Among the 485 women who participated in the study, the number of vitrified oocytes and the rates of ongoing pregnancy per cycle were higher in patients who had not undergone surgery (6.2–5.8). This study showed a considerable impact on the ovarian response to COS in patients under 35 years of age who had had surgery. The cumulative live birth rate in this population was 70% in conservative treatment versus 50% in operated patients [1].

This study contradicts the logical reasoning that younger women would be the best candidates for surgical intervention for endometriosis because they have a better ovarian reserve. Though it may seem a reasonable theory, this population was the one that suffered the most with the negative impact of surgery. Despite having a larger pool of antral follicles, the removal of healthy ovarian tissue along with the endometriomas had a negative impact on their treatment; the recommendation, therefore, is to perform the surgical procedure (when necessary) after the capture of oocytes [1].

Another retrospective cohort study published in 2016 analyzed more than 400,000 cycles of in vitro fertilization and showed that patients with endometriosis represented 11% of those who were treated for infertility, which in 22% of them was associated with a low ovarian reserve. The vast majority of these women also had other diagnoses that could cause infertility, with only 4% of them being diagnosed exclusively of endometriosis [20].

A curious finding of this publication is that patients with an exclusive diagnosis of endometriosis had an equal rate of live births compared to patients with other diagnoses, despite a smaller number of retrieved oocytes. Patients with endometriosis associated with another pathology causing infertility had lower pregnancy and live birth rates than patients free of the disease. These results were in line with a Norwegian study that was carried out over a 20-year period and also found equal cumulative live birth rates in patients undergoing IVF when comparing patients with endometriosis (regardless of stage) to patients with other causes of infertility [20].

Some authors have found significantly greater impacts on the ovarian reserve of patients with bilateral lesions compared to patients without endometriosis, but AMH levels do not seem to differ between patients with uni- versus bilateral lesions. A 2020 study showed fewer mature oocytes rescued from patients with bilateral lesions compared to unilateral (5.1 vs. 3.3) after COS to preserve fertility. COS was performed before the surgical excision of the lesions [23]. These populations should be advised on the freezing of eggs and their unfavorable prognosis, with the purpose of making them participate in the decisions regarding their treatment, so they can have their eggs frozen before the surgical intervention [5].

Therefore, from a practical point of view, current evidence suggests that the surgical removal of ovarian endometriotic lesions should be performed only after the extraction of oocytes to preserve fertility, given the possible impairment of the ovarian reserve caused by the surgery and the high return rate of these patients to assisted reproduction clinics to use their previously vitrified oocytes.

22.4 Strategies for COS in Patients with Endometriosis

One of the issues that undoubtedly deserves special attention is the choice of the COS protocol implemented to preserve the fertility of patients with endometriosis. The quest to optimize results in these women, who often have a low ovarian reserve, is a major challenge for contemporary reproductive medicine. Obtaining a higher number of oocytes and mature oocytes for vitrification is directly related to the likelihood of future pregnancy [28].

One of the pioneering works on this topic was published by Bastu et al., who compared COS protocols with GnRH agonists and antagonists in infertile patients who underwent ovarian endometrioma exeresis. Patients who used the agonist protocol obtained higher amounts of mature oocytes and good quality embryos, but the pregnancy and live birth rates did not differ between groups. This study was limited by its small sample size; nevertheless, when it comes to oocyte vitrification for preservation of fertility, the use of protocols with GnRH agonists should be considered [29].

Another more recently published study compared three COS protocols (long and short agonist and GnRH antagonist) in patients with a compromised ovarian reserve after cystectomy due to ovarian endometriomas. Among the 342 participating women, no significant differences in the number of oocytes obtained or in the fertilization rates were found between the groups. With an average of four oocytes aspirated per patient, the three protocols proved to be equally effective [30].

Considering the pathophysiology of endometriosis and its estrogen-dependent character, a Canadian retrospective study sought to compare clinical results in patients who underwent COS cycles with 2 months of previous preparation with a GnRH agonist and patients who followed this same treatment combined with 5 mg of letrozole orally daily [31].

The study showed that the combined therapy group had a higher AFC (10.3 vs. 6.4), more mature oocytes (9.1 vs. 4.0) and a considerable decrease in the size of ovarian endometriomas (1.8 cm vs. 3.2 cm). The good results of this combination therapy were attributed to a significant decrease in the ovarian and pelvic inflammatory process, which was now strongly blocked by both medications [31].

The results were even more expressive if we compare this same population with IVF cycles performed without any prior preparation, with a mean AFC of 6.2 and 3.2 mature oocytes obtained per patient, and an average endometrioma size of 3.5 cm [31].

Taking into account previously published work on therapy with GnRH agonists prior to COS in patients with endometriosis, an Italian study published in 2020 proved that the use of dienogest for 3 months prior to COS in women with previous failure in IVF also brought benefits in pregnancy and live birth rates. Among the 63 patients who used the therapy, an important increase in the number of oocytes obtained and embryos generated was evidenced [20].

Trying to elucidate this issue, another study this year (2020) in patients with endometriosis also evaluated the use of progesterone in COS cycles by comparing it with cycles with an antagonist. Fifty-four women were included in each group, with similar characteristics and an average age of 30. The number of oocytes obtained (8.1) and vitrified (6.4) after COS were the same in both groups. The use of progesterone (P4) to suppress the LH peak proved to be effective, cheap, and more convenient than cycles with antagonists, since many of these patients already used P4 to treat endometriosis prior to stimulation, and only continued its use [3].

Similar results had been published in 2017, when patients with endometriomas undergoing COS with progesterone had a higher number of mature oocytes and good quality morulae per stimulation cycle when compared to the group that used GnRH analogues. No premature LH surges were reported in the 147 cases analyzed and the implantation, pregnancy, fertilization, and cycle cancellation rates did not differ between protocols. This study confirmed the viability of COS with progesterone for endometriotic patients and suggests a possible reduction of pelvic inflammation during its use, which may explain the good results presented by this protocol [27].

When analyzing the chronic inflammatory processes of patients with endometriomas and their possible impacts on fertility, already mentioned throughout this chapter, the administration of GnRH, progesterone or letrozole agonists during or prior to COS can be considered, since the results they produced were equivalent to or even better than those of the protocols usually implemented. These findings can be explained by the anti-inflammatory properties of these drugs. Therefore, the recommendation is to personalize and individualize treatment in each case, and analyze the drug and financial tolerance of each patient.

22.5 Fertility Preservation by Cryopreservation of Ovarian Tissue

Cryopreservation of ovarian tissue has more than 20 years of history, and was initially developed to preserve the fertility and functionality of the gonads in cancer patients [32, 33]. Over 100 confirmed births in patients who underwent autotransplantation confirmed the feasibility of the technique and encouraged scientific societies to stop regarding it as experimental, a step taken in 2020 by the American Society for Reproductive Medicine (ASRM).

Removing a small portion of the ovarian cortex for freezing would preserve the thousands of follicles present there, which could undergo maturation/activation in vitro or in COS in cases of reimplantation in the remaining ovary, in the ovarian cave or in other anatomical locations. There are currently no published works on the use of the technique to preserve the fertility of patients with endometriosis, probably due to the cost, its invasive character and the high rates of follicular apoptosis reported, which make the freezing of oocytes or embryos preferable. High rates of ischemic stress are reported with the freezing/thawing of this tissue, which can compromise its viability [34, 35].

With regard to the removal of the cortex via laparoscopy, the surgical risks inherent to the procedure itself must be considered. Therefore, the technique should be indicated mostly in cases where waiting for COS is not a viable option (which is infrequent due to the existence of protocols for immediate initiation) and in patients with an indication for oophorectomy [32, 33].

Unpleasant experiences with neoplastic tissue reimplantation after ovarian tissue transplantation should also make us reflect on the risk of reimplanting ovarian endometriosis in postsurgical patients, given the severe nature of the disease [35, 36].

Therefore, the use of the technique as a fertility preservation measure indicated for other reasons, such as endometriosis or social motivation, still needs to be discussed [34, 35].

22.6 Conclusion

Endometriosis patients should be educated on the possibility of freezing oocytes to preserve fertility. When these women have ovarian endometriomas, response to controlled ovarian stimulation is observed, with fewer oocytes and mature oocytes obtained. The impact of endometriosis on oocyte quality is not fully understood, and similar rates of aneuploidy among patients with and without the pathology suggest similar quality. Surgical removal of endometriotic foci, especially ovarian (endometriomas), compromises the ovarian reserve and justifies the freezing of eggs prior to surgery.

References

1. Cobo A, Giles J, Paolelli S, Pellicer A, Remohí J, García-Velasco JA. Oocyte vitrification for fertility preservation in women with endometriosis: an observational study. Fertil Steril. 2020;113(4):836–44.
2. Garcia-Fernandez J, García-Velasco JA. Endometriosis and reproduction: what we have learned. Yale J Biol Med. 2020;93:571–7.
3. Mathieu d'Argent E, Ferrier C, Zacharopoulou C, Ahdad-Yata N, Boudy AS, Cantalloube A, Levy R, Antoine JM, Daraï E, Bendifallah S. Outcomes of fertility preservation in women with endometriosis: comparison of progestin-primed ovarian stimulation versus antagonist protocols. J Ovarian Res. 2020;13:18.
4. Gupta S, Agarwal A, Agarwal R, de Mola JR. Impact of ovarian endometrioma on assisted reproduction outcomes. Reprod Biomed Online. 2006;13(3):349–60.
5. Llarena NC, Falcone T, Flyckt RL. Fertility preservation in women with endometriosis clinical medicine insights. Reprod Health. 2019;13:1–8.
6. Busacca M, Riparini J, Somigliana E, Oggioni G, Izzo S, Vignali M, Candiani M. Postsurgical ovarian failure after laparoscopic excision of bilateral endometriomas. Am J Obstet Gynecol. 2006;195:421–5.
7. Younis JS, Shapso N, Fleming R, Ben-Shlomo I, Izhaki I. Impact of unilateral versus bilateral ovarian endometriotic cystectomy on ovarian reserve: a systematic review and meta-analysis. Hum Reprod Update. 2019;25:1–17.
8. Calagnaa G, Della Corte L, Giampaolino P, Maranto M, Perino A. Endometriosis and strategies of fertility preservation: a systematic review of the literature. Eur J Obstet Gynecol Reprod Biol. 2020;254:218–25.
9. Sanchez AM, Vanni VS, Bartiromo L, Papaleo E, Zilberberg E, Candiani M, Orvieto R, Viganò P. Is the oocyte quality affected by endometriosis? A review of the literature. J Ovarian Res. 2017;10:43.
10. Benaglia L, Somigliana E, Vercellini P, Abbiati A, Ragni G, Fedele L. Endometriotic ovarian cysts negatively affect the rate of spontaneous ovulation. Hum Reprod. 2009;24:2183–6.
11. Nakahara K, Saito H, Saito T, Ito M, Ohta N, Takahashi T, Hiroi M. Ovarian fecundity in patients with endometriosis can be estimated by the incidence of apoptotic bodies. Fertil Steril. 1998;69(5):931–5.
12. Orazov MR, Radzinsky VY, Ivanov II, Khamoshina MB, Shustova VB. Oocyte quality in women with infertility associated endometriosis. Gynecol Endocrinol. 2019;35(suppl 1):24–6.
13. Kitajima M, Dolmans MM, Donnez O, Masuzaki H, Soares M, Donnez J. Enhanced follicular recruitment and atresia in cortex derived from ovaries with endometriomas. Fertil Steril. 2014;101(4):1031–7.
14. Hsu AL, Townsend PM, Oehninger S, Castora FJ. Endometriosis may be associated with mitochondrial dysfunction in cumulus cells from subjects undergoing in vitro

fertilization-intracytoplasmic sperm injection, as reflected by decreased adenosine triphosphate production. Fertil Steril. 2015;103:347–52.
15. Garcia-Velasco JA, Arici A. Is the endometrium or oocyte/embryo affected in endometriosis? Hum Reprod. 1999;14:77–89. https://doi.org/10.1093/humrep/14.suppl_2.77.
16. Boucret L, Bouet P-E, Riou J, Legendre G, Delbos L, El Hachem H, Descamps P, Reynier P, May-Panloup P. Endometriosis lowers the cumulative live birth rates in IVF by decreasing the number of embryos but not their quality. J Clin Med. 2020;9:2478. https://doi.org/10.3390/jcm9082478.
17. Nieweglowska D, Hajdyla-Banas I, Pitynski K, Banas T, Grabowska O, Juszczyk G, Ludwin A, Jach R. Age-related trends in anti-Mullerian hormone serum level in women with unilateral and bilateral ovarian endometriomas prior to surgery. Reprod Biol Endocrinol. 2015;13:128.
18. Lemos NA, Arbo E, Scalco R, Weiler E, Rosa V, Cunha-Filho JS. Decreased anti-Mullerian hormone and altered ovarian follicular cohort in infertile patients with mild/minimal endometriosis. Fertil Steril. 2008;89(5):1064–8.
19. Sanchez AM, Vigano P, Somigliana E, Panina-Bordignon P, Vercellini P, Candiani M. The distinguishing cellular and molecular features of the endometriotic ovarian cyst: from pathophysiology to the potential endometrioma-mediated damage to the ovary. Hum Reprod Update. 2014;20(2):217–30.
20. Barra F, Laganà AS, Scala C, Garzon S, Ghezzi F, Ferrero S. Pretreatment with dienogest in women with endometriosis undergoing IVF after a previous failed cycle. Reprod Biomed Online. 2020;41(5):859–68.
21. Pluchino N, Roman H. Oocyte vitrification offers more space for a tailored surgical management of endometriosis. Reprod Biomed Online. 2020;41(5):753–5.
22. Marcoux S, Maheux R, Bérubé S. Laparoscopic surgery in infertile women with minimal or mild endometriosis. N Engl J Med. 1997;337:217–22. https://doi.org/10.1056/NEJM199707243370401.
23. Kim SJ, Kim SK, Lee JR, Suh CS, Kim SH. Oocyte cryopreservation for fertility preservation in women with ovarian endometriosis. Reprod Biomed Online. 2020;40(6):827–34.
24. Benaglia L, Busnelli A, Biancardi R, Vegetti W, Reschini M, Vercellini P, Somigliana E. Oocyte retrieval difficulties in women with ovarian endometriomas. Reprod Biomed Online. 2018;37(1):77–84.
25. Romero B, Aibar L, Navarro LM, Fontes J, Calderón MA, Mozas J. Pelvic abscess after oocyte retrieval in women with endometriosis: a case series. Iran J Reprod Med. 2013;11(8):677–80.
26. Younis JS, Ezra Y, Laufer N, Ohel G. Late manifestation of pelvic abscess following oocyte retrieval, for in vitro fertilization, in patients with severe endometriosis and ovarian endometriomata. J Assist Reprod Genet. 1997;14(6):343–6.
27. Guo H, Wang Y, Chen Q, Chai W, Sun L, Ai A, Fu Y, Lyu Q, Kuang Y. Use of medroxyprogesterone acetate in women with ovarian endometriosis undergoing controlled ovarian hyperstimulation for in vitro fertilization. Sci Rep. 2017;7(1):1–10.
28. Drakopoulos P, Blockeel C, Stoop D, Camus M, de Vos M, Tournaye H, Polyzos NP. Conventional ovarian stimulation and single embryo transfer for IVF/ICSI. How many oocytes do we need to maximize cumulative live birth rates after utilization of all fresh and frozen embryos? Hum Reprod. 2016;31(2):370–6.
29. Bastu E, Yasa C, Dural O, Mutlu MF, Celik C, Ugurlucan FG, Buyru F. Comparison of ovulation induction protocols after endometrioma resection. JSLS. 2014;18(3):e2014.
30. Zhao F, Lan Y, Chen T, Zhimin Xin Y, Liang YL, Wang S, Zhang J, Yang X. Live birth rate comparison of three controlled ovarian stimulation protocols for in vitro fertilization-embryo transfer in patients with diminished ovarian reserve after endometrioma cystectomy: a retrospective study. J Ovarian Res. 2020;13:23.
31. Cantor A, Tannus S, Son WY, Tan SL, Dahan MH. A comparison of two months pretreatment with GnRH agonists with or without an aromatase inhibitor in women with ultrasound-diagnosed ovarian endometriomas undergoing IVF. Reprod Biomed Online. 2019;38(4):520–7.
32. Lantsberg D, Fernando S, Cohen Y, Rombauts L. The role of fertility preservation in women with endometriosis: a systematic review. J Minim Invasive Gynecol. 2019;27(2):362–72.

33. Diaz-Garcia C, Domingo J, Garcia-Velasco JA, Herraiz S, Mirabet V, Iniesta I, Cobo A, Remohí J, Pellicer A. Oocyte vitrification versus ovarian cortex transplantation in fertility preservation for adult women undergoing gonadotoxic treatments: a prospective cohort study. Fertil Steril. 2017;109(3):478–85.
34. Kristensen SG, Andersen CY. Cryopreservation of ovarian tissue: opportunities beyond fertility preservation and a positive view into the future. Front Endocrinol. 2018;9:347.
35. Andersen CY, Mamsen LS, Kristensen SG. Fertility preservation: freezing of ovarian tissue and clinical opportunities. Reproduction. 2019;158(5):F27–34.
36. Suzuki N, Yoshioka N, Takae S, Sugishita Y, Tamura M, Hashimoto S, Morimoto Y, Kawamura K. Successful fertility preservation following ovarian tissue vitrification in patients with primary ovarian insufficiency. Hum Reprod. 2015;30(3):608–15.

Malignancy Risks Associated with Endometriosis: Epidemiology

23

Marina Kvaskoff and Stacey A. Missmer

Contents

The original version of the chapter has been revised. A correction to this chapter can be found at https://doi.org/10.1007/978-3-030-97236-3_45

M. Kvaskoff (✉)
Exposome and Heredity Team, Centre for Research in Epidemiology and Population Health, Inserm (French National Institute for Health and Medical Research), Villejuif, France
e-mail: marina.kvaskoff@inserm.fr

S. A. Missmer
Department of Obstetrics, Gynecology, and Reproductive Biology, College of Human Medicine, Michigan State University, Grand Rapids, MI, USA

E. Oral (ed.), *Endometriosis and Adenomyosis*, https://doi.org/10.1007/978-3-030-97236-3_23

23.1 Introduction

The association between endometriosis and cancer has had a long-lasting interest in the literature [1]. Since the publication of a first case report in 1946 [2], close to 10,000 scientific papers were published on this topic up to 2020; this interest increased starkly in the 2010s, with ~300 entries per year for "endometriosis and cancer" in the PubMed database.

This interest stemmed from several observations. While non-malignant, endometriosis exhibits features that are similar to cancer, including abnormal tissue growth, resistance to apoptosis, and development of local and distant foci with invasion of other tissues [3]. In addition, the disease is associated with chronic local and systemic inflammation [4] and has been reported to be associated with several cancer risk factors [5].

Several epidemiologic studies have explored whether women with endometriosis are at higher risk of cancer and have attempted to quantify this risk [6, 7]. Knowledge on cancer risk among women with endometriosis is indeed essential in terms of public health, in order to inform cancer screening and prevention. It is important also in the clinical setting for the long-term management of endometriosis patients. With regards to research, the exploration of the link between endometriosis and cancer is crucial to improve our understanding of endometriosis pathophysiology.

This chapter reviews the epidemiological evidence on the links between endometriosis and cancer, discusses methodologic considerations for this topic and the potential mechanisms underlying these associations, and provides recommendations for information to patients, cancer screening, and long-term patient management with regards to cancer risk.

23.2 Epidemiological Evidence on the Associations Between Endometriosis and Malignancy

A systematic review and meta-analysis of epidemiological studies published up to October 24, 2019, reported on the links between endometriosis and the risk of several types of cancer [7]. Based on a systematic search of the PubMed and Embase databases, the study identified 17,878 records, of which 636 full-text articles were assessed for eligibility, including 204 articles that were relevant to the epidemiological association between endometriosis and cancer. Of these, a total of 49 publications (38 studies) were included in quantitative synthesis, including 19 case-control studies and 19 cohort studies. The data were synthesized and analysed through random-effects meta-analysis using standard methodology, and the quality of the included studies and risk of bias were assessed through the ROBINS-I tool [8]. The study involved subgroup analyses by methodologic characteristics in order to investigate potential sources of heterogeneity among studies.

The meta-analysis included five studies that provided estimates on the risk of overall cancer, yielding a very small and non-statistically significant association between endometriosis and overall cancer risk (summary relative risk (SRR) = 1.07,

95% confidence interval (CI) = 0.98–1.16). However, the study showed substantial heterogeneity among studies ($I^2 = 88\%$, $P < 0.0001$), i.e. a high level of variation in study methodology and characteristics that may lead to invalid summary estimates.

The review details meta-analytic findings according to cancer type. Most prior research has focused on gynaecological cancers (ovarian cancer: $n = 24$ studies; breast cancer: $n = 20$ studies; endometrial cancer: $n = 17$ studies); research on other cancer sites being more limited ($n = 2–7$ studies).

23.2.1 Gynaecological Cancers

23.2.1.1 Ovarian Cancer

Based on 24 studies, the meta-analysis produced a SRR of 1.93 (95% CI = 1.68–2.22) for the association between endometriosis and ovarian cancer risk [7]. Importantly, there was significant evidence of publication bias, implying that positive, statistically significant results were more likely to be published, which biased the results towards an overestimation of the relation between endometriosis and ovarian cancer. In addition, there was a high level of heterogeneity among studies ($I^2 = 78\%$, $P < 0.0001$). Subgroup analyses revealed stronger associations among higher-quality studies, i.e. those involving a prospective cohort design, medical record confirmation of endometriosis (vs. self-report), or meeting the temporality criterion (i.e. ensuring that endometriosis preceded cancer diagnosis by at least 12 months in the analysis), although a high level of heterogeneity remained in these subgroups.

However, study heterogeneity disappeared in analyses by ovarian cancer histotype, associations being stronger for the clear-cell (SRR = 3.44, 95% CI = 2.82–4.20) and endometrioid (SRR = 2.33, 95% CI = 1.82–2.98) histotypes. There was also a modest positive association with serous tumours (SRR = 1.17, 95% CI = 1.03–1.32), which was restricted to low-grade serous tumours (SRR = 2.33, 95% CI = 1.64–3.31, $n = 2$ studies; high-grade tumours: SRR = 1.08, 95% CI = 0.88–1.32, $n = 3$ studies; P for heterogeneity <0.0001). Although publication bias was not detected in this sub-analysis, the authors warn that it cannot be ruled out given the small number of studies providing estimates by tumour histotype.

Only four studies provided estimates of the association between endometriosis and ovarian cancer according to the type of endometriosis. Of those, three focused on endometrioma only, irrespectively of other subtypes. Based on these four studies, the SRR for the association between endometrioma and ovarian cancer risk was 5.41 (95% CI = 2.25–13.00).

One retrospective study reported risk estimates for the association between endometriosis and ovarian cancer according to both macro-phenotype of endometriosis and histotype of ovarian cancer [9]. Endometrioma was associated with the clear cell (standardized incidence ratio (SIR) = 10.1), endometrioid (SIR = 4.7), and serous (SIR = 1.62) histotypes; similar associations were reported for superficial peritoneal endometriosis, but with a lower magnitude of effect (SIRs of 2.67, 2.03, and 1.32, respectively); while there was no association between deep endometriosis and ovarian cancer risk (SIRs of 0.00, 3.35, and

1.41, respectively, although power was limited given the small number of ovarian cancer cases with deep endometriosis).

Several important points should be noted regarding the interpretation of the association between endometrioma and ovarian cancer risk. First, only a small number of studies investigated this link. There was a high level of heterogeneity among them ($I^2 = 82\%$, $P = 0.001$) and a high level of imprecision given the wide confidence interval. Two studies included selected samples, one involving subfertile women [10] and the other one women with endometriosis only [11]. In addition, none of these studies was able to quantify the association with endometrioma exclusively. Only one study provided estimates for each endometriosis macro-phenotype: endometrioma (SRR = 2.56, 95% CI = 1.98–3.27), superficial peritoneal (SRR = 1.32, 95% CI = 0.99–1.72), and deep endometriosis (SRR = 1.41, 95% CI = 0.29–4.10) [9], and although the association was stronger for endometrioma than other subtypes, the groups were not mutually exclusive and the findings are thus difficult to interpret. However, exclusive subgroups should be considered not only for endometrioma, but also for the superficial peritoneal and deep endometriosis macro-phenotypes, since these subtypes are associated with a cancer-prone hyper-inflammatory environment also [12]. Many ovarian cancers have a non-ovarian origin [13]. Future studies should thus provide results among both exclusive and non-exclusive macro-phenotypic subgroups of endometriosis in order to have a clearer picture of the subtype-specific associations of endometriosis with ovarian cancer risk.

Importantly, since diagnosis is more straightforward for endometrioma than for other subtypes [14], studies may be more likely to include cases with this macro-phenotype, yielding a diagnostic bias specific to endometrioma, which is critical to explore in further research. In addition, endometrioma is also more likely to be visualized in women diagnosed with ovarian cancer, which induces a bias when the temporality of the association is not taken into account. Thus, while endometrioma has been proposed to be the main macro-phenotype of endometriosis that could lead to malignant transformation [15, 16], the methodologic points highlighted above show that many uncertainties remain on this pathway.

Moreover, some pathologists have suggested that endometrioma should be considered a pre-cancerous lesion. However, although endometrioma shares common molecular alterations with ovarian cancer [17], molecular studies have shown that the prevalence of cancer-driver mutations in deep endometriosis is identical to that of endometrioma [18]. However, a significantly higher prevalence of these mutations could be expected in endometriomas versus deep endometriosis since deep endometriosis is not associated with ovarian cancer risk [9], and the eutopic endometrium of healthy women carries cancer driver mutations in high proportions also [16]. More research will therefore be needed in order to answer the question "Is endometrioma a pre-cancerous lesion?". To have a clearer answer, future research efforts should be focused on endometriosis macro-phenotypic subtypes and on the ovarian cancer histotypes that have been associated with endometriosis.

23.2.1.2 Breast Cancer

Based on 20 studies on breast cancer included in the meta-analysis [7], there was a very small association between endometriosis and breast cancer risk (SRR = 1.04, 95% CI = 1.00–1.09). Only two studies provided estimates by breast cancer subtype: one US study showed no association with breast cancer overall, but a positive association that was restricted to oestrogen receptor-positive (ER+)/progesterone receptor-negative (PR-) tumours (hazard ratio (HR) = 1.90, 95% CI = 1.44–2.50; P for heterogeneity = 0.001) [19]. The study showed no difference in association according to menopausal status or type of menopause among post-menopausal women. In addition, a Danish study reported no differences according to breast cancer subtype [20]. No previous study has reported estimates of the association between endometriosis and breast cancer by endometriosis macro-phenotype. Given the known differences in associations for breast cancer risk factors according to breast cancer subtype [21, 22], it is critical that future research reports associations with endometriosis within subgroups of breast cancers.

23.2.1.3 Endometrial Cancer

The meta-analysis yielded a SRR of 1.23 (95% CI = 0.97–1.57) for the association between endometriosis and endometrial cancer, based on 17 studies, with a high heterogeneity level among studies ($I^2 = 81\%$, $P < 0.0001$) [7]. In subgroup analyses, it was observed that among studies using a prospective cohort design, which ensures rigorous temporality (i.e. endometriosis precedes endometrial cancer diagnosis), the association was null with no heterogeneity among studies (SRR = 0.99, 95% CI = 0.72–1.37, $I^2 = 0\%$, $P = 0.51$, $n = 5$ studies), while the association remained among retrospective cohort studies (SRR = 1.40, 95% CI = 1.00–1.96, $I^2 = 87\%$, $P < 0.0001$). In addition, the SRR varied greatly in sensitivity analyses according to the methodologic characteristics of the studies.

The stark differences in the findings according to the temporality associated with each study design suggest a potential diagnostic bias resulting from the higher detection of endometriosis among women undergoing evaluation for endometrial cancer. These differences call for further research in this area in order to better understand the link between endometriosis and endometrial cancer.

Only two studies explored the association according to endometrial cancer subtype. One reported a higher association for type I (SIR = 1.54, 95% CI = 1.20–1.96) versus type II tumours (SIR = 1.06, 95% CI = 0.28–2.71) [20], and the other reported a higher association with uterine sarcomas (relative risk (RR) = 2.72) than for indolent types (RR = 1.14) [23]. Only one study performed subgroup analyses by macrophenotype of endometriosis, reporting a higher risk of endometrial cancer associated with adenomyosis (hazard ratio (HR) = 4.38, 95% CI = 1.22–15.72) but no statistically significant association with endometrioma (HR = 3.23, 95% CI = 0.54–19.27). While power was insufficient to examine associations with endometrioma exclusively, the association was strengthened in the subgroup including adenomyosis exclusively, although confidence intervals were wide (HR = 5.13, 95%

CI = 1.36–19.40). Again, further research by disease subtype will be essential to increase our understanding of these associations in the future.

23.2.2 Other Types of Cancer

23.2.2.1 Skin Cancer

Seven studies on the associations between endometriosis and cutaneous melanoma were included in the meta-analysis [7]. The resulting SRR estimate was of 1.17 (95% CI = 0.97–1.41). The moderate level of heterogeneity among studies ($I^2 = 51\%$, $P = 0.05$) was substantially reduced in subgroup analyses by ROBINS-I risk of bias, with a SRR of 1.71 (95% CI = 1.24–2.36) in studies with low/moderate risk of bias, versus 1.08 (95% CI = 0.87–1.26) in those with critical or serious risk of bias (P for heterogeneity = 0.07). The substantial increase in magnitude of effect and statistical significance in higher-quality studies suggests that for this cancer type, biases may strongly mask a true association. The sole study reporting estimates by histotype of melanoma reported no statistically significant differences [24].

A meta-analysis of the sole two studies evaluating the association between endometriosis and basal-cell carcinoma resulted in a SRR of 1.18 (95% CI = 1.11–1.25) with no evidence of heterogeneity ($I^2 = 0\%$, $P = 0.89$) [24, 25].

23.2.2.2 Thyroid Cancer

Five studies were included on the associations between endometriosis and thyroid cancer, yielding a SRR of 1.39 (95% CI = 1.24–1.57) with no evidence of heterogeneity ($I^2 = 0\%$, $P = 0.69$) [7].

23.2.2.3 Colorectal Cancer

The five included studies that evaluated the associations between endometriosis and colorectal cancer produced a SRR of 1.00 (95% CI = 0.87–1.16), with a low level of heterogeneity among studies ($I^2 = 40\%$, $P = 0.16$) [7]. However, there was a positive association among studies with low/moderate risk of bias (SRR = 2.29, 95% CI = 1.00–5.26), suggesting an impact of bias in the overall results here also, although confidence intervals were wide.

23.2.2.4 Cervical Cancer

Four studies were included in the meta-analysis of the studies assessing the association between endometriosis and cervical cancer [7], resulting in a robust and statistically significant SRR of 0.68 (95% CI = 0.56–0.82) with no heterogeneity among studies ($I^2 = 0\%$, $P = 0.76$). However, it should be noted that all studies were conducted in Europe and were based on self-reported endometriosis.

The 32% lower risk of cervical cancer associated with endometriosis reported in this meta-analysis is consistent with the results from two previous meta-analyses, reporting reduced risks of 33% [26] and 22% [27]. However, these results need careful interpretation: while this inverse association is unlikely to reflect causality, it implies probable diagnostic and treatment biases linked to the higher exposure of endometriosis patients to the healthcare system [5]. Women with endometriosis are indeed more likely to be routinely screened for cervical hyperplasia and to receive treatment if positive than women without endometriosis or gynaecological conditions. This reinforces the importance of considering the potential impact of access to care overlaying the associations between endometriosis and cancer risk in general. Another potential pathway that could explain this inverse association is the impact of dyspareunia and chronic pelvic pain on sexual relationships, which could lead to a lower prevalence of human papillomavirus infection among women with endometriosis. This hypothesis remains to be explored in future research.

23.2.2.5 Other Cancers

The meta-analysis examined the risks associated with endometriosis for several other cancer types, based on <4 studies [7]. There were small associations between endometriosis and the risks of lymphatic and haematopoietic cancers (SRR = 1.09, 95% CI = 1.00–1.19, $n = 2$ studies), non-Hodgkin lymphoma (SRR = 1.18, 95% CI = 1.00–1.41, $n = 3$ studies), and brain cancer (SRR = 1.18, 95% CI = 1.02–1.36, $n = 2$ studies). However, it should be noted that the number of studies was low and mostly used a retrospective design, limiting the ability to adjust for potential confounders. More research will need to be conducted in order to inform our knowledge of the associations between endometriosis and the risk of other cancers.

23.3 Research Methodology Considerations

The meta-analysis on endometriosis and cancer risk [7] and previous work [6] have identified a number of methodologic complexities that need to be carefully considered in the study of the associations between endometriosis and the risk of cancer or any other type of disease. Given the risk of bias reported in the meta-analysis, showing severe or critical risk of bias in a majority (53%) of included studies, the following methodologic issues are critical to consider in order to perform high quality research in this field.

23.3.1 Temporality

To discuss the impact of endometriosis as a potential risk factor for cancer, studies need to ensure that endometriosis *precedes* the diagnosis of cancer. For this, the use of a prospective cohort design, enabling time-varying analysis of covariates over a sufficiently long duration of follow-up, in order to allow for initiation and promotion of cancer following endometriosis onset, is recommended. However, retrospective designs may also ensure this temporal order by restricting the definition of endometriosis diagnosed at least 1 year before cancer diagnosis. The meta-analytic findings on endometrial cancer showed that considering temporality can dramatically modify the conclusions on an association.

23.3.2 Misclassification and Population Sampling

Misclassification of endometriosis is a likely bias in epidemiologic research, given the requirement of surgical visualization for diagnosis, the existence of asymptomatic disease, and the known diagnostic delays associated with the disease [28]. Endometriosis is likely over-reported in clinical-based studies and under-reported in population-based studies [29]. In the absence of a non-invasive diagnostic tool, diagnostic biases are likely to be driven by the characteristics of the women who are able to achieve diagnosis and their symptoms.

This misclassification has the potential to attenuate the associations under study. Associations are driven towards the null also in studies basing the comparison group on a selected sample (e.g. infertile patients or women who have undergone hysterectomy), since potential underlying pathology in these women may also be associated with cancer risk [30]. It is thus important to use a population-based sample and to interpret the results considering this methodologic issue that is inherent to endometriosis research.

23.3.3 Confounding and Mediation

Studies evaluating the association between endometriosis and cancer risk should assess if these associations are driven by common risk factors, whether these factors precede endometriosis and cancer (confounders) or are along the causal pathway between endometriosis and cancer (mediators). Few of the studies included in the meta-analysis were able to adjust for potential confounders, and even fewer explored potential mediators of the associations.

23.3.4 Study Robustness and Study Heterogeneity

The assessed quality of evidence in the meta-analysis showed that more than half (53%) of the included studies evaluating associations between endometriosis and cancer were at serious or critical risk of bias, and statistically significant heterogeneity was observed for a large portion of cancer types [7]. Part of this heterogeneity was driven by the methodologic limitations of many studies (as listed in the points above), potentially leading to inaccurate or invalid estimates. Heterogeneity among studies also pertained to differences in the characteristics of the studied populations, which may lead to true differences in associations.

23.3.5 Endometriosis and Cancer Disease Heterogeneity

As reviewed above, extremely few studies were able to study associations between endometriosis and cancer risk by macro-phenotype of endometriosis and/or by cancer subtype. While the subgroup analyses in the meta-analysis confirmed that the association with ovarian cancer was restricted to specific histotypes (clear cell and endometrioid), only four studies were able to provide estimates according to the macro-phenotype of endometriosis, and only one by both type of endometriosis and histotype of ovarian cancer, none of which provided estimates for each type exclusively [7]. Only one study reported risk estimates for endometrioma and adenomyosis in exclusive subgroups, which showed a stronger association with endometrial cancer in the exclusive subgroup with adenomyosis [11], thereby reinforcing the need to explore mutually exclusive groups of macro-phenotype of endometriosis. Beyond the study of the endometriosis and cancer association, the lack of routine standardized reporting of endometriosis characteristics currently hampers analyses to this level of detail. Therefore, the record and use of such data is critical in endometriosis research as it has a high potential to provide new insights into the aetiology of the disease [12].

23.3.6 Publication Bias

As reported in the meta-analysis, there was statistically significant evidence of publication bias in the evaluation of the association between endometriosis and ovarian cancer risk, which likely overestimated the true association [7]. This highlights the need for high-quality studies to be published irrespectively of the direction, magnitude, or statistical significance of their results, in order to not mislead interpretation of these associations.

23.4 Potential Pathophysiological Mechanisms Underlying the Associations Between Endometriosis and Cancer

While the exact pathophysiology underlying the associations between endometriosis and cancer is unknown, several mechanisms may be hypothesized to be at play.

First, associations between endometriosis and cancer may be driven by shared risk factors (e.g. genetic susceptibility, patient characteristics, or environmental exposures). With regards to genetics, while cross-disease genetic correlation studies reported loci common to endometriosis and ovarian cancer [31, 32] or endometrial cancer [33], it should be mentioned that these studies did not examine variations in associations according to method of endometriosis assessment or consider the potential impact of diagnostic bias. Other factors (such as demographics, menstrual characteristics, anthropometry, lifestyle, or exposure to environmental toxicants) may act as confounders of the associations between endometriosis and cancer; however, too few studies were able to adjust for such factors or to examine potential mediating effects.

Beyond overlapping risk factors raising the risk of malignancy through various pathways, it is possible that endometriosis is causally associated with cancer risk. In this regard, mediation analysis is likely to provide insights into the pathways involved in these associations, which may include infertility, stress, anxiety and depression, or lifestyle changes associated with endometriosis symptoms (e.g. decreased physical activity). Mediators may also include treatment of endometriosis lesions and associated symptoms (medication use: analgesics, hormonal treatments; surgery: lesion ablation/excision, hysterectomy, bilateral salpingo-oophorectomy), which have also been associated with the risk of several cancer types.

Through mediators or through direct pathways, the presence of endometriosis may induce systemic changes that create a cancer-prone milieu, such as chronic inflammation, aberrant hormonal milieu, or aberrant immune response [4], which may underlie the associations with distal cancers, such as breast cancer, cutaneous melanoma, or thyroid cancer. Further research is warranted to enhance our understanding of the pathways underlying the associations between endometriosis and cancer, and to elucidate why associations are observed with some cancer types but not others. The –omics technologies are likely to help increase our knowledge and understanding of these associations in the future.

23.5 How Should Clinicians Inform Women with Endometriosis Regarding Their Cancer Risk?

The reported links between endometriosis and cancer may raise concerns in women with endometriosis, who need to be accurately informed and reassured about their long-term cancer risk. For clinicians, these links raise a number of practical questions on the long-term management of women with endometriosis.

The most robust positive association between endometriosis and cancer is that with ovarian cancer risk. While the absolute risk of developing ovarian cancer in the general female population is 1.3% [34], the SRR reported in the meta-analysis (SRR = 1.93) [7] translates to an absolute risk of 2.5% in the population of women with endometriosis, which remains very low. Although small, this absolute risk is likely even smaller given the identified publication bias that is likely to overestimate this association. Given the differential associations observed according to endometriosis or ovarian cancer subtype, studies including data on these subtypes are critically needed to provide more detailed absolute risk calculations.

Regarding other cancer types, the absolute risk of developing breast cancer in a woman's lifetime increases from 12.8% in the general female population [34] to 13.3% in women with endometriosis, after applying the meta-analytic result (SRR = 1.04) [7]. For thyroid cancer, this risk increases from 1.3% in the general female population to 1.8% in women with endometriosis, considering the reported SRR of 1.39 in the meta-analysis.

In an attempt to provide communication tools to clinicians on the link between endometriosis and ovarian cancer, a panel of key messages was proposed to put the quantified relative risks into perspective [35]. In addition to the translation into absolute risk, other messages included the comparison of absolute ovarian cancer risks in women inheriting a harmful *BRCA1* (39%) or *BRCA2* (11–17%) mutation, and comparison of the low absolute risk of ovarian cancer in women with endometriosis with the higher absolute risks of other cancer types in the general female population (breast (13%), lung (6%), and bowel (4%) cancers). Finally, given the low absolute risks of ovarian, breast, and thyroid cancers and the uncertainty regarding other cancer types, the panel points to general prevention messages that may be delivered to endometriosis patients, such as recommendations of avoiding smoking, maintaining a healthy weight, exercising regularly, having a balanced diet with high intakes of fruits and vegetables and low intake of alcohol, and using sun protection.

23.6 Cancer Screening and Monitoring Recommendations

The report of a higher risk of cancer in endometriosis patients could lead clinicians to direct patients to more frequent cancer screening. However, the results from the meta-analysis [7], and their translation into up to 1.2% increase in absolute risk of cancer compared with the general population, suggest that cancer screening recommendations should not differ in women with endometriosis compared with those in the general population of females. Thus, heightened screening is only recommended in those with known non-endometriosis specific risk factors (i.e. family history of cancer or germline mutation predisposing to cancer risk). While regular screening is recommended for breast, cervical, and colorectal cancers based on evidence showing that these screenings save lives [36], regular screening for ovarian cancer through serum CA-125 or transvaginal ultrasound is not recommended, since randomized-controlled trials have shown no benefit of screening on early ovarian cancer detection or mortality reduction [37, 38]. In fact, these trials have shown that false positive test results for ovarian cancer resulted in significant harms (e.g. unnecessary surgery, surgical complications, infections, and cardiovascular or pulmonary complications).

In addition, radical preventive measures to reduce ovarian cancer risk, such as bilateral salpingo-oophorectomy (BSO), are not recommended as a systematic measure to prevent ovarian cancer risk in women with endometriosis [39]. Here again, while BSO was recommended as an effective approach to reduce risk in women at high-risk of ovarian cancer (i.e. family history of cancer or germline mutation predisposing to cancer risk) [40], this procedure is associated with long-term health risks [41] of remarkably higher incidence than ovarian cancer in women with average lifetime absolute risk. These risks include, in premenopausal women, a higher risk of cardiovascular disease [42], depression, arthritis, asthma, chronic obstructive pulmonary disease, and osteoporosis [43]. In postmenopausal women, BSO also has adverse effects on cardiovascular risk, anxiety, and sexual function [44], risk of bone fracture [45], and neurologic disease and cognitive impairment [46]; in addition, it does not save quality-adjusted life years (QALYs) and is not cost-effective [47]. The low absolute risk of ovarian cancer in women with endometriosis thus does not justify performing this important procedure that has irreversible adverse effects on long-term health.

These conservative recommendations may be altered if future research shows quality evidence that some subtypes of endometriosis constitute a high-risk group for ovarian cancer. However, the current evidence suggests that no systematic procedure or screening is to be recommended. Of course, long-term management decisions must vary according to endometriosis patients' medical history, characteristics, other risk factors, and patient preferences after receiving full information on the current evidence and benefit/risk ratio [7].

23.7 Conclusion

In conclusion, endometriosis has been associated with a 93% increased risk of ovarian cancer, particularly the clear-cell (244%) and endometrioid (133%) histotypes. However, evidence of publication bias suggests that these associations are overestimated. Endometriosis was also associated with a very small (4%) increase in breast cancer risk, and with a 39% increase in thyroid cancer risk. An inverse association was consistently reported between endometriosis and cervical cancer (32% decreased risk), most likely reflecting diagnostic and treatment bias. Data on other cancer types were either too scarce or variable to sensitivity analyses to allow robust conclusions.

Given the low methodologic quality of most studies in this field, the current epidemiological evidence on the links between endometriosis and cancer is mostly not reliable. Future research efforts to investigate the association between endometriosis and cancer should take into account the critical methodological complexities in this field (i.e. temporality, misclassification, confounding and mediation, robustness, disease heterogeneity, publication bias), use a prospective design with a long duration of follow-up, a population-based sample with standardized collection of data and recognized criteria for the definition of endometriosis, and evaluate potential confounding and mediation. Importantly, to increase our understanding of endometriosis and cancer pathophysiology, it is crucial that research in this area explores the heterogeneity of endometriosis and cancer by examining results within subgroups of macro-phenotype of endometriosis, within subtypes of each type of cancer, and by cross-tabulating endometriosis and cancer types. Regarding macro-phenotypes of endometriosis in particular, the potential diagnostic bias linked to endometrioma must be explored further.

The close-to-double in risk of ovarian cancer in women with endometriosis translates into a very low increase in absolute risk – from 1.3% in the general female population to 2.5% in endometriosis patients. Absolute risk increases are even smaller with regards to breast or thyroid cancers (from 12.8% and 1.3% in the general female population, to 13.3% and 1.8% in women with endometriosis, respectively). Thus, no specific screening or preventive measure can be recommended in women with endometriosis compared with the general female population. Endometriosis patients should be fully informed and reassured, where appropriate, about their long-term cancer risk.

References

1. Missmer SA. Commentary: endometriosis--epidemiologic considerations for a potentially 'high-risk' population. Int J Epidemiol. 2009;38(4):1154–5.
2. Mc CK, Froats ER, Falk HC. Epidermoid carcinoma arising in an endometrial cyst of the ovary. Arch Pathol (Chic). 1946;41:335–7.
3. Garry R. Endometriosis: an invasive disease. Gynecol Endoscop. 2001;10:79–82.
4. Zondervan KT, et al. Endometriosis. Nat Rev Dis Primers. 2018;4(1):9.
5. Shafrir AL, et al. Risk for and consequences of endometriosis: a critical epidemiologic review. Best Pract Res Clin Obstet Gynaecol. 2018;51:1–15.
6. Kvaskoff M, et al. Endometriosis: a high-risk population for major chronic diseases? Hum Reprod Update. 2015;21(4):500–16.
7. Kvaskoff M, et al. Endometriosis and cancer: a systematic review and meta-analysis. Hum Reprod Update. 2020;27:393.
8. Sterne JA, et al. ROBINS-I: a tool for assessing risk of bias in non-randomised studies of interventions. BMJ. 2016;355:i4919.
9. Saavalainen L, et al. Risk of gynecologic cancer according to the type of endometriosis. Obstet Gynecol. 2018;131(6):1095–102.
10. Buis CC, et al. Increased risk for ovarian cancer and borderline ovarian tumours in subfertile women with endometriosis. Hum Reprod. 2013;28:3358.
11. Kobayashi H, et al. Risk of developing ovarian cancer among women with ovarian endometrioma: a cohort study in Shizuoka, Japan. Int J Gynecol Cancer. 2007;17(1):37–43.
12. Zondervan KT, Becker CM, Missmer SA. Endometriosis. N Engl J Med. 2020;382(13):1244–56.
13. Vaughan S, et al. Rethinking ovarian cancer: recommendations for improving outcomes. Nat Rev Cancer. 2011;11(10):719–25.
14. Dunselman GA, et al. ESHRE guideline: management of women with endometriosis. Hum Reprod. 2014;29(3):400–12.
15. Lac V, et al. Iatrogenic endometriosis harbors somatic cancer-driver mutations. Hum Reprod. 2019;34(1):69–78.
16. Lac V, et al. Oncogenic mutations in histologically normal endometrium: the new normal? J Pathol. 2019;249(2):173–81.
17. Ruderman R, Pavone ME. Ovarian cancer in endometriosis: an update on the clinical and molecular aspects. Minerva Ginecol. 2017;69(3):286–94.
18. Anglesio MS, et al. Cancer-associated mutations in endometriosis without cancer. N Engl J Med. 2017;376(19):1835–48.
19. Farland LV, et al. Laparoscopically confirmed endometriosis and breast cancer in the Nurses' Health Study II. Obstet Gynecol. 2016;128(5):1025–31.
20. Mogensen JB, et al. Endometriosis and risks for ovarian, endometrial and breast cancers: a nationwide cohort study. Gynecol Oncol. 2016;143(1):87–92.
21. Mavaddat N, et al. Polygenic risk scores for prediction of breast cancer and breast cancer subtypes. Am J Hum Genet. 2019;104(1):21–34.
22. Glynn RJ, et al. Comparison of questionnaire-based breast cancer prediction models in the Nurses' Health Study. Cancer Epidemiol Biomark Prev. 2019;28(7):1187–94.
23. Brinton LA, et al. Relationship of benign gynecologic diseases to subsequent risk of ovarian and uterine tumors. Cancer Epidemiol Biomark Prev. 2005;14(12):2929–35.
24. Farland LV, et al. Endometriosis and the risk of skin cancer: a prospective cohort study. Cancer Causes Control. 2017;28:1011.
25. Saavalainen L, et al. A Nationwide Cohort Study on the risk of non-gynecological cancers in women with surgically verified endometriosis. Int J Cancer. 2018;143:2725.
26. Li J, et al. Impact of endometriosis on risk of ovarian, endometrial and cervical cancers: a meta-analysis. Arch Gynecol Obstet. 2019;299(1):35–46.
27. Gandini S, et al. The risk of extra-ovarian malignancies among women with endometriosis: a systematic literature review and meta-analysis. Crit Rev Oncol Hematol. 2019;134:72–81.

28. Nnoaham KE, et al. Impact of endometriosis on quality of life and work productivity: a multicenter study across ten countries. Fertil Steril. 2011;96:366.
29. Ghiasi M, Kulkarni MT, Missmer SA. Is endometriosis more common and more severe than it was 30 years ago? J Minim Invasive Gynecol. 2020;27(2):452–61.
30. Missmer SA. Why so null? Methodologic necessities to advance endometriosis discovery. Paediatr Perinat Epidemiol. 2019;33(1):26–7.
31. Lee AW, et al. Evidence of a genetic link between endometriosis and ovarian cancer. Fertil Steril. 2016;105(1):35–43 e1-10.
32. Lu Y, et al. Shared genetics underlying epidemiological association between endometriosis and ovarian cancer. Hum Mol Genet. 2015;24(20):5955–64.
33. Painter JN, et al. Genetic overlap between endometriosis and endometrial cancer: evidence from cross-disease genetic correlation and GWAS meta-analyses. Cancer Med. 2018;7(5):1978–87.
34. National Cancer Institute. SEER cancer statistics review (CSR) 1975–2014. 2017; Available from: https://seer.cancer.gov/csr/1975_2014 (accessed June 26, 2017).
35. Kvaskoff M, Horne AW, Missmer SA. Informing women with endometriosis about ovarian cancer risk. Lancet. 2017;390(10111):2433–4.
36. American Cancer Society. American Cancer Society Guidelines for the Early Detection of Cancer: Cancer Screening Guidelines | Detecting Cancer Early. 2018 15 September 2020];. Available from: www.cancer.org/healthy/find-cancer-early/cancer-screening-guidelines/american-cancer-society-guidelines-forthe-early-detection-of-cancer.html.
37. Buys SS, et al. Effect of screening on ovarian cancer mortality: the Prostate, Lung, Colorectal and Ovarian (PLCO) cancer screening randomized controlled trial. JAMA. 2011;305(22):2295–303.
38. Jacobs IJ, et al. Ovarian cancer screening and mortality in the UK Collaborative Trial of Ovarian Cancer Screening (UKCTOCS): a randomised controlled trial. Lancet. 2016;387(10022):945–56.
39. Mallen A, et al. Surgical prevention strategies in ovarian cancer. Gynecol Oncol. 2018;151(1):166–75.
40. Berek JS, et al. Prophylactic and risk-reducing bilateral salpingo-oophorectomy: recommendations based on risk of ovarian cancer. Obstet Gynecol. 2010;116(3):733–43.
41. Parker WH, et al. Effect of bilateral oophorectomy on women's long-term health. Womens Health (Lond). 2009;5(5):565–76.
42. Atsma F, et al. Postmenopausal status and early menopause as independent risk factors for cardiovascular disease: a meta-analysis. Menopause. 2006;13(2):265–79.
43. Rocca WA, et al. Accelerated accumulation of multimorbidity after bilateral oophorectomy: a population-based Cohort Study. Mayo Clin Proc. 2016;91(11):1577–89.
44. Chen X, Guo T, Li B. Influence of prophylactic oophorectomy on mood and sexual function in women of menopausal transition or postmenopausal period. Arch Gynecol Obstet. 2013;288(5):1101–6.
45. Melton LJ 3rd, et al. Fracture risk after bilateral oophorectomy in elderly women. J Bone Miner Res. 2003;18(5):900–5.
46. Parker WH. Bilateral oophorectomy versus ovarian conservation: effects on long-term women's health. J Minim Invasive Gynecol. 2010;17(2):161–6.
47. Manchanda R, et al. Defining the risk threshold for risk reducing salpingo-oophorectomy for ovarian cancer prevention in low risk postmenopausal women. Gynecol Oncol. 2015;139(3):487–94.

Malignancy Risks Associated with Endometriosis: Clinical Aspects

24

Rasmus Schmaedecker and Uwe Andreas Ulrich

Contents

24.1 Introduction

Although endometriosis is generally regarded as a histologically benign condition [1, 2], by factors such as local invasion, tissue damage, neoangiogenesis, genomic instability, resistance to apoptosis, and elevation of CA-125 levels, it has been shown to share some characteristics with malignant tumors [3–6]. Overall, patients with endometriosis are not generally at higher risk to develop cancer [7, 8]. Yet, epidemiologic studies in endometriosis show an increased risk by 1.3- to 1.9-fold to develop ovarian cancer [7, 8]. Furthermore, other studies suggest endometriosis as a moderate risk factor to develop endometrial cancer, breast cancer, colorectal cancer, non-Hodgkin lymphoma as well as melanoma [9, 10]. With the non-genital carcinomas, however, the association to endometriosis remains unclear [7], which is why it is important to differentiate them from the carcinomas *arising* from

R. Schmaedecker (✉) · U. A. Ulrich
Department of Gynecology and Obstetrics, Martin Luther Krankenhaus, Berlin, Germany
e-mail: rasmus.schmaedecker@jsd.de

E. Oral (ed.), *Endometriosis and Adenomyosis*,
https://doi.org/10.1007/978-3-030-97236-3_24

endometriosis, most importantly ovarian cancer [7]. Clinical evidence suggests a transformation of endometriosis into malignant tissue through "atypical endometriosis" [11–13]. Some authors go as far as to call endometriosis a "precancerous lesion" [12] or "precursor lesion" [14, 15], although most scientific evidence does not back this theory [16, 17].

24.2 Background

Of all *endometriosis-associated malignancies* (EAMs), 80% are located in the ovary and 20% at extragonadal sites [18, 19]. Ongoing studies suggest an even higher rate of ovarian involvement with a rate of 90–100%. In general, endometriotic lesions may transform into cancer at any anatomic site that could potentially harbor that tissue (Fig. 24.1). The rectosigmoid colon and the rectovaginal septum are the most common sites of occurrence of extragonadal EAMs [20]. Apart from that, EAMs may arise in the parametrium, the gastrointestinal tract, the abdominal wall, umbilicus, pleura, and other organs [21]. Table 24.1 shows the location of extragonadal malignant tumors arising from endometriosis (adapted from *Ulrich* et al.) [20].

So clinically, the most relevant associated carcinoma to endometriosis seems to be ovarian cancer. *Sampson* suggested as early as 1925 that ovarian endometrial implants may give rise to an endometroid carcinoma of the ovary [22]. His definition of *endometriosis-associated ovarian carcinoma* (EAOC) stated three conditions [22]:

1. Evidence of endometriosis in close proximity to the tumor
2. Another source of invasion must be excluded
3. Presence of endometrial stroma should be clearly evident

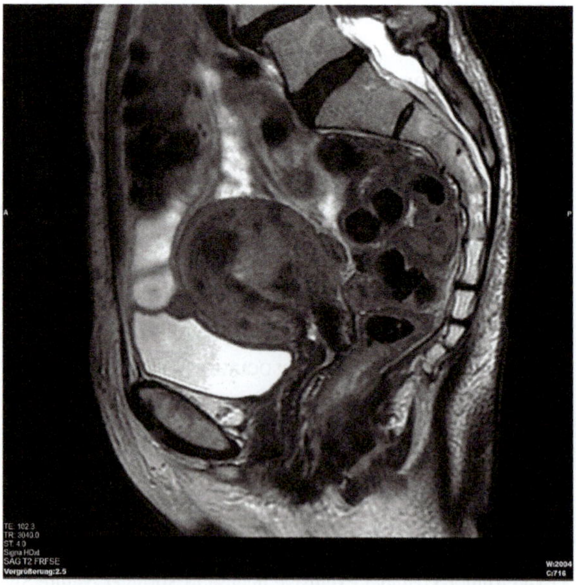

Fig. 24.1 A 79-year-old patient with endometriosis-associated intramural carcinosarcoma of the uterus (arising from adenomyosis) (Department of Radiology, Martin Luther Krankenhaus Berlin)

Table 24.1 Location of extragonadal EAM [20]

Location of extragonadal EAMs	Number of cases
Bowel	40 (78% in rectum and sigmoid colon)
Rectovaginal	18
Uterus (i.e., arising from adenomyosis)	12
Peritoneum	8
Broad ligament and parametrium	6
Urinary bladder	4
Vagina	3
Fallopian tube	2
Cervix	2
Others (umbilicus, pleura, vulva, omentum)	44
Total	139

Over time, another criterion became part of that definition [23]:

4. Histological proof of the transition from benign endometriosis to malignant change

This definition of the EAOC remains valid, even today. Histologically, EAOCs may also present as seromucinous borderline tumors, adenosarcomas, or endometrial stromal sarcomas, but most commonly they are of the clear-cell or endometrioid type [6, 19, 20, 24]. An association to the occurrence of mucinous and high-grade serous ovarian cancer has not been found [19, 25].

24.3 Clinic

24.3.1 Risk Factors

Various risk factors for the development of an EAM) have been identified. Hyperestrogenism, exogenous as well as endogenous (through obesity), administration of unopposed estrogens after hysterectomy and the use of tamoxifen are statistically significant risk factors for developing an EAM [17, 26, 27]. Furthermore, postmenopausal status and endometrioma size have been shown to be a risk factor for the development of ovarian cancer [28]. A size of 9 cm or larger has been identified as risk factor in one prospective cohort study [28]. Protective factors, on the other hand, seem to be hysterectomy, tubal ligation, childbearing, and oral hormonal contraceptive use [29, 30].

24.3.2 Diagnosis

The diagnosis of an EAOC can be quite challenging. Transvaginal ultrasonography by the experienced clinician is the essential clinical tool. The *International Ovarian Tumor Analysis* (IOTA) work group developed a practical guideline in 2010 to

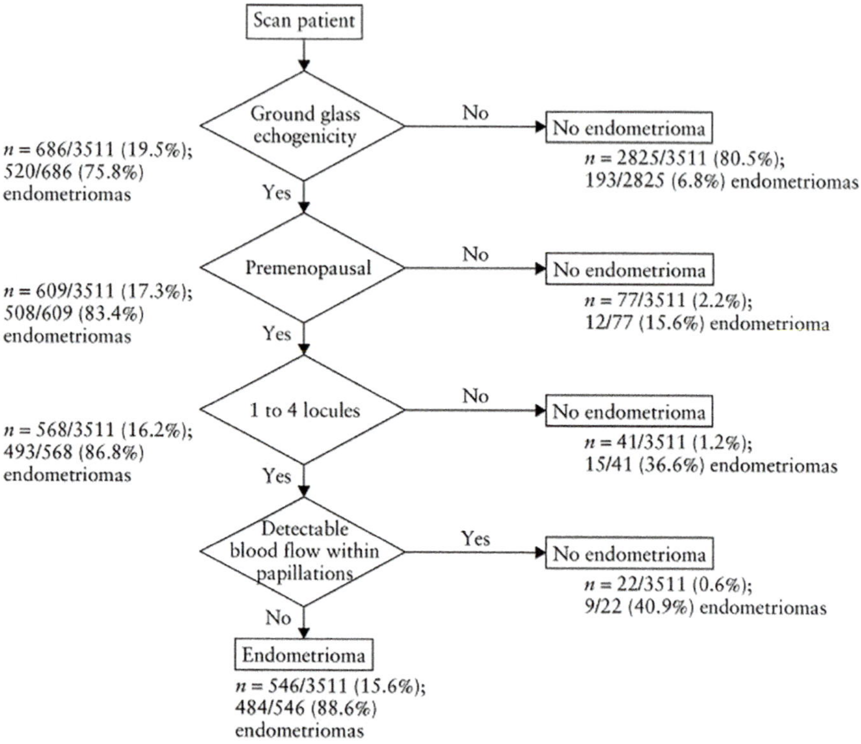

Fig. 24.2 Decision tree with consecutive conditions for predicting an endometrioma. Diamonds are decision nodes. Rectangles are prediction nodes [31]

detect endometrioma and differentiate it from malignant ovarian masses [31] (Fig. 24.2). Basically, they describe *"4 Rules of endometrioma"*

1. Premenopausal status
2. Ground-glass echogenicity of the cyst fluid
3. One to four locules
4. No solid parts

Ultimately, *pattern recognition* by the experienced oncological gynecologic clinician plays the most important part in diagnosing an EAOC. Nevertheless, we think these rules offer a solid guideline for clinical diagnostics.

24.3.3 Clinical Presentation

Patients with EAOC seem to present about 5.5 years earlier than high-grade serous ovarian cancer, with a mean age of 48.3 ± 10.8 years [32, 33]. Another study shows

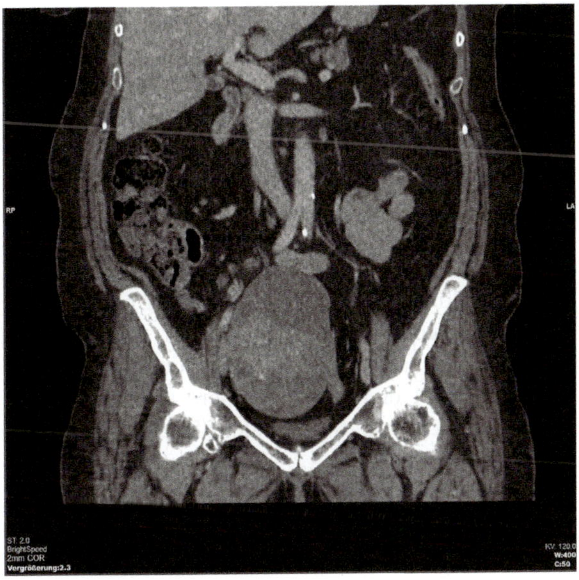

Fig. 24.3 A 66-year-old patient with endometriosis-associated endometrioid adenocarcinoma of the right ovary, history of abdominal hysterectomy (Department of Radiology, Martin Luther Krankenhaus Berlin)

patients with clear cell ovarian cancer being about 10 years younger than patients with non-endometriosis-associated ovarian cancers [34].

Also, endometrioid EAOC presents at lower stages (FIGO I or II) and with lower grading (grade 1 or 2) (Fig. 24.3) [35]. Clear cell EAOCs are, by definition, high-grade tumors (grade 3). On initial presentation, ascites is a rare clinical feature [36]. There is contradicting evidence regarding prognosis and overall survival. Some authors claim that EAOC is associated with a better prognosis [37], while other groups, after control for age, treatment, grade, and stage find no difference for overall survival between the EAOC and non-EAOC patient groups [35, 38, 39]. Ultimately, the better clinical outcomes of monophasic clear cell and endometrioid EAOC might be explained by more early-stage tumors rather than by the association with endometriosis [35, 36, 38, 40, 41].

24.3.4 Therapy

Oncologically sound removal with tumor-free margins is the treatment of choice for EAOC and extragonadal EAM [21]. In case of extragonadal EAMs, there is a lack of clear guidelines for classification and treatment of these tumors [21]. In the absence of clinical studies, treatment of EAOC is the same as treatment for ovarian cancer [42]. EAOC will be treated with postoperative chemotherapy according to the guideline for ovarian cancer [42], although there has been debate as to the efficacy in these patients due to EAOCs mostly being of low- or intermediate grade [43, 44]. In patients with endometrioid extragonadal EAM, especially involving the rectum or rectovaginal septum, complete surgical resection followed by adjuvant pelvic radiotherapy might be the better option [20, 43, 45].

24.3.5 Clinical Implications

The surgical concept of therapy for premenopausal patients with endometriosis should generally not be influenced by the slightly higher risk for ovarian cancer [7]. Some studies show a lower risk for developing ovarian cancer after oophorectomy plus resection of all lesions, while other studies show no benefit [46]. Nevertheless, good clinical diagnosis is crucial, and there are some important clinical implications of what we know about EAM and EAOC that should be taken into account when counseling patients. For example, patients with a history of endometriosis should, even after hysterectomy, not be treated with unopposed estrogens. A postmenopausal recurrence of symptoms or change in sonographic features of a known endometrioma should alert the physician for a possible EAM or EAOC. As there seems to be an association to Lynch syndrome, especially patients under 55 years with endometrioid or clear cell EAOC should be screened [7, 42, 47–49].

Note A similar article on the subject has been published by Prof. Ulrich in "Endometriosis – A Concise Practical Guide to Current Diagnosis and Treatment" (see Ref. 21).

References

1. Berkley KJ, Rapkin AJ, Papka RE. The pains of endometriosis. Science. 2005;308(5728):1587–9.
2. Kurman RJ, Hedrick Ellenson L, Ronnett BM, Blaustein A, editors. Blaustein's pathology oft he female genital tract: with 125 tables. 6th ed. New York: Springer; 2011.
3. Gazvani R, Templeton A. New considerations for the pathogenesis of endometriosis. Int J Gynaecol Obstet. 2002;76(2):117–26.
4. Horn LC, Hentschel B, Meinel A, Alexander H, Leo C. Cyclooxygenase-2 expression, Ki-67 labeling index, and perifocal neovascularization in endometriotic lesions. Ann Diagn Pathol. 2009;13(6):373–7.
5. Maiorana A, Cicerone C, Niceta M, Alio L. Evaluation of serum CA 125 levels in patients with pelvic pain related to endometriosis. Int J Biol Markers. 2007;22(3):200–2.
6. Schmidt D, Ulrich U. Endometrioseassoziierte Tumorerkrankungen des Ovars [Endometriosis-related ovarian tumors]. Pathologe. 2014;35(4):348–54.
7. Diagnosis and therapy of endometriosis. Guideline of the DGGG, SGGG and OEGGG (S2k-Level, AWMF Registry No. 045/015, August 2020). http://www.awmf.org/leitlinien/detail/ll/015-045.html
8. Somigliana E, Vigano P, Parazzini F, Stoppelli S, Giambattista E, Vercellini P. Association between endometriosis and cancer: a comprehensive review and a critical analysis of clinical and epidemiological evidence. Gynecol Oncol. 2006;101:331–41.
9. Melin A, Sparen P, Persson I, Bergqvist A. Endometriosis and the risk of cancer with special emphasis on ovarian cancer. Hum Reprod. 2006;21:1237–42.
10. Gandini S, Lazzeroni M, Peccatori FA, Bendinelli B, Saieva C, Palli D, Masala G, Caini S. The risk of extra-ovarian malignancies among women with endometriosis: a systematic literature review and meta-analysis. Crit Rev Oncol Hematol. 2019;134:72–81.

11. Ness RB. Endometriosis and ovarian cancer: thoughts on shared pathophysiology. Am J Obstet Gynecol. 2003;189(1):280–94.
12. Siufi Neto J, Kho RM, Siufi DF, Baracat EC, Anderson KS, Abrão MS. Cellular, histologic, and molecular changes associated with endometriosis and ovarian cancer. J Minim Invasive Gynecol. 2014;21(1):55–63.
13. Tanase Y, Furukawa N, Kobayashi H, Matsumoto T. Malignant transformation from endometriosis to atypical endometriosis and finally to endometrioid adenocarcinoma within 10 years. Case Rep Oncol. 2013;6(3):480–4.
14. del Carmen MG. Evidence for the relationship between endometriosis and epithelial ovarian cancer. Obstet Gynecol Surv. 2015;70(9):587–95.
15. Prowse AH, Manek S, Varma R, Liu J, Godwin AK, Maher ER, Tomlinson IP, Kennedy SH. Molecular genetic evidence that endometriosis is a precursor of ovarian cancer. Int J Cancer. 2006;119(3):556–62.
16. Fukunaga M, Nomura K, Ishikawa E, Ushigome S. Ovarian atypical endometriosis: its close association with malignant epithelial tumours. Histopathology. 1997;30(3):249–55.
17. Worley MJ, Welch WR, Berkowitz RS, Ng SW. Endometriosis-associated ovarian cancer: a review of pathogenesis. Int J Mol Sci. 2013;14(3):5367–79.
18. Heidemann LN, Hartwell D, Heidemann CH, Jochumsen KM. The relation between endometriosis and ovarian cancer – a review. Acta Obstet Gynecol Scand. 2014;93(1):20–31.
19. Kim HS, Kim TH, Chung HH, Song YS. Risk and prognosis of ovarian cancer in women with endometriosis: a meta-analysis. Br J Cancer. 2014;110(7):1878–90.
20. Ulrich U, Rhiem K, Kaminski M, Wardelmann E, Trog D, Valter M, Richter ON. Parametrial and rectovaginal adenocarcinoma arising from endometriosis. Int J Gynecol Cancer. 2005;15(6):1206–9.
21. Ulrich U, Schmidt D. Endometriosis associated malignant neoplasms. In: Alkatout I, Meinhold-Heerlein I, Keckstein J, Mettler L, editors. Endometriosis: a concise practical guide to current diagnosis and treatment. 1st ed. Tuttlingen: EndoPress; 2017. p. 367–73.
22. Sampson JA. Endometrial carcinoma of the ovary, arising in endometrial tissue in that organ. Arch Surg. 1925;10(1):1–72.
23. Scott RB. Malignant changes in endometriosis. Obstet Gynecol. 1953;2(3):283–9.
24. Vlahos NF, Kalampokas T, Fotiou S. Endometriosis and ovarian cancer: a review. Gynecol Endocrinol. 2010;26(3):213–9.
25. Pearce CL, Templeman C, Rossing MA, Lee A, Near AM, Webb PM, Nagle CM, Doherty JA, Cushing-Haugen KL, Wicklund KG, Chang-Claude J, Hein R, Lurie G, Wilkens LR, Carney ME, Goodman MT, Moysich K, Kjaer SK, Hogdall E, Jensen A, Goode EL, Fridley BL, Larson MC, Schildkraut JM, Palmieri RT, Cramer DW, Terry KL, Vitonis AF, Titus LJ, Ziogas A, Brewster W, Anton-Culver H, Gentry-Maharaj A, Ramus SJ, Anderson AR, Brueggmann D, Fasching PA, Gayther SA, Huntsman DG, Menon U, Ness RB, Pike MC, Risch H, Wu AH, Berchuck A, Ovarian Cancer Association Consortium. Association between endometriosis and risk of histological subtypes of ovarian cancer: a pooled analysis of case-control studies. Lancet Oncol. 2012;13(4):385–94.
26. McCluggage WG, Bryson C, Lamki H, Boyle DD. Benign, borderline, and malignant endometrioid neoplasia arising in endometriosis in association with tamoxifen therapy. Int J Gynecol Pathol. 2000;19(3):276–9.
27. Zanetta GM, Webb MJ, Li H, Keeney GL. Hyperestrogenism: a relevant risk factor for the development of cancer from endometriosis. Gynecol Oncol. 2000;79(1):18–22.
28. Kobayashi H, Sumimoto K, Kitanaka T, Yamada Y, Sado T, Sakata M, Yoshida S, Kawaguchi R, Kanayama S, Shigetomi H, Haruta S, Tsuji Y, Ueda S, Terao T. Ovarian endometrioma–risks factors of ovarian cancer development. Eur J Obstet Gynecol Reprod Biol. 2008;138(2):187–93.
29. Merritt MA, De Pari M, Vitonis AF, Titus LJ, Cramer DW, Terry KL. Reproductive characteristics in relation to ovarian cancer risk by histologic pathways. Hum Reprod. 2013;28(5):1406–17.

30. Modugno F, Ness RB, Allen GO, Schildkraut JM, Davis FG, Goodman MT. Oral contraceptive use, reproductive history, and risk of epithelial ovarian cancer in women with and without endometriosis. Am J Obstet Gynecol. 2004;191(3):733–40.
31. Van Holsbeke C, Van Calster B, Guerriero S, Savelli L, Paladini D, Lissoni AA, Czekierdowski A, Fischerova D, Zhang J, Mestdagh G, Testa AC, Bourne T, Valentin L, Timmerman D. Endometriomas: their ultrasound characteristics. Ultrasound Obstet Gynecol. 2010;35(6):730–40.
32. Machado-Linde F, Sánchez-Ferrer ML, Cascales P, Torroba A, Orozco R, Silva Sánchez Y, Nieto A, Fiol G. Prevalence of endometriosis in epithelial ovarian cancer. Analysis of the associated clinical features and study on molecular mechanisms involved in the possible causality. Eur J Gynaecol Oncol. 2015;36(1):21–4.
33. Aris A. Endometriosis-associated ovarian cancer: a ten-year cohort study of women living in the Estrie region of Quebec, Canada. J Ovarian Res. 2010;19(3):2.
34. Orezzoli JP, Russell AH, Oliva E, Del Carmen MG, Eichhorn J, Fuller AF. Prognostic implication of endometriosis in clear cell carcinoma of the ovary. Gynecol Oncol. 2008;110(3):336–44.
35. Davis M, Rauh-Hain JA, Andrade C, Boruta DM 2nd, Schorge JO, Horowitz NS, May T, del Carmen MG. Comparison of clinical outcomes of patients with clear cell and endometrioid ovarian cancer associated with endometriosis to papillary serous carcinoma of the ovary. Gynecol Oncol. 2014;132(3):760–6.
36. Scarfone G, Bergamini A, Noli S, Villa A, Cipriani S, Taccagni G, Vigano' P, Candiani M, Parazzini F, Mangili G. Characteristics of clear cell ovarian cancer arising from endometriosis: a two center cohort study. Gynecol Oncol. 2014;133(3):480–4.
37. Acién P, Velasco I, Acién M, Capello C, Vela P. Epithelial ovarian cancers and endometriosis. Gynecol Obstet Investig. 2015;79(2):126–35.
38. Kumar S, Munkarah A, Arabi H, Bandyopadhyay S, Semaan A, Hayek K, Garg G, Morris R, Ali-Fehmi R. Prognostic analysis of ovarian cancer associated with endometriosis. Am J Obstet Gynecol. 2011;204(1):63.e1–7.
39. Melin A, Lundholm C, Malki N, Swahn ML, Sparen P, Bergqvist A. Endometriosis as a prognostic factor for cancer survival. Int J Cancer. 2011;129(4):948–55.
40. Cuff J, Longacre TA. Endometriosis does not confer improved prognosis in ovarian carcinoma of uniform cell type. Am J Surg Pathol. 2012;36(5):688–95.
41. Denschlag D, Manns M, Woll J, Ulrich U. Endometriose und ovarielle malignome. Frauenarzt. 2013;54:570–2.
42. Wagner U, Harter P, Hilpert F, Mahner S, Reuß A, du Bois A, Petru E, Meier W, Ortner P, König K, Lindel K, Grab D, Piso P, Ortmann O, Runnebaum I, Pfisterer J, Lüftner D, Frickhofen N, Grünwald F, Maier BO, Diebold J, Hauptmann S, Kommoss F, Emons G, Radeleff B, Gebhardt M, Arnold N, Calaminus G, Weisse I, Weis J, Sehouli J, Fink D, Burges A, Hasenburg A, Eggert C. S3-guideline on diagnostics, therapy and follow-up of malignant ovarian tumours: short version 1.0 – AWMF registration number: 032/035OL, June 2013. Geburtshilfe Frauenheilkd. 2013;73(9):874–89.
43. Heaps JM, Nieberg RK, Berek JS. Malignant neoplasms arising in endometriosis. Obstet Gynecol. 1990;75(6):1023–8.
44. Ulrich U, Wunschel A, Reichert VM, Darb-Esfahani S, Denschlag D, Horn L, et al. Endometriose-assoziierte maligne Tumoren. Gynakologe. 2015;48(3):221–7.
45. Erzen M, Rakar S, Klancnik B, Syrjänen K. Endometriosis-associated ovarian carcinoma (EAOC): an entity distinct from other ovarian carcinomas as suggested by a nested case-control study. Gynecol Oncol. 2001;83(1):100–8.
46. Melin AS, Lundholm C, Malki N, Swahn ML, Sparen P, Bergqvist A. Hormonal and surgical treatments for endometriosis and risk of epithelial ovarian cancer. Acta Obstet Gynecol Scand. 2013;92:546–54.
47. Fadare O, Parkash V. Pathology of endometrioid and clear cell carcinoma of the ovary. Surg Pathol Clin. 2019;12:529–64.

48. Gras E, Catasus L, Arguelles R, Moreno-Bueno G, Palacios J, Gamallo C, Matias-Guiu X, Prat J. Microsatellite instability, MLH-1 promoter hypermethylation, and frameshift mutations at coding mononucleotide repeat microsatellites in ovarian tumors. Cancer. 2001;92:2829–36.
49. Vierkoetter KR, Ayabe AR, VanDrunen M, Ahn HJ, Shimizu DM, Terada KY. Lynch syndrome in patients with clear cell and endometrioid cancers of the ovary. Gynecol Oncol. 2014;135:81–4.

Psychological Considerations in Endometriosis

25

Valentina Lucia La Rosa, Elena Commodari, and Salvatore Giovanni Vitale

Contents

25.1 Introduction

The chronic nature of endometriosis, together with its potential impact on fertility and relationships and the problematic treatment and treatment experiences, ensure that this disease has a significant impact on the quality of life and the psychological and social functioning of women affected [1, 2]. In this sense, in recent years, the scientific literature on the subject has progressively focused on the importance of assessing the quality of life of women with endometriosis. The symptoms can cause a progressive impairment of the woman's ability to carry out particular daily activities and, consequently, a worsening of the perceived state of health and the general

V. L. La Rosa (✉) · E. Commodari
Department of Educational Sciences, University of Catania, Catania, Italy
e-mail: valarosa@unict.it

S. G. Vitale
Obstetrics and Gynecology Unit, Department of General Surgery and Medical Surgical Specialties, University of Catania, Catania, Italy

E. Oral (ed.), *Endometriosis and Adenomyosis*,
https://doi.org/10.1007/978-3-030-97236-3_25

sense of well-being. The impact of these symptoms on patients' quality of life has been partially investigated and therefore needs further clinical studies and research [1, 3, 4].

Furthermore, endometriosis is associated with high costs, both from an economic and social point of view. In this respect, a recent study by Simoens et al. [5] has shown that endometriosis is associated with high direct and indirect costs, comparable to those of major chronic diseases globally, such as diabetes. In addition, endometriosis disorders substantially interfere with the working behavior of women, leading in many cases to job losses. Consequently, it is estimated that the indirect costs of endometriosis linked to this loss of productivity are even twice as high as the health costs associated with the clinical management of the disease [1].

In addition, sexuality is a crucial issue for women with endometriosis who should be adequately cared for in the clinical management of the disorder [6]. Indeed, since endometriosis affects about 5–10% of women of reproductive age, it can be estimated that about 2–4% of sexually active women may suffer from sexual dysfunction caused by endometriosis itself [7–9].

Therefore, in the light of these considerations, it is essential not to overlook the effects of endometriosis on the general quality of life, sexuality, and psychological well-being of women affected. This chapter aims to provide a general overview of the psychological and social impact of the disease and the effects of the different therapeutic options on the quality of life and general well-being of patients.

25.2 Endometriosis and Quality of Life

Endometriosis is now widely recognized to impact women's quality of life in various ways [10, 11]. In particular, endometriosis has been shown to significantly interfere with the quality of life due to the stress related to infertility and pain, adversely affecting social, sexual, and professional aspects. The disorder is also associated with depression, anxiety, and high stress levels [12–14].

It is important to stress that the endometriosis stage does not necessarily correspond with the severity of the symptoms. Consequently, a woman with endometriosis may experience a greater or lesser degree of symptomatology, which is not always related to the extent or severity of the disease. In addition, a significant proportion of women are in many cases asymptomatic [15]. For this reason, endometriosis is often misdiagnosed or detected late, and this inevitably has repercussions on stress levels and the overall quality of life of women [11, 16].

The most common clinical signs of endometriosis include menstrual irregularities, chronic pelvic pain, dysmenorrhea, dyspareunia, and infertility [17]. Such symptoms can often substantially affect the overall functioning and quality of life of patients [13, 18].

In recent years, several studies have been conducted to assess the quality of life outcomes in patients with endometriosis [1, 19–21] and have amply demonstrated that endometriosis is accompanied by a significant reduction in quality of life [1, 13].

In particular, according to data from the study by Simoens et al. [5], a small but not negligible percentage of women with endometriosis consider their current state of health "worse than death".

Women with endometriosis report worse scores in different domains of quality of life. Studies conducted through the SF-36 and the SF-12 show significant differences in the areas of physical activity, physical role and health, physical pain, social and emotional functioning, vitality, and mental health [22].

In particular, the pain has a very destructive impact on patients' lives [20, 23]. Endometriosis is, in fact, one of the most frequent causes of chronic pelvic pain [12, 19]. Women with endometriosis may suffer from a wide range of pelvic pain that includes dysmenorrhea, dyspareunia, chronic pelvic pain, pain during ovulation, dyschezia, and dysuria [24, 25]. As previously noted, pain seems to be independent of endometriosis, so women with mild endometriosis may experience intense pelvic pain, while women with more severe endometriosis may suffer less acute or chronic pain. This data suggests that psychological factors may influence the experience of pain in women with endometriosis [12, 26].

Many authors report a negative correlation between pain and quality of life. Women suffering from pelvic pain report high levels of anxiety and depression, loss of working capacity, and limitations in social activities [12, 20]. Patients with endometriosis also report significantly limited performance in all physical activities, and pain symptoms are significantly related to both the physical and mental components of quality of life [1]. Between 16% [5] and 61% [27] of women experience difficulties concerning mobility, daily activities, and self-care. It has also been found that sleep quality is adversely affected by endometriosis symptoms [19].

Domestic activities are negatively affected by endometriosis. A significant proportion of women report that the symptoms negatively affect the quality of family relationships and child care [1, 10, 11].

Energy and vitality levels are also compromised in women with endometriosis [28]. Fourquet et al. [27] show that 27% of women with endometriosis report low energy levels. Similarly, Petrelluzzi et al. observe low scores in the vitality domain of SF-36 in a sample of patients with endometriosis. Pain also has a strong negative impact on the performance of sports and physical exercise [29].

Another critical dimension of the general quality of life, negatively affected by this disorder, is social relations [11]. Petrelluzzi et al. showed lower scores in social functioning of women with endometriosis and chronic pelvic pain of moderate grade compared to a control group of women not affected by the disease [29]. Similarly, according to data reported by Gilmour et al. [30] and Jones et al. [28], women with endometriosis have a significant reduction in social activities due to pain, fatigue and the need to use toilets frequently. Women also feel less able to socialize due to concerns about their condition, resulting in a reduction in confidence and self-esteem levels [28].

Finally, only a few studies in the literature have deepened the impact of endometriosis on the study and training paths of affected women [1]. In this regard, the results are quite controversial: indeed, while some authors report a significant percentage of interruption of studies due to the discomfort caused by endometriosis symptoms [30, 31], others report only a few cases of women in which endometriosis has led to negative consequences as regards education and studies [10].

According to Fourquet et al. [27], women who have endometriosis lose on average 7.4 working hours per week and are absent from work on average for 19 days a year. In addition, the symptoms of endometriosis, particularly pain, have a significant negative impact on productivity levels, leading to a reduction in the ability to perform work tasks ranging between 23% and 66% [27]. Precisely, menstrual pain, disabling pain, and chronic pelvic pain predict more unsatisfactory performance at work. In addition, women report a reduction in the quality of their work and a loss in efficiency levels of around 64% [27]. For these reasons, endometriosis is a pathology with high economic and social costs: in fact, the economic costs linked to the loss of productivity due to endometriosis can be quantified in EUR 6298 per woman [5, 19].

An important aspect to consider is the difficulty of women in informing employers of their status [1]. On one hand, the woman considers it is a private condition, on the other, it is important to be able to receive support from the employer. Women can decide not to communicate their diagnosis for various reasons, including fear of possible consequences or difficulty in talking about a disorder affecting the intimate sphere of a woman in the case of a male employer [30].

25.3 Psychological and Emotional Impact of Endometriosis

The scientific literature on this topic has confirmed a significant association between endometriosis and psychological and emotional disorders [12].

Pope et al. [32, 33] pointed out that endometriosis is related to a wide range of psychopathological disorders, particularly depression, anxiety, psychosocial stress and poor quality of life. According to the most recent literature, depression and anxiety are the disorders most frequently associated with endometriosis [12, 34].

In this regard, Low et al. [35] considered the possibility of identifying a specific psychological profile of women with endometriosis compared to those suffering from other gynecological diseases. Based on the results of this study, patients with endometriosis report higher scores of psychoticism, introversion and anxiety than those of women suffering from other gynecological disorders [35].

In total agreement with these data, Sepulcri Rde and Amaral [36] evaluated depressive symptoms, anxiety, and quality of life in 104 women diagnosed with pelvic endometriosis. The authors used a battery of psychometric tests to evaluate anxiety-depressive symptoms and the WHOQOL-BREF to assess the quality of life. In the study, 86.5% participants had depressive symptoms, and 87.5% had anxiety, and, above all, psychiatric symptoms were not associated with the endometriosis stage [36]. In this study, age was positively correlated with depressive symptoms, while there was no association between age and anxious symptoms [36]. However, other authors found that only 29% of women with endometriosis showed moderate to severe anxiety symptoms, while depression was present in 14.5% of cases [37].

These apparently contradictory results may be due to the different methodologies used to identify psychiatric symptoms or to errors in selecting the study sample (in particular, the inclusion of other comorbidities that may seriously affect mental health) [12]. Furthermore, as women with endometriosis report high levels of alexithymia, which is a severe difficulty in identifying and describing emotions, this may make it further difficult to detect other psychiatric comorbidities [34].

In short, the literature confirms a significant incidence of anxiety, depression, and psychopathological symptoms among women with endometriosis. These comorbidities could affect the severity of the symptoms and the health-related quality of life of women affected by this disorder [4, 13, 38].

As for evaluating the possible anxiety and depressive symptoms related to endometriosis, several standardized psychometric tools are available in the literature for a correct diagnosis of the patient.

25.4 Endometriosis and Sexuality

Dyspareunia is undoubtedly the most frequent sexual dysfunction among women with endometriosis [39, 40], especially in the most severe cases, such as deep infiltrating endometriosis (DIE) [41–43]. It is generally associated with deep infiltration of the cardinal and uterosacral ligaments, the Douglas cavity, the anterior rectal wall and the posterior vaginal fornix [41]. Several studies have shown that dyspareunia is related, in particular, to endometriotic lesions that infiltrate the uterus-sacral ligaments. It is known that the uterus-sacral ligaments contain a considerable amount of nerve fibers; as a result, the tension at the level of these ligaments (infiltrated by endometriosis) during sexual intercourse can determine the triggering of painful symptoms [44].

Therefore, sexual activity is severely impaired among women with DIE. Ferrero et al. [44] have shown that women with DIE of uterosacral ligaments have the most severe impairments of sexual function. In addition, Montanari et al. [45] have clearly shown that women with DIE have a significant impairment of sexual function, related to a reduction in overall well-being levels. In addition, the presence of dyspareunia and endometriosis vaginal lesions appears to play an essential role in the onset of sexual dysfunction [45].

More specifically, the association between DIE and dyspareunia is related to a lower frequency of sexual intercourse and/or to their interruption and a reduced sexual functioning, feelings of fear before or during sexual intercourse, and feelings of guilt toward the partner [39, 46]. In addition, women with DIE frequently suffer from significant impairments of their female identity and body image as well as alexithymia (defined as the difficulty in recognizing and processing emotions). These problems may further exacerbate the severity of sexual dysfunction in women with endometriosis [41].

It is important to consider some fundamental elements about the effects of pain on the sexual function of women with endometriosis. First, other clinical conditions such as interstitial cystitis may overlap endometriosis (10–50% of cases), making sexual activity more painful [47, 48]. In addition, endometriosis lesions are associated with central and peripheral hyperalgesia, probably caused by local neuroinflammation, neuroangiogenesis, and sensory and autonomic fiber dysregulation. Finally, dyspareunia in women with endometriosis is often associated with chronic pelvic pain [6].

Although the literature available on the topic has focused more on dyspareunia and chronic pelvic pain in patients with endometriosis, it is also important to evaluate the overall sexual function of the woman and the quality of the relationship with the sexual partner.

The results of studies investigating the sexual function of women with endometriosis are available. The first study of this type is that by Waller and Shaw in 1995, which shows an increase in sexual avoidance in a group of 17 patients with mild or moderate endometriosis [49]. The avoidance of sexuality is also confirmed by other studies according to which women suffering from endometriosis tend to avoid or reduce sexual intercourse [39, 46, 50].

Ferrero et al. [44] assessed the sexual well-being of a cohort of patients suffering from sexual dysfunction caused by various genital disorders. This study shows that patients with deep endometriosis infiltrating the uterosacral ligaments have lower scores for overall sexual satisfaction than patients with peritoneal endometriosis and those not affected by the disease [44].

Vercellini et al. [51] also highlight the complexity of the relationship between endometriosis, pain, and sexual function. In particular, patients with rectovaginal endometriosis had a three times greater risk of being sexually dissatisfied or experiencing little or no sexual pleasure. In addition, the risk of engaging in limited or absent sexual activities and reduced ability to reach orgasm was about twice as high as women not suffering from endometriosis [51].

Other studies confirm the high prevalence of sexual dysfunction in women with endometriosis with a significant correlation between the stage of the disorder, painful symptoms and score specific questionnaires [52, 53].

Based on the available data, although still relatively limited, it is, therefore, possible to conclude that endometriosis hurts all domains of sexual function (desire/arousal, orgasm, satisfaction, and pain) and is associated with sexual disorders in 70–75% of patients, especially those with the most severe or chronic forms of endometriosis [6]. According to the cycle of sexual response based on motivation and incentives, the repeated painful sexual experiences and the absence of reward (negative outcome) probably cause a change in the sexual response from the dimension of motivation/arousal to that of hypervigilance and from the desire to fear and avoidance, thus causing significant sexual discomfort in patients with endometriosis [37, 54].

Although dyspareunia is the first step in developing sexual dysfunction, multiple variables contribute to influencing the sexuality of the woman and, consequently, the relationship with the partner. Some of these factors are related to the course and evolution of the disease toward more advanced stages with the consequent worsening of painful symptoms and chronic pelvic pain. Others are linked to the more specific characteristics of endometriosis, including frequent association with fertility problems, delayed diagnosis and possible recurrence after treatment [6].

At present, the scientific literature available on the topic has not exhaustively explored the impact on the quality of the relationship with the partner and the impact of the disease on the sexual function of the partner.

It has long been widely underlined that dyspareunia, comorbidity with other female sexual dysfunctions, and fertility problems (or concerns about possible infertility) have a strong destructive impact on the relationship with the partner as well as on his sexual function, especially in younger couples [11]. In fact, there is no doubt that the sexual discomfort of one inevitably affects the partner. However, it is expected that only one member of the couple requires a specialist consultation to recover an optimal quality of sex life. In the specific case of endometriosis, the woman generally requires help, and the gynecologists need to deal with both partners because of issues involving the intimate and sexual sphere.

Several international studies on patients with endometriosis have shown a significant reduction in the quality of communication between partners regarding sexuality [39, 44, 51]. In this regard, the results of the WERF EndoCost study report that 67% of the women involved reported significant problems with the partner due to endometriosis and that 19% of women with endometriosis considered the disease as a cause of the end of the relationship with the partner [55]. The study by Fagervold et al. [10] also confirms the same trend: in particular, according to the results of this study, 15% of patients with endometriosis, over 15 years, has had severe problems in their relationship with their partners due to the disorder while 7.7% of women have ended their relationship due to endometriosis symptoms [19].

Generally, the end of a relationship with the partner and divorce is mainly linked to the progressive social and relational closure determined by the discomfort created by the symptoms and the poor emotional support from the partner that the woman experiences [6].

As previously shown, many women avoid or interrupt sexual intercourse when it becomes too painful. In addition, some women experience pain even long after sexual intercourse [46, 56]. For this reason, the woman tends to experience feelings of guilt concerning her partner for the avoidance of sexual intercourse and feels unease with her own female identity and body image [41, 50, 53].

More specifically, younger women who are not engaged in stable relationships live the relationship with their partner with more significant discomfort and suffering [11, 56]. On the contrary, women who have more stable and lasting relationships tend to focus on other aspects of their relationship with their partners. In particular, these women tend to attribute relatively minor importance to an active sex life with their partner compared with other aspects of the relationship, including communication and sharing common goals and projects. This trend, however, varies according to the age of the woman and the length of the relationship [11, 56].

Women with endometriosis usually judge the partner as emotionally supportive, but it is also important to consider the impact the symptoms have on the emotional and sexual functioning of the man when the couple is diagnosed with endometriosis [6].

In this regard, the available data are still relatively limited. Most studies have focused on the experience of women with endometriosis, while the experience of their partners is almost absent from the literature on the subject. However, it is possible to find some exceptions that provide us with interesting data to consider. A study by Fernandez et al. [57] explored the experiences of 16 men, partners of women with endometriosis, using as a reference model that of the five stages of grief developed by the Swiss psychiatrist Elisabeth Kübler Ross. The results of this study show that the emotional responses of these men to their partners' disorders are entirely comparable to a process of grief, including, specifically, reactions of shock and denial, anger, anxiety, isolation and impotence, deflection of mood tone, and finally also acceptance and growth of relationship [57].

Similar results are reported in a study by Strzempko Butt and Chesla [58] on 13 couples in which the woman presents a diagnosis of endometriosis. The authors highlight a significant impact of endometriosis symptoms on sexuality and intimate relationships as well as on the daily life of the couple [58].

Although according to recent studies, the sexual function of the partner is not adversely affected by the presence of endometriosis [59], it is always important to take into account the severity of the pathology and the presence or absence of painful symptoms.

To confirm this, other studies show that male partners of women with induced vestibulodynia suffer from the consequences of partner pain, developing significant psychological discomfort, increased prevalence of sexual difficulties (e.g., erectile dysfunction), and a decrease in the degree of sexual satisfaction [60–62]. Therefore, it can be assumed that the quality of the relationship, the psychosocial functioning of man, and the male response to pain are related to painful symptoms, the sexual functioning, and the emotional and cognitive processing of pain by the woman [6].

In the specific case of endometriosis, it is important to remember that the ESHRE guidelines on the management of women with endometriosis stress the need to explore the psychosocial repercussions of the disorder on both the patient and her partner [63]. In this regard, the ENDOPART study conducted a qualitative analysis on the impact of endometriosis on the well-being of women, men and couples [64]. This study shows that the experiences of endometriosis patients' partners are often overlooked and not taken into account. Therefore, it is essential to recognize more the impact that this disease has on the male partner and implement further support and help for the couple [64].

Finally, we must not forget the fundamental importance that the effects of endometriosis on fertility take on within the couple. It is estimated that about 50% of women with infertility problems have endometriosis [38, 65]. As the literature on the topic has extensively documented, the experience of infertility has a significant impact on the psychological well-being of the woman and partner, and it is frequent to encounter problems such as anxiety, depression, low self-esteem, frustration, emotional stress and relational difficulties within the couple [66, 67]. In addition, psychological factors may affect the success of medically assisted procreation techniques, and the failure of infertility therapies may further impair the psychological state of the couple [68–70].

In the specific case of women with endometriosis, it is common for some of them to bear the pain experienced during intercourse because the desire for a pregnancy is a priority. For these women, the most critical consequence of endometriosis is the actual or perceived impact on their fertility [11].

In this case, the anxiety and stress related to difficulties in conceiving are aggravated by the diagnosis of endometriosis and significantly affect the relationship [65]. As a result, sexual self-esteem is impaired, and the couple perceives the failure to meet social and cultural expectations related to procreation [6].

Therefore, it is essential to provide an integrated treatment that focuses not only on the sexuality of women with endometriosis but also on the partner. The discomfort of one of the partners has essential effects on the sexuality of the other in a perspective of complementarity [71].

In conclusion, assessing the sexuality of the couple, the expectations and experiences of both partners, as well as the quality of the relationship of the couple, is of considerable help to the specialist in order to propose targeted diagnostic and therapeutic paths that suited to the needs of the individual couple [71].

25.5 Endometriosis Treatments and Quality of Life Assessment

The treatment of endometriosis can be complex and, in choosing the most suitable treatment for the individual patient, it is crucial to consider several factors such as side effects, the anatomical type of endometriosis, the role of any previous surgery, infertility, and desire for procreation [24, 63].

In particular, the primary purpose of the treatments should be pain control, improvement of quality of life, prevention of recurrence of disease, preservation of fertility, and reduction of anatomical damage [38, 72].

In this scenario, the assessment of the quality of life and psychological outcomes in patients undergoing different types of endometriosis treatment is important to identify the most effective therapeutic option for each patient, thus reducing the impact of the disease on women's well-being [12].

Surgery has always played a central role in treating endometriosis and was the primary approach to this disease in the past [24]. However, although surgery plays an important role, especially in the most severe cases, good results have been obtained in analgesic control also through medical therapy, which uses drugs with different actions (analgesics, estroprogestins, GnRH analogues, androgens, aromatase inhibitors) [63].

The effects of medical therapy on the quality of life of patients with endometriosis have been evaluated in the context of pharmacological treatments that include GnRH agonists (nafarelin, goserelin, and leuprolide), anastrozole, medroxyprogesterone, levonorgestrel, GnRH agonists plus estrogen and progestin, and chorionic gonadotropin [21]. However, the choice of the most appropriate hormonal therapy depends on several factors such as therapeutic efficacy, tolerability, the cost of the drug, the experience of the doctor, and the compliance of the patient [63]. In particular, although GnRH agonists are effective in reducing endometriosis symptoms, they are often associated with anxiety and depression during treatment [6]. In general, pharmacological therapies significantly improve psychological functioning, pain, vitality, physical functioning, and general health [21].

A prospective, randomized, double-blind study by Bergqvist and Theorell [73] evaluated painful symptoms and quality of life of women with endometriosis treated with naphthalene or medroxyprogesterone acetate for 6 months. Patients were also followed for a further 6 months after the end of treatment. The study results showed that, at the end of the follow-up, both treatments had improved anxiety-depressive symptoms and quality of life scores. In particular, the authors highlighted significant improvements in leisure, sex life, and domestic activities following treatment [73].

Another interesting study by Zupi et al. [74] assessed the benefits of combined therapy with GnRH agonists, estrogen and progesterone. In particular, women undergoing leuprolide acetate therapy combined with estrogen and progesterone reported significant improvements in the overall well-being ratios assessed through SF-36. In addition, compared to patients treated only with leuprolide acetate or estroprogestin, patients in combined therapy have achieved significantly better scores in the vitality domain of SF-36. Finally, treatment with leuprolide acetate combined with estroprogestins effectively improves physical function and painful symptoms compared to therapy with estroprogestins only [74].

Intrauterine levonorgestrel-releasing systems and human chorionic gonadotropin have been shown to effectively reduce pain levels in patients with endometriosis. In this regard, a study by Petta et al. [75] assessed the impact of the use of an intrauterine levonorgestrel-releasing system and the GnRH agonist on quality of life, suggesting that both therapies are associated with a significant reduction in visual-analogue scale (VAS) for pain as well as an overall improvement in the psychological well-being of patients. Huber et al. [76] have demonstrated the benefits of using chorionic gonadotropin to reduce painful endometriosis symptoms.

Surgery is the primary treatment for the most severe forms of endometriosis, such as deep infiltrative endometriosis (DIE) [77]. In the surgical treatment of endometriosis, there is a tendency to modulate the radicality of the treatment based on the desire for procreation and the future quality of life of the patient [12]. To date, the data available in the literature on quality of life and levels of anxiety and depression in women undergoing surgery for endometriosis treatment are still rather limited. Specifically, the types of surgery considered by these studies include laparoscopic laser treatment with carbon dioxide, radical resection of rectovaginal endometriosis, laparoscopic radical excision with or without resection of the uterosacral ligament and hysterectomy. Overall, surgery effectively improves the psychological functioning, pain, physical function, and general well-being of patients with endometriosis [21]. However, these treatments may be associated with adverse events, limiting their application in some patients.

A review of Deguara et al. [78] pointed out that laparoscopic surgery is associated with a more significant improvement in quality of life and emotional wellbeing than medical therapies.

A prospective cohort study by Van den Broeck et al. [79] assessed the levels of depression, the quality of the relationship, and the sexual functioning of 203 women undergoing laparoscopic surgery for moderate or severe endometriosis. The results showed that radical endometriosis surgery significantly improves patients' depression levels and sexual functioning [79].

Another interesting study by Low and colleagues [80] assessed the psychological functioning and perceived pain levels in a group of 37 women diagnosed with endometriosis and subjected to laparoscopic laser treatment with carbon dioxide. The authors pointed out that surgery resulted in a significant improvement in the levels of pain experienced, state and tract anxiety, and psychiatric comorbidity [80].

Vercellini et al. [81] have taken into account the psychological and quality of life outcomes in patients with endometriosis undergoing laparoscopic surgery with or without resection of the uterosacral ligament, highlighting a significant improvement in all quality of life domains assessed through SF-36, except for physical and emotional functioning in the group of women undergoing uterosacral ligament resection and perception of general well-being, vitality, and mental health in the group undergoing conservative surgery. In both groups, there was also a significant improvement in anxiety and depression levels as well as sexual functioning [81].

Regarding hysterectomy, an important international study that evaluated the quality of life of women with endometriosis undergoing this type of surgery is the Maine Women's Health Study [82]. The quality of life of the women involved in this study was evaluated through three indices: Mental Health Index, General Health Index, and Activity Index. For all three indices, the overall score is between 0 and 100, with higher scores corresponding to a better quality of life outcomes [82]. It is interesting to note that patients undergoing hysterectomy have significantly lower scores in Mental Health Index and General Health Index. At 6 months and 1 year after hysterectomy, all indices showed a significant increase compared to pre-surgery [82].

25.6 Effects of Endometriosis Treatments on Sexual Function

In recent years, research has increasingly focused on the impact of different therapeutic options for endometriosis on the sexual function of women. As noted above, the primary objective of endometriosis treatment is to reduce the intensity of symptoms (in particular pain) and improve the quality of life of the patient [6]. One possible option is pharmacological treatment, which seems to have a limited efficacy regarding the control of dyspareunia and the improvement of sexual function [9, 41]. Medical therapy for endometriosis is primarily based on hormonal contraceptives, progestins, danazol, GnRH agonists and antagonists, and aromatase inhibitors. The aim is to control the pain associated with endometriosis and to prevent any relapses [63]. Pharmacological and hormonal treatments, besides acting on the nociceptive processes at the level of the central and peripheral nervous system, also affect the brain areas involved in the sexual response (desire, arousal, libido), emotional and behavioral changes (mood, anxiety, fear), and peripheral genital response to sexual stimuli [6].

At present, no literature data on the effectiveness of GnRH analogues in improving the sexual function of women with endometriosis are available. Other studies, however, show an effective reduction in deep dyspareunia but at the same time a significant decline in libido and vaginal lubrication [6].

Combined hormonal contraceptives (COCs) and progestins effectively reduce the painful symptoms associated with endometriosis and improve the quality of life and sexual function, as widely demonstrated by several studies conducted on this topic [83, 84].

Since 2000, several studies have assessed the sexual function of women with endometriosis treated with estroprogestin. In particular, the studies related to the use of dienogest, a new progestin specifically proposed in the treatment of endometriosis, are particularly interesting. Morotti et al. [85] evaluated the sexual function of a group of women with rectovaginal endometriosis and persistent painful symptoms after 6 months of treatment with dienogest. Patients showed, overall, increased lubrication, decreased pain, and an overall improvement in sexual functioning. Treatment with Dienogest was also generally well tolerated, with no reported serious side effects [85]. These results are also confirmed by Vercellini et al. [86] and Caruso et al. [87, 88]. The first compared the sexual functioning of 90 patients with endometriosis treated with norethindrone acetate and 90 treated with dienogest. After 6 months of therapy, all participants reported substantial improvements in sexual function but no significant differences between the two patient groups [86]. The second study assessed the quality of life and sexual functioning of 54 women with endometriosis associated with pelvic pain after a 6-month treatment with 2 mg/day of dienogest. The results show a significant reduction in pain and an improvement in sexual function in women treated with dienogest compared to the control group consisting of women with endometriosis and pelvic pain who had refused hormonal treatment and were only treated with non-steroidal anti-inflammatory drugs [87, 88].

In light of these elements, hormonal treatments for endometriosis can be considered a valid option concerning sexuality. They significantly reduce the signs and symptoms of endometriosis and are associated with a significant improvement in women's quality of life and sexual function [83, 84].

In particular, the literature data seem to identify the Dienogest as a good option for the pharmacological treatment of endometriosis, also concerning the improvement of sexual function [89, 90]. Further studies will undoubtedly be needed to confirm these encouraging results.

A further option for treating endometriosis is surgery, especially suitable for women who do not respond adequately to pharmacological treatments, who wish to be pregnant or who have anatomical distortions, such as rectal stenosis, sigmoidal, or urethral [41]. Surgical treatment should aim at the complete excision of all macroscopic endometriotic lesions and requires a high level of technical expertise in case of extended disease [91, 92].

In particular, surgery for the most severe forms of endometriosis is subject to higher rates of complications such as perforation of the intestine and ureter and rectovaginal and uretero-vaginal fistulas, which may require additional surgical procedures. It is estimated that such complications occur in 4–6% of cases with a significant impact on the patient's quality of life [41, 93].

The potential benefits of radical surgery on deep dyspareunia have been extensively described in both retrospective and prospective studies. Garry et al. [94] assessed the impact of laparoscopic radical excision on various quality of life indicators, including sexual outcomes, noting a significant improvement in sexual function 4 months after surgery. The study of Abbott et al. [95] showed a better sexual function and reduced discomfort during sexual intercourse in a cohort of 176 women with endometriosis subjected to laparoscopic excision and evaluated 5 years after surgery. However, it should be noted that in 36% of cases, it was necessary to resort to additional surgery. Ferrero et al. [96] also showed a significant reduction of the deep dyspareunia to 6 and 12 months after the total excision of the endometriotic lesions through laparoscopic surgery. The study of Ceccaroni et al. [97] compared two different surgical techniques for the treatment of deep endometriosis (laparoscopic approach "nerve-sparing" and classic laparoscopic approach).

Regarding sexual function indicators, the study did not report any significant differences between the two surgical techniques concerning the frequency of sexual intercourse after surgery and the number of patients with dyspareunia, psychological stress, and vaginal dryness. Patients subjected to a classic laparoscopic approach presented more vaginal bleeding and decreased sex drive. Surprisingly, patients subjected to the "nerve-sparing" approach reported a reduced sexual pleasure compared to patients undergoing classical laparoscopy [97]. A recent study by Morelli et al. [98] analyzed the outcomes of radical surgery with a robotic approach in ten patients with deep endometriosis with colon-rectal involvement. The results showed a worsening of sexual functioning 1 month after surgery, with levels comparable to preoperative sexual functioning only 12 months after surgery. One year after the intervention, a statistically significant improvement was observed only in the area of inequality.

About postoperative treatment, it is now widely recognized that hormonal therapies should be systematically proposed to patients who do not intend to conceive due to the potential risk of recurrence of endometriosis [77]. In this regard, Seracchioli et al. [99] point out that therapy with oral contraceptives is associated with a significant reduction in the rate of anatomical recurrence to 1 year from the surgical treatment of endometriosis. The authors also point out that postoperative contraceptive therapy is associated with a significant reduction in the frequency and intensity of relapses of dysmenorrhea [99]. Mabrouk et al. have also confirmed that sexual desire, satisfaction, and pelvic pain impact on sexual activity significantly improve at 6 months after laparoscopic excision associated with postoperative therapy with COC [100].

In conclusion, endometriosis surgical and pharmacological treatments can undoubtedly improve the sexual function of the patient in the medium- and long-term but do not necessarily lead to a definitive resolution of sexual problems. For this reason, the ideal treatment should be conducted by a multidisciplinary team to improve overall sexual functioning and not only to reduce painful symptoms during intercourse [9].

In this sense, the involvement of a psychologist in the team that deals with the clinical management of patients with endometriosis indeed represents an added value in the diagnostic and therapeutic path of the pathology [71, 101].

These data suggest the importance of psychological factors and an adequate assessment of the quality of life and sexuality of patients with endometriosis, not only concerning the severity of the symptoms but also in the management of the disease and the choice of the most appropriate therapy [1, 21].

References

1. Culley L, Law C, Hudson N, Denny E, Mitchell H, Baumgarten M, et al. The social and psychological impact of endometriosis on women's lives: a critical narrative review. Hum Reprod Update. 2013;19(6):625–39. https://doi.org/10.1093/humupd/dmt027.
2. Dancet EA, Apers S, Kluivers KB, Kremer JA, Sermeus W, Devriendt C, et al. The ENDOCARE questionnaire guides European endometriosis clinics to improve the patient-centeredness of their care. Hum Reprod (Oxford, England). 2012;27(11):3168–78. https://doi.org/10.1093/humrep/des299.
3. Soliman AM, Coyne KS, Zaiser E, Castelli-Haley J, Fuldeore MJ. The burden of endometriosis symptoms on health-related quality of life in women in the United States: a cross-sectional study. J Psychosom Obstet Gynaecol. 2017;38(4):238–48. https://doi.org/10.1080/0167482X.2017.1289512.
4. Vitale SG, La Rosa VL, Rapisarda AMC, Laganà AS. Impact of endometriosis on quality of life and psychological well-being. J Psychosom Obstet Gynaecol. 2017;38(4):317–9. https://doi.org/10.1080/0167482x.2016.1244185.
5. Simoens S, Dunselman G, Dirksen C, Hummelshoj L, Bokor A, Brandes I, et al. The burden of endometriosis: costs and quality of life of women with endometriosis and treated in referral centres. Hum Reprod (Oxford, England). 2012;27(5):1292–9. https://doi.org/10.1093/humrep/des073.
6. Pluchino N, Wenger JM, Petignat P, Tal R, Bolmont M, Taylor HS, et al. Sexual function in endometriosis patients and their partners: effect of the disease and consequences of treatment. Hum Reprod Update. 2016;22(6):762–74. https://doi.org/10.1093/humupd/dmw031.
7. Vercellini P, Somigliana E, Buggio L, Barbara G, Frattaruolo MP, Fedele L. "I can't get no satisfaction": deep dyspareunia and sexual functioning in women with rectovaginal endometriosis. Fertil Steril. 2012;98(6):1503–11 e1. https://doi.org/10.1016/j.fertnstert.2012.07.1129.
8. Vercellini P, Meana M, Hummelshoj L, Somigliana E, Vigano P, Fedele L. Priorities for endometriosis research: a proposed focus on deep dyspareunia. Reprod Sci (Thousand Oaks, Calif). 2011;18(2):114–8. https://doi.org/10.1177/1933719110382921.
9. Barbara G, Facchin F, Meschia M, Berlanda N, Frattaruolo MP, Vercellin IP. When love hurts. A systematic review on the effects of surgical and pharmacological treatments for endometriosis on female sexual functioning. Acta Obstet Gynecol Scand. 2017;96(6):668–87. https://doi.org/10.1111/aogs.13031.
10. Fagervold B, Jenssen M, Hummelshoj L, Moen MH. Life after a diagnosis with endometriosis – a 15 years follow-up study. Acta Obstet Gynecol Scand. 2009;88(8):914–9. https://doi.org/10.1080/00016340903108308.
11. Denny E. The experience of living with endometriosis. Deep pelvic endometriosis. 2011. Springer, Milano. p. 79–92.

12. Laganà AS, La Rosa VL, Rapisarda AMC, Valenti G, Sapia F, Chiofalo B, et al. Anxiety and depression in patients with endometriosis: impact and management challenges. Int J Women's Health. 2017;9:323–30. https://doi.org/10.2147/ijwh.S119729.
13. La Rosa VL, De Franciscis P, Barra F, Schiattarella A, Torok P, Shah M, et al. Quality of life in women with endometriosis: a narrative overview. Minerva Med. 2020;111(1):68–78. https://doi.org/10.23736/S0026-4806.19.06298-0.
14. Laganà AS, La Rosa V, Petrosino B, Vitale SG. Comment on "risk of developing major depression and anxiety disorders among women with endometriosis: a longitudinal follow-up study". J Affect Disord. 2017;208:672–3. https://doi.org/10.1016/j.jad.2016.07.016.
15. Revised American Society for Reproductive Medicine classification of endometriosis: 1996. Fertil Steril. 1997;67(5):817–21. https://doi.org/10.1016/s0015-0282(97)81391-x.
16. Brasil DL, Montagna E, Trevisan CM, La Rosa VL, Lagana AS, Barbosa CP, et al. Psychological stress levels in women with endometriosis: systematic review and meta-analysis of observational studies. Minerva Med. 2020;111(1):90–102. https://doi.org/10.23736/S0026-4806.19.06350-X.
17. Vitale SG, Capriglione S, Peterlunger I, La Rosa VL, Vitagliano A, Noventa M, et al. The role of oxidative stress and membrane transport systems during endometriosis: a fresh look at a busy corner. Oxidative Med Cell Longev. 2018;2018:7924021. https://doi.org/10.1155/2018/7924021.
18. Laganà AS, Vitale SG, Salmeri FM, Triolo O, Ban Frangež H, Vrtačnik-Bokal E, et al. Unus pro omnibus, omnes pro uno: a novel, evidence-based, unifying theory for the pathogenesis of endometriosis. Med Hypotheses. 2017;103:10–20. https://doi.org/10.1016/j.mehy.2017.03.032.
19. Della Corte L, Di Filippo C, Gabrielli O, Reppuccia S, La Rosa VL, Ragusa R, et al. The burden of endometriosis on women's lifespan: a narrative overview on quality of life and psychosocial wellbeing. Int J Environ Res Public Health. 2020;17(13):4683. https://doi.org/10.3390/ijerph17134683.
20. Facchin F, Barbara G, Saita E, Mosconi P, Roberto A, Fedele L, et al. Impact of endometriosis on quality of life and mental health: pelvic pain makes the difference. J Psychosom Obstet Gynaecol. 2015;36(4):135–41. https://doi.org/10.3109/0167482X.2015.1074173.
21. Gao X, Yeh YC, Outley J, Simon J, Botteman M, Spalding J. Health-related quality of life burden of women with endometriosis: a literature review. Curr Med Res Opin. 2006;22(9):1787–97. https://doi.org/10.1185/030079906X121084.
22. Marinho MCP, Magalhaes TF, Fernandes LFC, Augusto KL, Brilhante AVM, Bezerra L. Quality of life in women with endometriosis: an integrative review. J Womens Health (2002). 2018;27(3):399–408. https://doi.org/10.1089/jwh.2017.6397.
23. Vitale SG, La Rosa VL, Rapisarda AM, Lagana AS. Comment on: "impact of endometriosis on quality of life and mental health: pelvic pain makes the difference". J Psychosom Obstet Gynaecol. 2017;38(1):81–2. https://doi.org/10.1080/0167482X.2016.1244183.
24. Kennedy S, Bergqvist A, Chapron C, D'Hooghe T, Dunselman G, Greb R, et al. ESHRE guideline for the diagnosis and treatment of endometriosis. Hum Reprod (Oxford, England). 2005;20(10):2698–704. https://doi.org/10.1093/humrep/dei135.
25. Porpora MG, Koninckx PR, Piazze J, Natili M, Colagrande S, Cosmi EV. Correlation between endometriosis and pelvic pain. J Am Assoc Gynecol Laparosc. 1999;6(4):429–34. https://doi.org/10.1016/s1074-3804(99)80006-1.
26. Eriksen HL, Gunnersen KF, Sorensen JA, Munk T, Nielsen T, Knudsen UB. Psychological aspects of endometriosis: differences between patients with or without pain on four psychological variables. Eur J Obstet Gynecol Reprod Biol. 2008;139(1):100–5. https://doi.org/10.1016/j.ejogrb.2007.10.002.
27. Fourquet J, Baez L, Figueroa M, Iriarte RI, Flores I. Quantification of the impact of endometriosis symptoms on health-related quality of life and work productivity. Fertil Steril. 2011;96(1):107–12. https://doi.org/10.1016/j.fertnstert.2011.04.095.

28. Jones G, Jenkinson C, Kennedy S. The impact of endometriosis upon quality of life: a qualitative analysis. J Psychosom Obstet Gynaecol. 2004;25(2):123–33. https://doi.org/10.1080/01674820400002279.
29. Petrelluzzi KF, Garcia MC, Petta CA, Grassi-Kassisse DM, Spadari-Bratfisch RC. Salivary cortisol concentrations, stress and quality of life in women with endometriosis and chronic pelvic pain. Stress. 2008;11(5):390–7. https://doi.org/10.1080/10253890701840610.
30. Gilmour JA, Huntington A, Wilson HV. The impact of endometriosis on work and social participation. Int J Nurs Pract. 2008;14(6):443–8. https://doi.org/10.1111/j.1440-172X.2008.00718.x.
31. Huntington A, Gilmour JA. A life shaped by pain: women and endometriosis. J Clin Nurs. 2005;14(9):1124–32. https://doi.org/10.1111/j.1365-2702.2005.01231.x.
32. Pope CJ, Sharma V, Sharma S, Mazmanian D. A systematic review of the association between psychiatric disturbances and endometriosis. J Obstet Gynaecol Can. 2015;37(11):1006–15. https://doi.org/10.1016/s1701-2163(16)30050-0.
33. Vitale SG, Petrosino B, La Rosa VL, Rapisarda AM, Lagana AS. A systematic review of the association between psychiatric disturbances and endometriosis. J Obstet Gynaecol Can. 2016;38(12):1079–80. https://doi.org/10.1016/j.jogc.2016.09.008.
34. Cavaggioni G, Lia C, Resta S, Antonielli T, Benedetti Panici P, Megiorni F, et al. Are mood and anxiety disorders and alexithymia associated with endometriosis? A preliminary study. BioMed Res Int. 2014;2014:786830. https://doi.org/10.1155/2014/786830.
35. Low WY, Edelmann RJ, Sutton C. A psychological profile of endometriosis patients in comparison to patients with pelvic pain of other origins. J Psychosom Res. 1993;37(2):111–6. https://doi.org/10.1016/0022-3999(93)90077-s.
36. Sepulcri Rde P, do Amaral VF. Depressive symptoms, anxiety, and quality of life in women with pelvic endometriosis. Eur J Obstet Gynecol Reprod Biol. 2009;142(1):53–6. https://doi.org/10.1016/j.ejogrb.2008.09.003.
37. Friedl F, Riedl D, Fessler S, Wildt L, Walter M, Richter R, et al. Impact of endometriosis on quality of life, anxiety, and depression: an Austrian perspective. Arch Gynecol Obstet. 2015;292(6):1393–9. https://doi.org/10.1007/s00404-015-3789-8.
38. Vitale SG, La Rosa VL, Rapisarda AMC, Laganà AS. Endometriosis and infertility: the impact on quality of life and mental health. J Endometr Pelvic Pain Disord. 2017;9(2):112–5. https://doi.org/10.5301/je.5000274.
39. Fritzer N, Haas D, Oppelt P, Renner S, Hornung D, Wolfler M, et al. More than just bad sex: sexual dysfunction and distress in patients with endometriosis. Eur J Obstet Gynecol Reprod Biol. 2013;169(2):392–6. https://doi.org/10.1016/j.ejogrb.2013.04.001.
40. Barbara G, Facchin F, Buggio L, Somigliana E, Berlanda N, Kustermann A, et al. What is known and unknown about the association between endometriosis and sexual functioning: a systematic review of the literature. Reprod Sci (Thousand Oaks, Calif). 2017;24(12):1566–76. https://doi.org/10.1177/1933719117707054.
41. Vitale SG, La Rosa VL, Vitagliano A, Noventa M, Laganà FM, Ardizzone A, et al. Sexual function and quality of life in patients affected by deep infiltrating endometriosis: current evidence and future perspectives. J Endometr Pelvic Pain Disord. 2017;9(4):270–4. https://doi.org/10.5301/jeppd.5000303.
42. La Rosa VL, De Franciscis P, Barra F, Schiattarella A, Tropea A, Tesarik J, et al. Sexuality in women with endometriosis: a critical narrative review. Minerva Med. 2020;111(1):79–89. https://doi.org/10.23736/S0026-4806.19.06299-2.
43. Noventa M, Scioscia M, Schincariol M, Cavallin F, Pontrelli G, Virgilio B et al. Imaging modalities for diagnosis of deep pelvic endometriosis: comparison between trans-vaginal sonography, rectal endoscopy sonography and magnetic resonance imaging. a head-to-head meta-analysis. Diagnostics (Basel). 2019;9(4). https://doi.org/10.3390/diagnostics9040225.
44. Ferrero S, Esposito F, Abbamonte LH, Anserini P, Remorgida V, Ragni N. Quality of sex life in women with endometriosis and deep dyspareunia. Fertil Steril. 2005;83(3):573–9. https://doi.org/10.1016/j.fertnstert.2004.07.973.

45. Montanari G, Di Donato N, Benfenati A, Giovanardi G, Zannoni L, Vicenzi C, et al. Women with deep infiltrating endometriosis: sexual satisfaction, desire, orgasm, and pelvic problem interference with sex. J Sex Med. 2013;10(6):1559–66. https://doi.org/10.1111/jsm.12133.
46. Di Donato N, Montanari G, Benfenati A, Monti G, Bertoldo V, Mauloni M, et al. Do women with endometriosis have to worry about sex? Eur J Obstet Gynecol Reprod Biol. 2014;179:69–74. https://doi.org/10.1016/j.ejogrb.2014.05.022.
47. Speer LM, Mushkbar S, Erbele T. Chronic pelvic pain in women. Am Fam Physician. 2016;93(5):380–7.
48. Patnaik SS, Laganà AS, Vitale SG, Butticè S, Noventa M, Gizzo S, et al. Etiology, pathophysiology and biomarkers of interstitial cystitis/painful bladder syndrome. Arch Gynecol Obstet. 2017;295(6):1341–59. https://doi.org/10.1007/s00404-017-4364-2.
49. Waller KG, Shaw RW. Endometriosis, pelvic pain, and psychological functioning. Fertil Steril. 1995;63(4):796–800. https://doi.org/10.1016/s0015-0282(16)57484-6.
50. Fritzer N, Tammaa A, Haas D, Oppelt P, Renner S, Hornung D, et al. When sex is not on fire: a prospective multicentre study evaluating the short-term effects of radical resection of endometriosis on quality of sex life and dyspareunia. Eur J Obstet Gynecol Reprod Biol. 2016;197:36–40. https://doi.org/10.1016/j.ejogrb.2015.11.007.
51. Vercellini P, Somigliana E, Consonni D, Frattaruolo MP, De Giorgi O, Fedele L. Surgical versus medical treatment for endometriosis-associated severe deep dyspareunia: I. Effect on pain during intercourse and patient satisfaction. Hum Reprod (Oxford, England). 2012;27(12):3450–9. https://doi.org/10.1093/humrep/des313.
52. Jia SZ, Leng JH, Sun PR, Lang JH. Prevalence and associated factors of female sexual dysfunction in women with endometriosis. Obstet Gynecol. 2013;121(3):601–6. https://doi.org/10.1097/AOG.0b013e3182835777.
53. Evangelista A, Dantas T, Zendron C, Soares T, Vaz G, Oliveira MA. Sexual function in patients with deep infiltrating endometriosis. J Sex Med. 2014;11(1):140–5. https://doi.org/10.1111/jsm.12349.
54. Basson R. Human sexual response. Handb Clin Neurol. 2015;130:11–8. https://doi.org/10.1016/B978-0-444-63247-0.00002-X.
55. De Graaff AA, D'Hooghe TM, Dunselman GA, Dirksen CD, Hummelshoj L, Consortium WE, et al. The significant effect of endometriosis on physical, mental and social wellbeing: results from an international cross-sectional survey. Hum Reprod (Oxford, England). 2013;28(10):2677–85. https://doi.org/10.1093/humrep/det284.
56. Denny E, Mann CH. Endometriosis-associated dyspareunia: the impact on women's lives. J Fam Plann Reprod Health Care. 2007;33(3):189–93. https://doi.org/10.1783/147118907781004831.
57. Fernandez I, Reid C, Dziurawiec S. Living with endometriosis: the perspective of male partners. J Psychosom Res. 2006;61(4):433–8. https://doi.org/10.1016/j.jpsychores.2006.06.003.
58. Strzempko Butt F, Chesla C. Relational patterns of couples living with chronic pelvic pain from endometriosis. Qual Health Res. 2007;17(5):571–85. https://doi.org/10.1177/1049732307299907.
59. Hammerli S, Kohl Schwartz AS, Geraedts K, Imesch P, Rauchfuss M, Wolfler MM, et al. Does endometriosis affect sexual activity and satisfaction of the man partner? A comparison of partners from women diagnosed with endometriosis and controls. J Sex Med. 2018;15(6):853–65. https://doi.org/10.1016/j.jsxm.2018.03.087.
60. Jodoin M, Bergeron S, Khalife S, Dupuis MJ, Desrochers G, Leclerc B. Male partners of women with provoked vestibulodynia: attributions for pain and their implications for dyadic adjustment, sexual satisfaction, and psychological distress. J Sex Med. 2008;5(12):2862–70. https://doi.org/10.1111/j.1743-6109.2008.00950.x.
61. Smith KB, Pukall CF. Sexual function, relationship adjustment, and the relational impact of pain in male partners of women with provoked vulvar pain. J Sex Med. 2014;11(5):1283–93. https://doi.org/10.1111/jsm.12484.

62. Boerner KE, Rosen NO. Acceptance of vulvovaginal pain in women with provoked vestibulodynia and their partners: associations with pain, psychological, and sexual adjustment. J Sex Med. 2015;12(6):1450–62. https://doi.org/10.1111/jsm.12889.
63. Dunselman GA, Vermeulen N, Becker C, Calhaz-Jorge C, D'Hooghe T, De Bie B, et al. ESHRE guideline: management of women with endometriosis. Hum Reprod (Oxford, England). 2014;29(3):400–12. https://doi.org/10.1093/humrep/det457.
64. Culley L, Law C, Hudson N, Mitchell H, Denny E, Raine-Fenning N. A qualitative study of the impact of endometriosis on male partners. Hum Reprod (Oxford, England). 2017;32(8):1667–73. https://doi.org/10.1093/humrep/dex221.
65. La Rosa VL, Barra F, Chiofalo B, Platania A, Di Guardo F, Conway F, et al. An overview on the relationship between endometriosis and infertility: the impact on sexuality and psychological well-being. J Psychosom Obstet Gynaecol. 2020;41(2):93–7. https://doi.org/10.1080/0167482X.2019.1659775.
66. El Kissi Y, Romdhane AB, Hidar S, Bannour S, Ayoubi Idrissi K, Khairi H, et al. General psychopathology, anxiety, depression and self-esteem in couples undergoing infertility treatment: a comparative study between men and women. Eur J Obstet Gynecol Reprod Biol. 2013;167(2):185–9. https://doi.org/10.1016/j.ejogrb.2012.12.014.
67. Gadarowski A. Procreative sex in infertile couples: the decay of pleasure? A letter to the editor. Health Qual Life Outcomes. 2013;11:52. https://doi.org/10.1186/1477-7525-11-52.
68. Maroufizadeh S, Karimi E, Vesali S, Omani SR. Anxiety and depression after failure of assisted reproductive treatment among patients experiencing infertility. Int J Gynaecol Obstet. 2015;130(3):253–6. https://doi.org/10.1016/j.ijgo.2015.03.044.
69. Barra F, La Rosa VL, Vitale SG, Commodari E, Altieri M, Scala C, et al. Psychological status of infertile patients who had in vitro fertilization treatment interrupted or postponed due to COVID-19 pandemic: a cross-sectional study. J Psychosom Obstet Gynaecol. 2020:1–8. https://doi.org/10.1080/0167482X.2020.1853095.
70. Vitale SG, La Rosa VL, Rapisarda AM, Laganà AS. Psychology of infertility and assisted reproductive treatment: the Italian situation. J Psychosom Obstet Gynaecol. 2017;38(1):1–3. https://doi.org/10.1080/0167482x.2016.1244184.
71. Leroy A, Azaïs H, Garabedian C, Bregegere S, Rubod C, Collier F. Psychologie et sexologie: une approche essentielle, du diagnostic à la prise en charge globale de l'endométriose. Gynecol Obstet Fertil. 2016;44(6):363–7. https://doi.org/10.1016/j.gyobfe.2016.03.017.
72. Bedaiwy MA, Allaire C, Yong P, Alfaraj S. Medical management of endometriosis in patients with chronic pelvic pain. Semin Reprod Med. 2017;35(1):38–53. https://doi.org/10.1055/s-0036-1597308.
73. Bergqvist A, Theorell T. Changes in quality of life after hormonal treatment of endometriosis. Acta Obstet Gynecol Scand. 2001;80(7):628–37.
74. Zupi E, Marconi D, Sbracia M, Zullo F, De Vivo B, Exacustos C, et al. Add-back therapy in the treatment of endometriosis-associated pain. Fertil Steril. 2004;82(5):1303–8. https://doi.org/10.1016/j.fertnstert.2004.03.062.
75. Petta CA, Ferriani RA, Abrao MS, Hassan D, Rosa ESJC, Podgaec S, et al. Randomized clinical trial of a levonorgestrelreleasing intrauterine system and a depot GnRH analogue for the treatment of chronic pelvic pain in women with endometriosis. Hum Reprod (Oxford, England). 2005;20(7):1993–8. https://doi.org/10.1093/humrep/deh869.
76. Huber AV, Huber JC, Kolbus A, Imhof M, Nagele F, Loizou D, et al. Systemic HCG treatment in patients with endometriosis: a new perspective for a painful disease. Wien Klin Wochenschr. 2004;116(24):839–43. https://doi.org/10.1007/s00508-004-0296-5.
77. Roman H, Vassilieff M, Gourcerol G, Savoye G, Leroi AM, Marpeau L, et al. Surgical management of deep infiltrating endometriosis of the rectum: pleading for a symptom-guided approach. Hum Reprod (Oxford, England). 2011;26(2):274–81. https://doi.org/10.1093/humrep/deq332.
78. Deguara CS, Pepas L, Davis C. Does minimally invasive surgery for endometriosis improve pelvic symptoms and quality of life? Curr Opin Obstet Gynecol. 2012;24(4):241–4. https://doi.org/10.1097/GCO.0b013e328355626f.

79. Van den Broeck U, Meuleman C, Tomassetti C, D'Hoore A, Wolthuis A, Van Cleynenbreugel B, et al. Effect of laparoscopic surgery for moderate and severe endometriosis on depression, relationship satisfaction and sexual functioning: comparison of patients with and without bowel resection. Hum Reprod (Oxford, England). 2013;28(9):2389–97. https://doi.org/10.1093/humrep/det260.
80. Low WY, Edelmann RJ, Sutton C. Short term psychological outcome of surgical intervention for endometriosis. Br J Obstet Gynaecol. 1993;100(2):191–2. https://doi.org/10.1111/j.1471-0528.1993.tb15223.x.
81. Vercellini P, Frontino G, De Giorgi O, Pietropaolo G, Pasin R, Crosignani PG. Endometriosis: preoperative and postoperative medical treatment. Obstet Gynecol Clin N Am. 2003;30(1):163–80. https://doi.org/10.1016/s0889-8545(02)00059-1.
82. Carlson KJ, Miller BA, Fowler FJ Jr. The Maine women's health study: I. Outcomes of hysterectomy. Obstet Gynecol. 1994;83(4):556–65. https://doi.org/10.1097/00006250-199404000-00012.
83. Caruso S, Agnello C, Intelisano G, Farina M, Di Mari L, Sparacino L, et al. Prospective study on sexual behavior of women using 30 microg ethinylestradiol and 3 mg drospirenone oral contraceptive. Contraception. 2005;72(1):19–23. https://doi.org/10.1016/j.contraception.2005.02.002.
84. Caruso S, Agnello C, Intelisano G, Farina M, Di Mari L, Cianci A. Sexual behavior of women taking low-dose oral contraceptive containing 15 microg ethinylestradiol/60 microg gestodene. Contraception. 2004;69(3):237–40. https://doi.org/10.1016/j.contraception.2003.11.001.
85. Morotti M, Sozzi F, Remorgida V, Venturini PL, Ferrero S. Dienogest in women with persistent endometriosis-related pelvic pain during norethisterone acetate treatment. Eur J Obstet Gynecol Reprod Biol. 2014;183:188–92. https://doi.org/10.1016/j.ejogrb.2014.10.036.
86. Vercellini P, Bracco B, Mosconi P, Roberto A, Alberico D, Dhouha D, et al. Norethindrone acetate or dienogest for the treatment of symptomatic endometriosis: a before and after study. Fertil Steril. 2016;105(3):734–43 e3. https://doi.org/10.1016/j.fertnstert.2015.11.016.
87. Caruso S, Iraci M, Cianci S, Casella E, Fava V, Cianci A. Quality of life and sexual function of women affected by endometriosis-associated pelvic pain when treated with dienogest. J Endocrinol Investig. 2015;38(11):1211–8. https://doi.org/10.1007/s40618-015-0383-7.
88. Caruso S, Iraci M, Cianci S, Fava V, Casella E, Cianci A. Comparative, open-label prospective study on the quality of life and sexual function of women affected by endometriosis-associated pelvic pain on 2 mg dienogest/30 microg ethinyl estradiol continuous or 21/7 regimen oral contraceptive. J Endocrinol Investig. 2016;39(8):923–31. https://doi.org/10.1007/s40618-016-0460-6.
89. Caruso S, Iraci M, Cianci S, Vitale SG, Fava V, Cianci A. Effects of long-term treatment with Dienogest on the quality of life and sexual function of women affected by endometriosis-associated pelvic pain. J Pain Res. 2019;12:2371–8. https://doi.org/10.2147/JPR.S207599.
90. Laganà AS, Vitale SG, Granese R, Palmara V, Ban Frangež H, Vrtačnik-Bokal E, et al. Clinical dynamics of Dienogest for the treatment of endometriosis: from bench to bedside. Expert Opin Drug Metab Toxicol. 2017;13(6):593–6. https://doi.org/10.1080/17425255.2017.1297421.
91. Vercellini P, Carmignani L, Rubino T, Barbara G, Abbiati A, Fedele L. Surgery for deep endometriosis: a pathogenesis-oriented approach. Gynecol Obstet Investig. 2009;68(2):88–103. https://doi.org/10.1159/000219946.
92. Laganà AS, Vitale SG, Trovato MA, Palmara VI, Rapisarda AM, Granese R, et al. Full-thickness excision versus shaving by laparoscopy for intestinal deep infiltrating endometriosis: rationale and potential treatment options. Biomed Res Int. 2016;2016:3617179. https://doi.org/10.1155/2016/3617179.
93. Mabrouk M, Montanari G, Guerrini M, Villa G, Solfrini S, Vicenzi C, et al. Does laparoscopic management of deep infiltrating endometriosis improve quality of life? A prospective study. Health Qual Life Outcomes. 2011;9:98. https://doi.org/10.1186/1477-7525-9-98.

94. Garry R, Clayton R, Hawe J. The effect of endometriosis and its radical laparoscopic excision on quality of life indicators. BJOG. 2000;107(1):44–54. https://doi.org/10.1111/j.1471-0528.2000.tb11578.x.
95. Abbott JA, Hawe J, Clayton RD, Garry R. The effects and effectiveness of laparoscopic excision of endometriosis: a prospective study with 2–5 year follow-up. Hum Reprod (Oxford, England). 2003;18(9):1922–7. https://doi.org/10.1093/humrep/deg275.
96. Ferrero S, Abbamonte LH, Giordano M, Ragni N, Remorgida V. Deep dyspareunia and sex life after laparoscopic excision of endometriosis. Hum Reprod (Oxford, England). 2007;22(4):1142–8. https://doi.org/10.1093/humrep/del465.
97. Ceccaroni M, Clarizia R, Bruni F, D'Urso E, Gagliardi ML, Roviglione G, et al. Nerve-sparing laparoscopic eradication of deep endometriosis with segmental rectal and parametrial resection: the Negrar method. A single-center, prospective, clinical trial. Surg Endosc. 2012;26(7):2029–45. https://doi.org/10.1007/s00464-012-2153-3.
98. Morelli L, Perutelli A, Palmeri M, Guadagni S, Mariniello MD, Di Franco G, et al. Robot-assisted surgery for the radical treatment of deep infiltrating endometriosis with colorectal involvement: short- and mid-term surgical and functional outcomes. Int J Color Dis. 2016;31(3):643–52. https://doi.org/10.1007/s00384-015-2477-2.
99. Seracchioli R, Mabrouk M, Manuzzi L, Vicenzi C, Frasca C, Elmakky A, et al. Post-operative use of oral contraceptive pills for prevention of anatomical relapse or symptom-recurrence after conservative surgery for endometriosis. Hum Reprod (Oxford, England). 2009;24(11):2729–35. https://doi.org/10.1093/humrep/dep259.
100. Mabrouk M, Montanari G, Di Donato N, Del Forno S, Frasca C, Geraci E, et al. What is the impact on sexual function of laparoscopic treatment and subsequent combined oral contraceptive therapy in women with deep infiltrating endometriosis? J Sex Med. 2012;9(3):770–8. https://doi.org/10.1111/j.1743-6109.2011.02593.x.
101. Lagana AS, La Rosa VL. Multidisciplinary management of endometriosis: current strategies and future challenges. Minerva Med. 2020;111(1):18–20. https://doi.org/10.23736/S0026-4806.19.06370-5.

Nutritional Interventions, Complementary and Alternative Medicine for Endometriosis

26

Maurizio Nicola D'Alterio, Stefano Angioni, Fabio Ghezzi, and Antonio Simone Laganà

Contents

26.1 Introduction

Alternative therapies for endometriosis are normally related to hormone therapy or surgical operations; however, these approaches are non-curative, do not comply with women's reproductive objectives, and sometimes result in the recurrence of the

The original version of the chapter has been revised. A correction to this chapter can be found at https://doi.org/10.1007/978-3-030-97236-3_45

M. N. D'Alterio · S. Angioni
Department of Surgical Sciences, University of Cagliari, Cagliari, Italy

F. Ghezzi · A. S. Laganà (✉)
Department of Obstetrics and Gynecology, "Filippo Del Ponte" Hospital, University of Insubria, Varese, Italy
e-mail: antoniosimone.lagana@uninsubria.it

E. Oral (ed.), *Endometriosis and Adenomyosis*,
https://doi.org/10.1007/978-3-030-97236-3_26

disease after discontinuation. Defining the factors that lead to lesion growth and progression is crucial to creating prevention opportunities and more successful therapeutic treatments. The discovery of changeable risk factors for endometriosis, such as diet and exercise, and the search for complementary and alternative therapies has become increasingly attractive. Diet is a key chronic disease risk factor [1]. The importance of nutrition in controlling the growth and development of endometriosis has lately emerged as a matter of study, mainly due to the finding that some of the disease-related physiological and pathological pathways, such as inflammatory response, estrogen production, menses succession, organochlorine influence, and prostaglandin secretion, may also be affected by nutrition and lifestyle [2]. In endometriosis, relevant habitual dietary habits tend to have a mild effect on certain inflammatory mechanisms [3].

Prostaglandin levels are one of the potential pathogenic factors causing both endometriosis and dysmenorrhea. Diet-derived omega-6 fatty acids are the integral components of pro-inflammatory prostaglandins, such as prostaglandin E2 (PGE2) and prostaglandin F2-α (PGF2-α), which are likely to exacerbate uterine cramps and to induce pain and discomfort [4]. Arachidonic acid (AA) is an omega-6 polyunsaturated fatty acid (PUFA) biosynthesized from linoleic acid, a key constituent of vegetable oil, and a substrate for the development of chemical messengers such as (PGE2) and leukotriene-4 (LTB4) that tend to be associated with the development of pain and endometriosis [4]. PGE2 affects cytokine and chemokine production, impacts steroidogenesis, induces angiogenesis, and enhances matrix metalloproteinases (MMPs). Estradiol, interleukin 1ß (IL-1ß), vascular endothelial growth factor (VEGF) affect cyclooxygenase-2 (cox-2) activity, contributing to continuous PGE2 generation through a persistent positive feedback loop [5]. However, prostaglandin E3 (PGE3), originating from omega-3 fatty acids, such as eicosapentaenoic acid (EPA) and docosahexaenoic acid (DHA), were related to decreased phlogosis and, therefore, reduced pain [4]. By contending with omega-6 PUFAs to generate anti-inflammatory lipid mediators, omega-3 PUFAs are crucial in regulating prostaglandins and cytokines, such as interleukin (IL)-1, −2, and −6 and tumor necrosis factor-α (TNF-α) [4]. EPA is a negative regulator of converting AA to PGE2 and LTB4. An unbalanced formulation of the appropriate omega-6 and omega-3 fatty acid ratio [1] can stimulate inflammatory pathways and may be correlated with intensified menstrual pain and autoimmune and hormonal dysfunctions [6].

Attaman et al. showed that in an endometriosis mouse model in which omega-6 fatty acids can be transformed into omega-3 fatty acids, the percentage of lesions induced in the mouse model was significantly lower compared to the controls, and pro-inflammatory cytokines such as IL-6 and inflammatory enzymes such as Cox-2 were decreased [7]. In a rabbit-endometriosis prototype surgically created, dietary ingestion of EPA and DHA caused decreased lesions and lower levels of PGE2 and prostaglandin F2 (PGF2) in the peritoneal fluid [8]. Trans-fatty acids (such as linoleic acid) are linked with higher systemic inflammation markers. A greater consumption is related to increased TNF system activity, higher TNF-receptor concentrations, and higher plasma levels of IL-6, C-reactive protein (CRP), and TNF-α [9].

Another risk factor for developing endometriosis could be elevated estrogen levels. Hence, we may presume that the dietary influence on the levels of circulating estrogen can also contribute to endometriosis etiology [2]. The inflammatory and proliferative features of endometriosis may be favored by estrogen upregulating prostaglandin synthesis [10]. Diet can affect the risk of endometriosis by its effect on steroid hormones. For example, red meat has been demonstrated to greatly reduce sex hormone-binding globulin (SHBG) and to enhance estradiol levels [11]. In contrast, fish oil has been correlated with reduced circulating concentrations of PGE2 and decreased inflammatory symptoms and reduced dysmenorrhea [12]. One of the main sources of pro-vitamin A, i.e., alpha-carotene, beta-carotene, and beta-cryptoxanthin, are fruits. Research shows that many women with endometriosis generally consume fewer Vitamin-A nutrients, compared to the women not suffering from the disease [13] Example cases include the presence of high concentrations of IL-6 in endometrial cells in humans, and especially in the affected women's peritoneal fluid. The experiments also prove the retinoic acid ability of reducing mRNA expression of IL-6 levels [14]. Furthermore, while VEGF has been proven to support the angiogenesis of endometriosis lesions, the stimulation of HL-60 cells using all-trans retinoic acid (atRA) reduces VEGF mRNA and proteins [14]. Other vitamins such as C and E with antioxidant properties also affect lipid peroxidation (LPO). The production of reactive oxygen species (ROS), which can come from several sources, may induce an LPO chain reaction causing chronic inflammatory diseases [15]. Free radicals, as well as reactive oxygen species (ROS) can regulate the development and adherence of endometrial cells in the abdominal cavity. Vitamin C is a known suppressant of free radicals and ROS [16].

Chemical substances from contaminated conditions, especially organochlorines, including polychlorinated biphenyls (PCBs) and pesticides/insecticides, may also be found in food. PCBs occur to bioaccumulate in the lipids found in meat, liver, and dairy products. Similarly, pesticides can be ingested with polluted fruits and vegetables. Among the risk factors for endometriosis, the above substances can also be listed, as they have been proven to achieve multiple effects through estrogen and androgen receptors, interacting with hormonal pathways [17, 18].

Additionally, vitamin D, calcium, and minerals such as magnesium and copper can also be involved in the pathogenesis and risk of developing endometriosis. Vitamin D and calcium activate T-regulatory cells and IL-10 secretion, decrease the concentrations of pro-inflammatory cytokines, such as IL-17, and mitigate the immune role of T-helper 1 [19]. Previous in vitro research explored the effects of calcitriol on human endometriotic stromal cells (ESCs), showing its effect on reducing IL-1 and TNF, and on suppressing viable ESCs numbers [20]. In addition, treatment with calcitriol significantly decreases VEGF and MMP-9 and significantly improves specific tissue inhibitors of metalloproteinase-2 (TIMP-2) concentrations in ectopic lesions, indicating that calcitriol may interact with the production and progress of endometriosis by repressing neovascularization and extracellular matrix remodeling, both of which are needed for invasive conditions contributing to advanced disease [21]. Additionally, in ESCs grown from ovarian endometriomas, an injection of 1,25(OH)-D3 induces an antiphlogistic result, expressed as decrements in IL-8, IL-6, and MMP-2/MMP-9 expression, prostaglandin production, and nuclear factor kappa-light-chain-enhancer of activated B cells (NF-κB) stimulation compared to untreated cells [20]. However, in a research including women with ovarian endometriosis, those with vitamin D deficiency (hypovitaminosis D) were more inclined to develop endometriosis than those with standard vitamin D serum concentrations [22]. Additionally, an inverse relationship between magnesium consumption and endometriosis risk was found in a prospective cohort study [23]. Lower concentrations of pro-inflammatory markers and endothelial dysfunction in postmenopausal women correlate with the dietary consumption of magnesium. Because the fallopian tubes of patients with endometriosis work more spasmodically, magnesium's soothing effect on the smooth muscles present in the tubes and uteri can help women with endometriosis [23]. In women with endometriosis, higher urinary and serous concentrations of copper have been detected. Moreover, the correlation observed between markers of copper, ceruloplasmin, and oxidative stress indicates their possible application for oxidative stress in endometriosis etiopathogenesis [24].

While a vast amount of the lay literature promotes dietary modifications to minimize endometriosis and related disorders, the scientific literature in this field remains scarce. Few human studies have studied the relationship between endometriosis and diet. Notably, most of the recorded researches supporting such a correlation was carried out using endometriosis animal models, with the results were merely deduced to humans. In addition, the analyses were primarily retrospective or case-control in the few studies of exposed women, which are susceptible to selection and/or recall bias and are usually too restricted in length to adequately illustrate the impact of nutritional interventions on the growth and expansion of lesions. An Italian case-control study by Parazzini et al. recorded that women with endometriosis had higher intakes of red meat and ham and lower consumption of fish, fresh fruits, and green vegetables compared to women without endometriosis [25]. On the contrary, a case-control study based in Washington documented no link between endometriosis diagnosis and increased consumption of red meat, fish, and vegetables, but instead, there was a higher intake of fruit among women with endometriosis. Trabert et al. hypothesized that exposure to pesticides through fruit ingestion might justify the higher risk of endometriosis in their research [26]. A major drawback in these studies was the retrospective compilation of nutritional data restricted to the analysis of diet in the year before the diagnosis of endometriosis. In a study by Harris et al., it was stated that the intake of citrus fruits rich in β-cryptoxanthin is protective against the development of endometriosis thanks to the noticeable increase in serum retinol. On the other hand, the intake of cruciferous vegetables has been related to an increased risk of endometriosis. Although rich in health benefits such as phytochemicals and nutrients, cruciferous vegetables may be difficult to digest and absorb. Some of these are rich in fermentable oligosaccharides, disaccharides, monosaccharides, and polyols (FODMAPs), which are strongly related to the exacerbation of irritable bowel syndrome (IBS) symptoms [27, 28].

A cohort study which explored the relationship between the consumption of red meat, poultry, fish, and seafood and the risk of endometriosis was published by Yamamoto et al. They found that the consumption of red meat (regardless of the type of animal fat), refined or unprocessed, is a major cause of an higher possibility of developing endometriosis. Meanwhile, red meat substitution with fish, shellfish, and eggs was correlated with a lower endometriosis risk [29]. The link between dietary fat consumption and the probability of developing endometriosis was investigated by Missmer et al., evaluating 12 years of prospective data from the Nurses' Health Study II that started in 1989. According to this broad, prospective study among premenopausal women, a considerably reduced incidence of laparoscopic endometriosis diagnosis was found among women with higher long-time consumption of omega-3 fatty acids. Contrarily, an increased risk was correlated with the intake of trans-unsaturated fat and, theoretically, a diet with a higher ingestion of animal fat [30]. Moreover, ligands of peroxisome proliferator-activated receptor gamma (PPAR-γ) cause regression in rodents and baboons with surgically induced endometriosis. The study's findings correlate with these models, as trans unsaturated fatty acids can decrease PPAR-γ expression by approximately 40%, contrary to the upregulating impact of polyunsaturated fatty acids (omega-3) that have been assumed to be natural PPAR-γ ligands [31].

Trabert et al. discovered an opposite association as regards dairy consumption and endometriosis. In contrast to women reporting <1 serving/day of milk products, the odds ratio for women with endometriosis reporting 1–2 servings/day was 0.6, while in women documenting >2 servings/day, it was 0.7 [26]. The general intake of milk and other low-fat dairy products was related to a lower probability of developing endometriosis in a 2013 study reported by Harris et al. The risk of endometriosis was 18% lower for women who ate more than three portions of dairy products daily than for women who consumed two or fewer portions of dairy products daily [23]. In adolescence, consuming dairy, precisely yogurt and ice cream intake, can lower the probability of consequent endometriosis [32].

Soy products include high levels of phytoestrogens, mainly the isoflavones genistein and daidzein, which are structurally comparable to estradiol and may interfere with estrogen receptors. It is believed that exposure to these substances during childhood raises the incidence of endometriosis in adulthood [33]. Mvondo et al. recently evaluated a diet on immature female rats with different soy formulations. At 13 weeks of age, the animals (except the normal control) underwent endometriosis transplantation. The severity of pelvic discomfort and the number of ectopic foci expanded in animals supplied a diet of more than 10% of soy. Consequently, these findings indicate that daily dietary intake containing more than 10% of soy from a prepubertal age may have facilitated endometriosis production by encouraging oxidative tissue stress and cell hypertrophy [34]. Early exposure to genistein has been shown to significantly raise uterine tumorigenesis in adulthood via an epigenetic pathway involving the decreased expression of the zest homologue 2 enhancer (EZH2) and histone 3 trimethylated lysine 27 (H3K27me3) enhancer. Decreasing H3K27me3 levels, a repressive mark for gene expression, in the development of the uterus, reconfigures estrogen-responsive genes to become ultra-responsive to estrogen in the adult uterus. The theory is that ectopic growth of the endometrium outside the uterine cavity could be caused by anomalies inherent in the eutopic endometrium not seen in women without endometriosis [35]. Conversely, either genistein or puerarin have been studied in animal models of endometriosis. It has been demonstrated that the size of endometriotic nodules decrease by suppressing aromatase and estrogen receptor activity and restricting of estrogen concentrations [36]. Overall, no variations in the levels of urinary phytoestrogen in women with or without endometriosis have been observed, independent of any discrepancies in the intake of soy supplements recorded [37].

A meta-analysis by Chiaffarino et al. reported that evidence is currently inadequate to indicate a strong link between caffeine intake and disease occurrence [38]. Caffeine has been indicated to act on the hepatic production of SHBG and to result in an associated decrease in bioavailable testosterone in women. Other studies have speculated on caffeine's involvement in the inhibition of aromatase, the main enzyme mediating the transition of androgens into estrogens. However, estrogen concentrations in the early follicular phase and oestrone levels have been shown to be superior in women with elevated caffeine consumption [39].

A fiber-rich diet improves the excretion and decreases the bioavailability of estrogens, while refined and whole grains impact the glycemic index and the demand for insulin. Insulin has been shown to induce endometrial stromal cell proliferation by reacting to its endometrial receptors. Furthermore, hyperinsulinemia can increase estrogen and insulin-like growth factor-1 (IGF-1) concentrations by decreasing SHBG concentrations and IGF-1 binding protein. Both estrogens and IGF-1 promote the proliferation of endometrial cells [40]. Based on these findings, the risk of endometriosis may be correlated with fiber and cereal intake. However, the published evidence does not support this correlation. In Trabert et al.'s analysis, there was no correlation between fiber intake and risk of endometriosis [26]; to the contrary, Savaris and do Amaral detected a significantly superior consumption of fiber in women with endometriosis, but the study had too many limitations to allow to draw any conclusions [41].

Patients with endometriosis suffer considerably from diet-related comorbidities, including food intolerances and allergies. Gastrointestinal symptoms, such as flatulence, swelling, constipation, and diarrhea, are also more frequent in the endometriosis community and appeared to worsen during the menstrual period [42]. There are numerous causes for these signs, ranging from the intestinal presentation of endometriotic lesions to the high incidence of food allergies or IBS. On the one hand, the overlap between endometriosis and IBS impedes an appropriate diagnosis; on the other hand, it provides new therapeutic opportunities for patients with both diseases [43, 44]. The diagnosis and management of diet-induced diseases, particularly food intolerances or allergies, through nutritional interventions can improve well-being and symptoms.

26.2 Nutritional Interventions

An online survey in Australia shows that approximately 76% of women suffering from endometriosis utilize several self-care techniques at home such as exercise, diet, and meditation. Close to half of the women had tried to treat endometriosis by changing diet, such as shifting to vegan and gluten-free diets. The study ranked the efficiency of the diet-change option as 6.4 out of 10 [45]. However, there is no scientific knowledge of the impact of diet on endometriosis [46]. The available researches investigating the impact of diet on endometriosis are more concerned diet as a risk for endometriosis rather than treatment.

26.2.1 Vitamin D and Fatty Acids

In a double-blind clinical trial, Almassinokiani et al. showed no variation in endometriosis-related pain between women taking 50.000 UI of vitamin D or placebo weekly for 12 weeks after surgical treatment [47].

In vivo and in vitro studies have shown that oral omega-3 PUFAs (i.e., EPA and DHA) have the potential to alleviate painful symptoms correlated with the disease, minimize lesion size, sustain patients' ability to conceive, and have no or minimal side effects [48]. However, the properties of omega-3 PUFAs to reduce the risk of endometriosis in women, focused on prospective results, are aligned with those derived from animal studies [7]. A specific example involves surgically-induced endometriosis rats that ingest omega-3 PUFAs, which causes major regression of endometriotic nodules, as well as the reduced IL-6, TNF-α, and VEGF peritoneal concentrations [8, 49]. In a recent study, Nodler et al., wanted to establish whether vitamin D and omega-3 can reduce pain or the need for pain medications, and thus improving the quality of life in women affected by endometriosis. The subjects received 2000 IU vitamin D3, 1000 mg fish oil, or a placebo as a control experiment. However, after 6 months of treatment, the study did not provide statistically relevant findings on the improvement of pain in the subjects, compared to those who took a placebo [50].

26.2.2 Antioxidant Diet

Oxidative stress, which is characterized by a disequilibrium in ROS generation and inactivation, is thought to be one of the triggering factors for endometriosis [51]. The finding is from laboratory experiments conducted on endometrial cell cultures from women with and without the disease. ESCs that have been cultured with antioxidants inhibit thymidine intake, while those subjected to oxidative stress inducers seem to support endometrial stromal growth [51]. The antioxidant pathway is one of the systems used to reduce oxidative stress, and works by eliminating free radicals. The system mainly consists of superoxide dismutase, and works by eliminating superoxide anion, thus getting rid of hydrogen peroxide. Patients of endometriosis generally have a reduced antioxidant system. The intracellular antioxidant system, comprising of glutathione, is crucial for endometrial detoxification and is an important factor in the endometriosis' pathophysiology [52].

A group of eight women with endometriosis showed positive improvement in the treatment of pain and bleeding using antioxidant diindolylmethane (DIM) and dienogest compared to those treated using dienogest alone. The antioxidant, DIM, is produced by acidic substances from indole-3-carbinol and is present in vegetables such as broccoli, cabbage, cardamom, and Brussel sprouts. In addition to influencing estrogen activity in cells by inhibiting the estrogen receptor, the compound also contains some anti-tumor effects [53].

Mier-Cabrera et al. suggested the intake of a high antioxidant diet (HAD) with variations of 150% of the daily recommended vitamin A nutrient (equivalent to 1050 μg of retinol), 660% of the recommended vitamin C (500 mg) nutrients, and at least 133% of the recommended ration of vitamin E (20 mg). The consumption of HAD in women affected by endometriosis led to an improvement in peripheral enzymatic superoxide dismutase and glutathione peroxidose. The diet also reduced the peripheral concentration in malondialdehyde as well lipid hydroperoxides within a period of 3 months [13].

In a multicenter, non-comparative clinical trial, 398 patients were managed for endometriosis-associated pelvic pain with antioxidant preparations of N-acetyl cysteine, alpha-lipoic acid, and bromelain. The formula was proven to have antioxidant properties upstream in the Cox-2 pathway, without the risk of affecting the patient's fertility, or having other adverse side effects, as is the case with many non-steroidal anti-inflammatory agents (NSAIDs). The experiment's success is undoubtedly attributed to N-acetyl cysteine, an important precursor of reduced glutathione. The study showed improvement in endometriosis-related pelvic pain and lower need for rescue analgesics in women with endometriosis who achieve pregnancy [54].

26.2.3 Combination of Nutrients

The results of a diet consisting of a mixture of vitamins (B6, A, C, and E), mineral salts (Ca, Mg, Se, Zn, and Fe), VSL3 lactic ferments (*Bifidobacterium breve, Bifidobacterium longum, Bifidobacterium infantis, Lactobacillus acidophilus, Lactobacillus casei, Lactobacillus bulgaricus*, and *Streptococcus thermophilus*), omega-3 fatty acids (fish oil), and omega-6 fatty acids (fish oil) were evaluated by Sesti et al. in a comparative randomized trial [55]. In their first research, the efficacy of endometriosis-related pain and quality of life outcomes of conservative surgery plus placebo were assessed in comparison with conservative surgery plus hormone suppression, such as gonadotrophin-releasing hormone agonists (GnRHa) or estro-progestin, or diet therapy. The results of their study support the hypothesis that GnRHa, oral contraceptives, or diet therapy, following conservative surgery for endometriosis is more effective than a placebo in obtaining the remission of endometriosis-associated pain and improved quality of life, especially in women suffering from non-menstrual pelvic pain or dysmenorrhea [55]. Adopting an identical dietary compound in a group of patients experiencing endometrioma cystectomy and adhesiolysis, the authors did not report any differences in endometrioma recurrence in women following the diet, whether using GnRH analogs or the placebo [56].

26.2.4 What About Nutrients to Avoid?

The introduction of a low-FODMAP diet has transformed the paradigm of IBS people management over the last decade. FODMAP is a category of short-chain carbohydrates present in many fruits, vegetables, and grains, which are improperly processed and rapidly fermentable by bacteria [57]. In patients with visceral hypersensitivity, their osmotic activities and gas formation induce intestinal luminal dilation, causing pain and bloating, with indirect impacts on gut motility. In women with endometriosis, visceral hypersensitivity, a characteristic of IBS, is also reported, indicating that the low FODMAP diet could be an advantageous strategy [58]. In a retrospective analysis by Moore et al., the FODMAP diet proved beneficial in women with IBS and endometriosis, showing a higher response than the group with IBS alone. According to specific intent-to-treat, a significantly higher percentage of patients with documented endometriosis responded to the diet (72%) compared to those without (49%) [28].

Borghini et al. speculated that women with endometriosis have a high prevalence of nickel allergy, and a low-nickel diet may be recommended. Nickel allergy can manifest in the form of allergic contact mucositis and may cause IBS-like and extra-intestinal symptoms. In this study, 90.3% of patients presented a positive test for nickel allergic contact mucositis. Both gastrointestinal and gynecological symptoms revealed a statistically significant decrease after 3 months of a low-nickel diet [59].

In a small clinical series, two women with endometriosis got rid of the pain by consuming soy-free diets. This effect is understandable since soya is rich in phytoestrogens, and considering that endometriosis is an estrogen-dependent illness. The quantity of phytoestrogens present in soya is however relatively low, so the impact of soya-elimination in the suppression of endometriosis symptoms is debatable [60].

One case report recorded that a woman with celiac disease had an endometrioma and became pregnant after a gluten-free diet. However, it was not clear if gluten removal could also be successful against endometriosis [61]. Gluten is the structural compound of protein found in wheat, consisting of gliadin and glutenin. Wheat intake can lead to chronic inflammation since gliadin and wheat germ agglutinin increase permeability in the intestines and stimulates the immune system. However, since there was only one case report showing a positive result in the effect of gluten reduction on fertility in a patient that suffered from endometriosis and was gluten-intolerant. Thus, it is still unclear whether the elimination of gluten in diet could be a suitable solution for women affected by endometriosis, especially since whole grains are an important part of diet [62]. The use of a gluten-free diets as a supplementary therapy with dienogest to treat deep infiltrating endometriosis was evaluated in a retrospective study by Marziali et al. The data revealed a statistically significant improvement in pelvic pain in patients treated with the gluten-free diet compared to those treated with dienogest alone [63].

26.3 Complementary and Alternative Medicine

Since endometriosis symptoms can significantly impact women's quality of life, while the short-term and particularly long-term therapeutic benefits of the at hand nowadays approaches are quite limited, there is increasing frustration among patients who undergo only hormonal and/or surgical intervention. Taking this into account, women with endometriosis also look for more alternative treatments to support their physical and psychological well-being, such as complementary health approaches (CHAs), the name used by the National Center for Complementary and Integrative Health (NCCIH), and home remedies (HRs) [64]. CHAs and HRs, both unconventional medical approaches developed outside of traditional western medicine suggest remedies such as; the use of topical heat, homeopathy, massage, relaxation, kinesiology, physiotherapy, movement, acupuncture, electrotherapy, yoga, osteopathic manipulative therapy, and traditional Chinese medicine [65]. Complementary and alternative medicine (CAM), also called as an option "apart from" traditional medicine varies from the medical standard and is globally recognized as a form of medical care. The practices include the entire health systems, procedures, theories, cultural attitudes, and modalities as described in the 1995 CAM Research Methodology Conference. The therapies can be subdivided into five categories which are biological treatments, mind-body therapies, muscle-joint stimulations, energy therapies, and alternative medical systems [65]. In a research survey of 574 women with a documented endometriosis diagnosis, 62.5% reported using some form of CHA and HR. In contrast to people without these features, women suffering from fatigue more frequently chose alternative therapies. Moreover, the above alternative solutions are more often preferred by women who are unsatisfied with their doctor's health care [66]. An Australian survey of 7427 women recorded an increased use of vitamins, yoga, minerals, acupuncture, or traditional Chinese medicine than women without endometriosis [67]. As traditional treatments may not be adequately efficient, the women's wishes should be carefully evaluated, and clinicians should explore and facilitate individual treatment options to offer the best possible complete and accurate treatment for endometriosis.

26.3.1 Chinese Medicine Decoctions

Various traditional decoctions, such as Xuefu Zhuyu decoction (XZD), Xiaochaihu decoction (XCHD), Qu Yi Kang (QYK), YiWei San (YWS), and Huoxue Xiaoyi decoction (HXD), are utilized to treat endometriosis in China. Several studies have found that XZD can alleviate dysmenorrhea, reduce ectopic lesions, and assist fertility [68]. In a rat endometriosis-induced model, XCHD may reduce serum estradiol concentration and may diminish the expression of P450 aromatase protein and Cox-2 protein in endometriotic tissue. In a rat prototype undergoing XCHD therapy, endometrial lesion volume was significantly reduced at the same time as the serum and peritoneal fluid concentrations of IL-8, TNF-α, and VEGF [69]. Some researchers have found that QYK might lessen the peritoneal fluid concentrations of IL-2 and IL-6, suppress endometrial tissue growth and proliferation in rat models, and remove new vascular connections on the ectopic endometrium by diminishing the VEGF proteins synthesis inside endometrial tissue [70]. By reducing the expressions of intercellular adhesion molecule-1 (ICAM-1), MMP-9, and VEGF, HXD and YWS may down-regulate the process of adhesion, invasion, and local angiogenesis of endometriosis [71]. In a retrospective study, Meissner et al. attempted to determine the efficacy of combination therapy with traditional Chinese medicine and hypnotherapy systemic autoregulation therapy (SART) as an innovative approach for endometriosis symptoms. Forty-seven patients with endometriosis who were managed with SART were monitored by phone surveys. The median follow-up period was 5 years. On a 0–10-point visual analog scale, the median severity of pain associated with endometriosis was reduced from eight to three points. Therapy of endometriosis using traditional Chinese medicine and hypnotherapy may lead to significant pain relief and higher birth rates in patients with medication-refractory endometriosis [72].

26.3.2 Herbal Medicines (Phytotherapy)

Medicinal plants and botanical extracts are also widely adopted to treat the symptoms of many gynecological diseases, such as endometriosis. Medicinal herbs and their effective ingredients have antiproliferative, antioxidant, analgesic, and anti-inflammatory effects. These features can aid in the treatment or regression of endometriosis [73]. Moreover, the various systems implicated in endometriosis etiopathogenesis may be the object of herbal medicines. Reduced apoptosis and enhanced cell survival are often documented in the eutopic and ectopic endometrium of patients suffering from endometriosis in comparison with healthy controls, and some studies have examined the effects of different plants on apoptosis and cell survival. In addition, there is evidence that particular herbs may affect the epigenome, which is a therapeutic technique to theoretically correct the aberrant epigenetic modifications recorded in endometriosis [73]. Similarly, other pathways that have a central role in the progression of endometriosis have been investigated as potential targets for phytotherapy, such as:

1. Angiogenesis mediated by VEGF: *Alchemilla* (family of Rosaceae) [74]; *Allium sativum* (garlic) [75]; *Salvia miltiorrhiza* [76]; *Aloe vera* (family of Xanthorrhoeaceae) [77]; *Viburnum* (family of Caprifoliaceae) [78]; *Viburnum opulus* (family of Adoxaceae) [78]; *Achillea biebersteinii* (family of Asteraceae) [79]; *Alchemilla mollis* (family of Rosaceae) [74].
2. Altered inflammatory microenvironment involving cytokines and immune cells: *Allium sativum* (garlic) suppresses the leukocyte production of IL-10 [75]; *Artemisia princeps* (family of Asteraceae) reduces interferon-γ (IFN-γ), IL-2, TNF-α, and IL-1β [80]; *Aloe vera* (family of Xanthorrhoeaceae) [77], *Viburnum* (family of Caprifoliaceae) reduces TNF-α and IL-6 [78]; *Andrographis paniculate* (family of Acanthaceae), decreases Cox-2 activity and the phosphorylation

of p50 and p65 [81]; *Viburnum opulus* (family of Adoxaceae), *Achillea biebersteinii* (family of Asteraceae), and *Alchemilla mollis* (family of Rosaceae) decrease the levels of TNF-α and IL-6 [82–84]; *Tenacetum parthenium* (family of Asteraceae) inhibits prostaglandin synthesis and mast cell degranulation [85].

3. Reduction of oxidative stress improving antioxidant enzymes: *Allium sativum* (garlic) [75]; *Aloe vera* (family of Xanthorrhoeaceae) [77]; *Echinacea sp.* (family of Asteraceae) [86].
4. Proapoptotic effect inducing caspase and proapoptotic proteins: *Allium sativum* (garlic) [75]; *Salvia miltiorrhiza* [76]; *Artemisia princeps* (family of Asteraceae) [80]; *Aloe vera* (family of Xanthorrhoeaceae) [77].
5. Reduction in proliferation and migration, attenuating the expression of vascular cell adhesion molecule 1 (VCAM-1) and ICAM-1: *Allium sativum* (garlic) [75]; *Salvia miltiorrhiza* [76]; *Artemisia princeps* (family of Asteraceae) [80].

26.3.3 Herbal Extracts Therapies

Epigallocatechin Gallate (EGCG) is a green tea catechin monomer with potent anti-angiogenic, antioxidant, and proapoptotic characteristics and is, unsurprisingly, associated with the inhibition of endometriosis lesions induced in mouse models. EGCG's inhibition of VEGF/VEGF receptor signaling occurring through interferon-γ, MMP-9, and chemokine ligand has been shown to mediate the restricted macrovascular structure in lesions [87]. Treatment that started 15 days after surgery has been shown to influence the development and persistence of previously known endometriotic-like lesions [88].

Curcumin is *a Curcuma longa* (Zingiberaceae) polyphenolic monomer extract. It promotes microcirculation and has many pharmacological characteristics, such as antioxidants, anti-inflammatory, and anti-proliferative. Angiogenesis is fundamental for the persistence of peritoneal endometriosis implants and the development of endometriosis. Many studies have shown that curcumin consumption decreases the amount of microvessels and VEGF protein synthesis in the ectopic endometrium of rat endometriosis-induced models [89]. Other studies have shown that curcumin administration inhibits the expression and activity of MMP-3, MMP-9, MMP-2, TNF-α, monocyte chemotactic protein-1 (MCP-1), IL-6, and IL-8, [90].

Puerarin is a common isoflavonoid product derived from *Radix puerariae*. It has a low estrogen effect through binding to estrogen receptors. Puerarin administration decreases the levels of MMP-9, ICAM-1, and VEGF proteins, but enhances the percentage of TIMP-1 in endometriotic stromal cells. Moreover, it controls the enrollment of nuclear receptors that suppress the mitogen-activated protein kinase (MAPK) signaling pathway and also inhibits local aromatase [91].

Xanthohumol is a prenylated flavonoid with anti-proliferative, anti-inflammatory, and antiangiogenic characteristics. Xanthohumol has been demonstrated to successfully minimize the concentration of phosphoinositide 3-kinase protein in a Bagg-Albino (BALB/c) mouse endometriosis model and also to considerably reduce the microvessel density (MVD) [92].

Resveratrol, a stilbenoid, is a polyphenol present in red grapes, pistachios, peanuts blueberries, and other berries. This substance has been shown to reduce ectopic lesion size in a mouse model of endometriosis while decreasing peritoneal fluid VEGF and peritoneal and plasma monocyte chemoattractant protein-1 (MCP-1) levels and lesion VEGF expression [93]. Resveratrol therapy might reduce the expression of IGF-1 and hepatocyte growth factor (HGF) in ectopic, which plays a key role in disease progression [94].

Polydatin is a natural resveratrol glucoside and is found in fruit, grapes, and peanuts, and it is sometimes co-micronized to palmitoylethanolamide (PEA) as an alternative or supplementary treatment of pain control for endometriosis patients [95]. Polydatin has anti-inflammatory, antioxidant and anti-chemotactic activities, reducing the inflammatory response by suppressing the production of releasing pro-inflammatory mediators and mast cell degranulation, as well as changing eicosanoid production [96].

Palmitoylethanolamide (PEA) is a component of the N-acylethanolamine family of fatty acid amides. It is a signaling molecule that can regulate the activation of mast cells and microglial cells' activity. It works peripherally on the intermodulation between mast cells and nociceptive nerve fibers, and in the central nervous system, decreasing the central pain hypersensitization correlated with microglial activation [97]. High concentrations of activated mast cells have been observed in endometriotic lesions and, specifically, in deep infiltrating nodules, proximal to nerves, indicating that mast cells may provide endometriotic pain by having a direct impact on nerve structures. In fact, mast cells' activation can stimulate the excessive secretion of pro-inflammatory products liable for peripheral neuronal sensitization processes, which are intensified by microglial stimulation at the central level, with the production of chronic pelvic pain. Furthermore, cytokines and secreted growth factors facilitate the infiltration and growth of ectopic endometrium, promoting proliferation and angiogenesis. Therefore, mast cells can be a revolutionary target for treatment options intended to limit inflammation and the subsequent hyperalgesia and allodynia in patients with endometriosis [82]. A meta-analysis in 2017 showed that a combination of micronized PEA (400 mg) and polydatin (40 mg) dispensed orally twice daily for 3 months in a heterogeneous population of endometriotic patients with endometriosis-related pain resulted in a clinically important improvement in the VAS score for chronic pelvic pain and dysmenorrhea, as well as a more limited decrease in deep dyspareunia and no clinical decrease in dyschezia [83]. Stochino-Loi et al. found that patients with symptomatic endometriosis managed with 600 mg of ultramicronized palmitoylethanolamide twice daily for 10 days accompanied by co-micronized palmitoylethanolamide (400 mg) and polydatin (40 mg) for 80 days experienced a significant decrease in painful symptoms (assessed with VAS score) and an improvement in quality of life (QoL) and psychological well-being (evaluated with SF-36 and SCL-90). The finding that these two compounds enhance women's quality of life and psychological well-being can be related to the drug's pain control properties. However, recent medical research has shown a correlation between inflammatory diseases and emotional disorders. In particular, as far as endometriosis patients are concerned, immunological changes have been observed, resulting in imbalances in pro-(IL-1, IL-2, IFN-γ) and anti-inflammatory (IL-4) cytokine production, associated with mood disorders such as depression and anxiety. Moreover, this therapy does not display any significant side effects, which are especially acceptable for women who are seeking pregnancy and without other infertility factors [84]. Another recent study explored the effects of alpha-lipoic acid, palmitoylethanolamide, and myrrh on endometriosis cyst volume and pain in women with endometriosis. Endometrioma measurements did not improve after administering this compound, but chronic pelvic pain and dysmenorrhea assessed with VAS score significantly reduced [98].

26.3.4 Acupuncture and Electrotherapy

Acupuncture is one of the most important types of traditional Chinese medicine (TCM). There are many distinct types of acupuncture, such as body acupuncture, electroacupuncture, auricular acupuncture, and scalp acupuncture. Auricular acupuncture is the most widely performed because of the following five auricular acupuncture points: Ting Zhong (center of cymba auriculae), Pi Zhi Xia (hypo-cortex), Nei Fen Mi (endocrine), Jiao Gan (sympathetic), and Nei Sheng Zhi Qi (internal genitals), which are typically adopted to alleviate pain and treat the reproductive system [99]. In China, acupuncture and moxibustion practitioners interpret the human body as a whole, focused on the meridians, viscera, and Qi-blood principles. Chinese medicine assumes that Qi is the essential manifestation of human material foundation. Qi and blood have distinct functions, but are interrelated, delivering nutrients to the organs and tissues to sustain life-saving activities. The meridians in TCM corresponds to the pathways of Qi and blood, and these pathways are intertwined. TCM believes the pain is caused by blood or Qi stagnation in the uterus. Acupuncture can stimulate the circulation of blood and Qi, relying on the energy transfer of meridian acupoints and the central and peripheral nervous system's activity. When the flow of Qi and blood is free from obstruction, there might be less pain [100]. While endometriosis has not been described as a specific entity in the classical text of TCM, symptoms are considered in the categories of dysmenorrhea, irregular menstruation, abdominal mass, and infertility. The key pathology of endometriosis is the inhibited flow of Qi and blood culminating in congestion of the Chong and Ren channels. The concept underlying acupuncture practice is to correct the lack of balance and remove the obstacle in the associated channels [101].

The benefits of acupuncture can be correlated with the stimulation of analgesic pathways, such as the secretion of neurohumoral factors (including beta-endorphin, adenosine, acetylcholine, nitric oxide, and noradrenaline serotonin) and the regulation of multiple processes such as anti-inflammatory and inhibitory control mechanisms, inducing analgesia, sedation, and motor function recovery [102].

Lin et al. found that the therapeutic influence of acupuncture on dysmenorrhea could be attributable to its effects on the concentration of prostaglandin PGF2-α in menstrual blood. The same authors suggested that acupuncture can play a role in ovarian stimulation and fertility treatment by modifying the hypothalamic–pituitary–ovarian axis [103]. Other studies have also shown that acupuncture can reduce serum estradiol concentrations, thereby inhibiting ectopic endometrium growth and alleviating pain [104]. In a systematic review in 2011, Zhu et al. found that the improvement rate did not vary significantly between auricular acupuncture and Chinese herbal medicine in mild-to-moderate dysmenorrhea, although auricular acupuncture significantly reduced pain in patients with severe dysmenorrhea [105]. Another meta-analysis in 2017 showed that acupuncture has a more positive impact on pain levels and decreases CA-125 levels than other therapies such as traditional Chinese medicine, medications, or placebo [106]. In 2018, a randomized, single-blind, multicenter, placebo-controlled study began comparing the effectiveness and safety of acupuncture on endometriosis-related pelvic pain using comfort needles. This trial is still ongoing, and participants assigned to the treatment group are being treated in Guanyuan (CV4), Sanyinjiao (SP6), Taichong (LR3), Zhaohai (KI6), and Qichong (ST30) with acupuncture treatment, as long as the control group is undergoing acupuncture at non-acupoints [107].

Electrotherapy through transcutaneous electrical nerve stimulation (TENS) is a cheap, non-invasive, and easy-to-use pain relief treatment. TENS works by spinal blocking and releasing endogenous opioids [108]. Two physical therapy methods, namely, TENS-like acupuncture and self-administered TENS, applied in the sacral region of women with endometriosis, were evaluated by Mira et al. for 8 weeks. The study revealed no differences in the effectiveness between the two treatment groups concerning the procedure, indicating that both approaches successfully relieve chronic pelvic pain and deep dyspareunia and improve the quality of life of patients affected by deep endometriosis [108]. Bi et al. examined the impact of neuromuscular electrical stimulation (NMES) on the treatment of endometriosis-associated pain in another retrospective study. Eighty-three patients were allocated to the treatment group and received NMES treatment, while 71 patients in the waiting list formed the control group. After 10 weeks of treatment, those who received NMES therapy reported improved pain scores (evaluated with NRS score) and quality of life (assessed with the SF-36 scale) performance in comparison with patients on the waiting list [109].

26.3.5 Osteopathic Manipulative Therapy and Yoga

Osteopathy refers to a method of diagnosis and treatment by the American, Andrew Taylor Still. Its main objective is concentrated with the musculo-fascial structures and the effects on somatic symptoms. There have been developed three modes of practice, namely: pariental osteopathy, craniosacral therapy, and visceral osteopathy. Osteopathy tries to explain the cause-and-effect of some symptoms and illnesses associated with facial interactions of the musculoskeletal system and the delicate internal organs. The phlogosis in the internal organs may trigger severe musculoskeletal symptoms and vice versa. Axial skeletal injuries, for example, can cause abdominal symptoms. Additionally, the impairment on one skeletal part can cause illness elsewhere. Such interconnections are referred to as “lesion chains”

[110]. The osteopathic model suggests that the body's structure and functions are interconnected. The method looks at the body's natural internal mechanisms to perform self-repair, by the use of the human hands. Techniques of visceral manipulation, such as pelvic mobility, abdominal diaphragm mobility, liver mobility, and motility techniques among others can cause pain reduction as well as enhance QoL, thus supporting the correct functioning and stability of the pelvic organs [111].

In a meta-analysis, which included four studies analyzing the role of high-velocity, low- amplitude manipulation, and one on Toftness manipulation strategies in women with dysmenorrhea, Proctor et al. documented an absence evidence that spinal manipulation (parietal osteopathic technique) was successful [112].

Sillem et al. examined in a pilot study of 28 gynecologic patients, 14 women with a diagnosis of endometriosis whose only clinical observation was intense pelvic floor muscle stiffness. A systematic approach was adopted, beginning with the discharge of musculoskeletal blocks, especially the sacroiliac joints, followed by the mobilization of the diaphragm and abdominal organs. All patients reported pelvic relaxation and improvement of dyspareunia. This study stated that osteopathy might be considered a useful complementary treatment as an element of a multimodal approach to treating endometriosis and chronic pelvic pain [113]. Daraï et al. utilized osteopathy to cure 20 women affected by deep endometriosis infiltration and colorectal infiltration. The assessment of QoL with SF-36 improved physical well-being in 80% of patients and improved psychological well-being in 60% of patients [114]. Another case report by Goyal et al. demonstrated that osteopathic therapy consisting of all visceral manipulation techniques (i.e., pelvic, abdominal diaphragm, and liver mobility) might improve irregular uterine bleeding, pain, and quality of life in patients with endometriosis [115].

Yoga, defined as a body–mind activity by the World Health Organization, includes a spectrum of contemplative exercises that strengthen muscles and alleviate tension, helping to integrate body and mind [116]. Chronic stress was correlated with impaired hypothalamus–pituitary–adrenal axis and autonomic nervous system stimulation. This mechanism is liable for the sympathetic and parasympathetic nervous system's stress reaction and impacts the respiratory, cardiac, and digestive functions. The hypothalamic–pituitary–adrenal axis also controls the metabolism, immune system, thyroid, and reproduction [117]. Relaxation used in yoga exercises can reduce negative stress effects by providing equilibrium to the autonomic nervous system and the hypothalamic–pituitary–adrenal axis. Yoga, meditation, and relaxation may also be adjuvant therapies in clinical practice [117].

Recent studies on yoga practice in women with dysmenorrhea have indicated that some yoga poses can alleviate pain during menstruation. The cobra position enhances spinal stability and reinforces the muscles of the back. The cat position begins with a movement from the core and coordinates movement and breathing. The fish position decreases the tension of the neck and shoulder muscles and increases the spine's flexibility. According to these study results, it can be assumed that yoga could be a good strategy to reduce not only menstrual pain but also the pain associated with endometriosis. The practice of yoga may regulate the pain gate's control in the spinal cord and the release of natural opioids in the body [118].

Gonçalves et al. compared chronic pelvic pain, menstrual cycles, and QoL in two groups of women with endometriosis: those who did and those who did not take part in a specific 8-week yoga intervention. The procedure consisted of relaxing exercises, breathing-related posture, and conversations with women before and after sessions. The technique demonstrated effectiveness in relieving pain and improving QoL, with no difference in the menstrual flow [119].

References

1. Harvie M, Howell A, Evans DG. Can diet and lifestyle prevent breast cancer: what is the evidence? Am Soc Clin Oncol Educ Book. 2015:e66–73. https://doi.org/10.14694/edbook_am.2015.35.e66.
2. Jurkiewicz-Przondziono J, Lemm M, Kwiatkowska-Pamula A, Ziółłko E, Wójtowicz MK. Influence of diet on the risk of developing endometriosis. Ginekol Pol. 2017;88:96–102. https://doi.org/10.5603/GP.a2017.0017.
3. Galland L. Diet and inflammation. Nutr Clin Pract. 2010;25:634–40. https://doi.org/10.1177/0884533610385703.
4. Fjerbæk A, Knudsen UB. Endometriosis, dysmenorrhea and diet-what is the evidence? Eur J Obstet Gynecol Reprod Biol. 2007;132:140–7. https://doi.org/10.1016/j.ejogrb.2006.12.006.
5. Wu MH, Lu CW, Chuang PC, Tsai SJ. Prostaglandin E2: the master of endometriosis? Exp Biol Med. 2010;235:668–77. https://doi.org/10.1258/ebm.2010.009321.
6. Simopoulos AP. The omega-6/omega-3 fatty acid ratio: health implications. Oléagineux Corps Gras Lipides. 2010;17:267–75. https://doi.org/10.1051/ocl.2010.0325.
7. Attaman JA, Stanic AK, Kim M, Lynch MP, Rueda BR, Styer AK. The anti-inflammatory impact of omega-3 polyunsaturated fatty acids during the establishment of endometriosis-like lesions. Am J Reprod Immunol. 2014;72:392–402. https://doi.org/10.1111/aji.12276.
8. Covens AL, Christopher P, Casper RF. The effect of dietary supplementation with fish oil fatty acids on surgically induced endometriosis in the rabbit. Fertil Steril. 1988;49:698–703. https://doi.org/10.1016/s0015-0282(16)59842-2.
9. Mozaffarian D. Trans fatty acids – effects on systemic inflammation and endothelial function. Atheroscler Suppl. 2006;7:29–32. https://doi.org/10.1016/j.atherosclerosissup.2006.04.007.
10. Laganà AS, Garzon S, Götte M, Viganò P, Franchi M, Ghezzi F, et al. The pathogenesis of endometriosis: molecular and cell biology insights. Int J Mol Sci. 2019;20. https://doi.org/10.3390/ijms20225615.
11. Brinkman MT, Baglietto L, Krishnan K, English DR, Severi G, Morris HA, et al. Consumption of animal products, their nutrient components and postmenopausal circulating steroid hormone concentrations. Eur J Clin Nutr. 2010;64:176–83. https://doi.org/10.1038/ejcn.2009.129.
12. Harel Z, Biro FM, Kottenhahn RK, Rosenthal SL. Supplementation with omega-3 polyunsaturated fatty acids in the management of dysmenorrhea in adolescents. Am J Obstet Gynecol. 1996;174:1335–8. https://doi.org/10.1016/S0002-9378(96)70681-6.
13. Mier-Cabrera J, Aburto-Soto T, Burrola-Méndez S, Jiménez-Zamudio L, Tolentino MC, Casanueva E, et al. Women with endometriosis improved their peripheral antioxidant markers after the application of a high antioxidant diet. Reprod Biol Endocrinol. 2009;7. https://doi.org/10.1186/1477-7827-7-54.
14. Sawatsri S, Desai N, Rock JA, Sidell N. Retinoic acid suppresses interleukin-6 production in human endometrial cells. Fertil Steril. 2000;73:1012–9. https://doi.org/10.1016/S0015-0282(00)00483-0.
15. Traber MG, Stevens JF. Vitamins C and E: beneficial effects from a mechanistic perspective. Free Radic Biol Med. 2011;51:1000–13. https://doi.org/10.1016/j.freeradbiomed.2011.05.017.

16. Jackson LW, Schisterman EF, Dey-Rao R, Browne R, Armstrong D. Oxidative stress and endometriosis. Hum Reprod. 2005;20:2014–20. https://doi.org/10.1093/humrep/dei001.
17. Gerhard I, Runnebaum B. The limits of hormone substitution in pollutant exposure and fertility disorders. Zentralbl Gynakol. 1992;114:593–602.
18. Grassi P, Fattore E, Generoso C, Fanelli R, Arvati M, Zuccato E. Polychlorobiphenyls (PCBs), polychlorinated dibenzo-p-dioxins (PCDDs) and dibenzofurans (PCDFs) in fruit and vegetables from an industrial area in northern Italy. Chemosphere. 2010;79:292–8. https://doi.org/10.1016/j.chemosphere.2010.01.028.
19. Chambers ES, Hawrylowicz CM. The impact of vitamin D on regulatory T cells. Curr Allergy Asthma Rep. 2011;11:29–36. https://doi.org/10.1007/s11882-010-0161-8.
20. Miyashita M, Koga K, Izumi G, Sue F, Makabe T, Taguchi A, et al. Effects of 1,25-Dihydroxy vitamin d3 on endometriosis. J Clin Endocrinol Metab. 2016;101:2371–9. https://doi.org/10.1210/jc.2016-1515.
21. Yildirim B, Guler T, Akbulut M, Oztekin O, Sariiz G. 1–Alpha, 25–Dihydroxyvitamin D3 regresses endometriotic implants in rats by inhibiting neovascularization and altering regulation of matrix metalloproteinase. Postgrad Med. 2014;126:104–10. https://doi.org/10.3810/pgm.2014.01.2730.
22. Ciavattini A, Serri M, Delli Carpini G, Morini S, Clemente N. Ovarian endometriosis and vitamin D serum levels. Gynecol Endocrinol. 2017;33:164–7. https://doi.org/10.1080/09513590.2016.1239254.
23. Harris HR, Chavarro JE, Malspeis S, Willett WC, Missmer SA. Dairy-food, calcium, magnesium, and vitamin D intake and endometriosis: a prospective cohort study. Am J Epidemiol. 2013;177:420–30. https://doi.org/10.1093/aje/kws247.
24. Turgut A, Özler A, Görük NY, Tunc SY, Evliyaoglu O, Gül T. Copper, ceruloplasmin and oxidative stress in patients with advanced-stage endometriosis. Eur Rev Med Pharmacol Sci. 2013;17:1472–8.
25. Parazzini F, Chiaffarino F, Surace M, Chatenoud L, Cipriani S, Chiantera V, et al. Selected food intake and risk of endometriosis. Hum Reprod. 2004;19:1755–9. https://doi.org/10.1093/humrep/deh395.
26. Trabert B, Peters U, De Roos AJ, Scholes D, Holt VL. Diet and risk of endometriosis in a population-based case-control study. Br J Nutr. 2011;105:459–67. https://doi.org/10.1017/S0007114510003661.
27. Harris HR, Eke AC, Chavarro JE, Missmer SA. Fruit and vegetable consumption and risk of endometriosis. Hum Reprod. 2018;33:715–27. https://doi.org/10.1093/humrep/dey014.
28. Moore JS, Gibson PR, Perry RE, Burgell RE. Endometriosis in patients with irritable bowel syndrome: specific symptomatic and demographic profile, and response to the low FODMAP diet. Aust N Z J Obstet Gynaecol. 2017;57:201–5. https://doi.org/10.1111/ajo.12594.
29. Yamamoto A, Harris HR, Vitonis AF, Chavarro JE, Missmer SA. A prospective cohort study of meat and fish consumption and endometriosis risk. Am J Obstet Gynecol. 2018;219:178.e1–178.e10. https://doi.org/10.1016/j.ajog.2018.05.034.
30. Missmer SA, Chavarro JE, Malspeis S, Bertone-Johnson ER, Hornstein MD, Spiegelman D, et al. A prospective study of dietary fat consumption and endometriosis risk. Hum Reprod. 2010;25:1528–35. https://doi.org/10.1093/humrep/deq044.
31. Lebovic DI, Mwenda JM, Chai DC, Mueller MD, Santi A, Fisseha S, et al. PPAR-gamma receptor ligand induces regression of endometrial explants in baboons: a prospective, randomized, placebo- and drug-controlled study. Fertil Steril. 2007;88:1108–19. https://doi.org/10.1016/j.fertnstert.2006.12.072.
32. Nodler JL, Harris HR, Chavarro JE, Frazier AL, Missmer SA. Dairy consumption during adolescence and endometriosis risk. Am J Obstet Gynecol, Mosby Inc. 2020;222:257.e1–257.e16. https://doi.org/10.1016/j.ajog.2019.09.010.
33. Jefferson WN, Patisaul HB, Williams CJ. Reproductive consequences of developmental phytoestrogen exposure. Reproduction. 2012;143:247–60. https://doi.org/10.1530/REP-11-0369.

34. Mvondo MA, Ekenfack JD, Minko Essono S, Saah Namekong H, Awounfack CF, Laschke MW, et al. Soy intake since the prepubertal age may contribute to the pathogenesis of endometriosis in adulthood. J Med Food. 2019;22:631–8. https://doi.org/10.1089/jmf.2018.0160.
35. Greathouse KL, Bredfeldt T, Everitt JI, Lin K, Berry T, Kannan K, et al. Environmental estrogens differentially engage the histone methyltransferase EZH2 to increase risk of uterine tumorigenesis. Mol Cancer Res. 2012;10:546–57. https://doi.org/10.1158/1541-7786.MCR-11-0605.
36. Chen Y, Chen C, Shi S, Han J, Wang J, Hu J, et al. Endometriotic implants regress in rat models treated with puerarin by decreasing estradiol level. Reprod Sci. 2011;18:886–91. https://doi.org/10.1177/1933719111398500.
37. Mumford SL, Weck J, Kannan K, Louis GMB. Urinary phytoestrogen concentrations are not associated with incident endometriosis in premenopausal women. J Nutr. 2017;147:227–34. https://doi.org/10.3945/jn.116.238840.
38. Chiaffarino F, Bravi F, Cipriani S, Parazzini F, Ricci E, Viganò P, et al. Coffee and caffeine intake and risk of endometriosis: a meta-analysis. Eur J Nutr. 2014;53:1573–9. https://doi.org/10.1007/s00394-014-0662-7.
39. Wedick NM, Mantzoros CS, Ding EL, Brennan AM, Rosner B, Rimm EB, et al. The effects of caffeinated and decaffeinated coffee on sex hormone-binding globulin and endogenous sex hormone levels: a randomized controlled trial. Nutr J. 2012;11. https://doi.org/10.1186/1475-2891-11-86.
40. Friberg E, Wallin A, Wolk A. Sucrose, high-sugar foods, and risk of endometrial cancer – a population-based cohort study. Cancer Epidemiol Biomark Prev. 2011;20:1831–7. https://doi.org/10.1158/1055-9965.EPI-11-0402.
41. Savaris AL, Do Amaral VF. Nutrient intake, anthropometric data and correlations with the systemic antioxidant capacity of women with pelvic endometriosis. Eur J Obstet Gynecol Reprod Biol. 2011;158:314–8. https://doi.org/10.1016/j.ejogrb.2011.05.014.
42. Schink M, Konturek PC, Herbert SL, Renner SP, Burghaus S, Blum S, et al. Different nutrient intake and prevalence of gastrointestinal comorbidities in women with endometriosis. J Physiol Pharmacol. 2019;70. https://doi.org/10.26402/jpp.2019.2.09.
43. Maroun P, Cooper MJW, Reid GD, Keirse MJNC. Relevance of gastrointestinal symptoms in endometriosis. Aust N Z J Obstet Gynaecol. 2009;49:411–4. https://doi.org/10.1111/j.1479-828X.2009.01030.x.
44. Lea R, Whorwell PJ. Irritable bowel syndrome or endometriosis, or both? Eur J Gastroenterol Hepatol. 2003;15:1131–3. https://doi.org/10.1097/00042737-200310000-00012.
45. Armour M, Sinclair J, Chalmers KJ, Smith CA. Self-management strategies amongst Australian women with endometriosis: a national online survey. BMC Complement Altern Med. 2019;19. https://doi.org/10.1186/s12906-019-2431-x.
46. Huijs E, Nap A. The effects of nutrients on symptoms in women with endometriosis: a systematic review. Reprod Biomed Online. 2020;41:317–28. https://doi.org/10.1016/j.rbmo.2020.04.014.
47. Almassinokiani F, Khodaverdi S, Solaymani-Dodaran M, Akbari P, Pazouki A. Effects of vitamin D on endometriosis-related pain: a double-blind clinical trial. Med Sci Monit. 2016;22:4960–6. https://doi.org/10.12659/MSM.901838.
48. Calder PC. Marine omega-3 fatty acids and inflammatory processes: effects, mechanisms and clinical relevance. Biochim Biophys Acta. 1851;2015:469–84. https://doi.org/10.1016/j.bbalip.2014.08.010.
49. Netsu S, Konno R, Odagiri K, Soma M, Fujiwara H, Suzuki M. Oral eicosapentaenoic acid supplementation as possible therapy for endometriosis. Fertil Steril. 2008;90:1496–502. https://doi.org/10.1016/j.fertnstert.2007.08.014.
50. Nodler JL, DiVasta AD, Vitonis AF, Karevicius S, Malsch M, Sarda V, et al. Supplementation with vitamin D or ω-3 fatty acids in adolescent girls and young women with endometriosis (SAGE): a double-blind, randomized, placebo-controlled trial. Am J Clin Nutr. 2020;112:229–36. https://doi.org/10.1093/ajcn/nqaa096.

51. Foyouzi N, Berkkanoglu M, Arici A, Kwintkiewicz J, Izquierdo D, Duleba AJ. Effects of oxidants and antioxidants on proliferation of endometrial stromal cells. Fertil Steril. 2004;82:1019–22. https://doi.org/10.1016/j.fertnstert.2004.02.133.
52. Szczepańska M, Koźlik J, Skrzypczak J, Mikołajczyk M. Oxidative stress may be a piece in the endometriosis puzzle. Fertil Steril. 2003;79:1288–93. https://doi.org/10.1016/S0015-0282(03)00266-8.
53. Morales-Prieto DM, Herrmann J, Osterwald H, Kochhar PS, Schleussner E, Markert UR, et al. Comparison of dienogest effects upon 3,3′–diindolylmethane supplementation in models of endometriosis and clinical cases. Reprod Biol. 2018;18:252–8. https://doi.org/10.1016/j.repbio.2018.07.002.
54. Lete I, Mendoza N, de la Viuda E, Carmona F. Effectiveness of an antioxidant preparation with N-acetyl cysteine, alpha lipoic acid and bromelain in the treatment of endometriosis-associated pelvic pain: LEAP study. Eur J Obstet Gynecol Reprod Biol. 2018;228:221–4. https://doi.org/10.1016/j.ejogrb.2018.07.002.
55. Sesti F, Pietropolli A, Capozzolo T, Broccoli P, Pierangeli S, Bollea MR, et al. Hormonal suppression treatment or dietary therapy versus placebo in the control of painful symptoms after conservative surgery for endometriosis stage III-IV. A randomized comparative trial. Fertil Steril. 2007;88:1541–7. https://doi.org/10.1016/j.fertnstert.2007.01.053.
56. Sesti F, Capozzolo T, Pietropolli A, Marziali M, Bollea MR, Piccione E. Recurrence rate of endometrioma after laparoscopic cystectomy: a comparative randomized trial between post-operative hormonal suppression treatment or dietary therapy vs. placebo. Eur J Obstet Gynecol Reprod Biol. 2009;147:72–7. https://doi.org/10.1016/j.ejogrb.2009.07.003.
57. Halmos EP, Power VA, Shepherd SJ, Gibson PR, Muir JG. A diet low in FODMAPs reduces symptoms of irritable bowel syndrome. Gastroenterology. 2014;146. https://doi.org/10.1053/j.gastro.2013.09.046.
58. Issa B, Onon TS, Agrawal A, Shekhar C, Morris J, Hamdy S, et al. Visceral hypersensitivity in endometriosis: a new target for treatment? Gut. 2012;61:367–72. https://doi.org/10.1136/gutjnl-2011-300306.
59. Borghini R, Porpora MG, Casale R, Marino M, Palmieri E, Greco N, et al. Irritable bowel syndrome-like disorders in endometriosis: prevalence of nickel sensitivity and effects of a low-nickel diet. An open-label pilot study. Nutrients. 2020:12. https://doi.org/10.3390/nu12020341.
60. Chandrareddy A, Muneyyirci-Delale O, McFarlane SI, Murad OM. Adverse effects of phytoestrogens on reproductive health: a report of three cases. Complement Ther Clin Pract. 2008;14:132–5. https://doi.org/10.1016/j.ctcp.2008.01.002.
61. Caserta D, Matteucci E, Ralli E, Bordi G, Moscarini M. Celiac disease and endometriosis: an insidious and worrisome association hard to diagnose: a case report. Clin Exp Obstet Gynecol. 2014;41:346–8.
62. De Punder K, Pruimboom L. The dietary intake of wheat and other cereal grains and their role in inflammation. Nutrients. 2013;5:771–87. https://doi.org/10.3390/nu5030771.
63. Marziali M, Capozzolo T. Role of gluten-free diet in the management of chronic pelvic pain of deep infiltranting endometriosis. J Minim Invasive Gynecol. 2015;22:S51–2. https://doi.org/10.1016/j.jmig.2015.08.142.
64. National Center for Complementary and Integrative Health. https://www.nccih.nih.gov/. Accessed 24 Oct 2020.
65. Kong S, Zhang YH, Liu CF, Tsui I, Guo Y, Ai BB, et al. The complementary and alternative medicine for endometriosis: a review of utilization and mechanism. Evid Based Complement Alternat Med. 2014;2014. https://doi.org/10.1155/2014/146383.
66. Schwartz ASK, Gross E, Geraedts K, Rauchfuss M, Wölfler MM, Häberlin F, et al. The use of home remedies and complementary health approaches in endometriosis. Reprod Biomed Online. 2019;38:260–71. https://doi.org/10.1016/j.rbmo.2018.10.009.
67. Fisher C, Adams J, Hickman L, Sibbritt D. The use of complementary and alternative medicine by 7427 Australian women with cyclic perimenstrual pain and discomfort: a

cross-sectional study. BMC Complement Altern Med. 2016;16:1–11. https://doi.org/10.1186/s12906-016-1119-8.
68. Zhang JY. Clinical observation of 79 endometriosis patients treated with Xuefu Zhuyu Decoction. Zhejiang J Tradit Chin Med. 2008;43:455.
69. Zhang WJ, Wang ZN, Zhen PE, Zheng H. The regulation of Xiaochaihu Decoction on interleukin-8 and tumor necrosis factor in endometriotic tissues. Shaanxi J Tradit Chin Med. 2004;5:468–70.
70. Yang JB, Xu C. Effects of Quyikang on IL-2 and IL-6 in peritoneal fluid of endometriosis rats. Yunnan J Tradit Chin Med Mater Med. 2007;28:36–9.
71. Zhao R, Yang Y, Li M, Xu C, Xia W. Influences of Huoxue Xiaoyi Fang on ICAM-1, MMP-9 and VEGF in rats with endometriosis [J]. J Beijing Univ Tradit Chin Med. 2012;35(12):826–99.
72. Meissner K, Böhling B, Schweizer-Arau A. Long-term effects of traditional Chinese medicine and hypnotherapy in patients with severe endometriosis – a retrospective evaluation. Forsch Komplementmed. 2010;17:314–20. https://doi.org/10.1159/000322890.
73. Ilhan M, Gürağaç Dereli FT, Akkol EK. Novel drug targets with traditional herbal medicines for overcoming endometriosis. Curr Drug Deliv. 2019;16:386–99. https://doi.org/10.2174/1567201816666181227112421.
74. Küpeli Akkol E, Demirel MA, Bahadır Acıkara O, Süntar I, Ergene B, Ilhan M, et al. Phytochemical analyses and effects of Alchemilla mollis (Buser) Rothm. and Alchemilla persica Rothm. in rat endometriosis model. Arch Gynecol Obstet. 2015;292:619–28. https://doi.org/10.1007/s00404-015-3665-6.
75. Bayan L, Koulivand PH, Gorji A. Garlic: a review of potential therapeutic effects. Avicenna J Phytomed. 2014;4:1–14. https://doi.org/10.22038/ajp.2014.1741.
76. Su CY, Ming QL, Rahman K, Han T, Qin LP. Salvia miltiorrhiza: traditional medicinal uses, chemistry, and pharmacology. Chin J Nat Med. 2015;13:163–82. https://doi.org/10.1016/S1875-5364(15)30002-9.
77. Bostanci MS, Bakacak M, Kizilkale Yildirim O, Yildirim G, Attar R, Özkan F, et al. Effects of aloe vera gel on the induction of endometriosis and regression of endometrial explants in a rat model. Clin Exp Obstet Gynecol. 2016;43:529–33.
78. Saltan G, Süntar I, Ozbilgin S, Ilhan M, Demirel MA, Oz BE, et al. Viburnum opulus L.: a remedy for the treatment of endometriosis demonstrated by rat model of surgically-induced endometriosis. J Ethnopharmacol. 2016;193:450–5. https://doi.org/10.1016/j.jep.2016.09.029.
79. Demirel MA, Suntar I, Ilhan M, Keles H, Kupeli AE. Experimental endometriosis remission in rats treated with Achillea biebersteinii Afan.: histopathological evaluation and determination of cytokine levels. Eur J Obstet Gynecol Reprod Biol. 2014;175:172–7. https://doi.org/10.1016/j.ejogrb.2014.01.011.
80. Kim JH, Jung SH, Yang YI, Ahn JH, Cho JG, Lee KT, et al. Artemisia leaf extract induces apoptosis in human endometriotic cells through regulation of the p38 and NFκB pathways. J Ethnopharmacol. 2013;145:767–75. https://doi.org/10.1016/j.jep.2012.12.003.
81. Zheng W, Cao L, Xu Z, Ma Y, Liang X. Anti-Angiogenic alternative and complementary medicines for the treatment of endometriosis: a review of potential molecular mechanisms. Evid Based Complement Alternat Med. 2018;2018. https://doi.org/10.1155/2018/4128984.
82. Skaper SD, Facci L. Mast cell-glia axis in neuroinflammation and therapeutic potential of the anandamide congener palmitoylethanolamide. Philos Trans R Soc Lond B Biol Sci. 2012;367:3312–25. https://doi.org/10.1098/rstb.2011.0391.
83. Indraccolo U, Indraccolo SR, Mignini F. Micronized palmitoylethanolamide/trans-polydatin treatment of endometriosis-related pain: a meta-analysis. Ann Ist Super Sanita. 2017;53:125–34. https://doi.org/10.4415/ANN_17_02_08.
84. Stochino-Loi E, Pontis A, Cofelice V, Pirarba S, Fais MF, Daniilidis A, et al. Effect of ultramicronized-palmitoylethanolamide and co-micronizedpalmitoylethanolamide/polydatin on chronic pelvic pain and quality of life in endometriosis patients: an open-label pilot study. Int J Women's Health. 2019;11:443–9. https://doi.org/10.2147/IJWH.S204275.

85. Pareek A, Suthar M, Rathore GS, Bansal V. Feverfew (Tanacetum parthenium L.): a systematic review. Pharmacogn Rev. 2011;5:103–10. https://doi.org/10.4103/0973-7847.79105.
86. Sharma M, Schoop R, Hudson JB. Echinacea as an antiinflammatory agent: the influence of physiologically relevant parameters. Phytother Res. 2009;23:863–7. https://doi.org/10.1002/ptr.2714.
87. Laschke MW, Schwender C, Scheuer C, Vollmar B, Menger MD. Epigallocatechin-3-gallate inhibits estrogen-induced activation of endometrial cells in vitro and causes regression of endometriotic lesions in vivo. Hum Reprod. 2008;23:2308–18. https://doi.org/10.1093/humrep/den245.
88. Ricci AG, Olivares CN, Bilotas MA, Bastón JI, Singla JJ, Meresman GF, et al. Natural therapies assessment for the treatment of endometriosis. Hum Reprod. 2013;28:178–88. https://doi.org/10.1093/humrep/des369.
89. Arablou T, Kolahdouz-Mohammadi R. Curcumin and endometriosis: review on potential roles and molecular mechanisms. Biomed Pharmacother. 2018;97:91–7. https://doi.org/10.1016/j.biopha.2017.10.119.
90. Kim KH, Lee EN, Park JK, Lee JR, Kim JH, Choi HJ, et al. Curcumin attenuates TNF-α-induced expression of intercellular adhesion molecule-1, vascular cell adhesion molecule-1 and proinflammatory cytokines in human endometriotic stromal cells. Phytother Res. 2012;26:1037–47. https://doi.org/10.1002/ptr.3694.
91. Wang D, Liu Y, Han J, Zai D, Ji M, Cheng W, et al. Puerarin suppresses invasion and vascularization of endometriosis tissue stimulated by 17β-estradiol. PLoS One. 2011;6:e25011. https://doi.org/10.1371/journal.pone.0025011.
92. Rudzitis-Auth J, Krbel C, Scheuer C, Menger MD, Laschke MW. Xanthohumol inhibits growth and vascularization of developing endometriotic lesions. Hum Reprod. 2012;27:1735–44. https://doi.org/10.1093/humrep/des095.
93. Ergenoğlu AM, Yeniel AÖ, Erbaş O, Aktuğ H, Yildirim N, Ulukuş M, et al. Regression of endometrial implants by resveratrol in an experimentally induced endometriosis model in rats. Reprod Sci. 2013;20:1230–6. https://doi.org/10.1177/1933719113483014.
94. Arablou T, Delbandi AA, Khodaverdi S, Arefi S, Kolahdouz-Mohammadi R, Heidari S, et al. Resveratrol reduces the expression of insulin-like growth factor-1 and hepatocyte growth factor in stromal cells of women with endometriosis compared with nonendometriotic women. Phytother Res. 2019;33:1044–54. https://doi.org/10.1002/ptr.6298.
95. Indraccolo U, Barbieri F. Effect of palmitoylethanolamide-polydatin combination on chronic pelvic pain associated with endometriosis: preliminary observations. Eur J Obstet Gynecol Reprod Biol. 2010;150:76–9. https://doi.org/10.1016/j.ejogrb.2010.01.008.
96. De La Lastra CA, Villegas I. Resveratrol as an anti-inflammatory and anti-aging agent: mechanisms and clinical implications. Mol Nutr Food Res. 2005;49:405–30. https://doi.org/10.1002/mnfr.200500022.
97. Cerrato S, Brazis P, della Valle MF, Miolo A, Puigdemont A. Effects of palmitoylethanolamide on immunologically induced histamine, PGD2 and TNFα release from canine skin mast cells. Vet Immunol Immunopathol. 2010;133:9–15. https://doi.org/10.1016/j.vetimm.2009.06.011.
98. De Leo V, Cagnacci A, Cappelli V, Biasioli A, Leonardi D, Seracchioli R. Role of a natural integrator based on lipoic acid, palmitoiletanolamide and myrrh in the treatment of chronic pelvic pain and endometriosis. Minerva Ginecol. 2019;71:191–5. https://doi.org/10.23736/S0026-4784.19.04384-3.
99. Xiang D, Situ Y, Liang X, Cheng L, Zhang G. Ear acupuncture therapy for 37 cases of dysmenorrhea due to endometriosis. J Tradit Chin Med. 2002;22:282–5.
100. Wang SM, Kain ZN, White P. Acupuncture analgesia: I. The scientific basis. Anesth Analg. 2008;106:602–10. https://doi.org/10.1213/01.ane.0000277493.42335.7b.
101. Liao XH, Zhang GM, Qi QY, Zhang YY. Overview of TCM research on endometriosis. Zhong Yi Yao Xin Xi (Inf Tradit Chin Med). 2008;25:24–5.
102. Leung L. Neurophysiological basis of acupuncture-induced analgesia-an updated review. J Acupunct Meridian Stud. 2012;5:261–70. https://doi.org/10.1016/j.jams.2012.07.017.

103. Lin LL, Liu CZ, Huang BY. Clinical observation on treatment of primary dysmenorrhea with acupuncture and massage. Zhongguo Zhong Xi Yi Jie He Za Zhi. 2008;28:418–20.
104. Ma J, Yun-guang H, Zhang DH. Effects of acupuncture on bone metabolism and serum estradiol level in ovariectomy-induced osteoporosis rats. Zhen Ci Yan Jiu (Chin J Integr Tradit West Med). 2008;33:235–9.
105. Zhu X, Hamilton KD, McNicol ED. Acupuncture for pain in endometriosis. Cochrane Database Syst Rev. 2011:CD007864. https://doi.org/10.1002/14651858.cd007864.pub2.
106. Xu Y, Zhao W, Li T, Zhao Y, Bu H, Song S. Effects of acupuncture for the treatment of endometriosis-related pain: a systematic review and meta-analysis. PLoS One. 2017;12. https://doi.org/10.1371/journal.pone.0186616.
107. Liang R, Li P, Peng X, Xu L, Fan P, Peng J, et al. Efficacy of acupuncture on pelvic pain in patients with endometriosis: study protocol for a randomized, single-blind, multi-center, placebo-controlled trial. Trials. 2018;19. https://doi.org/10.1186/s13063-018-2684-6.
108. Mira TAA, Giraldo PC, Yela DA, Benetti-Pinto CL. Effectiveness of complementary pain treatment for women with deep endometriosis through transcutaneous electrical nerve stimulation (TENS): randomized controlled trial. Eur J Obstet Gynecol Reprod Biol. 2015;194:1–6. https://doi.org/10.1016/j.ejogrb.2015.07.009.
109. Bi XL, Xie CX. Effect of neuromuscular electrical stimulation for endometriosis-associated pain. Medicine (United States). 2018;97. https://doi.org/10.1097/MD.0000000000011266.
110. Haas NP, Hoppe JD, Scriba PC. Wissenschaftliche Bewertung osteopathischer Verfahren. Bekanntgabe Der Herausgeber Dtsch Ärztebl. 2009;106:A2325–34.
111. Licciardone JC, Buchanan S, Hensel KL, King HH, Fulda KG, Stoll ST. Osteopathic manipulative treatment of back pain and related symptoms during pregnancy: a randomized controlled trial. Am J Obstet Gynecol. 2010;202:43.e1–8. https://doi.org/10.1016/j.ajog.2009.07.057.
112. Proctor M, Hing W, Johnson TC, Murphy PA, Brown J. Spinal manipulation for dysmenorrhoea. Cochrane Database Syst Rev. 2006;2006. https://doi.org/10.1002/14651858.cd002119.pub3.
113. Sillem M, Juhasz-Böss I, Klausmeier I, Mechsner S, Siedentopf F, Solomayer E. Osteopathy for endometriosis and chronic pelvic pain – a pilot study. Geburtshilfe Frauenheilkd. 2016;76:960–3. https://doi.org/10.1055/s-0042-111010.
114. Daraï C, Deboute O, Zacharopoulou C, Laas E, Canlorbe G, Belghiti J, et al. Impact of osteopathic manipulative therapy on quality of life of patients with deep infiltrating endometriosis with colorectal involvement: results of a pilot study. Eur J Obstet Gynecol Reprod Biol. 2015;188:70–3. https://doi.org/10.1016/j.ejogrb.2015.03.001.
115. Goyal K, Goyal M, Narkeesh K, John Samuel A, Sharma S, Chatterjee S, et al. The effectiveness of osteopathic manipulative treatment in an abnormal uterine bleeding related pain and health related quality of life (HR-QoL) – a case report. J Bodyw Mov Ther. 2017;21:569–73. https://doi.org/10.1016/j.jbmt.2016.08.010.
116. World Health Organization. Traditional medicine strategy 2002–2005. 2002 (WHO/EDM/TRM/2002.1). http://www.who.int/medicines/publications/traditional/policy/en/. Accessed 24 Oct 2020.
117. Jeter PE, Slutsky J, Singh N, Khalsa SBS. Yoga as a therapeutic intervention: a bibliometric analysis of published research studies from 1967 to 2013. J Altern Complement Med. 2015;21:586–92. https://doi.org/10.1089/acm.2015.0057.
118. Rakhshaee Z. Effect of three yoga poses (cobra, cat and fish poses) in women with primary dysmenorrhea: a randomized clinical trial. J Pediatr Adolesc Gynecol. 2011;24:192–6. https://doi.org/10.1016/j.jpag.2011.01.059.
119. Gonçalves AV, Barros NF, Bahamondes L. The practice of hatha yoga for the treatment of pain associated with endometriosis. J Altern Complement Med. 2017;23:45–52. https://doi.org/10.1089/acm.2015.0343.

Prevention of Endometriosis: Is It Possible?

27

Sebastian Daniel Schäfer

Contents

27.1 Defining Prevention

Prevention in the context of health care is defined as the sum of purposeful measures and activities meant to prevent diseases or health damages, measures meant to reduce risks associated with a disease or measures meant to delay onset of a disease. Depending on the timing of preventive measures, those are summarized to be part of primary, secondary or tertiary prevention.

Primary prevention is meant to prevent the onset of diseases. Examples of primary prevention are healthy nutrition, physical activities and positive coping strategies with regard to stress in order to prevent the onset of type II diabetes or heart attack. Another example would be vaccination against influenza or other infectious diseases. In order to be able to implement primary preventive measures disease etiology needs to be known. This would allow for treatment of underlying causes before the disease occurs in the first place.

S. D. Schäfer (✉)
Department of Gynecology and Obstetrics, University Hospital Münster, Münster, Germany
e-mail: sd.schaefer@ukmuenster.de

E. Oral (ed.), *Endometriosis and Adenomyosis*,
https://doi.org/10.1007/978-3-030-97236-3_27

Secondary prevention is used in order to be able to diagnose an occuring disease as early as possible. Differentiation between primary and secondary prevention is not always easily possible. Examples are screening programs against colorectal cancer or cervical cancer. If those programs lead to diagnosis of precursor lesions and those are removed, these measures belong to primary prevention. If those programs lead to early diagnosis of invasive lesions, these screening measures belong to secondary prevention.

Tertiary prevention is used in order to alleviate disease sequelae, prevent recurrence of a disease which has already been there and prevent exacerbation of an ongoing disease.

27.2 Primary Prevention of Endometriosis

Different theories have been put forward in order to explain development of endometriosis and underlying causes. The most popular theories include implantation theory [1], coelomic metaplasia theory [2], and concept of tissue injury and repair [3, 4]. So far none of those theories can sufficiently explain the development of endometriosis. Presently the combination of these theories in addition with genetic defects and epigenetic phenomenons and other influencing factors is used to explain disease pathogenesis. Important factors seem to be hyperperistalsis [4], hyperestrogenism, inflammatory and immunological processes, prostaglandin biosynthesis, angiogenesis, oxidative stress, and other factors [5–7]. Several potential risk factors have been studied identifying cycle length of less than and equal to 27 days [8], duration of menstruation, number of pregnancies and miscarriages as influencing factors. Data on other potential risk factors such as age at menarche, oral contraceptive use, BMI [9, 10], smoking [11], caffeine consumption [12], nutrition [13] and physical activity [14] is not clear or even conflicting [15]. Additionally certain environmental factors such as polychlorated biphenyls, bisphenol A, and phthalates seem to be associated with genetic mutations and inflammatory processes [7, 16]. In summary, etiology is unclear. Therefore no causal therapy exists [17]. As etiological factors are unclear, also primary preventive measures do not exist or only do so in theory. For a more detailed description of the topic of pathogenesis see also Chap. 4.

In order to prevent endometriosis from developing according to the combined theories above, hysterectomy before menarche would possibly constitute a primary preventive operation. Quite clearly this is not a realistic option in adolescents or even girls as it most likely would prevent them from fulfilling their future family planning or even disrupting pubertal changes leading to further psychosocial side effects even in light of the experimental option of uterus transplantation. Also hysterectomy would not cure etiologically relevant genetic alterations. Even if hysterectomy would be performed as suggested, these alterations might still lead to development of endometriosis i.e., by way of metaplasia of coelomic epithelium in the abdominal or thoracic cavity.

Hyperperistalsis and hyperestrogenism could be addressed as a primary preventive measure by ovarian suppression leading to amenorrhea using combined oral contraceptives, progestogen monotherapy, or GnRH analogue therapy. In order for these measures to clearly constitute primary preventive measures they would need to be implemented with or before menarche. As these treatments are associated with potentially severe side effects such as thromboembolism, development of breast cancer or osteoporosis and only a minority of subjects would be expected to develop endometriosis in the future this strategy would constitute overtherapy for most adolescents treated and would have to be seen as disproportionate. In addition hormonal treatment is known to alleviate symptoms without safely preventing new lesions from developping [18]. Therefore, effectiveness of hormonal treatment as a primary preventive measure even if administered generally with menarche has to be called in question.

Inflammatory and immunological processes, prostaglandin biosynthesis, angiogenesis, and oxidative stress could also be targeted as a primary preventive measure in theory using immunomodulators, immunosuppression, COX-2-inhibitors, or antiangiogenic substances such as anti-VEGF-antibodies. As all of these mechanisms are important not only for the development of endometriosis, but also in order for the organism to be able to exist and defend itself against infection and trauma, general preventive use of the substances mentioned above also has to be considered disproportionate.

As data on other potentially causal factors such as BMI, smoking, caffeine intake, nutrition, and physical activity is unclear at best, no recommendations can be made with regard to prevention.

The same can be said about the role of pregnancies as a preventive measure. Some studies have shown pregnancies to be protective against development of endometriosis [15]. Therefore, early onset family planning should probably be advised. As it will be unclear if endometriosis has already developped in most cases, it is by definition also unclear, if achieving a pregnancy would serve as primary or tertiary prevention.

In summary primary prevention cannot be considered feasible as potential measures are either disproportionate in nature or of doubtful effectiveness.

27.3 Secondary Prevention of Endometriosis

Secondary prevention is aimed at early diagnosis of the disease. This should be possible to achieve as effective diagnostic measures exist and are readily available at least to large parts of the world population. Still even in developed countries time until diagnosis is reported to be around 8 to 10 years from onset of symptoms [19, 20].

The first step to early diagnosis of the disease is widespread knowledge about the disease in the general population and the medical community. National and international endometriosis societies such as European Endometriosis League (EEL) or World Endometriosis Society (WES) may play a key role in transporting knowledge and providing political support, social media outreach and cooperation, and support with self help organisations.

Educational programs for the general population are effective [21] and should be implemented starting at school age, as reported, i.e., by Bush et al. [22]. Endometriosis Awareness Month can also be used for this purpose. Another measure to facilitate early diagnosis should be education of pediatricians and general practitioners who are not as familiar with the disease as gynecologists but might still be the first or only health care professional with whom the patients are in contact [23]. Educational programs for gynecologists should aim at spreading knowledge about the disease in all and leading to subspecialization in some of them. In order to achieve this goal congresses, webinars, and one- or two-day-courses are implemented as well as the possibility of absolving specialist courses such as the EEL Masterclass which has been developed in recent years.

Early diagnosis of endometriosis can be achieved by optimizing diagnostic workup. The use of specific endometriosis questionnaires can help in early diagnosis of recurrences [24]. As first line diagnostic measures, gynecological examination including inspection of all fornices, rectovaginal palpation, and transvaginal ultrasound [25] are established. As second line, diagnostic measures such as MRI and transrectal endosonography have to be taken into account. Early diagnosis is then achieved by laparoscopy.

For a more detailed description of diagnostic options see also Chap. 6.

27.4 Tertiary Prevention of Endometriosis

Tertiary prevention is used in order to alleviate disease sequelae, prevent recurrence of endometriosis, and prevent exacerbation of ongoing endometriosis.

Considering this definition tertiary prevention of endometriosis can be achieved by medical or surgical treatment of the disease. These treatment options are effective at least in most cases in preventing disease progression and development of irreversible sequelae such as infertility and chronic pain syndromes.

Hormonal treatment can be considered as a tertiary preventive measure if amenorrhea can be achieved. This also means that in order for this preventive treatment to be effective in the long run, it needs to be implemented as a long-term treatment without interruption [18, 26]. In consequence preventive treatment should only be limited by severe side effects which cannot be handled or dealt with, wish for conception or menopause.

Systemic hormonal treatment options which can be used also as a preventive treatment after surgical removal of endometriosis include oral progestogens such as dienogest or norethisterone acetate [27, 28] and combined oral contraceptives (COC). These measures lead to hypoestrogenism by influencing the hypothalamic hypophysical axis causing decrease in proliferation, reduction of lesion size and activity. These effects can also be achieved by GnRH analogue treatment. As these substances lead to osteoporosis in case of longterm treatment they are of limited value as a potential preventive treatment. Still there is some data on postoperative use. A 6 month treatment using GnRH analogues led to a reduction of risk of recurrence [29]. If used GnRH analogues should be administered together with an add back therapy. As such progestogens and COCs can be used. Add back therapy leads to elevation of estrogen levels resulting in decrease of hypoestrogenic side effects without compromising effectiveness of GnRH analogue treatment [30, 31]. One RCT demonstrated that COCs should be used preferentially as add back therapy [32]. Prevention by COCs is controversial, as there is data that the estrogen included in this treatment might increase risk of recurrence [33]. If used estrogen progestogen combinations should be used nonstop as opposed to cyclic use [34–36]. It is unclear which estrogen-progestogen combination should be preferred [35, 37]. In conclusion tertiary preventive systemic hormonal therapy should preferentially be done by progestogen only treatment. In case of endometrioma, recurrence can be specifically prevented by COC [38] or dienogest [39] while a recent study did not confirm this [40]. A recent systematic review and metaanalysis confirmed effectiveness of recurrence prevention for all forms of hormonal therapy [41].

Local hormonal treament options can also be used such as progestogen releasing intrauterine devices (IUD) which lead to endometrial atrophy and stromal decidualization [18]. Levonorgestrel releasing IUDs have proven to be effective in recurrence prevention [42].

For details concerning hormonal therapy of endometriosis see also Chaps. 33 and 34.

Surgical removal of endometriosis naturally leads to regression or remission of symptoms and prevents complications such as hydronephrosis or bowel obstruction. Therefore surgical interventions constitute also tertiary prevention. Complete resection of symptomatic endometriotic manifestations should be the aim of endometriosis surgery [43] keeping in mind that improvement of quality of life should be the main goal of endometriosis treatment. Therefore sometimes compromises need to be made if complete resection of lesions would otherwise lead to decrease of quality of life. In case of ovarian endometriotic cysts, cystectomy is superior to other surgical treament options with regard to probability of recurrences [44–46].

27.5 Conclusion

In conclusion primary prevention of endometriosis is not possible. Secondary prevention can be achieved by implementing educational programs for health care professionals and the general population as well as optimizing diagnostic work up. Especially dedicated gynecological sonography increases probability of early diagnosis of endometriosis. Tertiary prevention can be realized by postoperative continuous hormonal therapy. Progestogen only therapy should be the treatment of first choice. In case of endometriotic ovarian cysts, prevention of recurrence is possible especially by COCs. Complete resection of symptomatic lesions especially in case of deep infiltrating endometriosis leads to tertiary prevention of disease progression and adverse sequelae. In response to this chapters headline question, primary prevention is not possible yet, secondary and tertiary prevention are definitively possible.

References

1. Sampson JA. Metastatic or embolic endometriosis, due to the menstrual dissemination of endometrial tissue into the venous circulation. Am J Pathol. 1927;3(93–110):143.
2. Meyer R. Über den Stand der Frage der Adenomyositis, Adenomyome im Allgemeinen und insbesondere über Adenomyositis seroepithelialis und Adenomyometritis sarcomatosa. Zentralbl Gynäkol. 1919;36:745–50.
3. Leyendecker G, Kunz G, Noe M, Herbertz M, Mall G. Endometriosis: a dysfunction and disease of the archimetra. Hum Reprod Update. 1998;4:752–62.
4. Leyendecker G, Wildt L, Mall G. The pathophysiology of endometriosis and adenomyosis: tissue injury and repair. Arch Obstet Gynecol Online. 2009;280:529–38.
5. Gordts S, Koninckx P, Brosens I. Pathogenesis of deep endometriosis. Fertil Steril. 2017;108(872–885):e871.
6. Koninckx PR, Ussia A, Adamyan L, Wattiez A, Gomel V, Martin DC. Pathogenesis of endometriosis: the genetic/epigenetic theory. Fertil Steril. 2019;111:327–40.
7. Parazzini F, Esposito G, Tozzi L, Noli S, Bianchi S. Epidemiology of endometriosis and ist comorbidities. Eur J Obstet Gynecol Reprod Biol. 2017;209:3–7.
8. Wei M, Cheng Y, Bu H, Zhao Y, Zhao W. Length of menstrual cycle and risk of endometriosis: a meta analysis of 11 case control studies. Medicine. 2016;95:e2922.
9. Backonja U, Buck Louis GM, Lauver DR. Overall adiposity, adipose tissue distribution and endometriosis: a systemativ review. Nurs Res. 2016;65:151–66.
10. Liu Y, Zhang W. Association between body mass index and endometriosis risk: a metaanalysis. Oncotarget. 2017;8:46928–36.
11. Bravi F, Parazzini F, Cipriano S, Chiaffarino F, Ricci E, Chiantera V, Vigano P, La Vecchia C. Tobacco smoking and risk of endometriosis: a systematic review and metaanalysis. BMJ Open. 2014;4:e006325.
12. Chiaffarino F, Bravi F, Cipriano S, Parazzini F, Ricci E, Vigano P, La Vecchia C. Coffee and caffeine intake and risk of endometriosis: a metaaanlysis. Eur J Nutr. 2014;53:1573–9.
13. Karacin O, Mutlu I, Kose M, Celik F, Kanat-Pektas M, Yilmazer M. Serum vitamin D concentrations in young Turkish women with primary dysmenorrhea: a randomised controlled study. Taiwanese J Obstet Gynecol. 2018;57:58–63.
14. Bonocher CM, Montenegro ML, Rosa ESJC, Ferriani RA, Meola J. Endometriosis and physical exercises: a systematic review. Reprod Biol Endocrinol. 2014;12:4.
15. Burghaus S, Klingsiek P, Fasching PA, Engel A, Haberle L, Strissel PL, Schmidt M, Jonas K, Strehl JD, Hartmann A, Lehmann J, Boosz A, Thiel FC, Müller A, Beckmann MW, Renner SP. Risk factors for endometriosis in a German case control study. Geburtshilfe Frauenheilkd. 2011;71:1073–9.
16. Roy D, Morgan M, Yoo C, Deoraj A, Roy S, Yadav VK, Garoub M, Assaggaf H, Doke M. Integrated bioinformatics, environmental epidemiologic and genomic approaches to identify environmental and molecular links between endometriosis and breast cancer. Int J Mol Sci. 2015;16:25285–322.
17. Hirsch M, Begum MR, Paniz E, Barker C, Davis CJ, Duffy J. Diagnosis and management of endometriosis: a systematic review of international and national guidelines. BJOG. 2018;125:556–64.
18. Nagandla K, Idris N, Nalliah S, Sreeramareddy CT, George SRK, Kanagasabai S. Hormonal treatment for uterine adenomyosis. Cochrane Database Syst Rev. 2014; https://doi.org/10.1002/14651858.CD011372.
19. Ballard K, Lowton K, Wright J. What's the delay? A qualitativ study of women's experiences of reaching a diagnosis of endometriosis. Fertil Steril. 2006;86:1296–301.
20. Hudelist G, Fritzer N, Thomas A, Niehues C, Oppelt P, Haas D, Tammaa A, Salzer H. Diagnostic delay for endometriosis in Austria and Germany: causes and possible consequences. Hum Reprod. 2012;27(12):3412–6.

21. Gombeski WR Jr, Briller S, Fishleder A, Bat-Cirjak E, Rothner AD, Secic M. Marketing impact of health education programs. J Hosp Mark. 1997;11(2):91–103.
22. Bush D, Brick E, East MC, Johnson N. Endometriosis education in schools: a New Zealand model examining the impact of an education program in schools on early recognition of symptoms suggesting endometriosis. Aust N Z J Obstet Gynecol. 2017;57:452–7.
23. Van der Zanden M, Nap AW. Knowledge of, and treatment strategies for, endometriosis among general practitioners. Reprod Biomed Online. 2016;32:527–31.
24. Ricci G, Castelpietra E, Romano F, Di Lorenzo G, Zito G, Ronfani L, Biffi S, Monasta L. Case-control study to develop and validate a questionnaire fort he secondary prevention of endometriosis. PLoS One. 2020;15(3):e0230828.
25. Guerriero S, Condous G, Van den Bosch T, Valentin L, Leone FPG, Van Schoubroeck D, Exacoustos C, Installé AJF, Martins WP, Abrao MS, Hudelist G, Bazot M, Alcazar JL, Goncalves MO, Pascual MA, Ajossa S, Savelli L, Dunham R, Reid S, Menakaya U, Bourne T, Ferrero S, Leon M, Bignardi T, Holland T, Jurkovic D, Benacerraf B, Osuga Y, Somigliana E, Timmerman D. Systematic approach to sonographic evaluation of the pelvis in women with suspected endometriosis, including terms, definitions and measurements: a consensus opinion from the International Deep Endometriosis Analysis (IDEA) group. Ultrasound Obstet Gynecol. 2016;48:318–32.
26. Li Q, Ding Y, Zhang XY, Feng WW, Hua KQ. Drug therapy for adenomyosis: a prospective, nonrandomized, parallel controlled study. J Int Med Res. 2018;46:1855–65.
27. Ferrero S, Barra F, Leone Roberti Maggiore U. Current and emerging therapeutics for the management of endometriosis. Drugs. 2018:1–18. https://doi.org/10.1007/s40265-018-0928-0.
28. Strowitzki T, Faustmann T, Gerlinger C, Schumacher U, Ahlers C, Seitz C. Safety and tolerabilits of dienogest in endometriosis: pooled analysis from the European clinical study program. Int J Women's Health. 2015;7:393–401.
29. Zheng Q, Mao H, Xu Y, Zhao J, Wei X, Liu P. Can postoperative GnRH agonist treatment prevent endometriosis recurrence? A meta-analysis. Arch Gyn Obstet. 2016;294:201–7.
30. Wu D, Hu M, Hong L, Hong S, Ding W, Min J, Fang G, Guo W. Clinical efficacy of add back therapy in treatment of endometriosis: a meta analysis. Arch Gyn Obstet. 2014;290:513–23.
31. Lee DY, Lee JY, Seo JW, Yoon BK, Choi DS. Gonadotropin-releasing hormone agonist with add back treatment is as effective and tolerable as dienogest in preventing pain recurrence after laparoscopic surgery for endometriosis. Arch Gyn Obstet. 2016;294:1257–63.
32. Di Vasta AD, Feldman HA, Sadler Gallagher J, Stokes NA, Laufer MR, Hornstein MD, Gordon CM. Hormonal add back therapy for females treated with gonadotropin releasing hormone agonist for endometriosis. Obstet Gynecol. 2015;126:617–27.
33. Casper CF. Progestin-only pills may be a better first-line treatment for endometriosis than combined estrogen-progestin contraceptive pills. Fertil Steril. 2017;107:533–6.
34. Edelman A, Micks E, Gallo MF, Jensen JT, Grimes DA. Continuous or extended cycle vs. cyclic use of combined hormonal contraceptives for contraception. Cochrane Database Syst Rev. 2014; https://doi.org/10.1002/14651858.CD004695. pub3: Cd004695
35. Jensen JT, Schlaff W, Gordon K. Use of combined oral contraceptives for the treatment of endometriosis-related pain: a systematic review of the evidence. Fertil Steril. 2018;110:137–152.e131.
36. Muzii L, Di Tucci C, Achilli C, Di Donato V, Musella A, Palaia I, Panici PB. Continuous versus cyclic oral contraceptives after laparoscopic excision of ovarian endometriomas: a systematic review and metaanalysis. AJOG. 2016;214:203–11.
37. Grandi G, Xholli A, Napolitano A, Palma F, Cagnacci A. Pelvic pain and quality of life of women with endometriosis during quadriphasic estradiol valerate/dienogest oral contraceptive: a patient preference prospective 24-week pilot study. Reprod Sci. 2015;22:626–32.
38. Zorbas KA, Economopoulos KP, Vlahos NF. Continuous versus cyclic oral contraceptives for the treatment of endometriosis: a systematic review. Arch Gynecol Obstet. 2015;292:37–43.
39. Adachi K, Takahashi K, Nakamura K, Otake A, Sasamoto N, Miyoshi Y, Shioji M, Yamamoto Y, Fujitani M, Wakimoto A, Tokuhira A, Kobayashi E, Yoshimura A, Sawada K, Kimura

T. Postoperative administration of dienogest for suppressing recurrence of disease and relieving pain in subjects with ovarian endometriomas. Gynecol Endocrinol. 2016;32:646–9.
40. Lee N, Seunggi M, Seyeon W, Yeon Jean C, Miseon K, Mi Kyoung K, Yong Wook J, Bo Seong Y, Seok JS, Mi-La K. The recurrence rate of ovarian endometrioma in women aged 40 – 49 years and impact of hormonal treatment after conservative surgery. Sci Reports. 2020;10:16461.
41. Zakhari A, Delpero E, McKeown S, Tomlinson G, Bougie O, Murji A. Endometriosis recurrence following post-operative hormonal suppression: a systematic review and meta-analysis. Hum Reprod Update. 2020:1–12. https://doi.org/10.1093/humupd/dmaa033.
42. Lee KH, Jung YW, Song SY, Kang BH, Yang JB, Ko YB, Lee M, Han HY, Yoo HJ. Comparison of the efficacy of dienogest and levonorgestrel-releasing intrauterine system after laparoscopic surgery for endometriosis. J Obstet Gynecol Res. 2018; https://doi.org/10.1111/jog.13703.
43. Bozdag G. Recurrence of endometriosis: risk factors, mechanisms and biomarkers. Womens Health. 2015;11(5):693–9.
44. Iwase A, Nakamura T, Nakahara T, Goto M, Kikkawa F. Assessment of ovarian reserve using anti-Mullerian hormone levels in benign gynecologic conditions and surgical interventions: a systematic narrative review. Reprod Biol Endocrinol. 2014;12:125.
45. Deckers P, Ribeiro SC, Simoes RDS, Miyahara C, Baracat EC. Systematic review and meta-analysis of the effect of bipolar electrocoagulation during laparoscopic ovarian endometrioma stripping on ovarian reserve. Int J Gynecol. 2018;140:11–7.
46. Moscarini M, Milazzo GN, Assorgi C, Pacchiarotti A, Caserta D. Ovarian stripping versus cystectomy: recurrence of endometriosis and pregnancy rate. Arch Gynecol Obstet. 2014;290:163–1.

Cost Estimates Associated with Diagnosis and Treatment of Endometriosis

28

Brintha Sivajohan, Tinya Lin, and Mohamed A. Bedaiwy

Contents

B. Sivajohan
Schulich School of Medicine & Dentistry, Western University, London, ON, Canada

T. Lin
Department of Obstetrics and Gynecology, The University of British Columbia, Vancouver, BC, Canada

M. A. Bedaiwy (✉)
Department of Obstetrics and Gynaecology, BC Women's Hospital and Health Center, Faculty of Medicine, The University of British Columbia, Vancouver, BC, Canada
e-mail: mohamed.bedaiwy@cw.bc.ca

E. Oral (ed.), *Endometriosis and Adenomyosis*,
https://doi.org/10.1007/978-3-030-97236-3_28

28.1 Introduction

28.1.1 What Is Endometriosis?

Endometriosis is a chronic condition characterized by the growth of endometrial-like tissue outside the uterus with varying degrees of severity and non-specific symptoms [1]. Endometriosis commonly presents in pelvic locations such as the ovaries as endometriomas, peritoneum, bowel, and bladder amongst other less common locations such as the lungs, liver, and inguinal region with a range of symptomatology affecting multiple organ systems [2, 3]. The broad spectrum of this disease can be classified as three predominant phenotypes (Fig. 28.1): superficial

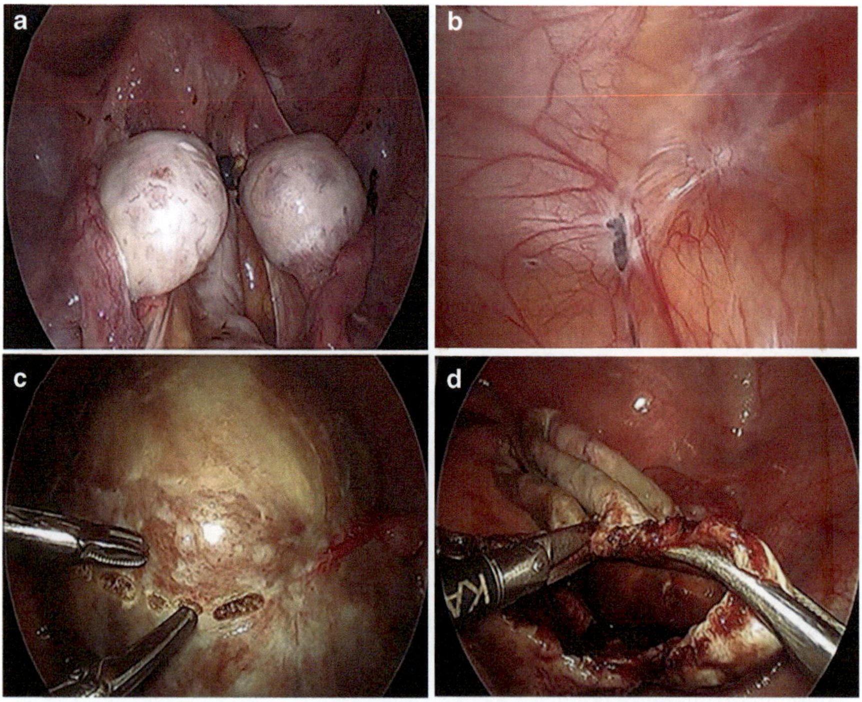

Fig. 28.1 Three different phenotypes of endometriosis. From left to right, starting from the top, the three different phenotypes of endometriosis are shown: (**a**) deeply infiltrating endometriosis (DIE), (**b**) superficial peritoneal endometriosis, and (**c**) ovarian endometriomas with (**d**) excision of the ovarian endometrioma cyst. Figures courtesy of Dr. Mohamed Bedaiwy

peritoneal, endometriomas, or deeply infiltrating endometriosis (DIE) [5]. DIE occurs when the endometrial-like tissue penetrates the peritoneal space either 5 mm or more [2]. Due to its clinical heterogeneity, symptoms range from dysmenorrhoea and dyspareunia to chronic pelvic pain and infertility [1]. Reproductive-age women between the ages of 35 and 44 have been shown to be at highest risk for this chronic condition [6]; however, cases have been documented in pre-menarcheal girls and post-menopausal women [3]. Despite significant strides in the field, the pathogenesis of this disease is still not clear. There is a growing body of literature pointing to the importance of immunological, inflammatory, genetic, and environmental factors and their interactions in the aetiology of endometriosis [7, 8].

28.1.2 What Is the Prevalence of Endometriosis?

It has been estimated that close to 176 million women globally are impacted by this disorder [9, 10], encompassing about 10% of reproductive-age women [10, 11]. Since definitive diagnosis is only established through surgical histopathology, the true prevalence is difficult to elucidate and likely significantly underreported [10]. Louis et al. [12] estimated that approximately 11% of American women may have endometriosis during their reproductive years despite being asymptomatic and presenting with no complaints.

The majority of prevalence studies are in women who are symptomatic. One US study found endometriosis in 23% of women undergoing diagnostic laparoscopy for dysmenorrhoea and infertility [13]. The prevalence of endometriosis amongst women exhibiting infertility and chronic pelvic pain has been estimated to be between 30% and 50% [14]. In infertile women with regular ovulatory cycles and partners with healthy sperm, the prevalence rate increases up to 50% [14]. Studies in adolescents with severe dysmenorrhoea demonstrate that about 50–70% of individuals receive a diagnosis of endometriosis [12]; however, there are very few studies that look specifically at adolescent populations. About 24–40% of women presenting with chronic pelvic pain are diagnosed with endometriosis making this condition the most common cause of chronic pelvic pain [15, 16]. In brief, between 35% and 50% of symptomatic women are impacted by endometriosis [17].

28.1.3 What Are the Signs and Symptoms of Endometriosis?

The documented signs and symptoms of endometriosis are non-specific and vary in degree of severity amongst patients. Table 28.1 illustrates some of the common signs and symptoms that are reported in patients with endometriosis. Due to its clinical heterogeneity, patients with endometriosis can present with a vast array of symptoms including chronic pelvic pain, dysmenorrhoea, and deep dyspareunia with variable intensity and combination of these symptoms. Patients can also present with bowel and urinary symptoms such as dyschezia, dysuria, haematuria, and abdominal pain [3] which can correlate with the anatomical location of endometriosis implants.

Table 28.1 Signs and symptoms of endometriosis

Signs and symptoms
Dysmenorrhoea
Heavy menstrual bleeding
Cyclical or non-cyclical abdominal pain
Chronic fatigue
Nausea, vomiting
Pelvic pain
Dyspareunia
Bowel symptoms:
Constipation
Diarrhoea
Dyschezia
Urinary symptoms:
Dysuria
Haematuria
Subfertility/Infertility

Reference: [3]

Some patients remain asymptomatic until they present with unexplained infertility. The vast majority of these symptoms are also present in patients with pelvic inflammatory disease, irritable bowel syndrome, adenomyosis, and overlap with many other chronic pain disorders such as pelvic floor dysfunction [18]. Non-specific symptoms in combination with a lack of healthcare provider awareness can lead to the misdiagnosis and under diagnosis of endometriosis.

28.1.4 What Are the Impacts of Endometriosis?

Due to the chronic and debilitating nature of this disease, there are various impacts on multiple domains across a patient's life course. The chronic symptoms of endometriosis, such as pelvic pain, dysmenorrhoea, and dyspareunia, increase healthcare resource utilization as well as negatively impact patients' health related quality of life and emotional well-being. The next section will breakdown the various impacts of endometriosis on patients and healthcare systems.

28.1.4.1 Impacts on Health-Related Quality of Life

Studies demonstrate that endometriosis contributes to significant impairments of psychosocial functioning and health-related quality of life (HRQoL) [19]. In comparison to asymptomatic controls with no diagnosis of endometriosis, physical HRQoL was significantly impaired in women with endometriosis [10], specifically on physical functioning and body pain scores. Physical HRQoL was more pronounced than mental HRQoL. Scores on the Short Form Health Survey Questionnaire in patients with endometriosis were similar to patients with cancer [10, 20]. Another study [21] used scores on the Endometriosis Health Profile (EHP-5) to demonstrate that 43% of patients with endometriosis reported that pain interfered with work substantially and 41% reported physical impairments (i.e. difficulties walking). Patients who experienced delays in receiving a diagnosis had even greater reduced

HRQoL, and this reduction remained significant after adjusting for the number of symptoms [10].

28.1.4.2 Impacts on Fertility

Approximately 30–50% of women diagnosed with endometriosis experience fertility issues, and about 20–50% of women presenting with concerns of infertility are diagnosed with endometriosis [22]. Senapati et al. [23] suggested that damage to the ovarian cortex can occur from endometriosis, or from surgical treatments (i.e. removal of endometriomas). This results in the need for increased gonadotrophin stimulation and fewer retrieved oocytes with stimulation for in vitro fertilization (IVF) [23]. The impacts of endometriosis on infertility often result in the need for more advanced reproductive planning, more visits to reproductive specialists, more invasive management options, higher stress on romantic relationships, and increased financial costs for patients.

28.1.4.3 Impacts on Psychosocial Functioning

Psychosocial functioning is significantly impacted by endometriosis, with studies demonstrating effects on general psychological well-being, sexual dysfunction, and relationships with partners. The most common symptoms of endometriosis include chronic pelvic pain and infertility which negatively impact psychological well-being in many patients. The stigma and social implications of endometriosis in combination with dealing with emotionally taxing symptoms are strong predictors of psychological distress in patients [24, 25]. Chronic pain in endometriosis associated with reproductive anatomy can carry a higher psychosocial cost attached to it due to the far-reaching impacts on infertility/subfertility, sexual discomfort, and interpersonal relationships as opposed to other chronic pain problems [26]. Endometriosis often leads to dyspareunia and sexual dysfunction which negatively impacts relationship adjustment and overall quality of life [26]. In addition, the chronic nature of this disease often demands the need for long-term treatment and is accompanied by a high risk of recurrence and progressive symptomatology which can exacerbate psychosocial functioning in patients.

Focus group studies have shown that aspects of psychosocial functioning such as everyday activities, life opportunities, and personal finances are extensively affected by having endometriosis [27, 28]. Future studies should explore how social support mitigates these real and perceived negative impacts.

28.1.4.4 Impacts on Employment and Work Productivity

Nnoaham et al. [10] found that women with endometriosis missed approximately 11 hours of employment per week. This loss was mainly due to presenteeism (reduced productivity while at work) rather than absenteeism (absence from work). The researchers noticed that patients' working capacity and capabilities were restricted due to their symptoms, and consequently, many opted to resign, switch roles, or use more allocated sick days resulting in loss of work productivity. These results align with prior findings demonstrating a strong correlation between pain severity and interference with work productivity [18]. Another study reported a significant association between adolescents experiencing severe dysmenorrhoea and absenteeism from school and work with 12% of individuals reporting monthly absences from school and work due to dysmenorrhoea [29]. Soliman et al. [30] reported an average weekly loss of 5.3 hours due to employment presenteeism and 1.1 hours lost due to employment absenteeism in women with endometriosis.

28.1.5 Why Are Costs of Endometriosis Important?

Endometriosis poses large direct and indirect costs to patients and society. In the USA, the annual economic burden of endometriosis was estimated to be $22 billion in 2002 [31] and climbed to $69.4 billion in 2009 [32]. Soliman et al. [33] conducted a systematic review of studies published from 2000 to 2013 and estimated direct costs to be close to $12,118 per patient annually while indirect costs were around $15,737 per patient annually. Despite these staggering numbers, they are likely an underestimate of the true costs to society due to the lack of data on direct non-healthcare costs (i.e. transportation for ambulatory visits, time off from work to attend appointments, and childcare costs during appointments) and indirect costs (i.e. reduced work productivity, caregiver costs, and short- and long-term disability).

Endometriosis is a complex, heterogeneous disease process that has significant financial impacts on healthcare systems. Healthcare systems are constantly under pressure to be as cost-efficient as possible in the face of spiralling healthcare costs and limited resources. There is a strong need for continued evaluation of indirect and direct cost estimates and economic evaluations of diagnostic and treatment methods. Given the prevalence of this disease and its far-reaching impacts on both healthcare and societal productivity, estimated costs of endometriosis burden can support appropriate resource allocation and the formation of cost-effective guidelines. This chapter outlines the cost studies that have identified the major contributors to diagnosis and treatment costs in endometriosis. It will also help inform future priorities in research to ensure that healthcare systems remain sustainable in the face of competing demands.

28.2 Costs Associated with the Diagnosis of Endometriosis

28.2.1 How Is Endometriosis Diagnosed?

The diagnosis of endometriosis is complex, with many challenges that result in additional costs to the patient and healthcare system. Endometriosis is traditionally diagnosed via laparoscopic visualization accompanied by the histologic confirmation of ectopic endometrial-like tissue [3]. Some forms of severe endometriosis such as DIE and endometriomas can be detected using imaging such as MRI or ultrasonography, but histological testing of excised lesions is historically recommended as the gold standard test [3]. Diagnostic procedures include laparotomy or laparoscopy, although the latter is more common [34] due to the benefit of reduced complications, length of hospital stay, and recovery times. A cost analysis study shows that laparotomy ($9533) is twice as expensive as laparoscopy ($5014) in direct healthcare costs [35] and has poorer outcomes. Laparoscopy also provides better visualization of the peritoneal cavity and has proven better for excising benign ovarian endometriomas [36]. As a result, laparoscopy has been favoured over laparotomy for the purposes of diagnosis [34].

Albeit these advantages, a laparoscopic diagnostic procedure still contributes heavily to the economic burden of endometriosis. Other than the direct healthcare costs associated with a surgical procedure, there is risk of post-operative complications such as surgery adhesion formation resulting in further complications that need management [37]. Currently, this gold standard test to diagnose endometriosis is invasive, costly, and poses some risks to the patient.

Other less invasive and inexpensive methods have been recently explored for the diagnosis of endometriosis. Ling [38] demonstrated that a 78–87% accuracy for a clinical diagnosis of endometriosis can be made using a history that documents symptoms of dysmenorrhoea, abnormal uterine bleeding, and dyspareunia and physical findings typical of uterosacral ligament nodularity. Alternatively, the rule-out method using history and physical evaluation to rule out other possible diagnoses and non-response to empirical treatment such as non-steroidal anti-inflammatory drugs (NSAIDs) and combined hormone contraceptives (CHCs) can be used to diagnose endometriosis accurately 80–90% of the time [38].

Despite research into less invasive methods of diagnosis, laparoscopic surgery followed by histology remains the gold standard diagnostic to detect and stage endometriosis. Due to the cost, potential complications, and invasiveness of laparoscopic diagnostics, it is usually recommended for patients where there is an intention to treat surgically concurrently [3].

28.2.2 What Are the Challenges Associated with Diagnosing Endometriosis?

Diagnosis of endometriosis is often missed in primary care due to non-specific symptoms resulting in delayed or missed diagnoses. Symptomatic women often have symptoms similar to those of other gynaecological, gastrointestinal, urinary, and other chronic pain conditions resulting in a long differential list [39]. Table 28.2 illustrates the many diagnoses commonly on a clinician's differential list when presented with a symptomatic patient. Additionally, a lack of consistent clinical guidelines for diagnosing endometriosis, especially in those with comorbidities, contributes to the difficulties in diagnosing this condition [43].

Another challenge in diagnosing endometriosis is the location of endometriotic growth. Most endometrial-like tissue growth are small lesions that tend to occur in pelvic regions and involve the parietal peritoneum and pelvic organs [3] as superficial endometriosis. As shown in Table 28.3, diagnostic methods such as ultrasound and magnetic resonance imaging (MRI) have not shown significant diagnostic power in detecting endometriosis [39], and diagnosis continues to rely on laparoscopic surgery.

An abnormal pelvic examination and clinical history compatible with common symptoms of endometriosis can be indicative of endometriosis; however, many women are also asymptomatic, and symptomatic women can present with a variety

Table 28.2 Differential diagnosis list for endometriosis

	Differential diagnoses
Gynaecologic causes	Primary dysmenorrhoea Adenomyosis Chronic pelvic pain Pelvic inflammatory disease Uterine fibroids Adnexal pathology Endometrial hyperplasia Endometritis Vaginal infections Cervical polyps Cervicitis Endometrial polyps Pelvic vascular congestion Other neoplasms (benign or malignant) Ovarian torsion
Urinary causes	Urinary tract infection Urethral syndrome Interstitial cystitis/bladder pain syndrome
Gastrointestinal causes	Constipation Irritable bowel syndrome
Other causes	Non-specific low back pain Medications (i.e. hypothalamic depressants) Coagulopathies

References: [3, 40–42]

Table 28.3 Specificity and sensitivity of physical exam, U/S, and MRI in the diagnosis of endometriosis

	Type of endometriosis	Sensitivity	Specificity
Physical exam [44]	Ovarian Endometriosis	23–41%	99%
	Pelvic endometriosis (vaginal, uterosacral ligament)	50–74%	78–100%
	Deeply infiltrating endometriosis (rectum, rectosigmoid, rectovaginal, bladder)	18–88%	54–100%
Ultrasound [45]	Pelvic endometriosis	79%	91%
	Ovarian endometriosis	93%	96%
	Deeply infiltrating endometriosis	79%	94%
MRI [45]	Pelvic endometriosis	79%	72%
	Ovarian endometriosis	95%	91%
	Deeply infiltrating endometriosis	94%	77%

of comorbidities resulting in challenges to diagnose. Prior research has shown that an abnormal pelvic examination correlates with a laparoscopic diagnosis of endometriosis about 70–90% of the time [38]. However, diagnosis should not be excluded on the basis of a normal pelvic exam because research has shown that more than 50% of women with a normal exam have been diagnosed with endometriosis after undergoing laparoscopic surgery [46]. A review by Taylor et al. [44] looked at the accuracy of physical exams as a method of diagnosis in patients with surgically confirmed endometriosis. The specificity, positive predictive value, and negative predictive value of a physical exam were in the range of 80 to 100%, especially for patients with a strong pretest probability of disease based on history. The sensitivity was much lower and more variable given the greater dependence on lesion location compared to other measures of diagnostic accuracy. Interestingly, studies have shown no correlation between depth and extent of lesions and the corresponding clinical symptoms and presenting complaints [3]. Thus, the ASRM has developed a staging system from stage I—mild to stage IV—severe disease that characterizes location, severity, and depth of endometriotic tissue but does not provide information on the severity of clinical symptoms. While clinicians should remain cautious of the validity of a non-surgical diagnosis of endometriosis, patients can still be managed presumptively while awaiting surgical confirmation.

28.2.2.1 Unnecessary Investigations and Lack of Reliable, Low-Cost Diagnostics for Endometriosis

The diagnostic delay in endometriosis is particularly important as it contributes significantly to the costs associated with diagnosis. Surgical diagnostic methods are invasive and costly, with debatable utility if there is no intent to treat the patient concurrently with surgical methods. The Society of Obstetricians and Gynaecologists Canada (SOGC) recommends using a cost-effective method which includes thorough history and physical evaluation along with transvaginal ultrasound as the first-line diagnostic method [47]. International guidelines also recommend empirical treatment using inexpensive and safe options such as CHCs and progestins when there is a high index of clinical suspicion for endometriosis [1, 47, 48], as 62 to 88% of patients will report improvement in symptoms [49]. Moreover, Frishman et al. [50] reported that only one-third of patients undergoing laparoscopy receive a definitive diagnosis of endometriosis. This demonstrates that a significant portion of diagnostic laparoscopies can be avoided in women with a clinical suspicion of endometriosis, with minimal impact on management, translating into a reduction in unnecessary invasive procedures and costs to the healthcare system.

Non-specific symptoms combined with a lack of healthcare provider awareness can often lead to high healthcare utilization and unnecessary investigations. In fact, women reported an average of seven visits to a primary care physician before receiving referrals to the appropriate specialist (i.e. gynaecologist) [10]. Women with endometriosis who present with urinary symptoms such as dysuria may undergo many unneeded cycles of empiric antibiotic therapy for urinary tract infections [3], adding to the economic burden of this disease and potentially contributing to future antibiotic resistance. Patients with gastrointestinal endometriosis are commonly misdiagnosed as having irritable bowel syndrome due to overlapping, non-specific symptoms, and this can lead to longer delays in receiving appropriate care and unnecessary tests [51]. Patients with higher BMIs also suffer diagnostic delays due to the difficulty in detecting abnormal pelvic pathology on physical examination [10]. However, this underscores the need for heightened awareness of endometriosis amongst primary care and faster referrals as opposed to initiating unnecessary investigations that are not cost-effective nor helpful in establishing a diagnosis.

A lack of non-invasive, reliable tests for first-line diagnostic use is a significant barrier to a cost-effective method for the diagnosis of endometriosis. Many clinical applications have been tested for their reliability and diagnostic power in detecting endometriosis. These include blood biomarkers, urinalysis markers, peritoneal fluid markers, and imaging techniques for the pelvic region. However, no one method has dominated in larger studies, and many have not shown reproducible results [45]. Better guidelines to approach diagnosis and more reliable diagnostic methods would help alleviate unwarranted costs between symptom onset and definitive diagnosis.

28.2.2.2 What Are the Impacts of a Delayed Diagnosis?

Challenges in diagnosing endometriosis often lead to long delays in patients receiving appropriate care and management. Both patient-centred factors such as stigma, embarrassment, lack of awareness regarding normal and abnormal symptoms, lack of symptoms and physician-centred causes such as inconsistent diagnostic guidelines and unnecessary investigations contribute to the long delays in receiving a definitive diagnosis [52]. Delays in diagnosis vary across the globe but demonstrate years of significant diagnostic delay. Women often have to wait between 6 and 12 years to receive a diagnosis [10, 53, 54], and there is considerable variability between countries in the time taken to receive an endometriosis diagnosis (Table 28.4). Untreated endometriosis during this period has been shown to impact quality of life, mental health, negatively interfere with employment and impact reproduction [19], leading to increased indirect costs and higher costs when treating patients. Studies have identified one main cause for this phenomenon as delays in receiving specialist referrals from primary care providers [10]. In the USA, Soliman et al. [57] documented an average delay of 4.4 years and noted that up to 89% of diagnoses were made only by trained specialists in endometriosis. These results may be indicative of a lack of healthcare provider awareness, and the need for improved diagnostic guidelines for generalists who represent the majority of first-line providers around the world.

In a study by Surrey et al. [58], healthcare resource utilization and endometriosis-related healthcare costs were examined in 11,793 patients with endometriosis who had experienced short, intermediate, and long diagnostic delays. All-cause healthcare costs were highest in patients who had a long diagnostic delay (average of $34460), followed by intermediate delay patients ($30,030), and were lowest in patients who experienced short diagnostic delays ($21,489). In an American,

Table 28.4 Diagnostic delay of endometriosis across different countries

Study	Country	Average diagnostic delay
Arruda et al. [55]	Brazil	Median time between onset of initial symptoms and definitive diagnosis is 7 years
Husby et al. [56]	Norway	Average diagnostic delay of 6.7 +/−6.2 years
Ballard et al. [52]	UK	Median diagnostic delay of 8.5 years
Nnoaham et al. [10]	Italy, China, Brazil, USA, UK, Spain, Nigeria, Belgium, Ireland, Argentina	Average diagnostic delay of 6.7 years across all 10 countries with a range of 3.3 years (China) to 10.7 years (Italy)
Prast et al. [53]	Austria	Average diagnostic delay of 10.4 years before receiving a conclusive diagnosis
Soliman et al. [57]	USA	Average diagnostic delay of 4.4 years

Medicaid-insured population, endometriosis patients showed higher all-cause healthcare resource utilization than age-matched controls during the pre-diagnosis period [59]. This was consistent with another study by Fuldeore et al. [60] which reported that patients with endometriosis spent $7028 more in healthcare utilization costs in comparison to matched controls in the 5 years leading up to diagnosis. Patients who had the longer delays had more endometriosis-related symptoms, endometriosis-related emergency visits, and in-patient hospitalizations in their pre-diagnosis period in comparison to those with shorter delays [58, 60]. The mean frequency of in-patient hospitalizations increased as a function of increasing diagnostic delay, further adding to increasing costs.

In a 60-month period prior to receiving a definitive diagnosis, patients who experienced longer diagnostic delays also reported more insurance claims for endometriosis symptoms and endometriosis-related comorbidities [58]. In the 5 years prior to diagnosis, patients with short delays spent $4298 per year on average on all-cause and endometriosis-related healthcare costs and patients with long delays spent $6892 per year—a 130% increase in endometriosis-related costs annually compared to patients with short delays [58]. Fuldeore et al. [60] used a claims database to report annual costs ranging from USD $3730 in the fifth year prior to diagnosis to USD $6649 in the year immediately prior to diagnosis—also demonstrating that costs incurred by patients and healthcare systems increase as the diagnostic delay gets longer.

Ambulatory visits appear to be a major driver of many of these direct costs during the delay period, as many patients visit ambulatory care multiple times between the time of initial symptom onset and the time of diagnosis. Ambulatory visits contributed for about 59.1% of total endometriosis-related costs, and researchers concluded that endometriosis-related costs were nearly twice as high in patients with intermediate and long diagnostic delays in comparison to those with shorter delays prior to a diagnosis of endometriosis [58]. Soliman et al. [61] looked at healthcare resource utilization during the year immediately prior to diagnosis and concluded that patients with endometriosis average 8 visits to physician offices, 1.8 visits to Ob/Gyn specialists, and 0.63 ER visits along with 20.2 prescriptions per patient in the 12-month period pre-diagnosis. All these outcomes were found to be significant when compared to utilization by matched controls. Fuldeore et al. [60] reported similar differences in emergency visits and physician visits for patients in the 5-year period before diagnosis. Patients with diagnostic delays therefore had a greater number of visits to emergency departments, visits to physicians, and visits to outpatient services which peaked in the year prior to diagnosis.

Pharmaceutical costs were also correlated with diagnostic delay and reported to average USD $568 for patients with short delays and USD $638 for those with long delays [58]. Baseline opioid prescription claims were significantly higher for cases (77.2%) than controls (40.6%) and close to double the number of claims was found for NSAIDs, antidepressants, and oestrogen/progestin CHCs amongst cases than controls. A lack of symptom control strategies before diagnosis along with long diagnostic delays contributes to increased prescription use for symptom management in patients with endometriosis, further contributing to direct costs associated with this disease. This cost difference is likely to be an underestimate as many studies that explore costs associated with endometriosis in the pre-index period lack cost data on over-the-counter pain management, naturopathic remedies, and other self-management methods used by patients. Future studies should explore the frequency and cost of these alternative management methods used by patients prior to diagnosis to fully understand how diagnostic delays are contributing to increasing costs.

The need for earlier diagnosis and the impact of delays on increasing economic burden is heavily highlighted by these studies. Diagnostic delays contribute to both direct and indirect costs through a variety of mechanisms. Using clinical algorithms and a high index of clinical suspicion surrounding women with pelvic symptoms and infertility, we can improve the diagnostic delay seen in endometriosis (both for superficial lesions, endometriomas, and DIE) using other methods (i.e. ultrasonography) whilst also reducing costs associated with diagnosis.

Interestingly, some studies have looked at the all-cause healthcare costs and endometriosis-related healthcare costs in the year following diagnosis to understand if there is a change in expenditures. One such study [60] demonstrated the most significant difference in healthcare expenditures between endometriosis patients and controls occurred in the year immediately prior to diagnosis and the year after diagnosis. In specific, all-cause cost differences peaked in the first year following diagnosis concurrently with a rise in in-patient visits, out-patient visits, and emergency room visits. All-cause medical service costs in the first year following diagnosis averaged $12,005 for endometriosis patients compared to $3115 for controls. Patients with endometriosis averaged total healthcare costs of $13,199 in the first year following diagnosis, but in following years, the average annual total healthcare costs ranged between $3389 and $6720. Soliman et al. [61] reported that up to 60% of total healthcare costs for endometriosis patients occur in the first 3 months after diagnosis but appear to decline significantly following the first year of diagnosis [60, 62, 63]. Future studies should focus on evaluating whether a shorter diagnostic delay can result in a reduction of costs in the first year following diagnosis.

28.2.3 Potential Investigations to Aid the Diagnosis of Endometriosis

28.2.3.1 Endometriosis Biomarkers

Research has been conducted on the role of diagnostic biomarkers in the diagnostic pathway. Their potential application includes risk screening in stratification of patients who would benefit from further investigations. In this clinical scenario, having a negative test could avoid costly, invasive tests and unnecessary investigations, thereby relieving a large economic burden [3]. A positive test would accelerate time to treatment and decrease diagnostic delay [3]. Biomarkers may also have a role in estimating recurrence risks and could reduce the unnecessary follow-up care in low-risk patients [3]. Finally, a biomarker could help identify the best management option for patients and reduce costs associated with unnecessary/ineffective treatments.

Table 28.5 List of some biomarkers studied in endometriosis (Nisenblat et al. [64])

Biologic group	Biomarkers	Sensitivity	Specificity
Angiogenesis & growth factors	Vascular Endothelial Growth Factor	0.50–0.93	0.61–0.97
Apoptosis markers	Survivin	0.07	0.90
Cell adhesion molecules	Laminin-1	0.72	0.70
Hormonal markers	Prolactin	0.2–0.44	0.94–1.00
Immune and inflammatory markers	Anti-endometrial antibodies	0.81–1.00	0.39–0.75
	Tumour necrosis factor alpha	0.68–0.89	0.35–0.87
	White blood cells	0.64	0.54
	Interleukin-4	0.64	0.65
	Interleukin-6	0.63	0.69
Tumour markers	Cancer antigen 19.9 (CA-19.9)	0.36	0.87
	Cancer antigen 125 (CA-125)	0.40–0.73	0.64–0.91

Identifying reliable biomarkers for endometriosis is particularly challenging due to the need for stability across the hormonal changes instituted by the menstrual cycle, or on hormonal treatment [3]. A series of Cochrane reviews determined that despite some promising candidates, there is currently no single biomarker or panel that demonstrates clinical relevance [64]. Table 28.5 illustrates some of the most commonly studied blood biomarkers for endometriosis. Thus, despite the potential cost-saving measures that biomarkers could provide, the current literature suggests that most biomarkers are of limited diagnostic value.

28.2.3.2 Imaging

Reliable imaging methods with sufficient diagnostic power can be used as a non-invasive tool to accelerate the time to receive a diagnosis and to potentially alleviate the need for an invasive surgical diagnosis. Imaging methods can additionally be used as surgical planning tools to reduce the costs associated with unexpected surgical findings such as greater operative time, resources, and rate of complications [45]. The most commonly used imaging tools include ultrasonography (U/S) and MRI. Typically, transvaginal U/S is used as a first-line method because it is more easily accessible than MRI and can accurately identify endometriomas [3]. MRI is used as a second-line method to reliably identify DIE but is associated with greater costs, and it is typically not as widely available [3].

The utility of U/S is limited to specific findings in endometriosis. Transvaginal U/S shows clinical utility in differentiating endometriomas from other forms of ovarian cysts [65, 66] with a sensitivity and specificity of 0.93 (95% CI 0.87–0.99) and 0.96 (95% CI 0.69–0.89), respectively [45, 48, 65, 66]. Dynamic markers such as the negative sliding-sign representing immobility of pelvic organs can also provide information on severe endometriotic adhesions and advanced-stage disease [3, 66]. For DIE, transvaginal ultrasound has been shown to have a sensitivity of 0.79 and specificity of 0.94 [45]. U/S is also unreliable in detecting pelvic endometriosis with a sensitivity of 0.65 and specificity of 0.95 [45]. Despite these values, there is great variability of U/S diagnostic ability between providers based on their level of experience. Studies report a sensitivity of 0.81 to 0.91 and specificity of 0.97 to 0.98

when ultrasonography was performed by an experienced specialist to diagnose DIE [67, 68]. As a result, normal findings on U/S does not rule out endometriosis in the presence of clinical symptoms due to the questionable diagnostic power of U/S especially for superficial implants, and its dependence on experienced clinicians.

MRI is not routinely used as the standard of care in the diagnostic pathway due to the high cost and limited accessibility. A Cochrane Database Review [45] showed that MRI was highly sensitive and specific for the detection of endometriomas at 0.95 (95% CI 0.90–1.00) and 0.91 (95% CI 0.86–0.97), respectively. Kinkel et al. [69] reported that while MRI is superior to U/S in detecting small endometriotic lesions, it still lacks reliability for superficial endometriosis with a sensitivity of 0.79 and specificity of 0.72. For DIE, the sensitivity is higher (0.94) with MRI, but specificity remains low (0.77) [45]. The majority of studies examining MRI in the diagnosis of endometriosis are limited by their small numbers and varying methodological quality, demonstrating a need for further research in this field [45].

Superficial and peritoneal endometriosis poses an interesting problem to clinicians as it remains highly undetectable to assess using non-invasive diagnostic methods [45, 64, 70] and largely depends on diagnostic laparoscopy to visualize [70]. Recently, Leonardi et al. [70] tested the diagnostic utility of a novel transvaginal U/S procedure called saline-infusion sonoPODography (SPG) for visualizing superficial endometriosis. The diagnostic accuracy of SPG for detecting superficial endometriosis was evaluated against direct visualization at laparoscopy and histology. For all participants, SPG had a sensitivity of 64.9% and specificity of 100.0%, and amongst participants without DIE or ovarian endometriomas or Pouch of Douglas obliteration, SPG had a sensitivity of 77.7% and specificity of 100.0%. For those with isolated superficial endometriosis, the overall accuracy of SPG for direct visualization of superficial endometriosis was 80.0%. This method shows promise in investigating endometriosis in patients without DIE, ovarian endometriomas, or Pouch of Douglas obliteration who present with chronic pain and infertility problems.

Thus, while imaging methods may have the potential to reduce the costs and invasive nature associated with the surgical diagnosis of endometriosis, its utility is predominately in assessing endometriomas and DIE. Currently, the field lacks a cost analysis on imaging methods in comparison to laparoscopy for diagnosis, but future research should survey the cost difference and how triaging with imaging can reduce both direct and indirect costs associated with diagnostic delays.

28.3 Costs Associated with the Treatment of Endometriosis

28.3.1 How Is Endometriosis Treated?

Treatments for endometriosis pose a substantial economic burden on patients and healthcare systems. Currently, the aims of therapy are to manage symptoms and reduce the presence and growth of extra-uterine endometriotic tissue. Treatment options primarily rely on medical or surgical intervention [2]. The type of treatment is selected based on the patient profile, disease location, severity, therapeutic goals, and desire for fertility. Early treatment has been shown to improve pain levels, quality of life, and daily functioning [71]. However, diagnostic delays significantly impede the ability to treat patients earlier and additionally contribute to increased costs in treatment.

The medical or surgical treatment options are thought to manage symptoms through reduction of inflammatory mechanisms and damage to nearby organs and tissues [72]. Currently, the mainstay of medical treatments are hormonal options [3]: CHCs, progestins, and gonadotropin-releasing hormone (GnRH) agonists and antagonists, as demonstrated in Table 28.6 [73]. While these treatments work to suppress oestrogen-induced growth of endometriotic tissue and relieve pain symptoms, they are each also associated with side effects [3, 73] and are not helpful when conception is a goal of treatment.

Table 28.6 Medical therapies for endometriosis

Drug category	Drug name	FDA-approved use
Combined hormone contraceptives (CHCs)	Monophasic oestrogen-progestin	FDA-approved treatment for endometriosis but may cause breakthrough bleeding
Gonadotropin-releasing hormone agonists (GnRH agonists)	Leuprolide depot Goserelin Nafarelin	FDA-approved treatment for endometriosis but may cause decreased bone density
Progestin-only contraceptives	Etonogestrel-releasing implant	Not FDA approved for treatment of endometriosis
	Norethindrone acetate	FDA-approved treatment for endometriosis
	Dienogest	Not FDA approved for treatment of endometriosis
	Depot medroxyprogesterone acetate (DMPA)	FDA-approved treatment for endometriosis but bone density loss is a concern with long-term use
	Levonorgestrel-releasing IUD	Not FDA approved for treatment of endometriosis but shown to be effective in reducing endometriosis-associated pain
Aromatase inhibitors	Letrozole Anastrozole	Not FDA approved for treatment of endometriosis and should be combined with CHCs, progestins, or GnRH agonists to prevent ovarian cyst development
Oral gonadotrophin-releasing hormone antagonists	Elagolix	Not FDA approved for treatment of endometriosis and may cause lipid abnormalities and bone density loss
Selective progesterone receptor modulators	Mifepristone Ulipristal acetate	Not FDA approved for treatment of endometriosis
Androgenic steroids	Danazol	FDA-approved treatment for endometriosis but seldom used due to undesirable androgenic side effects (i.e. acne, hirsutism)

Reference: [1]

The extent of surgical management depends on the goal of treatment. When fertility preservation is a primary goal, patients can undergo laparoscopic removal of endometriotic lesions through excision, cautery, or laser to improve the success of assisted-reproductive technologies [1]. When fertility preservation is not a concern, surgery can also concurrently include hysterectomy with or without bilateral salpingo-oophorectomy [1, 74], as this may reduce the risk of recurrent disease [75]. However, surgical complications and longer recovery times are associated with higher healthcare costs, poorer quality of life, and delayed return to employment.

Due to the chronic nature of the disease, endometriosis often requires long-term management depending on the patient's age, desire for conception, and disease severity. This section will focus on evaluating the costs associated with the various management options available to patients with endometriosis. It will also evaluate whether economic savings can be attributed to non-surgical approaches to care in primary care settings, while accounting for recurrence risk and associated complications.

Management for endometriosis is typically built on a "step-up" approach where patients are started on first-line therapies before progressing to more expensive options with higher risks of complications. This strategy is based on safety profile, cost-effectiveness, and patient-specific factors [76] as it limits the number of individuals who are placed on expensive medical therapy or who undergo surgery. Studies have shown that up to 75% of patients can receive effective symptom control from first-line therapy options including continuous use of CHC or progestins, thereby reducing the need for further treatment or surgery [76]. Surgical interventions such as excision or cautery of endometriosis or hysterectomy are typically reserved for patients who have not significantly improved with medical therapy or who have contraindications for medical options [77]. There is also evidence that a multidisciplinary approach with specific symptoms such as chronic pelvic pain is highly effective in conjunction with either medical or surgical management [78]. This hierarchical model for symptom management in endometriosis promotes the use of widely tolerated, low-risk therapies before escalating to the use of more invasive, riskier options.

28.3.2 Cost of Medical Treatments for Endometriosis

Patients who are medically treated for endometriosis suffer from high out-of-pocket prescription costs. Average annual costs range from USD $478 to $953 for controls without endometriosis compared to USD $608 to $1444 for patients with endometriosis [60]. The higher costs likely reflect the need for hormonal therapies such as CHCs, progestins, GnRH agonists and antagonists, in addition to the cost of analgesics. Many also use more than one medication at any given time for endometriosis symptoms, which can contribute to pill burden in addition to financial burden [32].

Several studies have contrasted costs for commonly prescribed medical treatments to determine the most cost-effective options with no clear result. A Scottish cost analysis [79] demonstrated that expectant management costs less at USD $697 compared to medical therapy at USD $1162 over the course of 6 months without significant differences in clinical and health outcomes [31, 79]. This conflicts with a decision analytic model suggesting that hormonal therapies were less expensive and provided more quality-adjusted life years in comparison to expectant treatment only with analgesics [80]. The increased costs associated with expectant management is attributed to increased healthcare utilization rates. Patients who exclusively used analgesics for symptom management had more frequent visits to their general practitioner in comparison to those using hormonal treatments [80]. In the UK, Pearson et al. [81] compared costs for 6 months of treatment on various medications for endometriosis. Treating patients with CHCs and progestins cost USD $8 and USD $11–$18, respectively, over 6 months [31, 81]. GnRH agonists, however, amounted to USD $1145 over the same period [31, 81]. Currently, the evidence comparing GnRH agonists to CHCs and progestins has demonstrated that there is limited utility and cost-effectiveness in using GnRH agonists as first-line treatments. Guzick et al. [82] demonstrated that there was no significant reduction in pain symptoms between patients administered a GnRH agonist and those using CHCs. Furthermore, the cost of treating patients for 48 weeks with the GnRH agonist was USD $8006 compared to USD $454 for CHCs. Due to the lack of data demonstrating significant improvements in symptoms, GnRH agonists have been commonly used as second-line treatments for patients who do not respond to CHCs or progestins or for those in which the former is contraindicated.

Many studies have also tried to draw cost comparisons between medical and surgical options. Empirical therapy with GnRH agonists has been shown to be less costly than surgical options when managing chronic pelvic pain in patients with endometriosis [83, 84]. A treatment protocol using a GnRH agonist as empirical therapy for endometriosis [85] and laparoscopy only for refractory cases projected cost savings of US $62,800 for the 22 patients enrolled in this trial. Although the upfront cost of GnRH agonists is significantly less than surgery [31, 83, 84], the reported 50% recurrence rate following treatment cessation should not be discounted [83]. Future research should explore the patient and disease factors of those who undergo surgery as a result of symptom recurrence once GnRH agonist therapy is terminated. This may help identify women who are better suited for surgery as opposed to GnRH agonist therapy earlier.

Currently, there is plenty of debate surrounding the cost-effectiveness of medical therapy in comparison to surgical intervention for patients that are appropriate candidates for both.

While there are reduced upfront costs for medical management compared to surgical management, it is important to consider side-effect profiles for medical therapies in addition to the financial burden of long-term medical management. At present, there are not enough high-quality studies to determine whether medical therapy is more cost-effective than surgery, given the high rates of symptom recurrence and potential need for surgical management following the end of the treatment course. There is also a lack of long-term prospective data describing the clinical efficacy of medical therapy in reducing recurrence rates and prevention of surgical intervention during the life course of a patient. These unanswered clinical questions pose significant barriers in the development of cost-effectiveness models that can assist in the production of clinical guidelines.

28.3.3 Costs Associated with Surgical Interventions for Endometriosis

Surgical treatments are often used for patients who are non-responders to medical therapy or for whom hormonal medications are contraindicated [86]. There are many surgical options available, and associated costs vary depending on the type of surgery, length of in-hospital stays, and risk of complications. Currently, laparoscopic surgery is favoured over laparotomy due to shorter recovery times and lower risk of complications [63].

Approximately 65.5% of patients diagnosed with endometriosis will undergo surgery within 1 year of their diagnosis as opposed to 1.5% of controls [63]. An international, multicentre study [32] determined that about 29% of endometriosis-specific healthcare costs are due to surgery. In Canada, hysterectomy accounted for about 30% of all surgical procedures for endometriosis patients. Hospital admissions and surgical procedures represented about 53% of total hospital-associated costs for endometriosis [87]. This comes at a significant cost burden as multiple studies have consistently demonstrated greater upfront direct costs for surgical management compared to medical management [83, 84, 88]. This section will explore the various costs associated with surgical methods and the many drivers of high costs.

28.3.3.1 Cost Differences Between Surgical Procedures

The choice between surgical procedures tends to vary based on patient preference, disease severity, and the desire to maintain fertility. For women who are looking to conceive, fertility-sparing conservative surgery such as laparoscopic excision, cautery, or laser of endometriotic lesions is appropriate [18]. The addition of hysterectomy with or without salpingo-oophorectomy is reserved for patients who do not desire fertility [86, 89]. For hysterectomy, costs also vary based on the surgical technique which can include laparotomy, vaginal, laparoscopy, or a combination of the above [90, 91]. Choice of technique depends on patient factors, disease severity, and surgeon comfort [74].

Fuldeore et al. [63] explored cost estimates for various surgical interventions and noted surgeries requiring hospital admissions, such as hysterectomies, were significantly more costly compared to procedures which usually took place in out-patient settings. In the USA, endometriosis-related surgical procedures had an average length of stay between 1.5 and 2.8 days, with longer stays associated with more invasive procedures such as laparotomy (2.33 days), abdominal hysterectomy (2.59 days), and hysterectomy with oophorectomy (2.81 days) [63]. It is now generally accepted that laparoscopic technique is associated with shorter hospital stay, reduced morbidity, and faster recovery compared to laparotomy for similar procedures [35]. One US study reported total direct costs of USD $3271 per patient in the laparoscopy group and USD $7075 per patient in the laparotomy group [35].

Robotic surgery in endometriosis has also gained popularity in recent years as an alternative method to standard laparoscopy. However, systematic reviews have demonstrated that robotic surgery has minimal additional benefits and is associated with increased expenditures and increased procedure length per patient [92, 93]. A randomized controlled trial performed in patients with endometriosis compared the use of conventional laparoscopy and robotic surgery and found that both methods had comparable clinical outcomes and improvement to quality of life [94]. Given the lack of significant advantages in using robotic methods over traditional laparoscopy, it is important to consider costs, accessibility, and economic burden to the healthcare system when opting to use robotic surgery.

Studies have also demonstrated that surgical treatment for endometriosis is costlier than the equivalent procedure for another benign gynaecologic cause. A Canadian study reported that the total hospital-related costs for all surgical interventions relating to endometriosis cost CAD $152,206,977 from 2008 to 2013 [87]. Hysterectomy for endometriosis carried the greatest cost burden, costing the public-payer system close to CAD $55,034,511, whereas ovarian endometriosis costs approximately CAD $45,230,906. On a case-by-case basis, non-hysterectomy surgical procedures for treating ovarian endometriosis cost CAD $3224, while hysterectomy for endometriosis costs CAD $2356 [87].

The potential for out-patient procedures also creates an area for potential healthcare savings. Out-patient hysterectomy procedures are now increasingly favoured over in-patient hysterectomy procedures due to the reduction with length of stay and subsequent cost savings. The increasing uptake of Enhanced Recovery After Surgery pathways for the standardization and optimization of peri-operative care has also been shown to reduce the cost burden in gynaecological procedures [95]. In conjunction, these studies demonstrate the large financial burden placed on individuals and healthcare systems when treating endometriosis surgically and brings into question the future of sustainable public healthcare systems with increasing costs for surgical interventions in settings with finite resources.

28.3.3.2 Cost Differences Between Medical and Surgical Treatment of Endometriosis

Soliman et al. [96] estimated that total direct healthcare costs for patients who underwent surgery was $19,203 per patient annually, whereas those who did not undergo surgery had average total direct healthcare costs of $6365 per patient annually [96]. This could be attributed to the increased healthcare resource utilization by surgical patients the following year after surgery [96]. In-hospital admissions were the main contributor to costs in the surgical cohort—which approximated 68.8% of the cost—followed by pharmaceutical claims. With an increasing number of practitioners opting for less invasive surgical options such as laparoscopy, the direct costs associated with the surgical procedure, length of stay, and in-hospital admissions can be controlled to various degrees. Cost-control measures could explore reducing this length of stay by choosing more minimally invasive approaches such as laparoscopy instead of laparotomy [87] and favouring out-patient pathways. The impact of indirect costs such as work absence and short-term disability due to surgery was also higher in patients who underwent surgery.

28.3.3.3 Hospital Admissions

In-patient stays and hospital admissions associated with endometriosis are large cost drivers for the healthcare system. In Canada, total hospital costs for endometriosis-related hospital admissions resulted in CAD $30.44 million annually (US $29.56 million), and on average, it costs CAD $3237 (US $3134) per admitted patient case [87]. In 2002, about $22 billion was spent on endometriosis-related costs in the USA of which $14.5 billion was spent on hospital care with admissions as the paramount cost driver [31]. In fact, endometriosis-related hospitalizations are the third leading cause of gynaecologic hospitalizations in the USA [97]. Interestingly, researchers found that different forms of endometriosis are associated with varying degrees of cost. Uterine endometriosis and ovarian endometriosis accounted for the bulk of hospital admissions, with uterine endometriosis being the most expensive to treat [CAD $4137 (US $4017) per case] followed by ovarian endometriosis [CAD $3506 (US $3404) per case].

28.3.3.4 Risk of Disease Recurrence

While surgical interventions can provide significant symptom relief and improvements in quality-adjusted life years, they are costly and have varying degrees of symptom recurrence associated with them. Fertility-sparing surgical interventions can improve fertility and reduce physical disease, but up to half of surgical patients will have recurrence at 2 to 5 years post-surgery [98, 99]. There is conflicting literature regarding rates of recurrence. Guo et al. [98] suggest that post-operative symptom recurrence can occur at a rate of 10% annually, whereas Sutton et al. [100] reported recurrence in approximately 44% of patients within 1 year of surgery. Similarly, Hornstein et al. [101] reported a 51% recurrence rate in patients who underwent laser ablation of endometriotic lesions. Although recurrence is more infrequent with hysterectomy and bilateral salpingo-oophorectomy [75], there is still a 5–10% probability that patients may continue to experience symptoms post-surgery [102]. The risk of recurrence carries negative impacts on patients' quality of life as well as consequences on healthcare expenditures. Patients who experience symptom recurrence may elect to undergo additional surgical procedures or may need to be placed on post-operative medical therapy to help control symptoms—both of which lead to further increasing costs in managing endometriosis.

There is some suggestion of higher symptom recurrence associated with medical management when compared to surgical treatment [102, 103]. Not many studies have evaluated recurrence rates with medical therapies, but one study reported recurrence rates at 1-year post-therapy cessation of 13% for patients on leuprolide acetate and 12% for goserelin acetate [104]. Another study [105] compared aromatase inhibitors (letrozole) with GnRH agonists (triptorelin) after a 2-month therapy period and found that the group on letrozole had a recurrence rate of 6.4%, whereas the group on triptorelin had a recurrence rate of 5%; however, there was no statistical significance between these therapies in symptom recurrence. A study exploring the benefits of nafarelin, another GnRH agonist, has also shown 26% of patients on either a 3- or 6-month therapy schedule experienced symptom recurrence [106].

Randomized controlled trials have explored the use combining medical therapy post-operatively to help with symptom recurrence. Specifically, the post-operative use of a levonorgestrel-releasing intrauterine device (LNG-IUD) has been shown to be effective in reducing the recurrence of dysmenorrhoea [107, 108]. However, the LNG-IUD does not inhibit ovulation and is consequently less effective in preventing the recurrence of endometrioma formation [108]. Prior research has also reported that pre-menopausal patients who undergo more conservative surgical procedures with ovarian or uterine preservation are at a six times greater risk for undergoing repeat surgical procedures due to the higher probability of disease recurrence [109–111].

It is clear that the risk of recurrence remains significant in both medical and surgical interventions for endometriosis and pose additional costs for patients in whom symptoms or endometriotic implants recur post-surgery. Studies that evaluate surgical cost-efficacy and report on cost estimates should also include costs associated with the risk of recurrence stratified by type of medical management or surgical procedure.

28.3.3.5 Costs Associated with Treating Endometriosis-Related Infertility/Subfertility

The impact of endometriosis on fertility is well documented in the literature. Options for women trying to conceive range from expectant management, surgical excision of lesions, or assisted reproductive technologies (ART) [3]. Hormonal medical therapies are contraindicated in these patients as they often suppress ovulation. Patients who are likely to succeed with expectant management often are younger, have normal ovarian reserve, regular ovulation, and uterine tube patency [3]. Older patients with more extensive disease are often treated with surgical therapy or ART [3].

While surgery may help stabilize the reproductive architecture and correct anatomical distortions from endometriotic implants, there is a correlation between surgical therapy and decreased ovarian reserve [3]. Patients with mild to moderate disease may benefit from surgery to increase their chances of spontaneous conception [112]. However, the improvement in fecundity is minor at 8%, with only marginal improvements in spontaneous conception [3, 113, 114]. In patients with moderate to severe disease, the estimated surgical benefit is smaller due to the presence of tubal adhesions, and ART is more often recommended [115]. Overall, the clinical utility in surgery for fertility is limited, as 25 patients would need laparoscopic surgical management to achieve one more live birth when compared to expectant management [112, 113, 116].

Patients with normal ovarian reserve may be eligible for multiple ART options such as superovulation or intrauterine insemination [116] which is less costly than in vitro fertilization (IVF). However, there are minimal benefits to using this approach in patients with endometriosis [117, 118]. IVF has been more associated with successful rates of pregnancy in patients with endometriosis, especially for those with diminished ovarian reserve [74]. Prolonged treatment with hormonal therapies such as GnRH agonists or CHCs has been shown to help improve pregnancy rates using ART [119, 120]. Outcomes using ART have also been shown to be superior to surgical therapy in patients with endometriosis to achieve conception [121].

The Endometriosis Fertility Index (EFI) has been used to predict the occurrence of spontaneous pregnancy following endometriosis surgery and plays an important role in helping physicians triage patients into expectant management or assisted reproductive technologies [122]. Ferrier et al. [122] conducted a cost-effectiveness analysis to determine the costs associated with different ART treatment pathways immediately after surgery for endometriosis-associated infertility. Specifically, they explored the use of the EFI to stratify patients and determine appropriate care pathways to study cost-effectiveness. Patients were channelled into three different care pathways to manage endometriosis-associated infertility using the EFI as a stratification tool: natural conception, immediate IVF-Intracytoplasmic sperm injection (IVF-ICSI), and delayed IVF-ICSI. The costs for patients who underwent IVF-ICSI amounted to €9509 per patient, €15,196 per pregnancy, and €18,235 per live birth with an incremental cost-effectiveness ratio of €31,469 per pregnancy over expectant management. Although immediate IVF-ICSI post-surgery is an appropriate method for attaining fertility in endometriosis patients, it presents significant costs for the healthcare system. Further research is needed in the role of expectant management for select patients after surgery (such as those with a good prognosis, normal ovarian reserve with high EFI score).

IVF, while demonstrating successful rates of conception in endometriosis patients, still poses a large financial burden on patients and healthcare systems. Apart from the costs associated with the procedure, there are also ancillary costs that are incurred by patients. These costs include medical costs, fertility counselling, time off work, and/or psychological support. Patients with diminished ovarian reserve often require egg donation which is also associated with significant logistical expenses incurred by the patient. A partially, publicly funded IVF model in Canada reported that 49% of patients still paid between CAD $5000 and CAD $10,000 in ancillary costs, with 18% paying between CAD $10,000 and CAD $20,000 to undergo IVF [123]. Collins [124] in 2002 found that the average cost per IVF-ICSI cycle was around $9547 in the USA and $3518 in 25 countries around the world. In fact, IVF costs ranged from 10% of annual household expenditure in European countries to 25% in Canada and the USA [124]. These studies explicitly display the large financial burden placed on individual patients and healthcare systems as a result of treating infertility, and these costs are compounded by the ART that is often needed to attain a pregnancy in patients with endometriosis.

28.4 Indirect Costs Associated with Endometriosis

Although direct costs have often taken the spotlight in cost-efficacy literature, indirect costs are equally as important to account for when creating true cost analyses for disease burden. Indirect costs are often left out of these estimates because of the difficulty and large variability in quantifying these costs. This often arises due to a large reliance on self-reported data to account for factors such as loss of work productivity, childcare, caregiver support as well as variable valuation of these factors [125]. The main demographic affected by endometriosis are of reproductive age, which constitutes the majority of working-age members of the population. In fact, patients between the ages of 18 and 44 years account for approximately 75% of all endometriosis hospital admissions [18]. In 2002, Simoens et al. [31] estimated the annual endometriosis-related healthcare cost burden in the USA to be close to $22 billion and 21% of this estimate ($4.7 billion) was due to indirect costs, mainly through a loss of productivity. In 2010, the annual societal burden of endometriosis in the USA was projected at $69.4 billion of which two-thirds was reportedly due to loss of productivity [32]. These studies demonstrate the significant role of indirect costs in the total economic burden of endometriosis.

28.4.1 What Are the Indirect Costs Associated with Work Absences and Productivity?

Work absences and productivity represent major contributors to the indirect costs associated with endometriosis. Missed hours of work annually due to endometriosis-related chronic pelvic pain range from 19.2 hours to 86.4 hours per patient [126, 127]. Mathias et al. [127] also noted that endometriosis caused patients to miss 1.6 hours of work every month in comparison to 0.05 hours missed by patients with other menstrual cycle–related diagnoses. Nnoaham et al. [10] showed that endometriosis resulted in equivalent work loss of approximately 6.4 hours per week due to presenteeism and 4.4 hours per week due to absenteeism across ten countries. In the USA, this would amount to approximately $3200 lost per year from absenteeism and $14,800 lost per year from presenteeism [10]. Levy et al. [128] quantified the loss of work productivity and leisure time costs to be close to $3854 per patient annually in Canada. It is evident from these studies that endometriosis-related pelvic pain severely impacts work productivity and patients' ability to maintain employment [129], thereby solidifying the further impact of endometriosis on economic burden.

There is also evidence that the work absences and productivity associated with endometriosis can have life-long negative effects. One matched case-control study demonstrated that women with endometriosis are significantly less likely to work in their desired profession, and more likely to consider health-related limitations in career choices, compared to a matched control group [130]. Similarly, those living with endometriosis can experience lower annual salary and salary growth compared to those without endometriosis [131]. The life-long cost implications are currently not well quantified in the literature.

28.4.2 What Are the Indirect Costs Associated with Surgery?

Surgical treatment plays a significant role in increasing indirect costs to patients. One study reported a productivity loss of $2236 per patient in the 6 months prior to surgery and $3686 in the 6 months post-surgery [132]. Indirect costs after surgery may be attributable to longer recovery times, absences from work, and post-surgical pain. These findings are aligned with the idea that pelvic pain and disease severity are major drivers of work productivity loss for endometriosis patients [10]. Another study demonstrated that absence claims were higher in patients who underwent surgical treatment for endometriosis, resulting in a loss of income close to $6237 for those in the surgery cohort compared to $4781 for those who were not in the surgery cohort [96]. Absenteeism, short-term disability, and long-term disability were also all reported significantly higher in the surgery cohort [96].

28.4.3 Why Are Indirect Costs Important?

Indirect costs are important contributors to the overall financial burden of endometriosis on the individual, healthcare systems, and society. The majority of economic literature has focused on direct costs, largely due to the difficult nature of reliable valuation of factors such as presenteeism, the lack of self-report data, or an inconsistency in what qualifies as an indirect cost. Most of the indirect costs to date have focused on factors such as absence claims, work productivity, and unemployment. There is a clear lack of research focusing on indirect costs such as childcare and transportation, in addition to the difficulty in quantifying costs of social withdrawal, psychological impacts, and loss of leisure time.

Indirect costs play a large role in the economic burden of endometriosis. Understanding these factors can provide strategies to mitigate the substantial productivity losses arising from endometriosis-related symptoms. The diagnostic and treatment delays also play a role in exacerbating productivity losses. These intangible costs are equally as important to study given the multifaceted impacts of endometriosis on patients' lives and the life-long impacts this can have.

28.5 Conclusions

28.5.1 What Is the Global Economic Burden of Endometriosis?

This chapter has highlighted the direct and indirect costs associated with endometriosis and the many ways these costs contribute to the economic burden of many societies and healthcare systems. Although it is difficult to draw direct comparisons between the cost estimates due to inherent differences in healthcare system structures and regional practices, the large global economic burden remains consistent. The cost-efficacy of practice and policy guidelines on the diagnosis and treatment of endometriosis must be taken into account to ensure sustainability of national healthcare systems.

The current available data are limited as the national economic burden varies from country to country depending on population size and the local guidelines for clinical practice for endometriosis. Differences in reported endometriosis prevalence rates can further the variations in the subsequent estimated economic burden.

Table 28.7 National economic burden by country

Country	National annual economic burden	Type of costs accounted for
Germany [133]	€40,708,716	Direct costs from in-patient treatments for endometriosis
Austria [53]	€328 million	Direct and indirect costs
Canada [128]	$1.8 billion	Treatment costs, quality of life, work absenteeism, and caregiver time
Denmark [32]	€0.8 million	Costs associated with endometriosis-related symptoms
Switzerland [32]	€1.3 billion	
Hungary [32]	€1.6 billion	
Belgium [32]	€1.7 billion	
Netherlands [32]	€2.6 billion	
Italy [32]	€9.3 billion	
France [32]	€9.5 billion	
UK [32]	€9.9 billion	
Germany [32]	€12.5 billion	
USA [32]	€49.6 billion	

Table 28.7 illustrates the variability in national economic burdens per country. In Europe, economic burdens range from €3114 to €9872 [32, 53, 134, 135] per patient annually, whereas US numbers range from USD $8417 to $18,881 per patient annually [18, 60, 63]. Endometriosis-associated costs appear to be highest in the USA, and this theme recurs quite often in the literature [18, 32, 60, 63, 87, 96]. Both the direct and indirect costs associated with endometriosis need to be included in these national cost analyses to identify potential interventions that can target these large hidden cost drivers.

It is clear that endometriosis has a large stake in national expenditures for many healthcare systems around the globe. There is a strong need to reduce the diagnostic delay using more consistent guidelines, increased awareness amongst general practitioners, and more reliable diagnostic tools. Timely diagnosis would help reduce both the unnecessary healthcare expenses and the indirect costs associated with loss of productivity. More cost-effectiveness studies need to be conducted regarding the treatment of endometriosis and its risk of recurrence. Finally, to ensure that healthcare systems remain sustainable, rising costs related to endometriosis should be monitored and its contributing factors should be studied for cost-efficacy and global economic impacts.

28.5.2 Limitations and Future Directions

28.5.2.1 Lack of Control Groups

There are many limitations to the cost analyses referenced in this chapter. One of the largest criticisms surrounding cost-effectiveness studies is the lack of control groups and matched controls to draw adequate comparisons. Control groups help delineate potential confounders, and a matched group of controls without endometriosis can help formulate better causal relationships about the economic burden of this disease on patients. A lack of control groups also biases cost estimates and makes it difficult for policy makers to understand the discrepancy in incurred costs for endometriosis patients compared to those living without endometriosis. Adequate control groups would also distinguish between costs incurred as a result of having endometriosis from costs incurred through endometriosis-related symptoms, such as pelvic pain and infertility, which are present in conditions outside of endometriosis [31]. This methodology would help better understand the costs arising from the disease itself as opposed to the related symptomatology.

28.5.2.2 Inclusion of Patient Profile Characteristics

Future studies should also attempt to understand how patient profile and disease characteristics impact endometriosis costs. Both direct and indirect costs may be influenced by patient factors and disease characteristics such as severity, symptoms, location, and type of endometriosis. Many studies did not list their patient profile or characterize individual disease, and this makes it difficult to generalize cost estimates to specific populations. This is especially relevant when comparing the heterogeneity of endometriosis, as more severe disease is likely to increase cost burden. There is also a lack of data focusing on endometriosis-related costs and economic burdens in Asian, Middle-Eastern, and African populations. Future research should focus on quantifying these costs in these populations and developing theoretical models to understand the global impact of endometriosis on health economics.

The presence of comorbidities is an important consideration when exploring costs associated with endometriosis as they ultimately inform treatment options and impact overall costs incurred. As endometriosis is commonly associated with other chronic pain disorders, its true economic burden may be underestimated when these comorbidities are not accounted for. Costs for comorbidities that are directly related to endometriosis should be included in cost analyses to capture the full spectrum of disease burden [33].

Another aspect that needs to be explored in cost estimates is the inclusion of suspected cases of endometriosis. Clinically suspected cases of endometriosis without histopathological diagnosis may benefit from inclusion in endometriosis studies to model the full extent of disease burden. These cases will provide valuable information regarding the true impact of the diagnostic delay and indirect costs such as productivity loss and unemployment. Inclusion of undiagnosed and misdiagnosed cases will also help explore costs incurred from unnecessary investigations and tests and multiple out-patient visits. Finally, many current studies tend to exclude adolescents and peri- or post-menopausal women and thereby, overlook the large costs specific to these groups. While the majority of endometriosis cases are in reproductive-age women [60], future studies should also explore hospitalizations for pelvic pain and endometriosis-related symptoms in women outside of this age range to accurately calculate cost estimates.

28.5.2.3 Costs Associated with Recurrence Risk

Despite its high prevalence, many studies do not account for costs following recurrence from cessation of medical therapy or post-surgery. Further research on the risk of recurrence could better estimate the costs associated with various risk factors to better understand their true effectiveness across a patient's life course. Recurrence rates and associated costs should also be assessed when conducting cost-effectiveness studies for various treatment interventions to be more reflective of the longitudinal and chronic nature of endometriosis.

28.5.2.4 Value-Based Care Studies

Future directions should also include the need for more value-based care studies on the impact of endometriosis expenditures [136]. Global guidelines for the diagnosis and treatment of endometriosis are inconsistent, producing a need for research that evaluates the merits of these varying interventions. These studies will help in reducing low-value care and unnecessary healthcare expenses. Value-based care studies should explore current screening, diagnostic options, and management options available to endometriosis patients to determine the optimal benefit associated with specific approaches to management. While it is difficult to draw parallels across different regions, there is utility to studying resource utilization rates to understand geographic variability in value-based care.

There is also a need for studies contrasting the cost-efficacy of different approaches to diagnosis and management. This will help policy makers stratify and prioritize diagnostic and treatment options while limiting the amount of unnecessary and costly tests and treatments. In particular, the cost-efficacy of medical versus surgical therapies need to be studied with a longitudinal approach across the lifespan of patients with endometriosis. Studies should aim to understand the utilization of healthcare resources, from the first initial visit with symptoms to the point of definitive diagnosis. There are usually multiple clinic and hospital visits with varying healthcare providers that occur during this window of time where many unnecessary tests are initiated in the pursuit of diagnosis. Similarly, the number of investigations and interventions from diagnosis to an improved quality of life need to be captured to study how patients with endometriosis utilize healthcare resources during their lifespan. To truly understand and help inform value-based care guidelines, unnecessary investigations and their utilization rates must be clearly studied. Furthermore, novel diagnostic tools and interventions should be assessed for their impact on reducing expenditures in conjunction with their ability to diagnose and treat endometriosis while improving quality of life for patients.

More comprehensive studies which document cost estimates, especially with regard to the direct and indirect costs of IVF and other forms of ART are needed. The literature is currently limited in identifying whether immediate ART post-surgery or delayed ART with expectant management is more cost-effective for treating fertility. Future research should also explore the overall financial burden related to treating endometriosis-associated infertility and subfertility, by calculating the total healthcare costs required to achieve a successful live birth per patient [18] and the number needed to treat to attain one more pregnancy.

28.5.2.5 Lack of Studies Quantifying Non-Healthcare Costs and Indirect Costs

The lack of research outlining the full spectrum of indirect costs associated with endometriosis is alarming and points toward conservative estimates of national economic burdens. The true financial impact of the diagnostic delay for endometriosis cannot be determined without the inclusion of indirect costs such as productivity loss and work absences during this period. Disease severity and level of impairment should also be studied to understand correlations between these factors and their impact on quality of life. Given that the majority of endometriosis patients are in the workforce, cost estimates and economic burden must take into account the various indirect costs. Of the studies that explore indirect costs, many studies focus on factors such as presenteeism, absenteeism, unemployment, and work productivity to quantify lost income. There is a lack of studies focusing on other forms of indirect costs such as caregiver support, transportation costs to appointments, and childcare costs. Other non-healthcare costs are also not studied such as the use of alternative medicine and supplemental care such as physiotherapy, chiropractic, or lifestyle interventions. Future studies need to focus on identifying and quantifying non-healthcare related costs and indirect costs.

28.5.3 Concluding Remarks

Healthcare resources are finite and given the current global climate, healthcare systems need to consider sustainability when faced with growing expenditures and disease burden. The cost-effectiveness of diagnostic procedures and treatments must be systematically reviewed to ensure that healthcare systems appropriately allocate care that is high impact, especially in publicly funded or administered models of care. This chapter highlights the enormous global economic burden associated with endometriosis, which likely remains a conservative estimate of the real costs posed to individuals, health systems, and society. There is substantial healthcare resource utilization which contributes to the economic burden of endometriosis, and this problem is compounded by the propensity of patients to undergo multiple unnecessary tests and interventions across a variety of settings before obtaining an appropriate diagnosis or treatment. Enormous endometriosis-related costs without the proportionate improvements in health outcomes threaten the sustainability of national healthcare systems. The numerous factors contributing to these rising costs have been explored thoroughly in this chapter, and this knowledge will help guide future healthcare providers, hospital administrators, and policy makers in curtailing expenditures while balancing patient outcomes.

References

1. American College of Obstetricians and Gynecologists. Management of endometriosis. ACOG Practice bulletin no. 114. Obstetr Gynecol. 2010;116(1):225–36.
2. Johnson NP, Hummelshoj L, Adamson GD, Keckstein J, Taylor HS, Abrao MS, et al. World Endometriosis Society consensus on the classification of endometriosis. Hum Reprod. 2017;32(2):315–24.
3. Zondervan KT, Becker CM, Koga K, Missmer SA, Taylor RN, Viganò P. Endometriosis (Primer). Nature Reviews: Disease Primers; 2018.
4. Santulli P, Marcellin L, Tosti C, Chouzenoux S, Cerles O, Borghese B, et al. MAP kinases and the inflammatory signaling cascade as targets for the treatment of endometriosis? Expert Opin Ther Targets. 2015;19(11):1465–83.
5. Reis FM, Santulli P, Marcellin L, Borghese B, Lafay-Pillet MC, Chapron C. Superficial peritoneal endometriosis: clinical characteristics of 203 confirmed cases and 1292 endometriosis-free controls. Reprod Sci. 2020;27(1):309–15.
6. Abbas S, Ihle P, Koster I, Schubert I. Prevalence and incidence of diagnosed endometriosis and risk of endometriosis in patients with endometriosis-related symptoms: findings from a statutory health insurance- based cohort in Germany. Eur J Obstet Gynecol Reprod Biol. 2012;160:79–83.
7. Zondervan KT, Cardon LR, Kennedy SH. The genetic basis of endometriosis. Curr Opin Obstet Gynecol. 2001;13(3):309–14.
8. Mihalyi A, Mutinda KC, Simsa P, Debrock S, Mwenda JM, D'Hooghe TM. Role of immunologic and inflammatory factors in the development of endometriosis: indications for treatment strategies. Clin Pract. 2005;2(4):623.
9. Adamson GD, Kennedy S, Hummelshoj L. Creating solutions in endometriosis: global collaboration through the World Endometriosis Research Foundation; 2010. p. 3–6.
10. Nnoaham KE, Hummelshoj L, Webster P, d'Hooghe T, de Cicco Nardone F, de Cicco Nardone C, et al. Impact of endometriosis on quality of life and work productivity: a multicenter study across ten countries. Fertil Steril. 2011;96(2):366–73.
11. Eskenazi B, Warner ML. Epidemiology of endometriosis. Obstet Gynecol Clin N Am. 1997;24(2):235–58.
12. Louis GM, Hediger ML, Peterson CM, Croughan M, Sundaram R, Stanford J, et al. Incidence of endometriosis by study population and diagnostic method: the ENDO study. Fertil Steril. 2011;96(2):360–5.
13. Barbieri RL. Etiology and epidemiology of endometriosis. Am J Obstet Gynecol. 1990;162(2):565–7.
14. Meuleman C, Vandenabeele B, Fieuws S, Spiessens C, Timmerman D, D'Hooghe T. High prevalence of endometriosis in infertile women with normal ovulation and normospermic partners. Fertil Steril. 2009;92(1):68–74.
15. Whitaker LH, Reid J, Choa A, McFee S, Seretny M, Wilson J, et al. An exploratory study into objective and reported characteristics of neuropathic pain in women with chronic pelvic pain. PLoS One. 2016;11(4):e0151950.
16. Mowers EL, Lim CS, Skinner B, Mahnert N, Kamdar N, Morgan DM, et al. Prevalence of endometriosis during abdominal or laparoscopic hysterectomy for chronic pelvic pain. Obstet Gynecol. 2016;127(6):1045–53.
17. Giudice LC, Kao LC. Endometriosis. Lancet. 2004;364:1789–99.
18. Gao X, Outley J, Botteman M, Spalding J, Simon JA, Pashos CL. Economic burden of endometriosis. Fertil Steril. 2006;86(6):1561–72.
19. Gao X, Yeh YC, Outley J, Simon J, Botteman M, Spalding J. Health-related quality of life burden of women with endometriosis: a literature review. Curr Med Res Opin. 2006;22(9):1787–97.
20. Surtees PG, Wainwright NW, Khaw KT, Day NE. Functional health status, chronic medical conditions and disorders of mood. Br J Psychiatry. 2003;183(4):299–303.

21. Fourquet J, Báez L, Figueroa M, Iriarte RI, Flores I. Quantification of the impact of endometriosis symptoms on health-related quality of life and work productivity. Fertil Steril. 2011;96(1):107–12.
22. Zhao SZ, Wong JM, Davis MB, Gersh GE, Johnson KE. The cost of inpatient endometriosis treatment: an analysis based on the Healthcare Cost and Utilization Project Nationwide Inpatient Sample. Am J Manag Care. 1998;4(8):1127–34.
23. Senapati S, Sammel MD, Morse C, Barnhart KT. Impact of endometriosis on in vitro fertilization outcomes: an evaluation of the Society for Assisted Reproductive Technologies Database. Fertil Steril. 2016;106(1):164–71.
24. Laganà AS, La Rosa VL, Rapisarda AM, Valenti G, Sapia F, Chiofalo B, et al. Anxiety and depression in patients with endometriosis: impact and management challenges. Int J Women's Health. 2017;9:323.
25. Facchin F, Barbara G, Dridi D, Alberico D, Buggio L, Somigliana E, et al. Mental health in women with endometriosis: searching for predictors of psychological distress. Hum Reprod. 2017;32(9):1855–61.
26. Aerts L, Grangier L, Streuli I, Dällenbach P, Marci R, Wenger JM, et al. Psychosocial impact of endometriosis: From co-morbidity to intervention. Best Pract Res Clin Obstet Gynaecol. 2018;50:2–10.
27. Culley L, Law C, Hudson N, Denny E, Mitchell H, Baumgarten M, et al. The social and psychological impact of endometriosis on women's lives: a critical narrative review. Hum Reprod Update. 2013;19(6):625–39.
28. Moradi M, Parker M, Sneddon A, Lopez V, Ellwood D. Impact of endometriosis on women's lives: a qualitative study. BMC Womens Health. 2014;14(1):123.
29. Zannoni L, Giorgi M, Spagnolo E, Montanari G, Villa G, Seracchioli R. Dysmenorrhea, absenteeism from school, and symptoms suspicious for endometriosis in adolescents. J Pediatr Adolesc Gynecol. 2014;27(5):258–65.
30. Soliman AM, Coyne KS, Gries KS, Castelli-Haley J, Snabes MC, Surrey ES. The effect of endometriosis symptoms on absenteeism and presenteeism in the workplace and at home. J Manag Care Spec Pharm. 2017;23(7):745–54.
31. Simoens S, Hummelshoj L, D'Hooghe T. Endometriosis: cost estimates and methodological perspective. Hum Reprod Update. 2007;13(4):395–404.
32. Simoens S, Dunselman G, Dirksen C, Hummelshoj L, Bokor A, Brandes I, et al. The burden of endometriosis: costs and quality of life of women with endometriosis and treated in referral centres. Hum Reprod. 2012;27(5):1292–9.
33. Soliman AM, Yang H, Du EX, Kelley C, Winkel C. The direct and indirect costs associated with endometriosis: a systematic literature review. Hum Reprod. 2016;31(4):712–22.
34. Yeung PP Jr, Shwayder J, Pasic RP. Laparoscopic management of endometriosis: comprehensive review of best evidence. J Minim Invasive Gynecol. 2009;16(3):269–81.
35. Luciano AA, Lowney J, Jacobs SL. Endoscopic treatment of endometriosis-associated infertility. Therapeutic, economic and social benefits. J Reprod Med. 1992;37(7):573–6.
36. Medeiros LR, Rosa DD, Bozzetti MC, Fachel JM, Furness S, Garry R, Rosa MI, Stein AT. Laparoscopy versus laparotomy for benign ovarian tumour. Cochrane Database Syst Rev. 2009;2:CD004751.
37. Chapron C, Cravello L, Chopin N, Kreiker G, Blanc B, Dubuisson JB. Complications during set-up procedures for laparoscopy in gynecology: open laparoscopy does not reduce the risk of major complications. Acta Obstet Gynecol Scand. 2003;82(12):1125–9.
38. Ling FW. Randomized controlled trial of depot leuprolide in patients with chronic pelvic pain and clinically suspected endometriosis. Obstet Gynecol. 1999;93(1):51–8.
39. Kennedy S, Bergqvist A, Chapron C, D'Hooghe T, Dunselman G, Greb R, et al. On behalf of the ESHRE Special Interest Group for Endometriosis and Endometrium Guideline Development Group. Hum Reprod. 2005;20(10):2698–704.
40. Heim LJ. Evaluation and differential diagnosis of dyspareunia. Am Fam Physician. 2001;63(8):1535.

41. Brenner PF. Differential diagnosis of abnormal uterine bleeding. Am J Obstet Gynecol. 1996;175(3):766–9.
42. Mounsey A, Wilgus A, Slawson DC. Diagnosis and management of endometriosis. Am Fam Physician. 2006;74(4):594–600.
43. Ay W. The significance of diagnostic delay in endometriosis. MOJ Womens Health. 2016;2:10–1.
44. Taylor HS, Adamson GD, Diamond MP, Goldstein SR, Horne AW, Missmer SA, et al. An evidence based approach to assessing surgical versus clinical diagnosis of symptomatic endometriosis. Int J Gynecol Obstet. 2018;142(2):131–42.
45. Nisenblat V, Bossuyt PM, Farquhar C, Johnson N, Hull ML. Imaging modalities for the non-invasive diagnosis of endometriosis. Cochrane Database Syst Rev. 2016;2:CD009591.
46. Eskenazi B, Warner M, Bonsignore L, Olive D, Samuels S, Vercellini P. Validation study of nonsurgical diagnosis of endometriosis. Fertil Steril. 2001;76(5):929–35.
47. Leyland N, Casper R, Laberge P, Singh SS, Allen L, Arendas K, et al. Endometriosis: diagnosis and management. J Endometr. 2010;2(3):107–34.
48. Practice Committee of the American Society for Reproductive Medicine. Treatment of pelvic pain associated with endometriosis: a committee opinion. Fertil Steril. 2014;101(4):927–35.
49. Vercellini P, Buggio L, Frattaruolo MP, Borghi A, Dridi D, Somigliana E. Medical treatment of endometriosis-related pain. Best Pract Res Clin Obstet Gynaecol. 2018;51:68–91.
50. Frishman GN, Salak JR. Conservative surgical management of endometriosis in women with pelvic pain. J Minim Invasive Gynecol. 2006;13(6):546–58.
51. Chiaffarino F, Cipriani S, Ricci E, Mauri PA, Esposito G, Barretta M, et al. Endometriosis and irritable bowel syndrome: a systematic review and meta-analysis. Arch Gynecol Obstet. 2020;303(1):17–25.
52. Ballard K, Lowton K, Wright J. What's the delay? A qualitative study of women's experiences of reaching a diagnosis of endometriosis. Fertil Steril. 2006;86(5):1296–301.
53. Prast J, Oppelt P, Shamiyeh A, Shebl O, Brandes I, Haas D. Costs of endometriosis in Austria: a survey of direct and indirect costs. Arch Gynecol Obstet. 2013;288(3):569–76.
54. Matsuzaki S, Canis M, Pouly JL, Rabischong B, Botchorishvili R, Mage G. Relationship between delay of surgical diagnosis and severity of disease in patients with symptomatic deep infiltrating endometriosis. Fertil Steril. 2006;86(5):1314–6.
55. Arruda MS, Petta CA, Abrão MS, Benetti-Pinto CL. Time elapsed from onset of symptoms to diagnosis of endometriosis in a cohort study of Brazilian women. Hum Reprod. 2003;18(4):756–9.
56. Husby GK, Haugen RS, Moen MH. Diagnostic delay in women with pain and endometriosis. Acta Obstet Gynecol Scand. 2003;82(7):649–53.
57. Soliman AM, Fuldeore M, Snabes MC. Factors associated with time to endometriosis diagnosis in the United States. J Women's Health. 2017;26(7):788–97.
58. Surrey E, Soliman AM, Trenz H, Blauer-Peterson C, Sluis A. Impact of endometriosis diagnostic delays on healthcare resource utilization and costs. Adv Ther. 2020;37(3):1087–99.
59. Soliman AM, Surrey ES, Bonafede M, Nelson JK, Vora JB, Agarwal SK. Health care utilization and costs associated with endometriosis among women with medicaid insurance. J Manag Care Spec Pharm. 2019;25(5):566–72.
60. Fuldeore M, Yang H, Du EX, Soliman AM, Wu EQ, Winkel C. Healthcare utilization and costs in women diagnosed with endometriosis before and after diagnosis: a longitudinal analysis of claims databases. Fertil Steril. 2015;103(1):163–71.
61. Soliman AM, Surrey E, Bonafede M, Nelson JK, Castelli-Haley J. Real-world evaluation of direct and indirect economic burden among endometriosis patients in the United States. Adv Ther. 2018;35(3):408–23.
62. Mirkin D, Murphy-Barron C, Iwasaki K. Actuarial analysis of private payer administrative claims data for women with endometriosis. J Manag Care Pharm. 2007;13:262–72.
63. Fuldeore M, Chwalisz K, Marx S, Wu N, Boulanger L, Ma L, et al. Surgical procedures and their cost estimates among women with newly diagnosed endometriosis: a US database study. J Med Econ. 2011;14(1):115–23.

64. Nisenblat V, Bossuyt PM, Shaikh R, Farquhar C, Jordan V, Scheffers CS, et al. Blood biomarkers for the non-invasive diagnosis of endometriosis. Cochrane Database Syst Rev. 2016;5:CD012179.
65. Moore J, Copley S, Morris J, Lindsell D, Golding S, Kennedy S. A systematic review of the accuracy of ultrasound in the diagnosis of endometriosis. Ultrasound Obstetr Gynecol. 2002;20(6):630–4.
66. Exacoustos C, Manganaro L, Zupi E. Imaging for the evaluation of endometriosis and adenomyosis. Best Pract Res Clin Obstet Gynaecol. 2014;28(5):655–81.
67. Testa AC, Timmerman D, Van Holsbeke C, Zannoni GF, Fransis S, Moerman P, et al. Ovarian cancer arising in endometrioid cysts: ultrasound findings. Ultrasound Obstet Gynecol. 2011;38(1):99–106.
68. Hudelist G, English J, Thomas AE, Tinelli A, Singer CF, Keckstein J. Diagnostic accuracy of transvaginal ultrasound for non-invasive diagnosis of bowel endometriosis: systematic review and meta-analysis. Ultrasound Obstet Gynecol. 2011;37(3):257–63.
69. Kinkel K, Frei KA, Balleyguier C, Chapron C. Diagnosis of endometriosis with imaging: a review. Eur Radiol. 2006;16(2):285–98.
70. Leonardi M, Robledo KP, Espada M, Vanza K, Condous G. SonoPODography: a new diagnostic technique for visualizing superficial endometriosis. Eur J Obstet Gynecol Reprod Biol. 2020;254:124–31.
71. Dmowski WP, Lesniewicz R, Rana N, Pepping P, Noursalehi M. Changing trends in the diagnosis of endometriosis: a comparative study of women with pelvic endometriosis presenting with chronic pelvic pain or infertility. Fertil Steril. 1997;67(2):238–43.
72. Vercellini P, Viganò P, Somigliana E, Fedele L. Endometriosis: pathogenesis and treatment. Nat Rev Endocrinol. 2014;10(5):261.
73. Johnson NP, Hummelshoj L, World Endometriosis Society Montpellier Consortium, Abrao MS, Adamson GD, Allaire C, Amelung V, Andersson E, Becker C, Birna Árdal KB, Bush D. Consensus on current management of endometriosis. Hum Reprod. 2013;28(6):1552–68.
74. Dunselman GA, Vermeulen N, Becker C, Calhaz-Jorge C, D'Hooghe T, De Bie B, et al. ESHRE guideline: management of women with endometriosis. Hum Reprod. 2014;29(3):400–12.
75. Clayton RD, Hawe JA, Love JC, Wilkinson N, Garry R. Recurrent pain after hysterectomy and bilateral salpingo-oophorectomy for endometriosis: evaluation of laparoscopic excision of residual endometriosis. BJOG Int J Obstet Gynaecol. 1999;106(7):740–4.
76. Vercellini P, Buggio L, Berlanda N, Barbara G, Somigliana E, Bosari S. Estrogen-progestins and progestins for the management of endometriosis. Fertil Steril. 2016;106(7):1552–71.
77. Olive DL, Schwartz LB. Endomeuiosis. N Engl J Med. 1993;328(24):1.
78. Allaire C, Long AJ, Bedaiwy MA, Yong PJ. Interdisciplinary teams in endometriosis care. In Seminars in reproductive medicine 2020. Thieme Medical Publishers.
79. Bodner C, Vale L, Ratcliffe J, Farrar S. Using economics alongside medical audit. A case study of the management of endometriosis. Health Bull. 1996;54(3):204–11.
80. Grand TS, Basarir H, Jackson LJ. The cost-effectiveness of oral contraceptives compared to 'no hormonal treatment for endometriosis-related pain: An economic evaluation. PLoS One. 2019;14(1):e0210089.
81. Pearson S, Pickersgill A. The costs of endometriosis. InGynaecol. Forum. 2004;9:23–7.
82. Guzick DS, Huang LS, Broadman BA, Nealon M, Hornstein MD. Randomized trial of leuprolide versus continuous oral contraceptives in the treatment of endometriosis-associated pelvic pain. Fertil Steril. 2011;95(5):1568–73.
83. Surrey E. An economically rational method of managing early-stage endometriosis. Med Interface. 1997;10(3):119.
84. Lindheim SR. Chronic pelvic pain: presumptive diagnosis and therapy using GnRH agonists. Int J Fertil Womens Med. 1999;44(3):131–8.
85. Kephart W. Evaluation of Lovelace Health Systems chronic pelvic pain protocol. Am J Manag Care. 1999;5(5 Suppl):S309.
86. Armstrong C. ACOG updates guideline on diagnosis and treatment of endometriosis. Am Fam Physician. 2011;83(1):84.

87. Chen I, Thavorn K, Yong PJ, Choudhry AJ, Allaire C. Hospital-associated cost of endometriosis in Canada: a population-based study. J Minim Invasive Gynecol. 2020;27(5):1178–87.
88. Winkel CA. Modeling of medical and surgical treatment costs of chronic pelvic pain: new paradigms for making clinical decisions. Am J Manag Care. 1999;5(5 Suppl):S276–90.
89. Bedaiwy MA, Barker NM. Evidence based surgical management of endometriosis. Middle East Fertil Soc J. 2012;17(1):57–60.
90. Cohen MM, Young W. Costs of hysterectomy: does surgical approach make a difference? J Women's Health. 1998;7(7):885–92.
91. Chapron C, Fernandez B, Dubuisson JB. Total hysterectomy for benign pathologies: direct costs comparison between laparoscopic and abdominal hysterectomy. Europ J Obstetr Gynecol Reprod Biol. 2000;89(2):141–7.
92. Liu H, Lu D, Wang L, et al. Robotic surgery for benign gynaecological disease. Cochrane Database Syst Rev. 2012;2:CD008978.
93. Kristensen SE, Mosgaard BJ, Rosendahl M, Dalsgaard T, Bjørn SF, Frøding LP, et al. Robot-assisted surgery in gynecological oncology: current status and controversies on patient benefits, cost and surgeon conditions–a systematic review. Acta Obstet Gynecol Scand. 2017;96(3):274–85.
94. Soto E, Luu TH, Liu X, Magrina JF, Wasson MN, Einarsson JI, et al. Laparoscopy vs. Robotic Surgery for Endometriosis (LAROSE): a multicenter, randomized, controlled trial. Fertil Steril. 2017;107(4):996–1002.
95. Pache B, Joliat GR, Hübner M, Grass F, Demartines N, Mathevet P, et al. Cost-analysis of Enhanced Recovery After Surgery (ERAS) program in gynecologic surgery. Gynecol Oncol. 2019;154(2):388–93.
96. Soliman AM, Taylor H, Bonafede M, Nelson JK, Castelli-Haley J. Incremental direct and indirect cost burden attributed to endometriosis surgeries in the United States. Fertil Steril. 2017;107(5):1181–90.
97. Missmer SA, Cramer DW. Epidemiology of endometriosis. In Endometriosis in clinical practice 2004. CRC Press. p. 79–94.
98. Guo SW. Recurrence of endometriosis and its control. Hum Reprod Update. 2009;15(4):441–61.
99. Vercellini P, Crosignani PG, Abbiati A, Somigliana E, Vigano P, Fedele L. The effect of surgery for symptomatic endometriosis: the other side of the story. Hum Reprod Update. 2009;15(2):177–88.
100. Sutton CJ, Ewen SP, Whitelaw N, Haines P. Prospective, randomized, double-blind, controlled trial of laser laparoscopy in the treatment of pelvic pain associated with minimal, mild, and moderate endometriosis. Fertil Steril. 1994;62(4):696–700.
101. Hornstein MD, Hemmings R, Yuzpe AA, Heinrichs WL. Use of nafarelin versus placebo after reductive laparoscopic surgery for endometriosis. Fertil Steril. 1997;68(5):860–4.
102. Winkel CA. Evaluation and management of women with endometriosis. Obstet Gynecol. 2003;102(2):397–408.
103. Wellbery C. Diagnosis and treatment of endometriosis. Am Fam Physician. 1999;60(6):1753.
104. Song JH, Lu H, Zhang J, Li B. Clinical study on the effectiveness and safety of combined laparoscopy and gonadotropin-releasing hormone agonist in the treatment of endometriosis. Zhonghua Fu Chan Ke Za Zhi. 2013;48(8):584–8. Chinese
105. Alborzi S, Hamedi B, Omidvar A, Dehbashi S, Alborzi S, Alborzi M. A comparison of the effect of short-term aromatase inhibitor (letrozole) and GnRH agonist (triptorelin) versus case control on pregnancy rate and symptom and sign recurrence after laparoscopic treatment of endometriosis. Arch Gynecol Obstet. 2011;284(1):105–10.
106. Hornstein MD, Yuzpe AA, Burry KA, Heinrichs LR, Buttram VL Jr, Orwoll ES. Prospective randomized double-blind trial of 3 versus 6 months of nafarelin therapy for endometriosis associated pelvic pain. Fertil Steril. 1995;63(5):955–62.
107. Tanmahasamut P, Rattanachaiyanont M, Angsuwathana S, Techatraisak K, Indhavivadhana S, Leerasiri P. Postoperative levonorgestrel-releasing intrauterine system for pelvic endometriosis-related pain: a randomized controlled trial. Obstet Gynecol. 2012;119(3):519–26.

108. Chen YJ, Hsu TF, Huang BS, Tsai HW, Chang YH, Wang PH. Postoperative maintenance levonorgestrel-releasing intrauterine system and endometrioma recurrence: a randomized controlled study. Am J Obstet Gynecol. 2017;216(6):582–e1.
109. Shuster LT, Rhodes DJ, Gostout BS, Grossardt BR, Rocca WA. Premature menopause or early menopause: long-term health consequences. Maturitas. 2010;65(2):161–6.
110. Gierach GL, Pfeiffer RM, Patel DA, Black A, Schairer C, Gill A, et al. Long-term overall and disease-specific mortality associated with benign gynecologic surgery performed at different ages. Menopause (New York, NY). 2014;21(6):592.
111. Faubion SS, Kuhle CL, Shuster LT, Rocca WA. Long-term health consequences of premature or early menopause and considerations for management. Climacteric. 2015;18(4):483–91.
112. Duffy JM, Arambage K, Correa FJ, Olive D, Farquhar C, Garry R, et al. Laparoscopic surgery for endometriosis. Cochrane Database Syst Rev. 2014;4:CD011031.
113. Practice Committee of the American Society for Reproductive Medicine. Endometriosis and infertility: a committee opinion. Fertil Steril. 2012;98(3):591–8.
114. Parazzini F, Di Cintio E, Chatenoud L, Moroni S, Ardovino I, Struzziero E, et al. Ablation of lesions or no treatment in minimal-mild endometriosis in infertile women: a randomized trial. Hum Reprod. 1999;14(5):1332–4.
115. Osuga Y, Koga K, Tsutsumi O, Yano T, Maruyama M, Kugu K, et al. Role of laparoscopy in the treatment of endometriosis-associated infertility. Gynecol Obstet Investig. 2002;53(Suppl. 1):33–9.
116. De Ziegler D, Borghese B, Chapron C. Endometriosis and infertility: pathophysiology and management. Lancet. 2010;376(9742):730–8.
117. Steures P, Van Der Steeg JW, Mol BW, Eijkemans MJ, Van Der Veen F, Habbema JD, et al. Prediction of an ongoing pregnancy after intrauterine insemination. Fertil Steril. 2004;82(1):45–51.
118. Eijkemans MJ, Kersten FA, Lintsen AM, Hunault CC, Bouwmans CA, Roijen L, et al. Cost-effectiveness of 'immediate IVF'versus 'delayed IVF': a prospective study. Hum Reprod. 2017;32(5):999–1008.
119. Benschop L, Farquhar C, van der Poel N, Heineman MJ. Interventions for women with endometrioma prior to assisted reproductive technology. Cochrane Database Syst Rev. 2010;11:CD008571.
120. de Ziegler D, Gayet V, Aubriot FX, Fauque P, Streuli I, Wolf JP, et al. Use of oral contraceptives in women with endometriosis before assisted reproduction treatment improves outcomes. Fertil Steril. 2010;94(7):2796–9.
121. Somigliana E, Vigano P, Benaglia L, Busnelli A, Berlanda N, Vercellini P. Management of endometriosis in the infertile patient. In Seminars in reproductive medicine 2017 (Vol. 35, No. 01, pp. 031-037). Thieme Medical Publishers.
122. Ferrier C, Boujenah J, Poncelet C, Chabbert-Buffet N, D'Argent EM, Carbillon L, et al. Use of the EFI score in endometriosis-associated infertility: a cost-effectiveness study. Eur J Obstetr Gynecol Reprod Biol. 2020;253:296–303.
123. Winsor SP, Ala-Leppilampi K, Spitzer K, Edney DR, Petropanagos A, Cadesky KI, et al. The affordability and accessibility of Ontario's publicly funded IVF program: a survey of patients. J Obstet Gynaecol Can. 2020;42(5):568–75.
124. Collins JA. An international survey of the health economics of IVF and ICSI. Hum Reprod Update. 2002;8(3):265–77.
125. Segel JE. Cost-of-illness studies—a primer. RTI-UNC Center of Excellence in Health Promotion Economics. 2006;1:39.
126. Kunz K, Kuppermann M, Moynihan C, Williamson A, Mazonson P. The cost of treatment of endometriosis in the California Medicaid population. Am J Managed Care. 1995;1(1):25–9.
127. Mathias SD, Kuppermann M, Liberman RF, Lipschutz RC, Steege JF. Chronic pelvic pain: prevalence, health-related quality of life, and economic correlates. Obstet Gynecol. 1996;87(3):321–7.

128. Levy AR, Osenenko KM, Lozano-Ortega G, Sambrook R, Jeddi M, Bélisle S, et al. Economic burden of surgically confirmed endometriosis in Canada. J Obstet Gynaecol Can. 2011;33(8):830–7.
129. Denny E. Women's experience of endometriosis. J Adv Nurs. 2004;46(6):641–8.
130. Sperschneider ML, Hengartner MP, Kohl-Schwartz A, Geraedts K, Rauchfuss M, Woelfler MM, et al. Does endometriosis affect professional life? A matched case-control study in Switzerland, Germany and Austria. BMJ Open. 2019;9(1):e019570.
131. Estes SJ, Soliman AM, Yang H, Wang J, Freimark J. A longitudinal assessment of the impact of endometriosis on patients' salary growth and risk of leaving the workforce. Adv Ther. 2020;37(5):2144–58.
132. Simoens S, Meuleman C, D'Hooghe T. Non-health-care costs associated with endometriosis. Hum Reprod. 2011;26(9):2363–7.
133. Oppelt P, Chavtal R, Haas D, Reichert B, Wagner S, Müller A, et al. Costs of in-patient treatment for endometriosis in Germany 2006: an analysis based on the G-DRG-Coding. Gynecol Endocrinol. 2012;28(11):903–5.
134. Taipale K, Leminen A, Räsänen P, Heikkilä A, Tapper AM, Sintonen H, et al. Costs and health-related quality of life effects of hysterectomy in patients with benign uterine disorders. Acta Obstet Gynecol Scand. 2009;88(12):1402–10.
135. Klein S, D'Hooghe T, Meuleman C, Dirksen C, Dunselman G, Simoens S. What is the societal burden of endometriosis-associated symptoms? A prospective Belgian study. Reprod Biomed Online. 2014;28(1):116–24.
136. Vercellini P, Giudice LC, Evers JL, Abrao MS. Reducing low-value care in endometriosis between limited evidence and unresolved issues: a proposal. Hum Reprod. 2015;30(9):1996–2004.

Part IV

Adenomyosis

What Is Adenomyosis?

29

Marwan Habiba and Giuseppe Benagiano

Contents

29.1 Introduction

In Chaps. 1 and 25 we explored the early history of the discovery of adenomyosis and endometriosis. It is notable that early writers described the presence of aberrant uterine mucosa with surrounding smooth muscle tissue present outside its normal

M. Habiba (✉)
Department of Health Sciences, University of Leicester and University Hospitals of Leicester, Leicester, UK
e-mail: mah6@leicester.ac.uk

G. Benagiano
Department of Maternal and Child Health, Gynaecology and Urology, Sapienza University of Rome, Rome, Italy

E. Oral (ed.), *Endometriosis and Adenomyosis*,
https://doi.org/10.1007/978-3-030-97236-3_29

location – namely, lining the uterine cavity – as one condition. Thus 'epithelial invasion' was clearly described towards the end of the nineteenth century by a number of authors [1–5] and was referred to as *adenomyoma*.

An early definition of adenomyoma was provided by Cuthbert Lockyer in 1918 [6], who wrote: "the term *adenomyoma* implies a new formation composed of gland-elements, hyperplastic cellular connective tissue, and smooth muscle".

Emge [7] reviewed the topic in 1962 and noted that only little advance had been made in understanding disease causation and in recognizing its clinical importance. For this reason, he referred to it as an "elusive disease". Emge emphasized the difficulty in diagnosis and the lack of concordance between clinical features and histological diagnosis and also highlighted the risk of over-diagnosis.

In 1972, Bird et al. [8] provided a definition of adenomyosis that remains currently recognized they defined adenomyosis as: "the benign invasion of endometrium into the myometrium, producing a diffusely enlarged uterus, which microscopically exhibits ectopic non-neoplastic, endometrial glands and stroma surrounded by hypertrophic-hyperplastic musculature". Bird et al. provided three reasons why they still viewed adenomyosis as an elusive disease. The first reason, they argued, was because its aetiology is unknown. The second, was because of the wide variation in reported incidence in surgical specimens and the third reason was because adenomyosis can be asymptomatic. It can be readily noted that these observations remain true 50 years later.

Today, more is known about the pathogenesis and a number of molecular investigations pointing to mechanism through which endometrial cells and stroma may penetrate through the myometrial junctional zone (JZ) and invade the uterine muscle. Nevertheless, much remains before we can achieve a full understanding of the disease.

As for the second argument of Bird et al. it remains the case that the reported incidence of adenomyosis in histologic specimens vary widely. This can be affected by factors not related to the disease itself. Finally, while early descriptions addressed the clinical manifestations purely as narrative cases histories of cases undergoing hysterectomy, this cannot provide a comprehensive account of disease impact. Bird et al. [8] made an important contribution as they introduced the notion of adenomyosis 'sub-basalis' (Grade 1), in which gland penetration within the myometrium is confined to one low power field (LPF) below the basal endometrium. According to this classification, adenomyosis was marked as Grade 2 or Grade 3 at a cut-off point at mid myometrium. They reported that menorrhagia was linked to Grade 1 adenomyosis and to cases where there was a marked degree of involvement (large areas affected). Dysmenorrhea was linked to higher depth of gland penetration within the myometrium and to the size of the area affected.

Adenomyosis is defined by the presence of heterotopic endometrial glands and stroma embedded within the myometrium. Diagnostic features that can clarify the extent of the disease are the depth of stromal and glandular presence within the muscle and the extent of uterine wall involvement. Often the myometrium is referred to as hypertrophic, but there are no objective definitions for the reported changes in smooth muscles. One typical histological feature of adenomyosis is its association with a degree of disruption to the normal endometrial-myometrial interface which becomes irregular with glands present within the myometrium. In addition, imaging techniques show that the inner myometrium, the so-called myometrial junctional zone (JZ), is increased in thickness [9]. A JZ of more than 12 mm has been taken as the threshold for a non-invasive diagnosis but this has recently been questioned [10]. Currently, the identification of adenomyosis relies on an assessment of whether features at the interface between the mucosal and the muscle layers deviate from the normal. This contrasts with historical descriptions of the disease which focused on grossly abnormal uteri with large lesions. Early descriptions were confined to case reports of large lesions and adenomyomas were considered rare. However, Cullen [11] noted that he was amazed by the frequency by which he encountered the disease.

During the second decade of the twentieth century, there was an exponential rise in diagnosis and, because of concern about over diagnosis, there were calls for the adoption of conservative cut-off points to distinguish adenomyosis from normal irregularity at the interface between the epithelium and myometrium. But such attempts will necessarily be hampered in the absence of clinical correlates. Pre-operative diagnosis faces the additional challenge because of the needs to prove high correlation with histological diagnosis [12].

29.2 From Adenomyoma to Adenomyosis: The Endometrial Myometrial Interface

At the core of the early debate about terminology is the desire to avert terms that imply an etiology. Frankl [13], who proposed the term adenomyosis to identify intra-myometrial ectopic endometrial foci, as well as many of his contemporaries, specifically rejected terms that implied a pathogenesis. Yet, current descriptions commonly refer to adenomyosis in term of gland 'invasion' and myometrial 'disruption'. Vercellini et al. [14] wrote: "it is generally agreed that adenomyosis occurs when the normal boundary between the endometrial basal layer and the myometrium is disrupted … as a consequence of this disruption, the endometrial glands invade the myometrium".

The *endometrial-myometrial interface* (EMI) has a unique characteristic because of the lack of a separating basement membrane. Thus, the endometrium sits directly on the myometrium. Understanding the factors that determine the alignment at the normal interface and their disruption become crucial to our understanding of the disease. Another important challenge arises because disruption at the EMI can be patchy. Histological mapping of the uterine affection is necessarily labor intensive. The diagnosis has been shown to be dependent on the number of histological sections examined. Consideration needs to be given to whether such effort is warranted outside a research setting given that it can have little, if any, impact post-hysterectomy.

Understanding the clinical significance of adenomyosis need to consider the impact of the depth, the spread and density of gland presence within the myometrium and their exact location. There is the additional question of how to address non-uniform distribution of these features. This lends support to the call for reports to detail the actual findings depth and distribution of glandular structures, rather than using a dichotomous classification as normal and adenomyosis. Better understanding the import of the different features is critical to the development of a classification system for the condition [12].

It is notable that there is no agreement on the cut-off point at which glands within the myometrium can be considered abnormal. Levgur et al. [15] regarded cases with glands within 2.5 mm from the EMI as normal. Glands <40%, 40–80%, and >80% were classed as superficial, intermediate, or deep adenomyosis, respectively. Sammour et al. [16] proposed four categories based on the depth of glands within the myometrium according to whether these are present at <25%, 26–50%, 51–75%, and >75% of myometrial thickness.

As already mentioned, Bird et al. [8] proposed three grades of adenomyosis based on the depth of invasion; Grade I or sub-basal lesions within one low power field, Grade II where glands are present up to mid-myometrium, and Grade III where glands are present beyond mid-myometrium. They also propsoed three degrees of involvemen; Slight in which there are 1–3 glands per LPF, Moderate in which there are 4–9 glands per LPF, and Marked where there are 10 or more glands per LPF. Other authors adopted similar criteria [17, 18]. Different functional characteristics between the inner and outer myometrium may have relevance to the development or progressions of adenomyosis through mechanisms involving recurrent tissue injury and repair (ReTIAR) [19].

29.3 Diagnosing Adenomyosis

Histology remains the gold standard for the diagnosis of adenomyosis, but there has been an increase in the use of ultrasound and MRI for the non-invasive diagnosis prior to hysterectomy and in women not undergoing surgery.

29.3.1 Clinical Diagnosis

Classically, the uterus with adenomyosis is described as tender, soft and symmetrically enlarged. Adenomyosis may be asymptomatic or linked to pelvic pain, abnormal and heavy menstrual bleeding or infertility. An important cofounding factor is that adenomyosis often coexists with fibroids or with endometriosis. Symptoms linked to adenomyosis are not pathognomonic. Curiously, Cullen [11] wrote that the disease could be diagnosed with great ease based on clinical features alone. He claimed that the diagnosis can even be made by the "hospital assistant". Even so, Lockyer [6] concluded that: "in many cases, if not in most, the diagnosis is made at the operation or by the microscope", this affirmation seems more in tune with our current understanding as the reported preoperative diagnosis remains poor (range of 2–26%) [17, 20, 21]. Thus, clinical features may be suggestive but are unreliable for diagnosis or as a basis of classification of adenomyosis.

29.3.2 Imaging Diagnosis

The use of two dimensional or three-dimensional ultrasound (US) and of magnetic resonance imaging (MR) provides a means to identify and to map the presence of adenomyosis prior to surgery. US and MR also enable the identification of coexistent pathology such as fibroids. This may enable conservative management and better understanding of the natural history of the disease in women not undergoing surgery.

29.3.2.1 Magnetic Resonance Imaging

MR imaging allows the identification of the uterine JZ and its alterations in the presence of adenomyosis. In 1983, Hricak et al. [22] were the first to describe three distinct uterine zones on T2-weighted MR images; the endometrium (high signal), the sub-endometrial myometrium or JZ (low signal), and the outer myometrium (intermediate signal). In contrast to histological diagnosis which relies on the identification of aberrant endometrium within the myometrium, MR focuses on features of the myometrium and, as such, provides indirect evidence of the condition. For two decades, a maximum thickness of the junctional zone (JZmax) ≥12 mm was considered as highly suggestive of adenomyosis and a guide for a non-invasive diagnosis. This has been challenged for a number of reasons. First, the JZ is not consistently identifiable and may be influenced by the menstrual cycle phase. Second, the JZ is not identifiable in a larger proportion of older women which limits its utility in women ≤35 years. A more reliable diagnosis requires the presence of additional features such as diffuse, low-intensity areas and high-intensity spots near the endometrium [10]. Increased JZ thickness is reproducible but can only be measured in 20–30% of women of reproductive age. Similar to the case with histological diagnosis, the appropriate cut-off point for a normal JZ remains controversial. In addition, interpretation of MR features can be influenced by clinical features and by the presence of concomitant pathology. It is also relevant to consider that the histologic transition from the inner to the outer myometrium is gradual, with no clear demarcation point that may corresponds to MR features [23]. Overall, the calculated pooled sensitivity, specificity, positive likelihood ratio and negative likelihood ratio for MR were reported as 0.77, 0.89, 6.5 and 0.2, respectively, for all subtypes of adenomyosis [10].

29.3.2.2 Ultrasound

Ultrasound features linked to adenomyosis include uterine enlargement in the absence of fibroids, asymmetric thickening of the anterior or posterior uterine wall, thickening of the junctional zone, lack of contour abnormality, lack of mass effect, heterogeneous poorly circumscribed areas within the myometrium, anechoic myometrial blood-filled cysts, increased echogenicity of the endometrium and sub-endometrial linear striations. Ultrasound could also detect adenomyosis as localized non-homogenous lesions within the myometrium. Diagnosis may be enhanced with the use of color Doppler. Whilst transvaginal ultrasound (TVU) improved sensitivity and specificity to >80%, there is disagreement on the diagnostic value of individual ultrasound features. Changes in the JZ in adenomyosis can also be assessed with reference to the ratio of maximum JZ ($JZ^{max}/_{total\ myometrium}$), and a difference between the maximum and the minimum thickness (JZ^{max}-JZ^{min}) but these can be affected by the hormonal status and the phase of menstrual cycle.

Recently, the existence of a distinct category coined 'JZ hyperplasia' was proposed. This is defined as partial or diffuse thickening of the JZ from ≥8 mm to <12 mm in the absence of additional imaging features of adenomyosis [24]. The histological correlates of this category remain to be fully understood.

Some studies compared the use of ultrasound with histological diagnosis. Reinhold et al. [25] reported a Kappa statistic of 0.69 indicating good agreement between TVU and histology in depicting the location of adenomyosis and a Kappa statistic of 0.81 in relation to the maximum depth of involvement. In the study by Bazot et al. [26], sonography and histopathology concurred in only 57% of cases when assessing the depth of presence of endometrium within the myometrium and in only 23% of cases when assessing the degree of involvement and lesion density. Three-dimensional ultrasound shows promise, but its role is affected by disease prevalence, clinician expertise, previous uterine surgery, and hormone treatment [27–29].

It is envisaged that standardization as suggested through the MUSA (Morphological Uterus Sonographic Assessment) criteria would enable better understanding of adenomyosis [30, 31]. Yet, despite recent advances, imaging has not challenged histopathology as the gold standard for diagnosis. Imaging-based diagnosis may not be uniformly available and inter-observer reproducibility remains a challenge.

29.3.3 Biomarker-Based Diagnosis

The CA125 protein is one of the earliest biomarkers to be studied in adenomyosis, but meta-analysis of published results concluded that it is of limited utility [32]. Concomitant use of CA125, CA19-9, and IL-6 did not add significantly to the value of CA125 alone [33]. Agic et al. [34] measured chemokine (C-C motif) receptor 1 mRNA (CCR1 mRNA) in peripheral blood leukocytes together with monocyte chemotactic protein-1 (MCP-1) and CA125 protein in serum of women with endometriosis and adenomyosis. No significant difference in CCR1/HPRT mRNA (Hypoxanthine-guanine phospho-ribosyl transferase) ratio was found between women with adenomyosis and the control group. Another approach is the use of proteomic analysis of serum samples [35–38] or gene expression array [39]. Mehasseb et al. [40] reported differential protein expression in co-cultures of myocytes and endometrial stromal cells in adenomyosis compared to normal controls and identified a number of candidate proteins. But these developments have not reached clinical applicability.

29.4 Mapping of Adenomyosis

Adenomyotic lesions can be divided into different categories based on their morphology and location. There is often preferential expression in one of the uterine walls compared to the other. This could be symmetric or asymmetric. Gordts et al. [41] suggested classification into three subcategories according to the depth of involvement and whether the lesions reach <1/3, <2/3, >2/3 of the myometrium. This contrasts with focal adenomyosis which could be uni- or multi-focal. This is again distinct from an adenomyoma, and is differentiated from fibroids which have distinct margins.

Several authors argued that 'internal' and 'external' adenomyosis are distinct. Internal adenomyosis being characterised by focal or multifocal intra-myometrial tiny cystic structures on MRI possibly accompanied by an increased JZ thickness [9] and can be superficial or deep, symmetric or asymmetric, diffuse or local. External adenomyosis is a term applied to lesions in the outer myometrium [10]. Lesions can affect the posterior, anterior, or lateral uterine wall and be associated with either posterior, anterior or lateral deep endometriotic lesions.

Kishi et al. [42] proposed a classification of adenomyosis into four subtypes. They refer to Subtype I, as *intrinsic* adenomyosis or that affecting the inner uterine layer; Subtype II, is referred to as *extrinsic* adenomyosis that affects the outer uterine layer in the presence of a normal junctional zone; and Subtype III comprises solitary adenomyosis that has no connection to the junctional zone or to the serosa. They referred to the remaining unclassified cases as Subtype IV, or as an indeterminate type. In another report, Kishi et al. [43] compared Subtypes I and II lesions using cytoskeletal proteins, type I and III collagen, TGF-β and its signalling molecules. They reported different staining characteristics between the subtypes using non-muscle myosin IIB, TGF-β and phosphorylated TGF-β type I receptors, and argued that this is indicative of a different origin. Using a similar approach, Khan et al. [44] compared staining characteristics of lesions from intrinsic and extrinsic adenomyosis from women who had co-existing deep infiltrating lesions in the pouch of Douglas. However, the relation between adenomyosis affecting different parts of the uterus cannot be established based on differences in the proportion of glands or stroma or in staining characteristics.

29.5 Attempts at Creating a Classification of Adenomyosis

In addition to the above-mentioned categories which were based on depth of glands present below the EMI, a number of additional factors were introduced into proposed classifications. Most published studies have relied on routine histology which was not concerned with thorough mapping of the disease. Thus, the degree of involvement has rarely been the focus of research and even where mentioned it has seldom been included in analyses linked to symptoms. Grimbizis et al. [45] distinguished diffuse adenomyosis which features extensive foci of endometrial mucosa scattered throughout the uterine musculature from focal adenomyosis which features localized area within the myometrium. Some studies reported more affection in the posterior wall, but this is not universally agreed. A controversial issue concerns the diagnosis of myometrial hyperplasia and whether its presence is essential for diagnosis.

Based on the consistency of tisue encountered during surgery, Pistofidis et al. [46] distinguished three variants: The 'diffuse' type which has a spongiform texture, the 'sclerotic' type characterized by irregular thickening of the myometrium and the 'nodular' type which features spherical well-defined lesions surrounded by smooth muscle hyperplasia. This distinction may have some relevance at the time of conservative surgery or when comparing outcomes, but the relation to symptoms and clinical presentation is not known.

The traditional definition of adenomyosis includes reference to endometrial invasion within the myometrium. This may have its roots in the earlier writings by Sampson who drew analogies between aberrant benign endometrial tissue and cancer. This theory may have had some support from evidence that the eutopic endometrium in women with adenomyosis, as well as endometriosis, possesses an invasive phenotype [40, 43, 44, 47]. But this evidence is fragmentary and incomplete. The relationship between external or extrinsic adenomyosis and variants of endometriosis has also attracted debate. One view is that deep infiltrating endometriosis and bladder endometriosis originate as adenomyotic nodules in the posterior uterine or cervical wall and invade the rectovaginal space, the digestive tract or the bladder. Alternatively, it was proposed that adenomyosis in the outer uterine myometrium results from invasion by endometriosis first implanted on the peritoneum. But there remain unresolved questions about the genesis of these lesions.

29.6 Adenomyosis in Young Women and After the Menopause

The study of adenomyosis across different age groups confirms it as a disease of the adult woman. Whereas endometriosis can manifest in young adolescents and even before menarche (see Chap. 8), the rare juvenile cases of adenomyosis feature localized cysts, rather than the classic features [48]. The variant of adenomyosis that seems specific to young women is the so-called myometrial cystic adenomyosis. Affected young patients present with severe dysmenorrhea that does not respond to treatment. Diagnosis which is usually delayed can be readily made by MRI. Cystic adenomyosis can reach up to 3 cm in diameter and has hemorrhagic content. Histologically, cysts are lined with an endometrial-like layer. The presence of adenomyosis in post-menopausal women receiving HRT or in women on tamoxifen is well documented and often represents reactivation of dormant lesions [48].

29.7 Variants with Similarities to Adenomyosis

When considering a classification for adenomyosis, it is necessary to consider the place of other variants containing a mixture of myometrium and endometrium, such as the typical and atypical polypoid adenomyomas as well as other rare forms, such as the endocervical and retroperitoneal variants. Up to 20% of cases of adenomyosis may also contain tubal type ciliated epithelium. Lesions that contain tubal and endocervical type epithelium are referred to as *endosalpingiosis* and *endocervicosis*, respectively; there is also a variety with mixed type epithelium that is often referred to as *Müllerianosis*.

A variety of benign tumors containing an admixture of endometrium and myometrium that are distinct from classic adenomyosis have been reported in literature. These include the Uterus like mass (U-LM), endomyometriosis, cystic adenomyoma, adenomyoma (including extrauterine adenomyoma) and adenomyomatous polyps. Most of these are rare and thus reported as case reports of individual or a small number of cases. Because they are more common, there are small case series of polypoid adenomyoma (PA) or atypical polypoid adenomyoma (APA) [49].

An adenomyoma is a circumscribed nodular aggregate of benign endometrial glands surrounded by endometrial stroma with leiomyomatous smooth muscle bordering the endometrial stroma. Adenomyoma may be within the myometrium or may involve or originate in the endometrium or form a polyp. The term polypoid adenomyoma appears infrequently in literature. It is often used synonymously with adenomyomatous polyp. Adenomyomatous polyp is characterized by the presence of smooth muscle cells within a polyp. The U-LM comprises a central cavity lined by endometriotic tissue and surrounded by a thick wall of smooth muscle cells similar to the myometrium. Extrauterine adenomyoma can resemble the U-LM but lacks a uterus like structure. Endomyometriosis comprises chocolate like material contained within the centre of the structure surrounded by smooth muscle. Atypical Polypoid Adenomyoma (APA) is a rare type of mixed Müllerian tumor that usually arises from the lower uterine segment [49].

The nomenclature used in case reports largely aimed at conveying the histological features and the tissue types contained within excised lesions, with less emphasis on macroscopic description or clinical features. The lesions may have been associated with abnormal bleeding, dysmenorrhea or mass effect but some may have been incidental findings. Many articles refer to the same lesion using different nomenclature which can create considerable confusion.

29.8 Conclusion

As mentioned above, the availability of non-invasive diagnostic tests provides an important enabler to the understanding of adenomyosis in cases not requiring surgery and for longitudinal follow-up of disease progress. An agreed system for classification and reporting can enhance our understanding of the disease and can enable research and treatment outcomes. In this context, there remain uncertainties about the classification of affections of the utero-vesical pouch, the pouch of Douglas and lesions in the outer myometrium. Previous attempts at producing a taxonomy is contained in a recent review [12], but this effort requires consideration of the clinical correlates of the various anatomical and histological features.

References

1. Rokitansky C. Lehrbuch der pathologischen anatomie. Wien: Wilhelm Braumüller; 1861.
2. von Recklinghausen F. Die Adenomyomata und Cystadenomata der Uterus und Tubenwandung: Ihre Abkunft von Resten des Wolffischen Körpers [*The adenomyomas and cystadenomas of the uterus and tube wall: their origin from remnants of the Wolffian body*]. Berlin: August Hirschwald Verlag; 1896.
3. Cullen TS. Adeno-myome des uterus [*Uterine adenomyoma*]. Berlin: Verlag von August Hirschwald; 1903.
4. Pick L. Die Adenomyome der leistengegend und des hinteren scheidengewölbes, ihre Stellung zu den paroophoralen adenomyomen der Uterus- und tubenwandung v. Recklinghausen's. Arch Gynakol. 1899;57:461–509.
5. Rolly F. Über einen fall von adenomyoma uteri mit übergang in karcinom und metastasenbildung. [*About a case of uterine adenomyoma with transition to carcinoma and metastasis*]. Archiv Pathol Anat Physiol Klin Med. 1897;150:555–82.
6. Lockyer C. Fibroids and allied tumours (myoma and adenomyoma). London: Macmillan; 1918.
7. Emge LA. The elusive adenomyosis of the uterus. Am J Obstet Gynecol. 1962;83:1541–63.
8. Bird CC, McElin TW, Manalo-Estrella P. The elusive adenomyosis of the uterus - revisited. Am J Obstet Gynecol. 1972;112(5):583–93.
9. Togashi K, Nishimura K, Itoh K, Fujisawa I, Noma S, Kanaoka M, Nakano Y, Itoh H, Ozasa H, Fujii S. Adenomyosis: diagnosis with MR imaging. Radiology. 1988;166:111–4.
10. Bazot M, Daraï E. Role of transvaginal sonography and magnetic resonance imaging in the diagnosis of uterine adenomyosis. Fertil Steril. 2018;109:389–97.
11. Cullen TS. Adenomyoma of the uterus. Philadelphia & London: WB. Saunders; 1908.
12. Habiba M, Gordts S, Bazot M, Brosens I, Benagiano G. Exploring challenges for a new classification of adenomyosis. Reprod Biomed Online. 2020;40:569–81.
13. Frankl O. Adenomyosis uteri. Am J Obstet Gynecol. 1925;10:680–4.
14. Vercellini P, Viganò P, Somigliana E, Daguati R, Abbiati A, Fedele L. Adenomyosis: epidemiological factors. Best Pract Res Clin Obstet Gynaecol. 2006;20:465–77.
15. Levgur M, Abadi MA, Tucker A. Adenomyosis: symptoms, histology, and pregnancy terminations. Obstet Gynecol. 2000;95:688–91.
16. Sammour A, Pirwany I, Usubutun A, Arseneau J, Tulandi T. Correlations between extent and spread of adenomyosis and clinical symptoms. Gynecol Obstet Investig. 2002;54:213–6.
17. Owolabi TO, Strickler RC. Adenomyosis: a neglected diagnosis. Obstet Gynecol. 1977;50:424–7.
18. Bergholt T, Eriksen L, Berendt N, Jacobsen M, Hertz JB. Prevalence and risk factors of adenomyosis at hysterectomy. Hum Reprod. 2001;16:2418–21.
19. Zhang Q, Duan J, Olson M, Fazleabas A, Guo SW. Cellular changes consistent with epithelial-mesenchymal transition and fibroblast-to-Myofibroblast trans-differentiation in the progression of experimental endometriosis in baboons. Reprod Sci. 2016;23:1409–21.
20. Azziz R. Adenomyosis: current perspectives. Obstet Gynecol Clin N Am. 1989;16(1):221–35.
21. Molitor JJ. Adenomyosis: a clinical and pathological appraisal. Am J Obstet Gynecol. 1971;110(2):275–84.
22. Hricak H, Alpers C, Crooks LE, Sheldon PE. Magnetic resonance imaging of the female pelvis: initial experience. Am J Roentgenol. 1983;141:1119–28.
23. Mehasseb MK, Bell SC, Brown L, Pringle JH, Habiba M. Phenotypic characterisation of the inner and outer myometrium in normal and adenomyotic uteri. Gynecol Obstet Investig. 2011;71(4):217–24.
24. Exacoustos C. Adenomyosis and ultrasound: the role of ultrasound and its impact on understanding the disease. In: Habiba M, Benagiano G, editors. Uterine Adenomyosis. Cham: Springer; 2016.
25. Reinhold C, McCarthy S, Bret PM, Mehio A, Atri M, Zakarian R, Glaude Y, Liang L, Seymour RJ. Diffuse adenomyosis: comparison of endovaginal US and MR imaging with histopathologic correlation. Radiology. 1996;199(1):151–8.

26. Bazot M, Cortez A, Darai E, Rouger J, Chopier J, Antoine JM, Uzan S. Ultrasonography compared with magnetic resonance imaging for the diagnosis of adenomyosis: correlation with histopathology. Hum Reprod. 2001;16(11):2427–33.
27. Luciano DE, Exacoustos C, Albrecht L, LaMonica R, Proffer A, Zupi E, Luciano AA. Three-dimensional ultrasound in diagnosis of adenomyosis: histologic correlation with ultrasound targeted biopsies of the uterus. J Minim Invasive Gynecol. 2013;20:803–10.
28. Exacoustos C, Brienza L, Di Giovanni A, Szabolcs B, Romanini ME, Zupi E, Arduini D. Adenomyosis: three dimensional sonographic findings of the junctional zone and correlation with histology. Ultrasound Obstet Gynecol. 2011;37:471–9.
29. Naftalin J, Hoo W, Nunes N, Mavrelos D, Nicks H, Jurkovic D. Inter- and intraobserver variability in three-dimensional ultrasound assessment of the endometrial- myometrial junction and factors affecting its visualization. Ultrasound Obstet Gynecol. 2012;39:587–91.
30. Van den Bosch T, Dueholm M, Leone FP, Valentin L, Rasmussen CK, Votino A, Van Schoubroeck D, Landolfo C, Installé AJ, Guerriero S, Exacoustos C, Gordts S, Benacerraf B, D'Hooghe T, De Moor B, Brölmann H, Goldstein S, Epstein E, Bourne T, Timmerman D. Terms, definitions and measurements to describe sonographic features of myometrium and uterine masses: a consensus opinion from the Morphological Uterus Sonographic Assessment (MUSA) group. Ultrasound Obstet Gynecol. 2015;46:284–98.
31. Van den Bosch T, de Bruijn AM, de Leeuw RA, Dueholm M, Exacoustos C, Valentin L, Bourne T, Timmerman D, Huirne JAF. Sonographic classification and reporting system for diagnosing adenomyosis. Ultrasound Obstet Gynecol. 2019;53:576–82.
32. Mol BW, Bayram N, Lijmer JG, Wiegerinck MA, Bongers MY, van der Veen F, Bossuyt PM. The performance of CA-125 measurement in the detection of endometriosis: a meta-analysis. Fertil Steril. 1998;70(6):1101–8.
33. Somigliana E, Viganò P, Tirelli AS, Felicetta I, Torresani E, Vignali M, Di Blasio AM. Use of the concomitant serum dosage of CA 125, CA 19-9 and interleukin-6 to detect the presence of endometriosis. Results from a series of reproductive age women undergoing laparoscopic surgery for benign gynaecological conditions. Hum Reprod. 2004;19(8):1871–6.
34. Agic A, Djalali S, Wolfler MM, Halis G, Diedrich K, Hornung D. Combination of CCR1 mRNA, MCP1, and CA125 measurements in peripheral blood as a diagnostic test for endometriosis. Reprod Sci. 2008;15(9):906–11.
35. Long X, Jiang P, Zhou L, Zhang W. Evaluation of novel serum biomarkers and the proteomic differences of endometriosis and adenomyosis using MALDI-TOF- MS. Arch Gynecol Obstet. 2013;288(1):201–5.
36. Jing J, Qiao Y, Suginami H, Taniguchi F, Shi H, Wang X. Two novel serum biomarkers for endometriosis screened by surface-enhanced laser desorption/ionization time-of-flight mass spectrometry and their change after laparoscopic removal of endometriosis. Fertil Steril. 2009;92(4):1221–7.
37. Ding X, Wang L, Ren Y, Zheng W. Detection of mitochondrial biomarkers in eutopic endometria of endometriosis using surface-enhanced laser desorption/ionization time-of-flight mass spectrometry. Fertil Steril. 2010;94(7):2528–30.
38. Kyama CM, Mihalyi A, Gevaert O, Waelkens E, Simsa P, Van de Plas R, Meuleman C, De Moor B. D'Hooghe TM. Evaluation of endometrial biomarkers for semi-invasive diagnosis of endometriosis. Fertil Steril. 2011;95(4):1338–43 e1–3.
39. Dechaud H, Haouzi D, Vincens C, Bersinger N, Mueller MD, Hamamah S. New biomarkers of adenomyosis in endometrium. Fertil Steril. 2014;102(Suppl):e49–50.
40. Mehasseb MK, Taylor AH, Pringle JH, Bell SC, Habiba M. Enhanced invasion of stromal cells from adenomyosis in a three-dimensional coculture model is augmented by the presence of myocytes from affected uteri. Fertil Steril. 2010;94:2547–51.
41. Gordts S, Brosens JJ, Fusi L, Benagiano G, Brosens I. Uterine adenomyosis: a need for uniform terminology and classification. Reprod Biomed Online. 2008;17:244–8.
42. Kish Y, Suginami H, Kuramori R, Yabuta M, Suginami R, Taniguchi F. Four subtypes of adenomyosis assessed by magnetic resonance imaging and their specification. Am J Obstet Gynecol. 2012;207:114.e1.

43. Kishi Y, Shimada K, Fujii T, Uchiyama T, Yoshimoto C, Konishi N, Ohbayashi C, Kobayashi H. Phenotypic characterization of adenomyosis occurring at the inner and outer myometrium. PLoS One. 2017;12:18e0189522.
44. Khan KN, Fujishita A, Koshiba A, Kuroboshi H, Mori T, Ogi H, Itoh K, Nakashima M, Kitawaki J. Biological differences between intrinsic and extrinsic adenomyosis with coexisting deep infiltrating endometriosis. Reprod Biomed Online. 2019;39:343–53.
45. Grimbizis GF, Mikos T, Tarlatzis B. Uterus sparing operative treatment for adenomyosis. Fertil Steril. 2014;101:472–87.
46. Pistofidis G, Makrakis E, Koukoura O, Bardis N, Balinakos P, Anaf V. Distinct types of uterine adenomyosis based on laparoscopic and histopathologic criteria. Clin Exp Obstet Gynecol. 2014;41:113–8.
47. García-Solares J, Donnez J, Donnez O, Dolmans MM. Pathogenesis of uterine adenomyosis: invagination or metaplasia? Fertil Steril. 2018;109:371–9.
48. Benagiano G, Brosens I, Habiba M. Adenomyosis: a life-cycle approach. Reprod Biomed Online. 2015;30:220–32.
49. Habiba M, Brosens I, Zannoni GF, Benagiano G. Uncommon mixed endometrial-myometrial benign tumors of the reproductive tract: literature review. Gynecol Obstet Investig. 2019;84(6):521–47.

A History of Adenomyosis

30

Giuseppe Benagiano, Donatella Lippi,
and Marwan Habiba

Contents

30.1 Introduction

In the first chapter of this book, we reconstructed the early work carried out in the second half of the nineteenth century, aimed at uncovering the presence of *mucosal invasions of peritoneal organs*. That description is very pertinent to the history of adenomyosis for the simple reason that, up to 1925, adenomyosis and endometriosis, both *mucosal invasions*, were considered as one condition, later coined adenomyoma. In recognition of the occurrence of tubal type epithelium in some lesions affecting the ovaries, Bailey [1] proposed that they be referred to as

G. Benagiano
Department of Maternal and Child Health, Gynaecology and Urology, Sapienza University of Rome, Rome, Italy

D. Lippi
Department of Experimental and Clinical Medicine, School of Sciences of Human Health, University of Florence, Florence, Italy

M. Habiba (✉)
Department of Health Sciences, University of Leicester and University Hospitals of Leicester, Leicester, UK
e-mail: mah6@leicester.ac.uk

E. Oral (ed.), *Endometriosis and Adenomyosis*,
https://doi.org/10.1007/978-3-030-97236-3_30

ectopic Müllerianoma. According to the comprehensive book on myomas and adenomyomas by Cuthbert Lockyer [2], the first detailed descriptions of an adenomyoma were made by Babes [3] who, in 1882, published a case of an intramural myoma containing cysts lined with low cubical epithelium derived from embryonic germs and by Diesterweg [4] who, in 1883, described two polypi of the posterior uterine wall containing cysts lined with ciliated epithelium and filled with blood. Then, in 1893 and in 1895, von Recklinghausen published two reports on adenomyomas [5, 6]. In these he refers to the publication by Babes [3] as having stimulated his interest in the origin of adenomyoma. He also acknowledged the work of Rokitansky [7], Kolb [8], and Röhrig [9] as relevant contributions to the knowledge of the disease.

In 1896 von Recklinghausen published an acclaimed book on the uterine and tube-wall adenomyoma and cysto-adenomyoma [10]. He divided adenomyomas into two classes:

1. Those situated at the periphery of the uterus and in the tubes
2. Those arising centrally (within the uterus)

von Recklinghausen argued that while it is possible to envisage that lesions close to the uterine cavity may originate from endometrial glands, he remained unconvinced that the same origin could apply to lesions nearer the peritoneum. He therefore favored for both a derivation from a *numerical increase of the Wolffian tubule*s which in his view can have similarities to the Müllerian structure. He described similarities between the glandular morphology of these growths and the mesonephros. These descriptions provided a basis for his theory of Wolffian origin which was held in esteem by some but strongly criticized by others including Kossmann [11] who argued that the aberrant glands originate from accessory Müllerian ducts.

In von Recklinghausen's opinion, adenomyomas arising within the myometrium (the variant we would today call adenomyosis) were prone to undergo malignant degeneration; he reported to have observed three such cases. Today, we know that such a malignant transformation is rare and that cancer is more likely to spread from the endometrium into adenomyotic foci than vice versa [12].

For the record, reference to adenomyoma appeared for the first time around the end of the nineteenth century when, in 1896, both von Recklinghausen and Cullen utilized the term [10, 13]. They were followed by Pick [14] and Rolly [15, 16] in 1897. However, the claim to have been the first to describe an adenomyoma was made by Ivanoff [17] who, illustrating his case in 1898, stated that he had already published a paper in Russian with a microscopic evaluation of the glands found in a "cystic myoma." As to the origin, he believed that the glands found in the tumor *were derived from the serosal epithelium.*

In contrast to the paucity of recorded cases in early literature, Cullen [18] commented on the high incidence of uterine adenomyomas which he calculated at 5.7%. In contrast, Breus [19] mentioned that 100 cases were described prior to 1884, with the earliest example described by John Hunter in 1793 [20–22]. It seems however that much of the early literature also included examples of what was termed cystofibroma of the uterus [23, 24]. These are often large lesions with multiple interconnected cavities that are perhaps best regarded as degenerated fibroids or unusual variants. At the beginning of the twentieth century, Bishop [25] outlined a clear distinction based on the presence of mucosal lining, and cystofibromas were considered a variant of myoma, not adenomyoma.

Initially, the attention of researchers focused on investigating the origin of glandular tissue in adenomyomas. In this respect, in 1860, Carl Rokitansky, in Vienna [7], found *fibrous polyps of the uterus* and asserted that *among them there are some, in which glandular tubes are found.* He went on to mention that: *In some rare cases the extension of the uterine glands occurred in both directions, i.e. both into the uterus cavity, as well as into the uterus parenchyma, such that the sloped bulge represents a plug of longitudinal fibrous appearance driven into, as it were, the uterine mass.* He describes one case where: *the thick-walled uterus of an aged female showed this inter alia. On the left-hand-side under the mouth of the tuba was a swollen, about 1–2" long, smoothly coated polyp of 1½" diameter in the pedunculus, from 4–5" on the free end. A similar bisecting perpendicular section continuing into the uterine mass shows that the pedunculus penetrates to a depth of 4" into the uterine mass and stores a wedge driven right in to the uterine tissue; on its section along its length it has a fibrous appearance and can be torn into fibres in this direction; the arrangement of the fibres is determined by numerous extremely long glandular tubes held together by means of a core-rich connective tissue.* Some take this to be the first description of a case of adenomyosis; however, it seems more consistent with what is recognized today as the rare adenomyomatous polyp.

Over 25 years after Rokitansky's description [7], Gusserow [26] seems to have been the first to refer to his work when, in discussing fibroid polyps, it was stated that lesions containing glandular structures are better viewed as lesions of the mucosa. In those days, pathologists and gynecologists, with few exceptions, rejected the hypothesis that the glands they observed were derived from the endometrium. In 1897 Ludwig Pick asserted that the *mesonephric origin of adenomyoma* had been definitely established by *fundamental proof* [14]. In 1903, Meyer [27] described a case of what we would call today secondary or implantation endometriosis around a silk ligatures of a laparotomy. He then elaborated his theory of *epithelial heterotopy*, which he considered to be a kind of healing process. He viewed adenomyomas as *epithelial invasion of inflammatory infiltrated tissue* and concluded that epithelial heterotopy can occur both in dystopic (embryonic) and orthotopic (mature) epithelium. In this way, he explained the findings of Orloff [28], who had described *glandular spaces under the serosa covering uterine myomata*, as derived from *embryonic cells*. Lockyer [2] discussed the various theories and collated five cases labeled adenomyoma of the ovarian ligament published prior to his 1918 book [18, 27, 29, 30]. He accepted von Recklinghausen [10] and Frankl's theory [31] that these tumors arose from parts of the Wolffian system (the medullary cord or duct). The mesonephric origin of what we probably would consider cases of endometriosis was accepted by most early researchers.

Schikele [32] was among the last to argue in favor of a mesonephric origin of mucosal growth. He wrote: *when I try to take an impartial view of published cases, I am compelled to state that the mucosal theory is not proved.*

Uncertainty continued and, in his book of 1918, Lockyer [2] stated that: *Nothing but the topography of the tumour, nothing but laborious research entailing the cutting of serial sections in great numbers, can settle the question as to the starting point of the glandular inclusions for many of the cases of adenomyoma.* Lockyer provided a comprehensive definition of an adenomyoma. He wrote: *the term 'adenomyoma' implies a new formation composed of gland-elements, hyperplastic cellular connective tissue, and smooth muscle. ... So far as the adenomatous elements are concerned, the same type of tumour-formation can be found also in the digestive tract (bowel and stomach), and some observers claim that analogous conditions can exist in the gall-bladder, in the kidney, and elsewhere.* Clearly under the term adenomyoma, early authors described both adenomyosis and endometriosis.

Lockyer includes a description of adenomyomas affecting the uterine wall (that we would today identify as adenomyosis), as well as extrauterine adenomyomas. Notable is Lockyer's reference to lesions in the recto-genital space. In his view, the condition should no longer be confused with malignancy because of the extensive literature available. This included the cases already mentioned, as well as a case by Pfannenstiel [33].

The work of Cullen enabled a renewed emphasis and a focus on adenomyomas and – more specifically – of what we today call adenomyosis. His work has a unique place in the history of adenomyosis as it enabled a clearer appreciation of the role and nature of the mucosa. It took some 20 years for this concept to take hold.

The reluctance of most of the early researchers into the origin of the islets of epithelial tissue observed in various abdominal organs to accept that they were transplants of uterine mucosa led to a long controversy. Illustrations of some of these uncommon lesions are contained in published literature of the time and have recently been reviewed [34]. The controversy continued until – as Lockyer [2] expressed it – there was a *gradual ascendancy of Cullen's mucosal theory*. Among the early supporters of Cullen's views was von Franqué [35] who believed that epithelial growths found in a number of abdominal organs derived from the *mature mucous membrane* of the uterus that had acquired the ability of infiltrating other organs as a consequence of a process of inflammation. Other early supporters of Cullen's theory were Baldy and Longcope [36], who not only refused von Recklinghausen's Wolffian hypothesis [10] but also rejected that put forward by Kossmann of an origin from accessory Müllerian ducts [11].

30.2 The Work of Thomas Cullen

Thomas Cullen presented his first case of adenomyoma of the uterus to the Johns Hopkins Hospital Medical Society in 1895 [13]. This was about 2 years after he completed his training in Germany and took his post in charge of gynecological pathology. Cullen's first important contribution to the field was published in German in 1903 as a tribute to Johannes Orth of Göttingen. In this, he acknowledges the support he received from von Recklinghausen. He included a description of known cases, including those of Paul Locksteadt who was able, through the introduction of

Prussian blue dye, to establish continuity between the glands in the myometrium and the uterine mucosa.

Then, in 1908, Cullen dedicated a monograph to *Adenomyoma of the Uterus* [18], and in it, he reconstructed the path that led him to identify the first case he came across: *One afternoon in October 1894, while making the routine examination of the material from the operating room I found a uniformly enlarged uterus about four times the natural size. On opening it I found that the increase in size was due to a diffuse thickening of the anterior wall. Professor William H. Welch, when consulted, said that the condition was evidently a most unusual one and suggested that sections be made from the entire thickness of the uterine wall. Examination of these sections showed that the increase in thickness was due to the presence of a diffuse myomatous tumor occupying the inner portion of the uterine wall, and that the uterine mucosa was at many points flowing into the diffuse myomatous tissue.*

Cullen then described all cases he had observed, providing astonishingly clear illustrations of the various types of adenomyoma known to him at the time. Although the vast majority consisted of myomatous tissue clearly infiltrated by uterine mucosa, the variant we would today call adenomyoma, he described a few cases in which there was no visible myoma; these we would today classify as adenomyosis.

He distinguished three types:

1. Adenomyomas in which the uterus preserves a relatively normal contour
2. Subperitoneal or intraligamentary adenomyomas
3. Submucous adenomyomas

Cullen was a gynecological surgeon and, for this reason, his book provides also a clinical picture of the condition. He reported the two main symptoms as *lengthened menstrual periods* that – as the disease progresses – *may be replaced by a continuous haemorrhagic discharge* and *a great deal of pain*. He claimed that *in the early and fairly advanced stages of the process, so definite are the symptoms that the hospital assistant now frequently comes and says that a given case has all the signs of an adenomyoma and that he feels sure that this is the cause of the bleeding.* This viewpoint is not currently accepted, and histological diagnosis, despite the availability of advanced imaging techniques, remains the gold standard.

Cullen also discussed treatment and concluded that *abdominal hysterectomy is indicated,* because *myomectomy is inapplicable, as the growth is so interwoven with the normal muscle that it cannot be shelled out.* It is notable, though, that some of the cases he described underwent resection of the lesion only.

In 1909, with HA Kelly, Cullen [37] detailed the characteristics of the condition we today call adenomyosis. They wrote: *In cases of adenomyoma of the uterus we usually find a diffuse myomatous thickening of the uterine muscle. This thickening may be confined to the inner layers of the anterior, posterior, or lateral walls, but in other cases the myomatous tissue completely encircles the uterine cavity. This diffuse myomatous tissue contains large or small chinks, and into these the normal uterine mucosa flows. If the chinks are small, there is only room for isolated glands, but where the spaces are goodly in size, large masses of mucosa flow into and fill them. We accordingly have a diffuse myomatous growth with normal mucosa flowing in all directions through it. The mucosa lining the uterine cavity is perfectly normal.*

Here, Kelly and Cullen first reiterated that the epithelial tissue is uterine mucosa, a position strengthened by their ability to trace in some cases a direct connection between the heterotopic endometrial nests and the mucosa of the uterine cavity. Secondly, as it had been first observed by Locksteadt [38], they described the presence in the myometrium of chinks, or fissures, through which the mucosa invades the underlying muscular tissue, thereby suggesting a mechanism through which the invasion occurs. Thirdly, they describe myomatous thickening of the uterine muscle. This was 75 years before Hricak et al. [39] described the junctional zone myometrium and almost a century before Tamai et al. [40] documented the importance of the thickening of the JZ myometrium for the noninvasive diagnosis of adenomyosis.

Cullen continued his interest in the subject in a seminal article first published in 1919 and reprinted in 1920 as part of a comprehensive summary of his work [41]. He wrote that he was *amazed at the widespread distribution of these tumours consisting of non-stripped muscle with islands of uterine mucosa scattered throughout them.* In his book on the distribution of adenomyomas containing uterine mucosa, Cullen elected to focus on his own cases. He described lesions under ten headings based on the site where they were identified: the body of the uterus, the rectovaginal septum, the uterine horn or the fallopian tube, the round ligament, the hilum of the ovary, the utero-ovarian ligament, the uterosacral ligament, the sigmoid flexure, the rectus muscle, and the umbilicus. There is similarity here with the classification provided in Lockyer's text which Cullen had received. The first case involving the round ligament was published in 1896 [13]. Cullen refers to the histological features that include striations with scattered chocolate-colored areas varying in diameter from 1 to 5 mm as the characteristic features of adenomyoma. Scattered endometrial glands were accompanied by stroma. Cullen observed the high incidence of uterine affection (73 cases out of 1283 patients of myomas, representing almost 6%). He classified uterine affection according to their site: interstitial, subperitoneal, and submucosal. The main focus of his monograph, however, was on affections of the rectovaginal septum. Importantly, he supported the view that the epithelial cells found were derived from the uterine mucosa. However, as already mentioned, many remained skeptical arguing that this theory is insufficient to explain mucosal invasion at all ectopic sites. Among the skeptics was Lockyer [2], who argued that theories pertinent to the etiology of adenomyoma needed to be adapted depending on the site.

Cullen's final major contribution to the field was the already mentioned comprehensive review, published in 1920 [41], of all his findings. Here the emphasis was on lesions found outside the uterus. He reported to have observed the presence of heterotopic uterine mucosa in a number of abdominal locations, including the ovary. Figure 30.1, taken from Cullen's paper, illustrates all the locations where he identified ectopic mucosa.

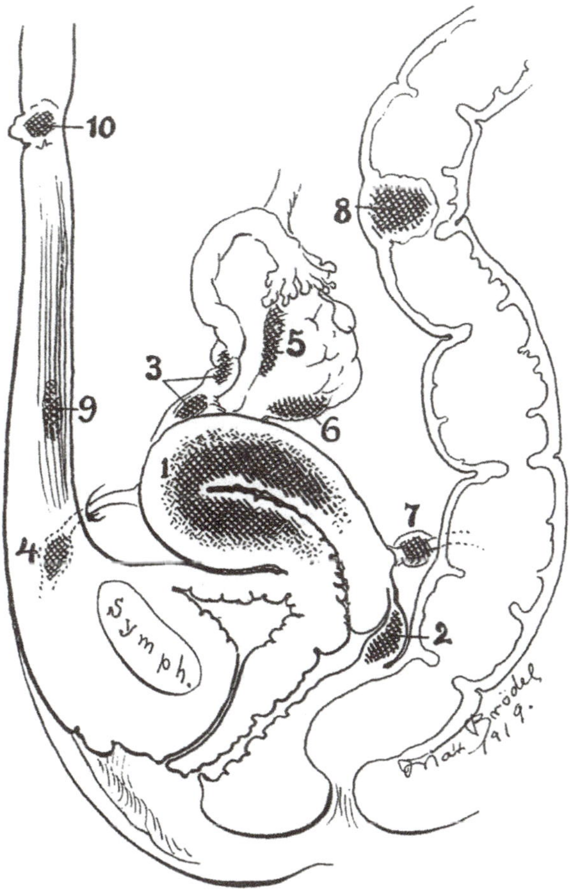

Fig. 30.1 The locations where Cullen identified uterine mucosa: (1) the body of the uterus; (2) the rectovaginal septum; (3) the uterine horn or fallopian tube; (4) the round ligament; (5) the hilum of the ovary; (6) the utero-ovarian ligament; (7) the uterosacral ligament; (8) the sigmoid flexure; (9) the rectus muscle; (10) the umbilicus. (From Cullen [41])

30.3 Otto Frankl and the Birth of Adenomyosis

In 1925, Otto Frankl [42] described anatomical features of the "intrauterine variety" of mucosal invasion, for which he coined the name *adenomyosis uteri* and explained: *I have chosen the name of adenomyosis, which does not suggest any inflammatory origin as do terms like adenometritis, adenomyositis, adenomyometritis, still employed. ... We were never able to find any trace of an inflammatory infiltration, either in the musculature or in the mucosa of this region. In the history of these patients, we did not find a single symptom suggesting a preceding puerperal or gonorrheal infection.*

In his description, Frankl also specified the criteria for differentiating adenomyosis from adenomyomas (what today we would call the various phenotypes of endometriosis). The main criterion, one we today cannot agree with, was that the glands of an adenomyoma originate independently within the myoma as an autochthonous growth, whereas in adenomyosis, there is always the possibility to establish a direct connection with the eutopic endometrium through serial sections. Frankl correctly pointed out similarities between his observations and those of Sampson, since he found the presence of blood in the glands within the myometrium and reported as: *An observation made only once should be mentioned, namely, the presence of blood in the glands within the myometrium. This finding was made in a woman of fifty years, who still was menstruating regularly. The last menstruation had occurred three weeks previous to operation. In a few glands, which were dilated cystically, we found only slightly changed blood.* Frankl pointed out that his observation was very similar to that of the *menstruating uterine mucosa on the surface of the ovary, first described by Sampson*. He concluded that, having studied Sampson's original slides, he became convinced that in his and in Sampson's case, *misplaced uterine glands were seen filled with blood, undoubtedly menstrual blood.*

Frankl also noted differences in the appearance of the mucosa in adenomyosis. He wrote: *The entire material from thirty cases shows in twelve instances the presence of myomas, mostly of very small size, a fact which should not be overlooked. Eleven times we found the mucosa in a hyperplastic condition. The coincidence of small myomas is not so striking inasmuch as they are quite common in general, but the presence of a hyperplastic mucosa eleven times is noteworthy. The penetration of a hyperplastic mucosa into the myometrium can be readily understood if we assume for it a more marked tendency toward proliferation.*

Clinically, Frankl described that in women suffering from adenomyosis, there is a sudden appearance, at the onset of the disease, of menorrhagia: *With the clinical picture of adenomyosis we must always associate a sudden onset of a very excessive haemorrhages, coincident with or independent of menstruation, and not one which gradually increases as is observed in a hemorrhagic metropathia.* He believed that the clinical picture might have a relationship with hormonal disturbances, although he concluded: *Not being able to prove or to disprove a hormonal cause for adenomyosis I am unwilling to consider the hemorrhages in this disease as having any connection with endocrine influences.*

These observations remained the cornerstone description of adenomyosis until, almost 50 years later, when, in 1972, Bird [43] provided the current definition: *Adenomyosis may be defined as the benign invasion of endometrium into the myometrium, producing a diffusely enlarged uterus which microscopically exhibits ectopic non-neoplastic, endometrial glands and stroma surrounded by the hypertrophic and hyperplastic myometrium.* Critically, Bird divided adenomyosis into grades based on the depth of gland invasion within the myometrium.

In this respect it is noteworthy that the lesions that brought the condition to early investigators were often those that acquired a large size or contained large fluid-filled cavities. The influential writings of Cullen and Lockyer focused the attention on the more common disease phenotypes which today constitute the vast majority of identified cases, whereas debate continues on whether the uncommon types should be viewed as variants of adenomyosis.

30.4 Conclusion

The present view of what we call adenomyosis emerged only after some 50 years of debate on the nature of mucosal invasions of peritoneal organs. Its history is one of the many examples of progress made by trial and error, where the "scientific truth" of today still leaves space for refinement, as well as change.

References

1. Bailey KV. The etiology, classification and life history of tumours of the ovary and other female pelvic organs containing aberrant Müllerian elements, with suggested nomenclature. J Obstet Gynaecol Br Emp. 1924;31:539–79.
2. Lockyer C. Fibroids and allied tumours (myoma and adenomyoma). London: Macmillan; 1918.
3. Babes G. Über epitheliale Geschwulste in Uterusmyomem [About epithelial tumors in uterine fibroids]. Allgem Wiener Med Ztschr. 1882;27:36–48.
4. Diesterweg B. Ein Fall von Cystofibrom uteri verum [A case of cystofibroma uteri verum]. Zeitschr Gebursthilfe. 1883;9:191.
5. von Recklinghausen F. Über die Adenocysten der Uterus-tumoren und über Reste des Wolfschen Organs [About the adenocysts of the uterine tumors and the remains of the Wolf organ]. Deutsche Med Wochenschr. 1893;46:824–6.
6. von Recklinghausen F. Über Adenomyome des Uterus und der Tuba [About the ademomyomas of the uterus and the tube]. Wiener klin Wochenschr. 1895;29:530–6.
7. Rokitansky C. Über Uterusdrüsen-Neubildung in Uterus- und Ovarial-Sarcomen. [On the neoplasm of uterus glands on uterine and ovarian sarcomas]. Zeitschr Gesellschaft der Aerzte in Wien. 1860;16:577–81.
8. Kolb JM. Pathologische Anatomie der weiblichen Sexualorgane [Pathological anatomy of the female sexual organs]. Vienna: Wilhelm Braumüller; 1864.
9. Röhrig A. Erfahrungen über verlauf und prognose der uterusfibromyome [Experience on the course and prognosis of uterine fibromyomas]. Zeitschrift für Geburtshulfe und Gynäkologie. 1880;5:265–316.
10. von Recklinghausen F. Die Adenomyomata und Cystadenomata der Uterus und Tubenwandung: Ihre Abkunft von Resten des Wolffischen Körpers [The adenomyomas and cystadenomas of the uterus and tube wall: their origin from remnants of the Wolffian body]. Berlin: August Hirschwald Verlag; 1896.
11. Kossman R. Die Abstammung der Drüseneinschlüsse in der Uterus und der Tuben [The lineage of the glandular inclusions in the uterus and tubes]. Arch Gynakol. 1897;54:359–81.
12. Habiba M, Pluchino N, Petignat P, Bianchi P, Brosens IA, Benagiano G. Adenomyosis and endometrial cancer: literature review. Gynecol Obstet Investig. 2018;83:313–28.
13. Cullen T. Adenomyoma of the round ligament. Johns Hopkins Hosp Bull. 1896;7:112–3.
14. Pick L. Ein neuer Typus des voluminösen paroophoralenAdenomyoms – zugleich über eine bisher nicht bekannte Geschwulst Form der Gebärmutter (Adenomyoma psammopapillare) und über totale Verdoppelung des Eileiters [A new type of voluminous paroophoral adenomyomas – both on a previously unknown form of tumor of the uterus (adenomyoma psammopapillare) and a total doubling of the oviduct]. Archiv Gynäkol. 1897;54:117–206.
15. Rolly F. Über einen Fall von Adenomyoma uteri mit Uebergang in Carcinom und Metastasenbildung. [About a case of uterine adenomyoma with transition to carcinoma and metastasis]. Archiv Pathol Anat Physiol Klin Med. 1897;150:555–82.
16. Rolly F. Über einen Fall von Adenomyoma uteri etc. [About a case of adenomyoma of the uterus, etc.] Virchow's Archiv Bd. 1897;150.

17. Ivanoff NS. Drüsiges cystenhaltiges Uterusfibromyom compliciert durch Sarcom und Carcinom (Adenofibromyoma cysticum sarcomatodes carcinomatosum) [Uterine fibromyoma containing glandular cyst complicated by sarcoma and carcinoma (Adenofibromyoma cysticum sarcomatodes carcinomatosum)]. Monatssch Gebursthilfe Gynäkol. 1898;7:295–300.
18. Cullen TS. Adenomyoma of the uterus. Philadelphia & London: WB Saunders; 1908.
19. Breus C. Über wahre epithel führende Cystenbildung in Uterusmyomen [Cyst formation in uterine fibroids leading to true epithelium]. Leipzig und Wien: Franz Deuticke; 1894.
20. Schröder O. Über cystofibroide des uterus speciell über einen fall von intra-uterinen cystofibroid [About cystofibroids of the uterus with special reference to a case of intra-uterine cystofibroid]. Strassburg: JH. ED. Heitz, Universitäts-Buchdrucker; 1873.
21. Heer O. Über fibrocysten des uterus [About fibrocysts of the uterus]. Druck von Zürcher und Furrer: Zurich; 1874.
22. Grosskopf C. (Thesis) Zur Kenntniss der cystomyome des uterus [On knowledge of cystomyomas of the uterus]. München; 1884.
23. Schuh F. Über die Erkenntniss der Pseudoplasmen [On the knowledge of pseudoplasms]. Vienna: LW. Siedel; 1851.
24. Wells T (Spencer). Diseases of the ovaries. Their diagnosis and treatment. London: J & A Churchill; 1872.
25. Bishop ES. Uterine fibromyomata: their pathology, diagnosis, and treatment. London: Rebman Ltd; 1901.
26. Gusserow A. Die neubildungen des uterus [The neoplasms of the uterus]. Stuttgart: Verlag von Ferdinand Enke; 1886.
27. Mayer R. Über eine adenomatose Wucherung der Serosa in einer Bauchnarde [On an adenomatous growth of the serosa around silk ligatures]. Zeitschr Gebursthilfe Gynäkol. 1903;49:32–41.
28. Orloff WN. Zür Genese der Uterusmyome [On the origin of uterine myomas]. Zeitschr Heilkunde. 1895;5:312–38.
29. Sitzenfrei A. Das übergreifen der adenomyome des uterus auf den mastdarm zugleichen beitrag zür klinik und histogenese des adenomyositis uteri et recti und des adenomyoma recti [The spreading of uterines adenomyomas to the rectum also contributes to the clinic and histogenesis of adenomyositis uteri and recti and of the adenomyoma recti]. Zeithschr Geburstshilfe Gynäkol. 1909;64:538–80.
30. Sitzenfrey A. Drei seltene geschwülste (epidermoid des antezervikalen Bindegewebes) [Three rare tumors (epidermoid of the antecervical connective tissue)]. Zeithschr Geburstshilfe Gynäkol. 1910;67:32–49.
31. Frankl O. Adenomyoma ligamenti ovarii. Arkiv Gynäkol. 1911;93:659–75.
32. Schikele G. Die lehre von den Mesonephrischen Geschülsten [The teaching of the Mesonephric Schools]. Zentralbl Allg Pathol Anat. 1904;15:261–302.
33. Pfannenstiel HJ. Über die Adenomyome des Genitalstranges [About the adenomyomas of the genital tract]. Verhandl Deutsch Gesellsch Gynäkol. 1897;7:195–9.
34. Habiba M, Brosens I, Zannoni GF, Benagiano G. Uncommon mixed endometrial-myometrial benign tumors of the reproductive tract: literature review. Gynecol Obstet Investig. 2019;19:1–27.
35. von Franqué O. Salpingitis nodosa isthmica und Adenomyoma tubae. Zeitschr Gebursthilfe Gynäkol. 1900;42:41–54.
36. Baldy JM, Longcope WT. Adenomyomata of the uterus. Am J Obstet Dis Women Child. 1903;45:78–92.
37. Kelly HA, Cullen TS. Myomata of the uterus. Philadelphia & London: WB Saunders; 1909.
38. von Lockstaedt P. Über Vorkommen und Bedeutung von Drüsenschläuchen in den Myomen des Uterus [About the occurrence and importance of glandular tubes in the fibroids of the uterus]. Monatssch. Geburtshilfe Gynäkol. 1898;7:188–232.

39. Hricak H, Alpers C, Crooks LE, Sheldon PE. Magnetic resonance imaging of the female pelvis: initial experience. Am J Roentgenol. 1983;141:1119–28.
40. Tamai K, Togashi K, Ito T, Morisawa N, Fujiwara T, Koyama T. MR imaging findings of adenomyosis: correlation with histopathologic features and diagnostic pitfalls. Radiographics. 2005;25:21–40.
41. Cullen TS. The distribution of adenomyomata containing uterine mucosa. Arch Surg. 1920;1:215–283 Reprinted from: Archives of Surgery 1920;1:215–83.
42. Frankl O. Adenomyosis uteri. Am J Obstet Gynecol. 1925;10:680–4.
43. Bird CC, McElin TW, Manalo-Estrella P. The elusive adenomyosis of the uterus. Am J Obstet Gynecol. 1972;112:583–93.

Insights on Adenomyosis Development

31

Silvia Vannuccini and Sara Clemenza

Contents

The original version of the chapter has been revised. A correction to this chapter can be found at https://doi.org/10.1007/978-3-030-97236-3_45

S. Vannuccini (✉) · S. Clemenza
Department of Experimental, Clinical and Biomedical Sciences, Careggi University Hospital, Florence, Italy
e-mail: silvia.vannuccini@unifi.it

E. Oral (ed.), *Endometriosis and Adenomyosis*,
https://doi.org/10.1007/978-3-030-97236-3_31

31.1 Introduction

Adenomyosis is a gynecological condition defined as the presence of endometrial glands and stroma deep within the myometrium, with associated myometrial hypertrophy, hyperplasia, and fibrosis [1]. Although the pathogenesis of adenomyosis remains unclear, two main theories have been proposed: (a) invagination of the endometrial basalis into the myometrium and (b) metaplasia of displaced embryonic pluripotent Müllerian remnants or differentiation of adult stem cells [2]. However, adenomyosis pathogenesis is elusive, and not a single theory may explain all of the different phenotypes of the disease [3]. Key pathogenic mechanisms of adenomyosis include estrogen dependence, progesterone resistance, inflammation, aberrant immune responses, cell migration, invasion and proliferation, fibrosis, and neuroangiogenesis [3] (Fig. 31.1).

Risk factors are also not fully understood. In the past, it was thought that adenomyosis affected almost exclusively women in their 40s and 50s, often multiparous. This belief was partially due to the fact that the diagnosis was generally confirmed upon hysterectomy [4]. Nowadays, by using imaging techniques such as transvaginal ultrasound (TVUS) and magnetic resonance (MRI), the epidemiological scenario has completely changed, and adenomyosis is increasingly identified in young women with pain, abnormal uterine bleeding (AUB), and infertility or as incidental finding in asymptomatic women undergoing imaging [3].

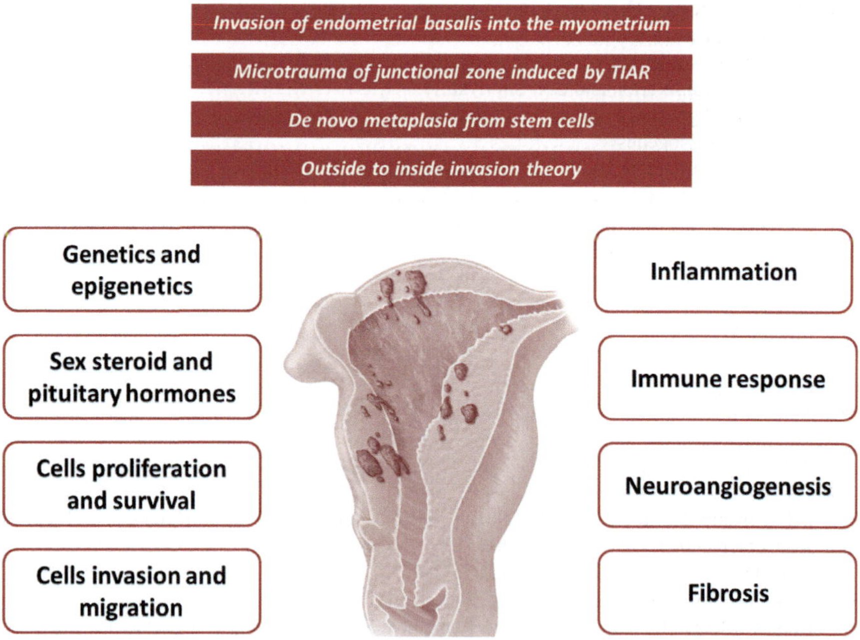

Fig. 31.1 Pathogenetic theories, mechanisms, and mediators for adenomyosis. TIAR: tissue injury and repair

31.2 Risk Factors for Adenomyosis

Prevalence and risk factors of adenomyosis are currently uncertain as the disease has historically been identified as a pathological entity from histological reports after hysterectomy. Thus, the available data show a higher prevalence of adenomyosis in patients in their late reproductive years or in perimenopausal women [1, 3]. Recent diagnostic advances have created the opportunity to detect adenomyosis with less invasive methods, such as TVUS and MRI. As imaging diagnostics improve, patients with adenomyosis, including women undergoing fertility evaluations and even adolescents, are being diagnosed earlier. This shift in diagnosis suggests that adenomyosis is not a condition affecting only older women [1].

Epidemiological findings also suggest that adenomyosis is found more often in multiparous than nulliparous women [5, 6]. The relationship between parity and adenomyosis may be biased since the diagnosis is typically made at hysterectomy. However, it was also suggested that foci of adenomyosis may be included in the myometrium due to the aggressive action of the trophoblast, and viable endometrium may be displaced during pregnancy and parturition. Alternatively, the hormonal milieu of pregnancy may favor the development of islands of ectopic endometrium [7]. Templeman et al. [6] reported that early menarche, short menstrual cycles, and obesity are risk factors for adenomyosis. In contrast, Vercellini et al. [7] and Parazzini et al. [8] found no association between age at menarche and the diagnosis of adenomyosis made at the time of hysterectomy.

Several studies have also suggested that dilation and curettage (D&C) and other prior uterine surgeries may be risk factors for adenomyosis [9, 10]. These surgical procedures in fact may disrupt the endo-myometrial interface and facilitate the invasion, implantation, embedding, and establishment of endometrial colonies within the myometrial wall, increasing the risk of adenomyosis [11].

Smoking is inconsistently shown to be a protective factor for adenomyosis. Since adenomyosis is an estrogen-dependent disorder, low concentrations of estrogens, such as those found in smokers, may reduce the risk of adenomyosis [8].

The association between adenomyosis and the past use of combined oral contraceptives (COCs) is also controversial. While Parazzini et al. [8] did not find any association between the risk of adenomyosis and COCs, Templeman et al. [6] reported higher rates of adenomyosis in patients who have used COCs. This correlation requires further investigation, as COCs constitute a common treatment for dysmenorrhea and heavy menstrual bleeding, which are common symptoms in patients with adenomyosis [2].

Finally, a higher prevalence of adenomyosis has been reported in women treated with tamoxifen for breast cancer [12, 13]. Although tamoxifen blocks estrogen receptors in breast tissue, in other tissues like endometrium, it may actually have an estrogenic effect and can promote proliferation and adenomyosis development or even reactivation of preexisting adenomyotic lesions [2].

Since the available evidence on epidemiological characteristics of women with adenomyosis is greatly biased by the type of population studied (i.e., women undergoing hysterectomy), noninvasive diagnostic methods should be used in future epidemiological studies in order to define incidence, prevalence, and risk factors of adenomyosis in the general population [7].

31.3 Pathogenic Theories on the Origin of Adenomyosis

31.3.1 Invasion from the Endometrium

According to the invasion theory, adenomyosis develops through invagination of the endometrium basalis into the myometrium through an altered or absent junctional zone (JZ). The JZ represents a highly specialized hormone-responsive structure located in the inner third of the myometrium, which can be identified using imaging techniques, such as ultrasound and MRI, but not histologically [3, 14].

The invagination theory was based largely on the tissue injury and repair (TIAR) theory proposed by Leyendecker et al. [15, 16]. The TIAR theory postulates that repeated and sustained overstretching due to hyperperistalsis and consequent increased intrauterine pressure may cause injury of the myocytes and fibroblasts in the JZ, leading to the invagination of the endometrial basal layer into the myometrium and thus to adenomyosis. This microtrauma promotes inflammation and local production of estradiol, which, in turn, cause more inflammation and more estrogen production, establishing a vicious circle [11]. Myometrial hyperperistalsis, induced by the local production of estrogen, has been considered the primary event in the disease process [17]. However, initial injury to the JZ may also result from iatrogenic trauma [4]. Thus, the invagination theory may be consistent with the epidemiological findings that multiparity and uterine surgery are risk factors for adenomyosis due to their potential to disrupt the JZ [3, 11].

31.3.2 Metaplasia

The metaplasia theory proposes that adenomyotic lesions may originate from the metaplasia of displaced embryonic pluripotent Müllerian remnants. It has been postulated that during Müllerian duct development, some remnants of the embryonic tissue may be misplaced in the myometrium [2, 18]. Intramyometrial embryonic pluripotent Müllerian remnants may undergo metaplastic changes in the adult uterine wall, leading to the establishment of de novo ectopic endometrial tissue within the myometrial wall, as adenomyotic foci [3]. Accordingly, the metaplasia theory could account for some cases of adenomyosis in the rudimentary muscular uterine wall of patients with Mayer-Rokitansky-Kuster-Hauser syndromes [4].

Alternatively, adenomyosis can differentiate from multipotent stem cells originated from bone marrow and other sources [17]. More recently, it has been demonstrated that adult stem cells are activated by tissue injury, promoting ectopic endometrial implants through endometrial stem/progenitor cell niche disruption [19]. However, more research is required to establish a role for endometrial stem/progenitor cells in the initiation and progression of adenomyosis.

Progenitor cells deposited in the peritoneal cavity by retrograde menstruation can possibly lead to the focal uterine adenomyosis [17]. Accordingly, Chapron et al. described "from outside to inside invasion" theory, hypothesizing the migration of ectopic endometrial cells from posterior endometriosis nodules into the myometrium. This theory was supported by the high prevalence of posterior focal adenomyosis of the outer myometrium found in patients with deep infiltrating endometriosis (DIE) nodules in the posterior compartment, diagnosed by MRI [20].

It was also suggested that diffuse and focal adenomyosis may result from different mechanisms: adenomyosis foci could originate from eutopic endometrium in diffuse adenomyosis lesions, whereas, for the focal form, adenomyosis foci could originate from functional ectopic endometrium derived from extrauterine endometriosis lesions in contact with the uterus. Therefore, different triggering factors (intrauterine triggers for diffuse forms and extrauterine triggers, such as DIE, for focal forms) may favor the development of these two different forms of adenomyosis [21].

31.4 Pathogenic Mechanisms

31.4.1 Genetics and Epigenetics

Current evidence supports genetics as a driver in the pathogenesis of adenomyosis [18]. Several mRNAs, involved in sex steroid signaling, inflammation, proliferation, apoptosis, extracellular matrix (ECM) remodeling, and angiogenesis, were found to be dysregulated in adenomyosis [4, 22, 23].

Many studies have shown that cytochrome P450 (CYP) genes and catechol-O-methyltransferase (COMT) gene variants, both involved in estrogen metabolism, could increase the risk of adenomyosis [24, 25]. Estrogen receptor (ER) and progesterone receptor (PR) gene polymorphisms may be also involved. Polymorphisms of the matrix metalloproteinases (MMPs) MMP-1 and MMP-2 were described in adenomyosis, supporting a role of ECM dysfunction in the pathogenesis of the disease [26, 27]. Variants of genes implicated in the angiogenesis process, such as fibroblast growth factors (FGF-1, FGF-2) [28] and vascular endothelial growth factor (VEGF) [29], were also associated with an increased susceptibility to adenomyosis. Moreover, genetic variation in the promoter region of cyclooxygenase 2 (COX-2) gene has been shown to heighten the risk of the disease [30]. A recent study based on next-generation sequencing technology identified recurrent Kirsten rat sarcoma viral oncogene homolog (KRAS) mutations in adenomyotic lesions and eutopic endometrium, concluding that adenomyosis might be an oligoclonal disease associated with mutations in the KRAS gene [31].

Epigenetic alterations have been also detected in adenomyosis. Compared with normal endometrium, the immunoreactivity to deoxyribonucleic acid methyltransferases (DNMTs), a family of enzymes that catalyze transfer of a methyl group to DNA, differs significantly in adenomyosis. DNMT1 and DNMT3B expressions have been shown to be higher in ectopic endometrium, while DNMT3A levels are reduced in both eutopic and ectopic endometria. Moreover, DNMT3B was associated with the severity of dysmenorrhea, suggesting that DNMTs may be involved in adenomyosis-related pain and its severity [32]. DNA hypomethylation and increased expression of CCAAT/enhancer-binding protein β (CEBPB), a transcription factor regulating gene expression to control cellular proliferation, differentiation, and metabolism, were also associated with the occurrence of adenomyosis [23]. Moreover, class I histone deacetylases (HDACs), known to play important roles in steroid hormone-dependent gene expression, endometrial differentiation, and implantation, were found to be aberrantly expressed in the ectopic endometrium of women with adenomyosis [33]. The potential role of HDACs in adenomyosis is also supported by the finding that the use of valproic acid (VPA), a histone deacetylase inhibitor (HDACI), resulted in the relief of dysmenorrhea and the reduction of uterus size in women with symptomatic adenomyosis [34]. Recently, Zhai et al. [35] have found that RNA methylation, especially N6-methyladenosine and its regulators, may be involved in the pathogenesis of adenomyosis through aberrant expression and actions in both the uterine endometrium and myometrium.

31.4.2 Sex Steroid Hormone Function

Steroid hormones play a central role in the pathogenesis of adenomyosis [17]. In particular, the disease is characterized by estrogen dependence and progesterone resistance. Elevated estradiol (E2) levels in menstrual blood of women with adenomyosis, but not in peripheral blood, compared with controls, suggest that local rather than systemic hyperestrogenism contributes to the development of the disease [18, 36].

Several gene polymorphisms causing increased production and decreased metabolism of estrogens were associated with a higher risk of adenomyosis development [24, 30]. The aromatase cytochrome P450, expressed in the eutopic endometrium of patients with adenomyosis, but not in the endometrium of women without the disease, may promote estrogen biosynthesis and higher estrogenic bioavailability due to local aromatization of circulating androgens into E2 [37, 38]. Furthermore, the altered regulation of 17ß-hydroxysteroid dehydrogenase type 2 (17β-HSD2) in the eutopic endometrium of women with adenomyosis may cause a decreased local estrogen metabolism [39].

Higher expression of ER-α and decreased expression of PR have also been reported in adenomyotic endometrium and lesions [40]. Considering that progesterone opposes estrogenic action via its receptors, decreased PR expression could favor progesterone resistance and hyperestrogenism in adenomyotic uteri [2, 41]. Moreover, the expression of G-protein-coupled estrogen receptor (GPER), a membrane estrogen receptor, structurally and genetically unrelated to ER-α and ER-β, was found to be significantly higher in women with adenomyosis compared to controls, both in the JZ and in the outer myometrium and both in the proliferative and in the secretory phases [42]. This finding confirms the notion that adenomyosis is associated with alteration in several different steroid receptors.

This hormonal status represents the "primum movens" of a chain of key events in the pathogenesis of adenomyosis. In fact, as mentioned above, local hyperestrogenism leads to increased peristalsis of the subendometrial myometrium and to microtrauma of the JZ, initiating TIAR and promoting a positive feed-forward cycle that facilitates the invasion of the endometrial basalis into the myometrium and eventually the establishment of adenomyotic lesions. Moreover, E2 is a potent stimulus of COX-2, which in turn leads to increased levels of prostaglandins (PGs) in the uterus and can potentiate the inflammation, inducing a vicious cycle [17, 18].

31.4.3 Pituitary Hormone Function

Oxytocin directly stimulates the contraction of smooth myocytes of the myometrium and its bloodstream by binding to its receptor (OTR). Studies have found that increased expression of OTR in the myometrium positively correlates with the amplitude of uterine contractions and can lead to the appearance of pathological and uncoordinated myometrial spasms, accompanied by severe dysmenorrhea and reduced fertility in women of reproductive age [43–46].

Compared with normal endometrium, the immunoreactivity of OTR is significantly increased in the ectopic endometrium of women with adenomyosis and is positively correlated with the severity of dysmenorrhea [47]. In normal uteri, the expression of OTR in the isthmus is significantly higher than in the fundus in the proliferative phase, but the opposite distribution pattern is observed in the secretory phase. Conversely, in adenomyosis uteri, the expression of OTR in the fundus was found to be significantly higher than in the isthmus in the proliferative phase [48]. The opposite expression pattern of OTR in isthmic and fundal regions may disturb the direction of the endometrial-myometrial interface (EMI) contractions, potentially interfering with sperm transport and fertility [18].

Besides causing uterine hyperactivity, OTR expression may also result in upregulation of COX-2, leading to overproduction of PGE2. Although the cause for OTR overexpression in adenomyosis is currently unclear, it has been shown that OTR expression increases in response to inflammatory cytokines and angiogenic factors. It is also possible that increased local estrogen production and constitutive activation of NF-kB may upregulate OTR in adenomyotic lesions [49].

Animal models have shown that increased uterine concentration of prolactin (PRL) may be a risk factor for adenomyosis. PRL is produced in the human endometrium and myometrium as well as in the pituitary gland and acts as a smooth muscle cell mitogen in vitro [50]. In murine uteri, minimal serum hyperprolactinemia is sufficient to cause adenomyosis [51, 52]. In humans, vaginal bromocriptine significantly decreased menstrual bleeding and pain and improved quality of life in women with the disease [50]. However, further studies are needed to establish mechanisms underlying the role of PRL in the pathogenesis of adenomyosis.

31.4.4 Inflammation

Adenomyosis is considered a chronic inflammatory disease. In fact, adenomyotic lesions, peripheral blood, and/or peritoneal fluid of women with adenomyosis is rich of inflammatory mediators [53]. IL-1β, IL-6, IL-8, corticotropin-releasing hormone (CRH), urocortin (Ucn), synaptophysin (SYN), and microtubule-associated protein 2 (MAP2) are highly expressed in adenomyotic nodules compared to eutopic endometrium and control [53–55].

COX-2 is overexpressed in eutopic and ectopic endometrium of adenomyosis and seems to play a key role in the pathogenesis of the disease. Since CRH and UCN have been shown to activate COX-2 in other tissues, the high expression of CRH and UCN in adenomyosis may also lead to increased PG synthesis [54]. Moreover, the mechanical stretching due to uterine peristalsis results in elevated IL-1β expression, which can also induce COX-2 [56]. This causes an increased production of PGE2 which, in turn, favors the expression of genes critical to estrogen production such as steroidogenic acute regulatory protein (StAR) and aromatase, resulting in a local hyperestrogenic state [11, 17]. According to this finding, PG levels are significantly increased in the peritoneal fluid of patients with adenomyosis and are positively associated with the degree of dysmenorrhea [53]. Furthermore, hyperestrogenism was shown to stimulate the production of IL-10, a cytokine with immunosuppressive abilities. High expression of IL-10 was demonstrated in both eutopic and ectopic endometria of women with adenomyosis [57]. This observation may explain the persistence of the ectopic foci within the myometrium without elimination by the immune system of the host [17].

Guo et al. [58] postulated that the TLR4 signaling pathway in stromal cells of the eutopic and ectopic endometrium may be essential for the pathogenesis of adenomyosis. TLR4-dependent signaling activated by endogenous ligands promoted the secretion of different cytokines and growth factors, stimulated endometrial cell proliferation, recruited and activated immune cells, triggered the local inflammatory response, and induced stromal cell proliferation and invasion, leading to the development of adenomyosis [17].

A decreased [59] and an increased [60] expression of the cannabinoid receptors CB1 and CB2 was found, respectively, in the endometrium and in the myometrium of patients with adenomyosis, suggesting that endocannabinoid system may participate in the pathogenesis of the disease [59]. Moreover, CB1 expression levels in JZ seem to be positively correlated with the severity of dysmenorrhea. The endocannabinoid system has long been known to have a role in inflammatory and immune regulation, fibrosis, angiogenesis, and neuroangiogenesis. However, additional investigations are needed to elucidate its role in adenomyosis.

31.4.5 Immune Response

Available data highlights the existence of aberrant immune responses in women with adenomyosis. In the uterus, a normal immune system serves a dual purpose.

On the one hand, it is essential to protect against pathogen invasion by way of an appropriate inflammatory reaction; on the other hand, a shift toward an immunosuppressive state is also required to allow successful embryonic implantation [21]. Several immune-related markers are altered in both eutopic and ectopic endometria of women with adenomyosis as well as at a systemic level. T-cell populations and macrophages are increased in the eutopic endometrium of women with adenomyosis, supporting the idea that both innate and adaptive immunities are involved in the development of the disease.

Macrophages are crucial to all physiological tissue repair processes, including inside the endometrium, where they release various pro- and anti-inflammatory chemokines, growth factors, MMPs, and adhesion factors, depending on the menstrual phase. Chronic trauma to the JZ would cause continuous infiltration by inflammatory macrophages which can lead to epithelial to mesenchymal transition (EMT) and fibrosis, while secreted inflammatory mediators in the uterus might interfere with other physiological functions, like embryo implantation [4].

It has been also suggested that immunotolerance of endometrial debris to natural killer (NK) cell cytolytic activity may be implicated in adenomyosis pathogenesis. HLA molecules should be involved in this process, as they play a key role in the establishment and maintenance of immune tolerance by inhibiting the functions of immunocompetent cells. Wang et al. [61] found that human leukocyte antigen-G (HLA-G) protein is expressed by eutopic and ectopic endometrium in adenomyosis patients, suggesting that these molecules may contribute to the resistance of endometrial cells to cytolysis. Another study argued for possible resistance of adenomyotic cells to NK cell activity, as levels of HLA class I and II expression were lower in endometrial specimens from women affected by adenomyosis compared to endometriosis and unaffected subjects [62]. Moreover, it was found that Indian hedgehog (Ihh) signaling, known to regulate autophagy, is suppressed in endometrial tissues of patients with adenomyosis, promoting aberrant survival of endometrial cells in ectopic sites [63].

Circulating B-cell-derived autoantibodies, mainly against phospholipids, have been detected in adenomyosis patients. These autoantibodies markedly decrease in women after hysterectomy for adenomyosis versus controls, suggesting an antigen-antibody response involving uterine antigens in adenomyosis [64]. However, further studies are needed to understand these observations and their possible physiologic relevance.

31.4.6 Proliferation and Cell Survival

Cell over-proliferation combined with impaired apoptosis are typical features of adenomyosis. Molecular mechanisms underlying decreased apoptosis and increased proliferation likely derive from excessive estradiol E2 in eutopic endometrium. In fact, it was found that treatment of human uterine smooth muscle cells of the JZ with E2 increases the expression of RhoA, a small guanosine triphosphatase involved in multiple cellular processes, including proliferation [65].

Myostatin, follistatin, and activin A, belonging to the transforming growth factor beta (TGF- β) superfamily, are highly expressed in adenomyotic nodules and may affect proliferation of endometrial glands/stroma and of surrounding myometrial cells [66]. Myocytes are the main target of myostatin, and their proliferative activity is modulated by these growth factors. Adenomyosis is characterized by hyperplasia of myometrial cells surrounding endometrial stroma and glands that may be linked to the myostatin/follistatin overexpression [17]. Furthermore, the mitogen-activated protein kinases/extracellular signal-regulated kinases (MAPKs/ERKs) and phosphoinositide 3-kinase/mammalian target of rapamycin/AKT (PI3K/mTOR/AKT) cell-signaling pathways appear to be involved in the proliferation of uterine smooth muscle cells of women with adenomyosis [67].

The B-cell lymphoma 2 (Bcl-2) protein, an apoptosis regulator, is abnormally expressed in adenomyosis. Overexpression of Bcl-2 enhanced the anti-apoptosis of endometrial cells, and the sensitivity of cells to apoptosis decreased, allowing cells to escape apoptosis resulting in implantation in the ectopic sites. In addition, Bcl-2 modulates other cellular functions such as autophagy, mitochondrial fusion, cell differentiation, senescence, cell migration, and angiogenesis, suggesting a key regulatory role in the development of adenomyosis [68].

The expression of the gene associated with retinoid-interferon-induced mortality 19 (*GRIM-19*), which promotes apoptosis, was found to be lower in the endometrial tissues of adenomyosis compared with normal endometrial tissue. Low levels of GRIM-19 may be caused by the polarization of M2 macrophages through TLR4 [69].

31.4.7 Migration, Invasion, and Fibrosis

Invasion of the myometrium by endometrial tissue is crucial for the establishment of adenomyosis. It has been suggested that EMT, a process where epithelial cells acquire an invasive and metastatic phenotype [18], is a key event boosting the migratory and invasive capacity of adenomyotic lesions [4]. The EMT events include the loss of expression or function of E-cadherin and a reduced abundance of tight junction proteins and cytokeratins, but an increase in the abundance of mesenchymal markers, such as vimentin, α-smooth muscle actin, and N-cadherin. This biological process implies that epithelial cells lose their polarity and cell-to-cell contacts to acquire a mesenchymal phenotype, which is crucial for cells to leave the epithelium and achieve the capacity to migrate [21].

In vitro experiments showed that changes to gene expression, along with acquisition of cell migration capacity, were estrogen-dependent, as blocking estrogen signaling completely eliminated these effects [70].

Several immune cells (platelets and macrophages) and inflammatory factors (TGF-β1, hepatocyte growth factor, focal adhesion kinase, integrin-linked kinase, Notch-1, and neuropilin-1) have been suggested as potential regulators of the EMT process in adenomyosis [71–75].

Activated macrophages co-cultured with both adenomyotic and unaffected endometrial cells induced EMT-like features, such as downregulation of the epithelial markers cytokeratin 7 and E- cadherin, upregulation of the mesenchymal markers vimentin and N-cadherin, and invasive capacities of semipermeable membranes [76].

EMT can also be induced via platelet activation, which has a role not only in hemostasis but also in immunological functions. Liu et al. [77] have demonstrated increased platelet aggregation in adenomyosis lesions, as well as an increase in TGF-β1 levels, concomitant with changes in EMT markers (reduction in E-cadherin and increase in vimentin) compared to controls. Moreover, antiplatelet treatment seems efficacious in suppressing myometrial infiltration by endometrial cells, improving generalized hyperalgesia, and reducing uterine hyperactivity in adenomyosis, providing a promising nonhormonal treatment for the disease [72].

Activin-related proteins are also key regulators of tissue remodeling and repair. Upregulation of these molecules in adenomyotic tissue may be related to myometrial response to ectopic endometrial cell invasion. There is strong evidence that myostatin, activin A, and TGF-β normally inhibit muscle growth and promote muscle protein loss in disease states, acting as powerful catabolic stimuli. Binding of these TGF-β ligands to muscle cell surface receptors leads to muscle proteolysis [78], which can further support the invagination theory. Such myometrium is able to produce soluble factors (cytokines, chemokines, or other soluble molecules) that enhance the migration of stromal cells [17].

To promote their invasiveness across the myometrium, adenomyotic cells acquire migratory properties such as loss of the cell-cell attachment or the capacity to degrade the ECM [2].

Chen et al. [79] observed an overexpression of the nuclear transcription factor Nrf2 (erythroid-E2-related factor 2) in the glandular epithelium of adenomyotic lesions compared with disease-free women. Overexpression of the nuclear factor Nrf2 could trigger intramyometrial migration of endometrial implants, through the regulation of MMP-9 which has an important role in extracellular matrix degradation. Other MMPs, such as MMP2 and MMP3, are also upregulated in eutopic endometrium of women with adenomyosis [80, 81].

Moreover, lysyl oxidase (LOX), an amine oxidase involved in the biogenesis of connective tissue matrices, is highly downregulated in eutopic endometrium of women with adenomyosis, resulting in a less rigid ECM [22]. Thus, the dysregulation of ECM function may promote invagination of endometrium into myometrium, resulting in adenomyosis.

Focal adhesion kinase (FAK) may also guide EMT in adenomyosis as the silencing of its expression inhibited adenomyosis cell migration in vitro [71].

Finally, adenomyosis is characterized by a certain degree of fibrosis, as a result of repeated cycles of TIAR. TGF-β signaling seems to play a major role in EMT and collagen production through cellular Smad2-/Smad3-dependent signaling pathway and connective tissue growth factor (CTGF) expression, leading to smooth muscle metaplasia and ultimately to fibrosis [18, 82].

31.4.8 Angiogenesis

Angiogenesis is the process of the outgrowth of new capillary blood vessels from existing blood vessels, which occurs in both physiological and pathological processes. It occurs during the proliferative phase of the menstrual cycle when the endometrium is regenerated and is essential for successful embryonic implantation [83].

Numerous studies have reported enhanced and abnormal vascularization in both eutopic and ectopic endometria from patients with adenomyosis, as well as its involvement in disease progression, heavy bleeding, and impaired embryo receptivity [4].

VEGF, one of the major mediators of angiogenesis, is thought to be a primary factor in adenomyosis pathogenesis [84]. VEGF is a potent endothelial cell mitogen secreted in the endometrium by epithelial, stromal, and perivascular cells. It is essential for normal endometrial repair in menstruation, but it has also been found to be upregulated in ectopic and eutopic endometrium of adenomyosis patients [83]. One of the most important transcription factors of VEGF in angiogenesis is hypoxia-inducible factor 1 alpha (HIF-1A) [84]. Hypoxia might be typical of adenomyosis, resulting from an injured JZ, with subsequent damage to vessels and loss of blood perfusion [4]. Goteri et al. [85] found that oxygen deficiency was responsible for the increasing levels of HIF-1A and in turn of VEGF, which might lead to increased angiogenesis in adenomyotic lesions. Moreover, the increased activin A mRNA expression observed in adenomyotic nodules may influence neoangiogenesis, as it stimulates the release of VEGF from endometrial stromal cells.

Increased microvessel density (MVD) is another marker of angiogenesis reported in adenomyotic lesions [4]. The MVD was evaluated in several studies by quantification of CD31, CD34, von Willebrand factor (vWF), or factor VIII antibody-stained microvessels. A significantly increased MVD in ectopic and eutopic endometrium compared with control endometrium was reported.

It is likely that increased angiogenesis leads to fragile and more permeable vessels resulting in adenomyosis-related AUB and possibly subfertility. However, this association has not been sufficiently studied, and future studies should investigate the exact role of angiogenesis in the etiology of adenomyosis and related AUB or subfertility in women with adenomyosis [83].

31.4.9 Neurogenic Factors and Neurogenesis

The functional layer of the endometrium is mainly innervated by sensory unmyelinated C nerve fibers [17]. Nerve endings of these fibers may be stimulated by various inflammatory substances, including histamine, serotonin, bradykinin, PGs, leukotriene, interleukin, acetylcholine, and growth factors (VEGF, epidermal growth factors, transforming growth factor-β, platelet, and nerve growth factor [NGF]) [86]. These algogenic factors are responsible for functional and structural changes of nociceptors, causing an increase in their excitability (peripheral sensitization) [87].

Neuroangiogenesis plays also a major role in the pathogenesis of adenomyosis [18]. In adenomyotic lesions, high expression of neurogenic factors, such as NGF, SYN, and MAP2, has been observed, indicating a possible role of neurogenesis in adenomyosis [54].

NGF is involved in pain generation, neural plasticity, immune cell aggregation, and release of inflammatory factors [17]. NGF levels are significantly increased by inflammatory mediators such as IL-1, TNF-α, or other cytokines. Ucn-induced NGF mRNA expression in cultured human endometrial stromal cells also confirms a link between inflammatory and neurogenic pathways [54]. In turn, NGF can induce hyperplasia and degranulation of mast cells, releasing additional inflammatory mediators such as serotonin which sensitize peripheral nociceptors. Moreover, local hyperestrogenism may favor NGF production which stimulated the proliferation and increased aromatase expression of endometrium stromal cells from adenomyosis foci, causing a vicious circle [88].

In a mouse model, NGF-β and its receptor levels increase as the disease worsens in terms of pain symptoms [89]. Orazov et al. [86] found that compared to the painless form of adenomyosis, the myometrial innervation apparatus of patients with pelvic pain is characterized by a significantly higher expression of NGF, which increases the area of the local innervation field and triggers the pain syndrome. Recent studies revealed that dienogest alleviate adenomyosis-related pain symptoms, reducing NGF expression and the density of nerve fibers [90, 91]. These findings confirm that NGF plays a pivotal role in the genesis of adenomyosis-associated pain.

31.5 Conclusions

Among the main hypotheses proposed to explain the pathogenesis of adenomyosis, the TIAR/invagination theory remains the most popular and the most widely investigated. However, a single theory may not explain all types of the disease. Sex hormones, inflammation, cell proliferation, apoptosis, migration, invasion, and neuroangiogenesis are involved in the development and maintenance of adenomyosis, but other pathogenetic mechanisms need to be further elucidated.

More research is needed to better understand the pathophysiology of adenomyosis in order to develop adequate therapeutic strategies.

References

1. Loring M, Chen TY, Isaacson KB. A systematic review of Adenomyosis: it's time to reassess what we thought we knew about the disease. J Minim Invasive Gynecol. 2020;28(3):644–55.
2. García-Solares J, Donnez J, Donnez O, Dolmans M-M. Pathogenesis of uterine adenomyosis: invagination or metaplasia? Fertil Steril. 2018;109(3):371–9.
3. Vannuccini S, Petraglia F. Recent advances in understanding and managing adenomyosis. F1000Res. 2019;8:F1000 Faculty Rev-283. https://doi.org/10.12688/f1000research.17242.1.
4. Stratopoulou CA, Donnez J, Dolmans MM. Origin and pathogenic mechanisms of uterine Adenomyosis: what is known so far. Reprod Sci. 2020;28(8):2087–97.

5. Weiss G, Maseelall P, Schott LL, Brockwell SE, Schocken M, Johnston JM. Adenomyosis a variant, not a disease? Evidence from hysterectomized menopausal women in the study of Women's Health Across the Nation (SWAN). Fertil Steril. 2009;91(1):201–6.
6. Templeman C, Marshall SF, Ursin G, Horn-Ross PL, Clarke CA, Allen M, et al. Adenomyosis and endometriosis in the California Teachers Study. Fertil Steril. 2008;90(2):415–24.
7. Vercellini P, Viganò P, Somigliana E, Daguati R, Abbiati A, Fedele L. Adenomyosis: epidemiological factors. Best Pract Res Clin Obstet Gynaecol. 2006;20:465–77.
8. Parazzini F, Vercellini P, Panazza S, Chatenoud L, Oldani S, Crosignani PG. Risk factors for adenomyosis. Hum Reprod. 1997;12(6):1275–9.
9. Panganamamula UR, Harmanli OH, Isik-Akbay EF, Grotegut CA, Dandolu V, Gaughan JP. Is prior uterine surgery a risk factor for adenomyosis? Obstet Gynecol. 2004;104(5):1034–8.
10. Taran FA, Weaver AL, Coddington CC, Stewart EA. Understanding adenomyosis: a case control study. Fertil Steril. 2010;94(4):1223–8.
11. Guo. The pathogenesis of Adenomyosis vis-à-vis endometriosis. J Clin Med. 2020;9(2):485.
12. Cohen I, Beyth Y, Shapira J, Tepper R, Fishman A, Cordoba M, et al. High frequency of adenomyosis in postmenopausal breast cancer patients treated with tamoxifen. Gynecol Obstet Investig. 1997;44(3):200–5.
13. Varras M, Polyzos D, Akrivis C. Effects of tamoxifen on the human female genital tract: review of the literature. Eur J Gynaecol Oncol. 2003;24(3–4):258–68.
14. Brosens I, Derwig I, Brosens J, Fusi L, Benagiano G, Pijnenborg R. The enigmatic uterine junctional zone: the missing link between reproductive disorders and major obstetrical disorders? Hum Reprod. 2010;25:569–74.
15. Leyendecker G, Wildt L. A new concept of endometriosis and adenomyosis: tissue injury and repair (TIAR). Horm Mol Biol Clin Investig. 2011;5(2).
16. Leyendecker G, Bilgicyildirim A, Inacker M, Stalf T, Huppert P, Mall G, et al. Adenomyosis and endometriosis. Re-visiting their association and further insights into the mechanisms of auto-traumatisation. An MRI study. Arch Gynecol Obstet. 2015;291(4):917–32.
17. Vannuccini S, Tosti C, Carmona F, Huang SJ, Chapron C, Guo SW, et al. Pathogenesis of adenomyosis: an update on molecular mechanisms. Reprod Biomed Online. 2017;35(5):592–601.
18. Zhai J, Vannuccini S, Petraglia F, Giudice LC. Adenomyosis: mechanisms and pathogenesis. Semin Reprod Med. 2020;38(2–3):129–43.
19. Gargett CE. Uterine stem cells: what is the evidence? Hum Reprod Update. 2006;13(1):87–101.
20. Chapron C, Tosti C, Marcellin L, Bourdon M, Lafay-Pillet MC, Millischer AE, et al. Relationship between the magnetic resonance imaging appearance of adenomyosis and endometriosis phenotypes. Hum Reprod. 2017;32(7):1393–401.
21. Bourdon M, Santulli P, Jeljeli M, Vannuccini S, Marcellin L, Doridot L, et al. Immunological changes associated with adenomyosis: a systematic review. Hum Reprod Update. 2021;27(1):108–29.
22. Herndon CN, Aghajanova L, Balayan S, Erikson D, Barragan F, Goldfien G, et al. Global transcriptome abnormalities of the Eutopic endometrium from women with Adenomyosis. Reprod Sci. 2016;23(10):1289–303.
23. Xiang Y, Sun Y, Yang B, Yang Y, Zhang Y, Yu T, et al. Transcriptome sequencing of adenomyosis eutopic endometrium: a new insight into its pathophysiology. J Cell Mol Med. 2019;23(12):8381–91.
24. Tong X, Li Z, Wu Y, Fu X, Zhang Y, Fan H. COMT 158G/A and CYP1B1 432C/G polymorphisms increase the risk of endometriosis and adenomyosis: a meta-analysis. Eur J Obstet Gynecol Reprod Biol. 2014;179:17–21.
25. Artymuk N, Zotova O, Gulyaeva L. Adenomyosis: genetics of estrogen metabolism. Horm Mol Biol Clin Investig. 2019;37(2):2–7.
26. Ye H, He Y, Wang J, Song T, Lan Z, Zhao Y, et al. Effect of matrix metalloproteinase promoter polymorphisms on endometriosis and adenomyosis risk: evidence from a meta-analysis. J Genet. 2016;95(3):611–9.

27. Kang S, Zhao X, Xing H, Wang N, Zhou R, Chen S, et al. Polymorphisms in the matrix metalloproteinase-2 and tissue inhibitor of metalloproteinase-2 and the risk of human adenomyosis. Environ Mol Mutagen. 2008;49(3):226–31.
28. Kang S, Li S-Z, Wang N, Zhou R-M, Wang T, Wang D-J, et al. Association between genetic polymorphisms in fibroblast growth factor (FGF)1 and FGF2 and risk of endometriosis and adenomyosis in Chinese women. Hum Reprod. 2010;25(7):1806–11.
29. Kang S, Zhao J, Liu Q, Zhou R, Wang N, Li Y. Vascular endothelial growth factor gene polymorphisms are associated with the risk of developing adenomyosis. Environ Mol Mutagen. 2009;50(5):361–6.
30. Wang Y, Qu Y, Song W. Genetic variation in COX-2 -1195 and the risk of endometriosis and adenomyosis. Clin Exp Obstet Gynecol. 2015;42(2):168–72.
31. Inoue S, Hirota Y, Ueno T, Fukui Y, Yoshida E, Hayashi T, et al. Uterine adenomyosis is an oligoclonal disorder associated with KRAS mutations. Nat Commun. 2019;10(1):5785.
32. Liu X, Guo S-W. Aberrant immunoreactivity of deoxyribonucleic acid methyltransferases in adenomyosis. Gynecol Obstet Investig. 2012;74(2):100–8.
33. Liu X, Nie J, Guo SW. Elevated immunoreactivity against class i histone deacetylases in adenomyosis. Gynecol Obstet Investig. 2012;74(1):50–5.
34. Liu X, Guo S-W. A pilot study on the off-label use of valproic acid to treat adenomyosis. Fertil Steril. 2008;89(1):246–50.
35. Zhai J, Li S, Sen S, Opoku-Anane J, Du Y, Chen ZJ, et al. m6A RNA methylation regulators contribute to Eutopic endometrium and myometrium dysfunction in Adenomyosis. Front Genet. 2020;11(July):1–16.
36. Rižner TL. The important roles of steroid sulfatase and sulfotransferases in gynecological diseases. Front Pharmacol. 2016;7:30.
37. Kitawaki J, Noguchi T, Amatsu T, Maeda K, Tsukamoto K, Yamamoto T, et al. Expression of aromatase cytochrome P450 protein and messenger ribonucleic acid in human endometriotic and adenomyotic tissues but not in normal endometrium. Biol Reprod. 1997;57(3):514–9.
38. Kitawaki J, Kusuki I, Koshiba H, Tsukamoto K, Fushiki S, Honjo H. Detection of aromatase cytochrome P-450 in endometrial biopsy specimens as a diagnostic test for endometriosis. Fertil Steril. 1999;72(6):1100–6.
39. Kitawaki J, Koshiba H, Ishihara H, Kusuki I, Tsukamoto K, Honjo H. Progesterone induction of 17beta-hydroxysteroid dehydrogenase type 2 during the secretory phase occurs in the endometrium of estrogen-dependent benign diseases but not in normal endometrium. J Clin Endocrinol Metab. 2000;85(9):3292–6.
40. Mehasseb MK, Panchal R, Taylor AH, Brown L, Bell SC, Habiba M. Estrogen and progesterone receptor isoform distribution through the menstrual cycle in uteri with and without adenomyosis. Fertil Steril. 2011;95(7):2228–35. 2235.e1
41. Nie J, Liu X, Guo S-W. Promoter hypermethylation of progesterone receptor isoform B (PR-B) in adenomyosis and its rectification by a histone deacetylase inhibitor and a demethylation agent. Reprod Sci. 2010;17(11):995–1005.
42. Li JJ, Duan H, Wang S, Sun FQ, Gan L, Tang YQ, et al. Expression pattern of G-protein-coupled Estrogen receptor in myometrium of uteri with and without Adenomyosis. Biomed Res Int. 2017;2017(1):5974693.
43. Jiang C, Cheng Z. Update of recent studies of adenomyosis-associated dysmenorrhea. Gynecol Minim Invasive Ther. 2016;5(4):137–40.
44. Mechsner S, Grum B, Gericke C, Loddenkemper C, Dudenhausen JW, Ebert AD. Possible roles of oxytocin receptor and vasopressin-1α receptor in the pathomechanism of dysperistalsis and dysmenorrhea in patients with adenomyosis uteri. Fertil Steril. 2010;94(7):2541–6.
45. Guo SW, Mao X, Ma Q, Liu X. Dysmenorrhea and its severity are associated with increased uterine contractility and overexpression of oxytocin receptor (OTR) in women with symptomatic adenomyosis. Fertil Steril. 2013;90:231–40.
46. Zhang Y, Yu P, Sun F, Li TC, Cheng J, mei, Duan H. Expression of oxytocin receptors in the uterine junctional zone in women with adenomyosis. Acta Obstet Gynecol Scand. 2015;94(4):412–8.

47. Nie J, Liu X, Guo SW. Immunoreactivity of oxytocin receptor and transient receptor potential vanilloid type 1 and its correlation with dysmenorrhea in adenomyosis. Am J Obstet Gynecol. 2010;202(4):346.e1–8.
48. Zhang Y, Yu P, Sun F, Li TC, Cheng JM, Duan H. Expression of oxytocin receptors in the uterine junctional zone in women with adenomyosis. Acta Obstet Gynecol Scand. 2015;94(4):412–8.
49. Guo SW, Mao X, Ma Q, Liu X. Dysmenorrhea and its severity are associated with increased uterine contractility and overexpression of oxytocin receptor (OTR) in women with symptomatic adenomyosis. Fertil Steril. 2013;99(1):231–40.
50. Andersson JK, Khan Z, Weaver AL, Vaughan LE, Gemzell-Danielsson K, Stewart EA. Vaginal bromocriptine improves pain, menstrual bleeding and quality of life in women with adenomyosis: a pilot study. Acta Obstet Gynecol Scand. 2019;98(10):1341–50.
51. Fiçicioğlu C, Tekin HI, Arioğlu PF, Okar I. A murine model of adenomyosis: the effects of hyperprolactinemia induced by fluoxetine hydrochloride, a selective serotonin reuptake inhibitor, on adenomyosis induction in Wistar albino rats. Acta Eur Fertil. 1995;26(2):75–9.
52. Singtripop T, Mori T, Park MK, Sakamoto S, Kawashima S. Development of uterine adenomyosis after treatment with dopamine antagonists in mice. Life Sci. 1991;49(3):201–6.
53. Li C, Chen R, Jiang C, Chen L, Cheng Z. Correlation of LOX-5 and COX-2 expression with inflammatory pathology and clinical features of adenomyosis. Mol Med Rep. 2019;19(1):727–33.
54. Carrarelli P, Luddi A, Funghi L, Arcuri F, Batteux F, Dela Cruz C, et al. Urocortin and corticotrophin-releasing hormone receptor type 2 mRNA are highly expressed in deep infiltrating endometriotic lesions. Reprod Biomed Online. 2016;33(4):476–83.
55. Carrarelli P, Yen CF, Funghi L, Arcuri F, Tosti C, Bifulco G, et al. Expression of inflammatory and neurogenic mediators in Adenomyosis. Reprod Sci. 2017;24(3):369–75.
56. Yang G, Im H-J, Wang JH-C. Repetitive mechanical stretching modulates IL-1beta induced COX-2, MMP-1 expression, and PGE2 production in human patellar tendon fibroblasts. Gene. 2005;363:166–72.
57. Wang F, Li H, Yang Z, Du X, Cui M, Wen Z. Expression of interleukin-10 in patients with adenomyosis. Fertil Steril. 2009;91(5):1681–5.
58. Guo J, Chen L, Luo N, Li C, Chen R, Qu X, et al. LPS/TLR4-mediated stromal cells acquire an invasive phenotype and are implicated in the pathogenesis of adenomyosis. Sci Rep. 2016;6:1–10.
59. Shen X, Duan H, Wang S, Gan L, Xu Q, Li JJ. Decreased expression of cannabinoid receptors in the eutopic and ectopic endometrium of patients with adenomyosis. Biomed Res Int. 2019;2019:5468954.
60. Shen X, Duan H, Wang S, Hong W, Wang YY, Lin SL. Expression of cannabinoid receptors in myometrium and its correlation with dysmenorrhea in Adenomyosis. Reprod Sci. 2019;26(12):1618–25.
61. Wang F, Wen Z, Li H, Yang Z, Zhao X, Yao X. Human leukocyte antigen-G is expressed by the eutopic and ectopic endometrium of adenomyosis. Fertil Steril. 2008;90(5):1599–604.
62. Baka S, Frangou-Plemenou M, Panagiotopoulou E, Makrakis E, Kaltsakas G, Hassiakos D, et al. The expression of human leukocyte antigens class I and II in women with endometriosis or adenomyosis. Gynecol Endocrinol Off J Int Soc Gynecol Endocrinol. 2011;27(6):419–24.
63. Zhou Y, Peng Y, Xia Q, Yan D, Zhang H, Zhang L, et al. Decreased Indian hedgehog signaling activates autophagy in endometriosis and adenomyosis. Reproduction. 2021;161(2):99–109.
64. Ota H, Maki M, Shidara Y, Kodama H, Takahashi H, Hayakawa M, Fujimori R, Kushima T, Ohtomo K. Effects of danazol at the immunologic level in patients with adenomyosis, with special reference to autoantibodies: a multi-center cooperative study. Am J Obstet Gynecol. 1992;167(2):418–6.
65. Sun FQ, Duan H, Wang S, Li JJ. 17β-Estradiol induces Overproliferation in Adenomyotic human uterine smooth muscle cells of the junctional zone through Hyperactivation of the Estrogen receptor-enhanced RhoA/ROCK signaling pathway. Reprod Sci. 2015;22(11):1436–44.

66. Carrarelli P, Yen CF, Arcuri F, Funghi L, Tosti C, Wang TH, et al. Myostatin, follistatin and activin type II receptors are highly expressed in adenomyosis. Fertil Steril. 2015;104(3):744–752.e1.
67. Streuli I, Santulli P, Chouzenoux S, Chapron C, Batteux F. Activation of the MAPK/ERK cell-signaling pathway in uterine smooth muscle cells of women with Adenomyosis. Reprod Sci. 2015;22(12):1549–60.
68. Li J, Yanyan M, Mu L, Chen X, Zheng W. The expression of Bcl-2 in adenomyosis and its effect on proliferation, migration, and apoptosis of endometrial stromal cells. Pathol Res Pract. 2019;215(8):152477.
69. Wang B, Yang Y, Deng X, Ban Y, Chao L. Interaction of M2 macrophages and endometrial cells induces downregulation of GRIM-19 in endometria of adenomyosis. Reprod Biomed Online. 2020;41(5):790–800.
70. Chen Y-J, Li H-Y, Huang C-H, Twu N-F, Yen M-S, Wang P-H, et al. Oestrogen-induced epithelial-mesenchymal transition of endometrial epithelial cells contributes to the development of adenomyosis. J Pathol. 2010;222(3):261–70.
71. Zheng D, Duan H, Wang S, Xu Q, Gan L, Li J, et al. FAK regulates epithelial-mesenchymal transition in adenomyosis. Mol Med Rep. 2018;18(6):5461–72.
72. Zhou W, Peng Z, Zhang C, Liu S, Zhang Y. ILK-induced epithelial-mesenchymal transition promotes the invasive phenotype in adenomyosis. Biochem Biophys Res Commun. 2018;497(4):950–6.
73. Khan KN, Kitajima M, Hiraki K, Fujishita A, Nakashima M, Masuzaki H. Involvement of hepatocyte growth factor-induced epithelial-mesenchymal transition in human adenomyosis. Biol Reprod. 2015;92(2):35.
74. Hu R, Peng G-Q, Ban D-Y, Zhang C, Zhang X-Q, Li Y-P. High-expression of Neuropilin 1 correlates to Estrogen-induced epithelial-mesenchymal transition of endometrial cells in Adenomyosis. Reprod Sci. 2020;27(1):395–403.
75. Qi S, Zhao X, Li M, Zhang X, Lu Z, Yang C, et al. Aberrant expression of Notch1/numb/snail signaling, an epithelial mesenchymal transition related pathway, in adenomyosis. Reprod Biol Endocrinol. 2015;13:96.
76. An M, Li D, Yuan M, Li Q, Zhang L, Wang G. Different macrophages equally induce EMT in endometria of adenomyosis and normal. Reproduction. 2017;154(1):79–92.
77. Liu X, Shen M, Qi Q, Zhang H, Guo S-W. Corroborating evidence for platelet-induced epithelial-mesenchymal transition and fibroblast-to-myofibroblast transdifferentiation in the development of adenomyosis. Hum Reprod. 2016;31(4):734–49.
78. Zhou S, Yi T, Liu R, Bian C, Qi X, He X, et al. Proteomics identification of annexin A2 as a key mediator in the metastasis and proangiogenesis of endometrial cells in human adenomyosis. Mol Cell Proteomics. 2012;11(7):M112.017988.
79. Chen N, Du B, Zhou H, Shen F, Li J, Xie Z. Abnormal expression of Nrf2 may play an important role in the pathogenesis and development of adenomyosis. PLoS One. 2017;12(8):e0182773.
80. Tokyol C, Aktepe F, Dilek FH, Sahin O, Arioz DT. Expression of cyclooxygenase-2 and matrix metalloproteinase-2 in adenomyosis and endometrial polyps and its correlation with angiogenesis. Int J Gynecol Pathol Off J Int Soc Gynecol Pathol. 2009;28(2):148–56.
81. Li T, Li Y-G, Pu D-M. Matrix metalloproteinase-2 and -9 expression correlated with angiogenesis in human adenomyosis. Gynecol Obstet Investig. 2006;62(4):229–35.
82. Cheong M-L, Lai T-H, Wu W-B. Connective tissue growth factor mediates transforming growth factor β-induced collagen expression in human endometrial stromal cells. PLoS One. 2019;14(1):e0210765.
83. Harmsen MJ, Wong CFC, Mijatovic V, Griffioen AW, Groenman F, Hehenkamp WJK, et al. Role of angiogenesis in adenomyosis-associated abnormal uterine bleeding and subfertility: a systematic review. Hum Reprod Update. 2019;25(5):647–71.
84. Yalaza C, Canacankatan N, Gürses İ, Aytan H, Taşdelen B. Altered VEGF, Bcl-2 and IDH1 expression in patients with adenomyosis. Arch Gynecol Obstet. 2020;302(5):1221–7.
85. Goteri G, Lucarini G, Montik N, Zizzi A, Stramazzotti D, Fabris G, et al. Expression of vascular endothelial growth factor (VEGF), hypoxia inducible factor-1alpha (HIF-1alpha), and

microvessel density in endometrial tissue in women with adenomyosis. Int J Gynecol Pathol Off J Int Soc Gynecol Pathol. 2009;28(2):157–63.
86. Orazov MR, Radzinsky VE, Nosenko EN, Khamoshina MB, Dukhin AO, Lebedeva MG. Immune-inflammatory predictors of the pelvic pain syndrome associated with adenomyosis. Gynecol Endocrinol. 2017;33:44–6.
87. Moalem G, Tracey DJ. Immune and inflammatory mechanisms in neuropathic pain. Brain Res Rev. 2006;51(2):240–64.
88. Anaf V, Simon P, El Nakadi I, Fayt I, Simonart T, Buxant F, et al. Hyperalgesia, nerve infiltration and nerve growth factor expression in deep adenomyotic nodules, peritoneal and ovarian endometriosis. Hum Reprod. 2002;17(7):1895–900.
89. Li Y, Zhang S, Zou S, Xia X, Bao L. Accumulation of nerve growth factor and its receptors in the uterus and dorsal root ganglia in a mouse model of adenomyosis. Reprod Biol Endocrinol. 2011;9(1):30.
90. Takeuchi A, Koga K, Miyashita M, Makabe T, Sue F, Harada M, et al. Dienogest reduces proliferation, NGF expression and nerve fiber density in human adenomyosis. Eur J Obstet Gynecol Reprod Biol. 2016;207:157–61.
91. Hirata T, Izumi G, Takamura M, Saito A, Nakazawa A, Harada M, et al. Efficacy of dienogest in the treatment of symptomatic adenomyosis: a pilot study. Gynecol Endocrinol. 2014;30(10):726–9.

Classification and Staging of Adenomyosis

32

George Pados and Angelos Daniilidis

Contents

32.1 Introduction

Various theories about the pathogenesis of adenomyosis have been reported. However, the precise pathophysiological pathway is not entirely known. It is commonly thought to originate from direct contact between the endometrium and the underlying myometrium, which allows the formation of ectopic endometrial glands and stroma. Reported risk factors for adenomyosis include previous uterine surgery and trauma of the endometrial junctional zone that promotes cell migration and invagination of the endometrial basalis [1–3]. The growth of ectopic endometrial glands and stroma into the myometrium due to injury of endometrial-myometrial border may explain ultrasound findings such as sub-endometrial lines, buds and cysts, and hyperechogenic islands in the myometrium. Some authors speculate that the number and type of layers involved might depend on the etiology of

G. Pados (✉)
School of Medicine, Aristotle University of Thessaloniki, 1st Dept. OB-GYN, "Papageorgiou" Hospital, Thessaloniki, Greece

Centre for Endoscopic Surgery, "Diavalkaniko" Hospital, Thessaloniki, Greece

A. Daniilidis
School of Medicine, Aristotle University of Thessaloniki, 2nd Dept. OB-GYN, "Hippokration" Hospital, Thessaloniki, Greece

E. Oral (ed.), *Endometriosis and Adenomyosis*,
https://doi.org/10.1007/978-3-030-97236-3_32

adenomyosis and be associated with the clinical presentation, the clinical features, and the severity, extent, and depth of adenomyosis [1, 4, 5]. However, several authors did not confirm speculations and proved that actually there were no significant differences in the prevalence of adenomyosis among women with or without a history of heavy menstrual bleeding [6–9]. Unfortunately, all these studies showed a great bias, since they were conducted postoperatively on the uteri of patients who had hysterectomy for severe symptoms, mostly older and with no fertility issues. In addition, clinical experience has indicated cases in which this classic hypothesis is unverifiable and direct relationship between adenomyosis and endometrium cannot be proved histologically. There are manifestations of the disease which appear to be more as a result of endometrial invasion from nearby endometriotic tissue outside the uterus or completely independently isolated from the uterine structural components [10]. Recent studies have proposed a mechanism of metaplastic process and de novo epithelial-mesenchymal transition among displaced embryonic Müllerian remnants or adult stem cells [11, 12]. Presumably, it could be postulated that adenomyosis is not a homogenous disease, but rather a composition of multiple heterogeneous subtypes. All these have made rather difficult to accurately stage and classify adenomyosis. As a result so far, the only classification proposed for the extension of the disease is based on the histologic findings after surgery.

This article aims to give briefly recent advances regarding up-to-date classification methods based on correlation between histology and imaging and discuss drawbacks and future perspectives.

32.2 What Is the Role of MRI and Ultrasound for an Accurate Classification?

Recent technological advances in imaging techniques and mainly in transvaginal ultrasound and MRI (magnetic resonance imaging) have improved substantially the accuracy of noninvasive diagnosis of adenomyosis (Table 32.1). Obviously, there are a variety of different morphological types on ultrasound examination which may manifest different histological types and stages in the development of the disease and even more may correspond to different clinical manifestation and significance.

The use of MUSA (Morphological Uterus Sonographic Assessment) has been considered to be the most accurate and standardized method of describing myometrial lesions seen on ultrasound assessment [13]. According to MUSA, typical features of adenomyosis include at least one of the following features: the presence of an enlarged globular uterus, the finding of asymmetrical thickening of the myometrium, the presence of myometrial cysts or echogenic sub-endometrial lines and hyperechogenic islands, the fan-shaped shadowing, the finding of an irregular or interrupted junctional zone, and the translesional vascularity [13]. Even though the terminology used is indeed straightforward and reasonably reliable to describe lesions of adenomyosis, nevertheless, it fails to provide any information regarding the classification of morphological subtypes of the disease. In 2019, there has been a consensus of experts regarding ultrasound-based

Table 32.1 Classification of adenomyosis based on imaging technology

Author	Year of publication	MRI or USG	Classification
Gordts et al. [27]	2008	MRI	JZ hyperplasia Adenomyosis Adenomyoma
Kishi et al. [21]	2012	MRI	Intrinsic Extrinsic Intramural All others
Grimbizis et al. [32]	2014	MRI	Diffuse Focal Polypoid Others
Bazot et al. [20]	2018	MRI	Internal Adenomyoma External
Lazzeri et al. [16]	2018	USG	Diffuse of the outer myometrium
Van den Bosch et al. [14]	*2019*		Diffuse of the inner myometrium or JZ
Exacoustos et al. [15]	*2020*		Focal of the outer myometrium Focal of the inner myometrium Adenomyoma

classification of adenomyosis [14]. It was then proposed that ultrasound classification should involve stepwise detailed description of the disease – starting with the MUSA criteria for the first step diagnosis and following (I) detailed determination of the location (anterior, posterior, lateral left, lateral right, or fundal to the uterine wall); (II) proper discrimination between focal and diffuse diseases (defined as focal if >25% of the circumference of the lesion or as diffuse if <25% of the lesion is surrounded by normal myometrium); (III) differentiation between cystic (with at least >2 mm diameter) and not cystic; (IV) mapping of layer involvement (type 1 for junctional zone, type 2 for inner myometrium, type 3 for outer close to serosa myometrium, and combinations for cases with more than one layer involved types 1–2, types 2–3, or types 1–3); (V) classification of the extent of the disease based on the proportion of uterine corpus affected, as mild (<25%), moderate (25–50%), and severe (>50%); and (VI) calculation of the size of lesion. This classification system although it is very descriptive fails to prove the correlation between histological, clinical, and ultrasound findings and severity of the disease. Combined oral contraceptive pills, other hormonal treatments might influence and mask ultrasound image. Studies are still lacking as to the real diagnostic value of using the transverse and/or coronal planes for discriminating between focal and diffuse adenomyoses. Finally, it is still to be clarified as to the clinical value in differentiating between the middle and the outer myometrium and how really feasible that might be in clinical settings.

In a recent multicenter, observational, prospective study, there has been an effort to overcome the problem of correlation between ultrasound findings and severity of the disease [15]. 108 patients with ultrasonographic signs of adenomyosis were classified according to the ultrasound scoring system described by Lazzeri et al. [16]. The same rules for ultrasound detection and classification applied as for the one already described by Van den Bosch et al. [14]. The main difference of this scoring system was on the detection of each type of adenomyotic lesion in the JZ and in the external myometrium, giving a more detailed score with four degrees of extension for each type of disease (diffuse and focal of inner and outer myometrium) and adenomyoma. For diffuse adenomyosis of the outer myometrium, the degree was assigned according to the thickness of the uterine wall (<20, >20<30, >30 mm) and the number of the uterine walls affected (anterior, posterior lateral left or right). For diffuse adenomyosis of the inner myometrium, a degree was assigned according to thickness (>6<8, >8) of the JZ and length of the infiltrated JZ (<20 mm, >20 mm, >50%<80% of the uterus, >80% total infiltration). For focal adenomyosis of the inner and outer myometrium, a degree was assigned according to the largest diameter of the focal lesion (<10 mm, >10<20 mm, >20 mm) and the number of foci (1, 2, 3,>3). Similarly, adenomyomas were divided into four degrees according to the size (largest diameter 20, 30, 40, >40 mm) and number of adenomyomas (1, 2, 3,>3). A score from 1 to 4 was attributed to each degree of disease considered. Finally, the ultrasound extent of the disease was calculated by the sum of the scores obtained and classified into three groups: mild (ranged, 1–3), moderate (4–6), and severe (≥7). According to the results, patients with ultrasound diagnosis of diffuse adenomyosis were older ($p = .04$) and had heavier menstrual bleeding ($p = .04$) than women with focal disease. There were no statistically significant differences regarding the presence and severity of dyspareunia and dysmenorrhea. The presence of ultrasound findings of focal disease was associated with a higher percentage of infertility than in those with diffuse disease, and the focal involvement of the junctional zone showed a higher percentage of at least one miscarriage than in those with diffuse adenomyosis. The study failed to prove any direct correlation between the ultrasound extension of adenomyosis within the uterus and the severity of symptoms. Perhaps the fact that there is no accurate proof until now about direct correlations of ultrasound findings and clinical manifestation of adenomyosis could be explained by other coexisting pathology like deep endometriosis. Moreover, adenomyosis is similar to endometriosis when small lesions might cause a lot of symptoms and severe disease is not related always with severe symptoms [17]. Another drawback of this type of rather extensive classification is that TVS has to be performed by dedicated subspecialized sonographers who are experts in endometriosis in order to achieve high accuracy in detecting/classifying this pathology, thus making general screening unfeasible.

MRI is proved to be highly accurate in the diagnosis of adenomyosis. Actually, large prospective studies have found a slightly higher sensitivity (70–93%) and specificity (86–93%) for diagnosing adenomyosis in comparison to transvaginal ultrasound, but of course it is costlier as an imaging method [18–20]. MRI has been used not only for diagnosis but also for categorization of subtypes of adenomyosis [21]. MRI findings from 163 patients who have been diagnosed with adenomyosis and have been treated either with laparoscopic hysterectomy or adenomyomectomy have been retrospectively evaluated. A stepwise logistic regression analysis was used in order to specify subtypes of the disease. According to authors, there are four discrete subtypes of adenomyosis based on the geographic interrelationship between the adenomyosis and other structural components of the uterus. Subtype I (intrinsic) has intimate relationship with the endometrium and the junctional zone. Subtype II (extrinsic) is present in the outer shell of the uterus disrupting the serosa but not affecting the inner components. Subtype III (intramural) is found solely in the myometrium. The remainder of the data comprised subtype IV (indeterminate) adenomyosis. Subtypes I–III were suggested as a product of direct endometrial invasion, endometriotic invasion from the outside, and de novo metaplasia, respectively. Subtype IV was a heterogeneous mixture of advanced disease [21]. According to authors, the first three subtypes are product of endometrial invasion, endometriotic invasion, and de novo metaplasia, respectively. The study failed to prove any relationship or difference between subtypes and symptoms. Also the classical hypothesis that the difference in MRI image was reflecting actually the progression of the disease in each patient has been confronted by the fact that the patients at the time of operation were younger in subtype III, followed by subtype II and subtype I. This last finding is arguing the logic of disease progression.

Both MRI and ultrasound have similar sensitivities and specificities for the basis of comparing imaging with histopathologic findings and for the diagnosis of adenomyosis. The skill of the sonographer appears to be more important for ultrasound than for MRI. It is still not clear whether 3D TVUS will provide enhanced utility as it was hoped for.

32.3 Difficulties with Classification: Correlation to Histology and Symptoms

The standard method for accurate diagnosis of adenomyosis is histology [22]. On histology, adenomyosis is classified as focal in case that circumscribed nodular aggregates of endometrial glands and stroma surrounded by normal myometrium are found on the specimen. Diffuse will be characterized if there are endometrial glands and stroma distributed throughout the myometrium. Adenomyomas are considered to be subgroup of focal adenomyosis which is surrounded by hypertrophic myometrium [6, 23]. A wide spectrum of histopathologic definitions of the disorder still exists though, typically based on the distance at which the endometrial-like tissue is present below the deepest level of the normal endometrium ranging from a measured depth of 2–8 mm below the last endometrial gland. A lot of times its presence has been defined by pathologists on the basis of the proportional involvement of the myometrium such as one-third or greater than of the thickness of the myometrium (Table 32.2). Lastly, there has been a variety of hypotheses for the presence of different pathogenic mechanisms to explain the pathogenesis of adenomyosis. It is more than likely that a combination of pathogenetic pathways is responsible for the wide spectrum of the disease phenotypes recognized in histology specimens and in clinical symptomatology [24].

Table 32.2 Histological classification of adenomyosis based on depth of invasion

Author	Year of publication	Classification according to depth of invasion
Bird et al. [4]	1972	Grade I (sub-basal lesions) Grade II (up to mid-myometrium) Grade III (beyond mid-myometrium)
Levgur et al. [1]	2000	2.5 mm depth as a cutoff from endometrial border Superficial: <40% Intermediate: between 40 and 80% wall thickness Deep: >80% wall thickness
Sammour et al. [17]	2002	Group A: up to 25% Group B: 26–50% Group C: 51–75% Group D: >75% of myometrial thickness
Hulka et al. [33]	2002	Category I: inner 1/3 of myometrium Category II: focal lesions Category III: affecting outer 2/3 of myometrium
Vercelini et al. [34]	2006	>2.5 mm from endometrial junction Mild: 1/3 of the uterine wall Moderate: 2/3 of the uterine wall Severe: >2/3 of the uterine wall

Several studies attempted to combine histologic and imaging findings into a reproducible classification with correlation to clinical manifestation of the disease. Bird et al. [4] was the first to present such a classification based on measuring the depth of myometrial invasion using histologic specimens after hysterectomy. Later on followed a classification scheme based on invasion with three distinct categories: deep (>80%), intermediate (40–80%), and superficial (<40%) by [1]. Advances on imaging techniques resulted to more complex classification schemes based on specific features like uterine size, detailed extent of disease, configuration of lesions (diffuse, focal, and nodular), and degree of junctional zone involvement [21, 25–27].

However, failure remains an ongoing challenge on correlating specific subtypes with degree of severity of symptoms; thus, no universal classification standard has been generally accepted. Like endometriosis, severity of clinical symptoms doesn't always correspond with imaging or histology expansion of the adenomyosis [28]. Also, severity of chronic pelvic pain has been confounded by the frequency with which both endometriosis and adenomyosis are present in the same patient.

Lazzeri in his prospective study evaluated the reproducibility of an MRI schematic mapping system based on the degree of myometrial involvement, junctional zone thickening, and size of the lesion [16]. Although the method was significantly accurate to the classification as focal, diffuse with or without JZ involvement, no correlation with histology or clinical symptoms has been evaluated. Another prospective observational study in 100 women undergoing hysterectomy evaluated a prediction model for diagnosing adenomyosis by using preoperatively 2-D and 3-D ultrasound, clinical questionnaires [29], and histopathology results. Authors reported sensitivity of 85% and specificity of 78% for diagnoses and significant correlation with symptoms, but this model needs a lot of clarifications and external validation.

The main disadvantage of the majority of studies is the fact that they have used a retrospective method of correlating symptoms, imaging and histology. Probably pathologists themselves may have shown variance in their diligence or interpretation, while frequently the diagnosis was probably limited by the extent to which the uterus was sectioned in a routine basis. Retrospective analysis of routine histology assessments implies no systematic investigation of the myometrium regarding the diagnosis of adenomyosis.

Most studies failed to use a properly defined, prospective methodology in order to compare imaging, clinical symptoms, and systematic microscopic evaluation of the uterine corpus [30]. Most authors seemed to focus on the endometrium and contiguous involvement of the myometrium, without really evaluating the rest of the myometrium separately, which have led to missed isolated myometrial disease. Lastly in all these studies, there is a potential selection bias because they would not include patients who are not undergoing hysterectomy.

32.4 Conclusion

This paper was designed to review the current status of classification systems of adenomyosis and to explore following pathways of consensus. Although histopathology is the "reference standard" for diagnosis of adenomyosis, there should be an alternative for women who wish to retain their uterus. In such a diverse disease like adenomyosis where the precise pathophysiological pathway is still not clearly established, it is more than obvious that international consensus on an accepted, uniform classification of adenomyosis is a difficult task [30]. Unfortunately, research is currently compromised by the absence of a universally accepted and validated system for categorizing the disorder. Different explanations for the pathogenesis might be one of the reasons for the lack of uniformity in classification of the disease. Presumably, adenomyosis manifests in a variety of ways, ranging from a complete lack of symptoms to combination in different extent of pain, infertility, and abnormal uterine bleeding [30].

On the basis of retrospective analyses of histopathologic reports describing hysterectomy specimens, even the relationship between adenomyosis and severity of symptoms has been challenged [6–8, 28]. Thus, an imaging-based disease phenotype will not adequately correlate with clinical manifestations [30]. From a diagnostic perspective and compared with histopathologic evaluation, MRI and TVUS seem to have similar sensitivity and specificity for the diagnosis of adenomyosis [14–16]. On the other hand, randomized prospective studies comparing imaging findings with posthysterectomy specimens to standardize a proper classification system are hard to be organized. Another issue to be clarified as debate still goes on and disagreements remain is the relationship and similarities between endometriosis and adenomyosis. Entities coexist quite often. Perhaps the classification system of adenomyosis should take into account possible connections and links in pathophysiology of deep endometriosis and adenomyosis [31]. Above all, such a system could offer real help to the clinician with regard to prognosis or efficacy of medical or surgical approach across the different subtypes of adenomyosis.

Research requires both an accurate diagnosis and a specific methodology on identification of disease phenotypes following standardized categorization. A consensus-building process of an appropriate reporting system would facilitate statistical comparison of outcomes in patients with similar disease characteristics including meta-analysis of studies. Perhaps the rapidly evolving technological field of ultrasound imaging and artificial intelligence might give a better utility and a more appropriate approach to improve interpretation of TVUS or MRI scans for adenomyosis and its classification in a harmonic fashion with histopathologic and clinical features of the disease [30].

References

1. Levgur M, Abadi MA, Tucker A. Adenomyosis: symptoms, histology, and pregnancy terminations. Obstet Gynecol. 2000;95:688–91.
2. Panganamamula UR, Harmanli OH, Isik-Akbay EF, Grotegut CA, Dandolu V, Gaughan JP. Is prior uterine surgery a risk factor for adenomyosis? Obstet Gynecol. 2004;104:1034–8.
3. Riggs JC, Lim EK, Liang D, Bullwinkel R. Cesarean section as a risk factor for the development of adenomyosis uteri. J Reprod Med. 2014;59:20–4.
4. Bird CC, McElin TW, Manalo-Estrella P. The elusive adenomyosis of the uterus—revisited. Am J Obstet Gynecol. 1972;112:583–93.
5. Nishida M. Relationship between the onset of dysmenorrhea and histologic findings in adenomyosis. Am J Obstet Gynecol. 1991;165:229–31.
6. Bergholt T, Eriksen L, Berendt N, Jacobsen M, Hertz JB. Prevalence and risk factors of adenomyosis at hysterectomy. Hum Reprod. 2001;16:2418–21.
7. Parazzini F, Vercellini P, Panazza S, Chatenoud L, Oldani S, Crosignani PG. Risk factors for adenomyosis. Hum Reprod. 1997;12:1275–9.
8. Weiss G, Maseelall P, Schott LL, Brockwell SE, Schocken M, Johnston JM. Adenomyosis a variant, not a disease? Evidence from hysterectomized menopausal women in the Study of Women's Health Across the Nation (SWAN). Fertil Steril. 2009;91:201–6.
9. Sakhel K, Abuhamad A. Sonography of adenomyosis. J Ultrasound Med. 2012;31:805–8.
10. Tana J, Yonga P, Bedaiwya MA. A critical review of recent advances in the diagnosis, classification, and management of uterine adenomyosis. Curr Opin Obstet Gynecol. 2019;31:212–21.
11. Vannuccini S, Tosti C, Carmona F, et al. Pathogenesis of adenomyosis: an update on molecular mechanisms. Reprod Biomed Online. 2017;35:592–601.
12. Chen N, Du B, Zhou H, et al. Abnormal expression of Nrf2 may play an important role in the pathogenesis and development of adenomyosis. PLoS One. 2017;12:e0182773.
13. Van den Bosch T, Dueholm M, Leone FP, Valentin L, Rasmussen CK, Votino A, Van Schoubroeck D, Landolfo C, Install'e AJ, Guerriero S, Exacoustos C, Gordts S, Benacerraf B, D'Hooghe T, De Moor B, Brolmann H, Goldstein S, Epstein E, Bourne T, Timmerman D. Terms, definitions and measurements to describe sonographic features of myometrium and uterine masses: a consensus opinion from the Morphological Uterus Sonographic Assessment (MUSA) group. Ultrasound Obstet Gynecol. 2015;46:284–98.
14. Van den Bosch T, De Bruin AM, De Leeuw RA, Dueholm M, Exacoustos C, Valentin L, Bourne T, Timmerman D, Huirne JAF. Sonographic classification and reporting system for diagnosing adenomyosis. Ultrasound Obstet Gynecol. 2019;53:576–82.
15. Exacoustos C, Morosetti G, Conway F, Camilli S, Martire FG, Lazzeri L, Piccione E, Zupi E. New sonographic classification of adenomyosis: do type and degree of adenomyosis correlate to severity of symptoms? J Minim Invasive Gynecol. 2020;27:1308–15.

16. Lazzeri L, Morosetti G, Centini G, et al. A sonographic classification of adenomyosis: interobserver reproducibility in the evaluation of type and degree of the myometrial involvement. Fertil Steril. 2018;110:1154–61.
17. Sammour A, Pirwany I, Usubutun A, Arseneau J, Tulandi T. Correlations between extent and spread of adenomyosis and clinical symptoms. Gynecol Obstet Investig. 2002;54:213–6.
18. Togashi K, Ozasa H, Konishi I, et al. Enlarged uterus: differentiation between adenomyosis and leiomyoma with MR imaging. Radiology. 1989;171:531–4.
19. Bazot M, Cortez A, Darai E, et al. Ultrasonography compared with magnetic resonance imaging for the diagnosis of adenomyosis: correlation with histopathology. Hum Reprod. 2001;16:2427–33.
20. Bazot M, Darai E. Role of transvaginal sonography and magnetic resonance imaging in the diagnosis of uterine adenomyosis. Fertil Steril. 2018;109:389–97.
21. Kishi Y, Suginami H, Kuramori R, Yabuta M, Suginami R, Taniguchi F. Four subtypes of adenomyosis assessed by magnetic resonance imaging and their specification. Am J Obstet Gynecol. 2012;207:114.
22. Garcia L, Isaacson K. Adenomyosis: review of the literature. J Minim Invasive Gynecol. 2011;18:428–37.
23. Tahlan A, Nanda A, Mohan H. Uterine adenomyoma: a clinicopathologic review of cases and a review of the literature. Int J Gynecol Pathol. 2006;25:361–5.
24. Garcıa-Solares J, Donnez J, Donnez O, Dolmans MM. Pathogenesis of uterine adenomyosis: invagination or metaplasia? Fertil Steril. 2018;109:371–9.
25. Munro MG, Critchley HO, Broder MS, Fraser IS. FIGO classification system (PALM-COEIN) for causes of abnormal uterine bleeding in nongravid women of reproductive age. Int J Gynaecol Obstet. 2011;113:3–13.
26. Exacoustos C, Zupi E. A new era in diagnosing adenomyosis is coming. Fertil Steril. 2018;110:858.
27. Gordts S, Brosens JJ, Fusi L, et al. Uterine adenomyosis: a need for uniform terminology and consensus classification. Reprod Biomed Online. 2008;17:244–8.
28. Vercellini P, Parazzini F, Oldani S, Panazza S, Bramante T, Crosignani PG. Adenomyosis at hysterectomy: a study on frequency distribution and patient characteristics. Hum Reprod. 1995;10:1160–2.
29. Tellum T, Nygaard S, Skovholt EK, et al. Development of a clinical prediction model for diagnosing adenomyosis. Fertil Steril. 2018;110(957):3–964.
30. Munro GM. Classification and reporting systems for adenomyosis. J Minim Invasive Gynecol. 2020;27:296–308.
31. Habiba M, Gordts S, Bazot M, Brosens I, Benagiano G. Exploring the challenges for a new classification of adenomyosis. Reprod Biomed Online. 2020;40(4):569–81.
32. Grimbizis GF, Mikos T, Tarlatzis B. Uterus-sparing operative treatment for adenomyosis. Fertil Steril. 2014;101:472–87.
33. Hulka CA, Hall DA, McCarthy K, Simeone J. Sonographic findings in patients with adenomyosis: can sonography assist in predicting extent of disease? Am J Roentgenol. 2002;179:379–83.
34. Vercellini P, Viganò P, Somigliana E, Daguati R, Abbiati A, Fedele L. Adenomyosis: epidemiological factors. Best Pract Res Clin Obstet Gynaecol. 2006;20:465–77.

Noninvasive Diagnosis of Adenomyosis: Ultrasonography

33

Caterina Exacoustos

Contents

33.1 Introduction

Adenomyosis is a common gynecologic disease characterized by the invasion of endometrial glands and stroma into the myometrium and is associated with smooth muscle hyperplasia and fibrosis. Adenomyosis is a heterogeneous disease that may present in different phenotypes in the myometrium: diffuse, focal, and adenomyoma. Furthermore, different myometrial layers could be impaired: the outer (neometra) or the inner (archimetra or junctional zone (JZ)) myometrium [24].

C. Exacoustos (✉)
University of Rome "Tor Vergata", Department of Surgical Sciences, Obstetrics and Gynecological Unit, University Hospital of Tor Vergata, Rome, Italy
e-mail: caterinaexacoustos@tiscali.it

E. Oral (ed.), *Endometriosis and Adenomyosis*,
https://doi.org/10.1007/978-3-030-97236-3_33

For more than a century after adenomyosis was first described, the diagnosis was only possible through pathological examination of hysterectomy specimens. This changed following the advent of transvaginal sonography (TVS) or magnetic resonance imaging (MRI), which enabled noninvasive diagnosis.

Young patients, reproducible, repeatable, less expensive, and widely available, better tolerate TVS compared to MRI. Several studies have illustrated that the sensitivity and specificity of 2D and 3D (two-/three-dimensional) TVS in diagnosing adenomyosis are comparable to those of MRI and/or histology ranging from 75% to 88% and from 67% to 93%, respectively [1, 8, 12, 13, 25, 40, 44]. However, all these studies regarding imaging and histopathological correlation have been done on hysterectomies mostly performed in patients over 40 years, and actually there is few information on the correlation of adenomyosis ultrasound findings to histological diagnosis in young patients. Except for adenomyomas that often underwent surgery, this correlation will be difficult, and therefore we should accept that TVS or MRI features of adenomyosis are nowadays diagnostic for this disease [9].

The quality of the ultrasound scanners in use today in clinical examination can identify a disease that previously had required the patient to undergo MRI. Today, a routine pelvic evaluation with a conventional two-dimensional (2D) transvaginal probe can easily identify whether a patient's uterus has adenomyotic signs [46]. In fact, the TVS 2D and 3D criteria for adenomyosis show a strong correlation with histological diagnosis [14, 26, 44, 52]. At the same time, these sonographic criteria facilitate the diagnosis of the disease at an earlier stage, in younger patients, at a lower cost, and with a technology with easier access for most patients [9].

33.2 Ultrasound Features of Adenomyosis

The presence of adenomyosis determines hyperplasia and hypertrophy of myocytes surrounding heterotopic endometrial tissue. The 2D sonographic findings of adenomyosis described in the literature are generally alterations of the outer myometrium. The 2D transvaginal sonographic evaluation of the junctional zone seems to be, also with high-frequency probes (5–10 MHz), difficult and imprecise due to the not always optimal sonographic differentiation of inner and outer myometrium. It is possible to visualize the junctional zone more clearly with some post-processing using coronal section of the uterus obtained with three-dimensional transvaginal sonography (3DTVS) [14, 18, 31, 34, 46].

33.2.1 2D TVS Features of Adenomyosis

Continuous improvements in the resolution of transvaginal ultrasound have enabled a more detailed assessment of uterine architecture. This has facilitated the detection of ultrasound myometrial features of adenomyosis, which could not have been seen with older ultrasound equipment.

According to several studies following 2D transvaginal sonographic features were considered associated with adenomyosis and defined as follows ([1, 6, 18, 19, 40, 46, 54] (Table 33.1):

Table 33.1 Definition and description of the typical ultrasound features in the myometrium correlated with adenomyosis

Ultrasound features for diagnosing adenomyosis	Definition	Additional ultrasound characteristics
Hyperechogenic islands	Hyperechogenic areas within the myometrium that have no connection with the endometrium. They may be regular, irregular or ill-defined	*Hyperechogenic islands do not have a minimum diameter, and need no minimum number* *There is no minimum distance from the endometrium*
Myometrial cysts	Rounded or oval lesions of any size within the myometrium. Contents may be anechoic, of low-level echogenicity, of ground-glass appearance. May be surrounded by a hyperechogenic rim	*Color Doppler should be used to differentiate between vessels and myometrial cysts*
Globular uterus	Typical spherical shape of a globular uterus with myometrial serosa diverges from the cervix in at least two directions (anterior/posterior/lateral) instead of following a trajectory parallel to the endometrium	*Globular uterus unrelated to leiomyoma, with diffuse minimal vascularity seen as diffuse spread of small vessels within the myometrium and not circular vascularization related typical to myomas*
Asymmetrical thickening	Asymmetrical thickening is present when the difference in thickness of the anterior and the posterior myometrial wall exceeds 5 mm or when the calculated ratio between the walls is well above or below 1	*Asymmetry unrelated to leiomyoma, with diffuse minimal vascularity seen as diffuse spread of small vessels within the myometrium and not circular vascularization related typical to myomas*
Hypoechogenic linear stripes	Presence of hypoechogenic stripes present behind the myometrial lesion, sometimes alternating with linear hyperechogenic stripes (fan-shaped shadowing)	*The presence of edge shadows and circular vascularization might indicate the presence of a fibroid*
Irregular junctional zone	The junctional zone can be irregular because of cystic areas, hyperechogenic dots, and hyperechogenic buds and lines	*There is no evidence of the relevance of measurements of JZ irregularities by ultrasonography. Only for research measurement of irregularity:* $Jz_{max} - Jz_{min} = Jz_{dif}$. *Extent of irregularity: % of JZ that is irregular (<50% or >50%)*
Interrupted junctional zone	There is interruption of the junctional zone when a proportion of JZ cannot be visualized in either 2D or 3D TVS in any plane	*The extent of interruption (JZ cannot be visualized <50% or >50%) can be evaluated but it is not mandatory*

JZ junctional zone; min, minimum, *max* maximum, *dif* difference, *3D* three-dimensional, *2D* two-dimensional, *TVS* transvaginal sonography

- Globally enlarged uterus: the fundus of the uterus appears enlarged (Fig. 33.1a, b).
- Asymmetrically enlarged uterus (one uterine wall thicker than others) unrelated to leiomyoma, with diffuse minimal vascularity seen as the diffuse spread of small vessels within the myometrium and not circular vascularization related typically to myomas (Fig. 33.2a, b). It is advisable to exclude the presence of transient uterine contractions, because they may modify the uterine wall's thickness and change the myometrial echotexture, making the uterus appear more globular and asymmetric [47].
- Inhomogeneous, irregular myometrial echotexture with:
  - Round cystic area within the myometrium surrounded by a hyperechoic halo
  - Hyperechogenic islands
  - Myometrial hypoechoic linear striations are seen as a radiating pattern of thin acoustic shadows not arising from echogenic foci or leiomyoma (fan-shaped shadowing) (Figs. 33.2 and 33.3).

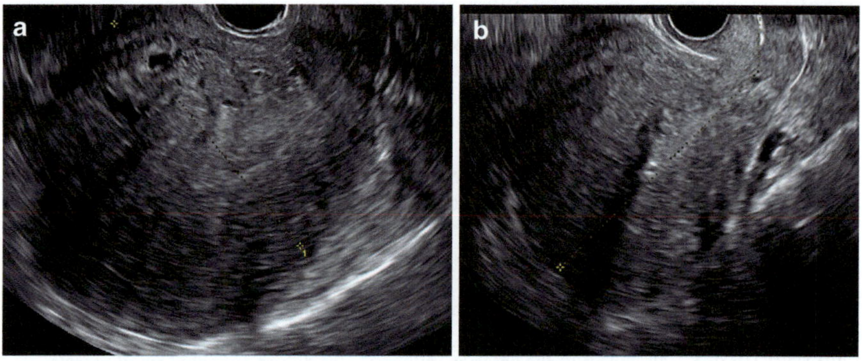

Fig. 33.1 (**a**, **b**) Two ultrasound images of a globular uterus with diffuse adenomyosis. Gray scale image showing a globally enlarged uterus, asymmetrically thickening of the uterine walls, and abnormal myometrial echogenicity

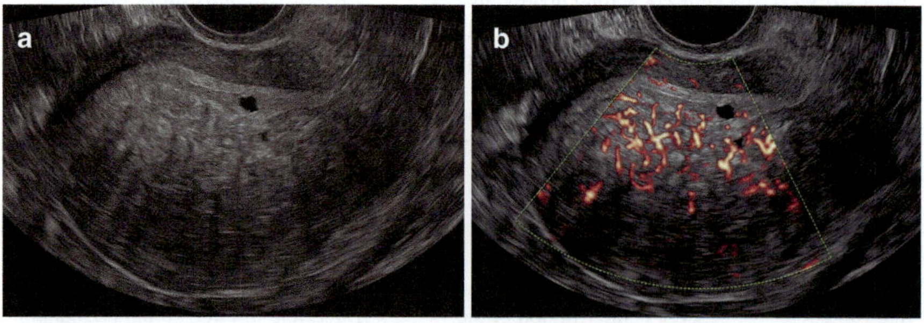

Fig. 33.2 (**a**, **b**) Ultrasound images of diffuse adenomyosis of the posterior uterine wall involving JZ and outer myometrium; note the hyperechoic striation and the cystic areas in the JZ. (**b**) Power Doppler image showing diffusely spread small vessels

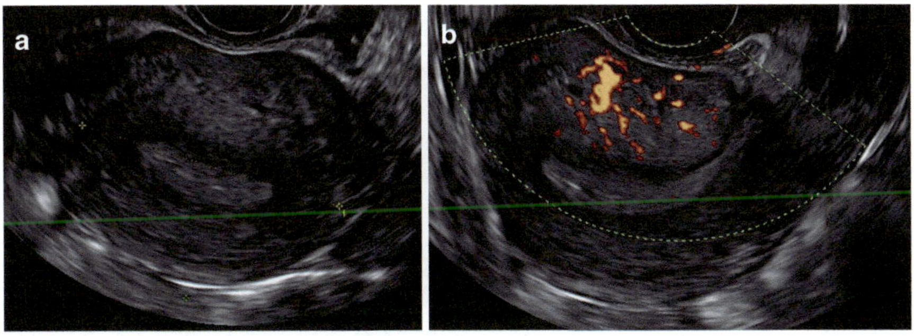

Fig. 33.3 (**a**, **b**) Ultrasound images of diffuse adenomyosis of the anterior uterine wall not involving JZ but only the outer myometrium; note the hyperechoic area and the intramyometrial cysts. (**b**) Power Doppler image showing diffusely spread small vessels

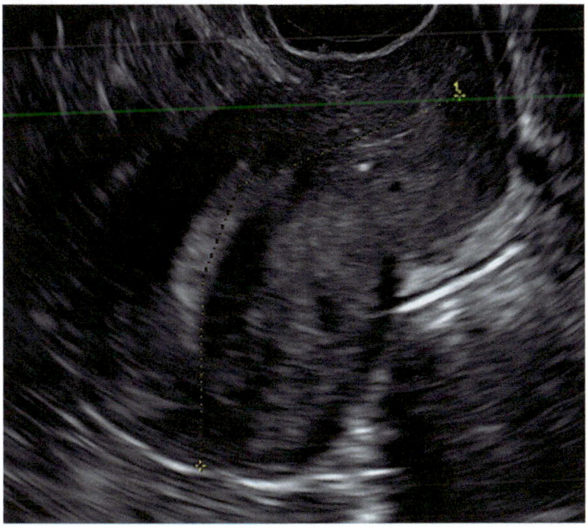

Fig. 33.4 Ultrasound images of diffuse adenomyosis of the posterior uterine wall with the typical question mark sign

- Indistinct, fuzzy endometrial-myometrial border (ill-defined endometrial stripe) (Fig. 33.1a, b).
- Presence of diffuse minimal vascularity seen as diffusely spread of small vessels which have not the normal course of the arcuate and radial arteries inside the myometrium.

Moreover, a new interesting sign called question mark form [11, 52] of uteri was reported recently. This is described when the corpus uterus was flexed backward, the fundus of uteri was facing the posterior pelvic compartment, and the cervix was directed frontally toward the urinary bladder (Figs. 33.4 and 33.5).

Power Doppler can be used to distinguish myometrial cysts from blood vessels and to discriminate between leiomyoma and focal adenomyosis (Fig. 33.6a, b). Uterine leiomyomas manifest a circular flow along the myoma capsule, while localized adenomyosis and adenomyomas are characterized by diffusely spread vessels inside the lesions.

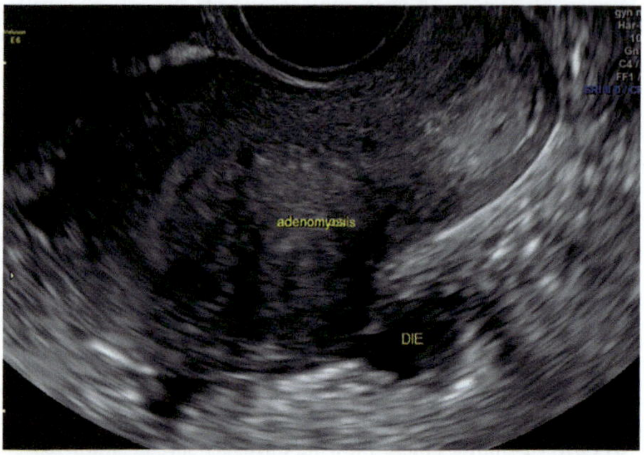

Fig. 33.5 Ultrasound images of diffuse adenomyosis of the posterior uterine wall with the typical question mark sign associated with posterior deep endometriosis of the rectal wall

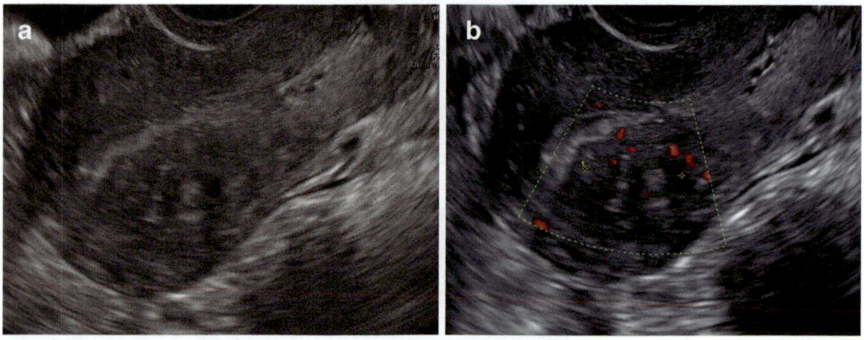

Fig. 33.6 (**a**, **b**) Ultrasound images of focal adenomyosis of the posterior uterine wall not involving JZ but only the outer myometrium; note the hyperechoic area and the intramyometrial cysts. (**b**) Power Doppler image showing diffusely spread small vessels

33.2.2 3D TVS Features of Adenomyosis

Although the junctional zone (JZ) can be visualized on 2D ultrasound, acquisition of a 3D volume enables a more complete assessment in the sagittal, transverse, and coronal plane as shown in a standardized multiplanar view [7, 14, 34, 46]. 3D transvaginal sonographic signs of adenomyosis are based on the evaluation of the junctional zone on the acquired volume of the uterus in order to obtain the coronal view. In the coronal view, the junctional zone appears as a hypoechoic zone around the endometrium. Using the volume contrast imaging (VCI) modality with 2–4 mm slices, the JZ can be seen clearer in all planes of the multiplanar view; this is also the case in the longitudinal and transverse uterine section where the anterior and posterior junctional zone could be evaluated [7, 14, 31, 32, 46].

The JZ may be regular, irregular, interrupted, not visible, and not assessable or may manifest more than one feature (e.g., irregular and interrupted). Any irregularity in the JZ can be described (e.g., cystic areas, hyperechogenic dots, hyperechogenic buds and lines) in each location in the uterus (anterior, posterior, lateral left, lateral right, fundus) [14, 31, 32, 46].

In order to avoid reliance on subjective morphological description of the JZ as irregularity and infiltration, objective parameters were proposed. These include measurements of the thickness of the JZ similar to those the radiologists generally use on MRI [14, 15, 26]. The JZ and the total myometrial wall thickness can be measured perpendicular to the endometrium on the same section through the uterus. The maximum thickness of the junctional zone (JZ_{max}) is measured at the area where the JZ appears to be at its thickest and the minimum thickness of the junctional zone (JZ_{min}) where it appears to be at its thinnest, after evaluation of the total three-dimensional volume of the uterus (Fig. 33.6). To define the ratio between the JZ and the total uterine wall thickness, both the JZ and the total uterine wall thickness should be measured on the same image [14, 26, 46]. The magnitude of a JZ irregularity is expressed as the difference between the maximal and the minimal JZ thickness: $(JZ_{max}) - (JZ_{min}) = JZ_{dif}$. The extent of JZ irregularity can be reported as the subjective estimation of the percentage of the JZ that is irregular (<50% or >50%) [14, 26, 46]. These measurements are actually proposed and relevant in the context of research protocols and had low application in the clinical practice.

Detailed morphological assessment of the JZ is currently proposed (Table 33.1):

- Irregular JZ: indistinct, poorly distinguishable endometrial-myometrial border (Fig. 33.7).
- Interrupted JZ: interruption of the JZ may be caused by focal or diffuse infiltration of the JZ by endometrial tissue. Contractions and changes within the JZ may also give rise to apparent JZ irregularities or influence JZ thickness. The extent of interruptions can be recorded as a subjective estimation of the percentage of the JZ that is interrupted (<50% or >50%), or it can be measured in length along the endometrial-myometrial border and in thickness [16, 23, 46].
- Junctional zone alterations due to subendometrial hyperechogenic lines and buds: infiltration of the JZ may be caused by focal adenomyosis [18] (Figs. 33.8 and 33.9).

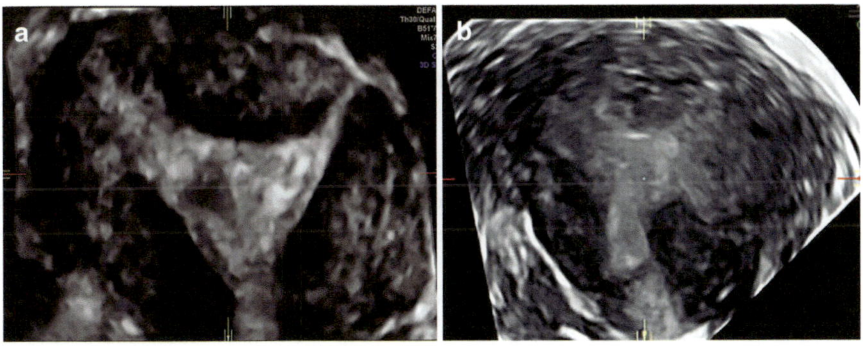

Fig. 33.7 (**a**, **b**) Two 3D ultrasound images of diffuse adenomyosis of the JZ in coronal view. (**a**) partial invasion, (**b**) total infiltration of the JZ

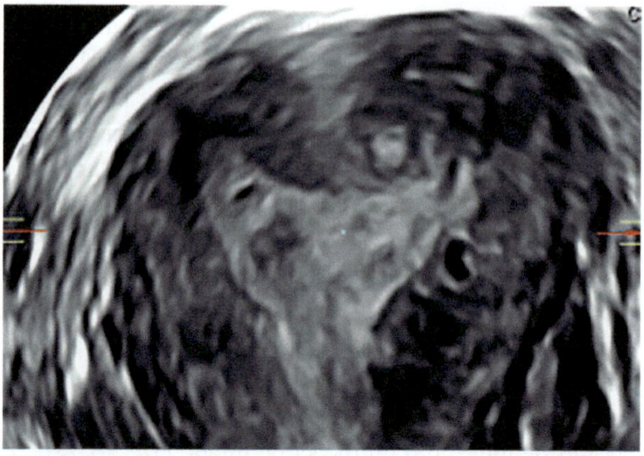

Fig. 33.8 Ultrasound images of focal adenomyosis of the JZ in 3D coronal view, note the buds and cystic areas inside the JZ

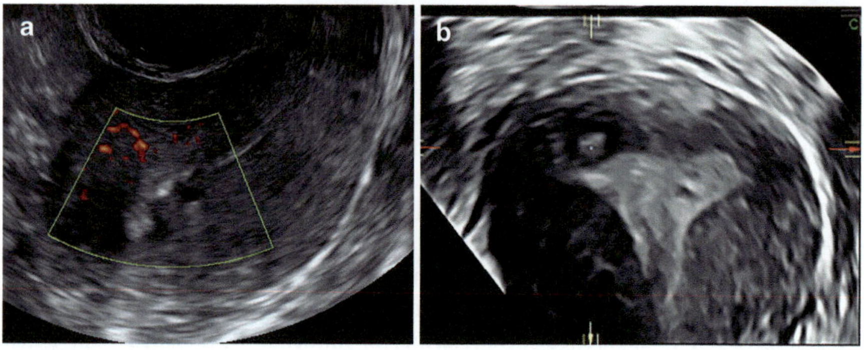

Fig. 33.9 (**a**, **b**) Ultrasound images of focal adenomyosis of the JZ. (**a**) 2D and power Doppler. (**b**) 3D coronal view, note the buds and cystic areas inside the JZ

33.3 Ultrasound Evaluation and Description of Adenomyosis

In the presence of the TVS criteria for adenomyosis, the disease showed different types and locations at the anatomical-histological evaluation but also at ultrasound. These adenomyosis characteristics should be described when the presence of the typical ultrasound features for adenomyosis is seen. Most of the studies utilizing TVS required the presence of at least two or three of ultrasound features for the diagnosis of adenomyosis [11, 14, 22, 31–33, 52]. The presence of only one of the typical TVS features of adenomyosis creates actually especially in young women some concerns. Recently, some more specific signs like intramyometrial cystic and hyperechoic areas and JZ bud and lines have been identified where only one of these features could be diagnostic [18]. The topographic distribution of adenomyotic lesions is variable and should be described.

Several attempts of classifying adenomyosis were performed by using the depth of myometrial penetration of adenomyotic foci at histological examination [5]; by grading the severity according to adenomyotic involvement of the inner third (superficial adenomyosis), two-thirds, and entire myometrium (deep adenomyosis) [43];

or according to the penetration ratio (depth of penetration/myometrial thickness) by representing the extent of the disease [42].

Vercellini et al. [50], based on the proposal of Siegler and Camilien [43], proposed to consider three different parameters: (i) depth of penetration (up to one-third, mild disease; between one- and two-thirds, moderate disease; more than two-thirds, severe disease), (ii) degree of spread defined by the number of foci per low-power field (1–3 islets, grade I; 4–10 islets, grade II; >10 islets, grade III), and (iii) configuration (diffuse versus nodular/focal). Actually we are waiting for new agreed histological system for classifying and reporting adenomyosis that will enhance our understanding of the disease and is envisaged to enable comparison of research studies and treatment outcomes [17]. TVS diagnosis based on the actual histopathological knowledge should include now not only the presence of adenomyosis features but also report type, location, and size of the disease (Tables 33.2 and 33.3).

Table 33.2 Definition and description of the ultrasound appearance of the different types of adenomyosis

2D US features	Diffuse adenomyosis	Focal adenomyosis	Adenomyoma
Serosal contour of the uterus	Often globally enlarged uterus	Often regular	Lobulated or regular
Definition of lesion	Ill-defined	Ill-defined or well-defined in case of cystic or hyperechoic lesions surrounded mostly by normal myometrium	May be well-defined surrounded by hypertrophic myometrium
Symmetry of uterine walls	Myometrial anterior-posterior or lateral asymmetry	Often symmetric	Asymmetrical in presence of well-defined lesion
Shape	Ill-defined	Ill-defined, oval in case of cystic lesions	Round, oval, lobulated
Contour	Ill-defined	Irregular or ill-defined	Regular or ill-defined
Shadowing	No edge shadows Fan-shaped shadowing Linear hypoechoic striation	No edge shadows Rarely fan-shaped shadowing or linear hypoechoic striation	Edge shadows may be present, internal often fan-shaped shadowing
Echogenicity	*Non-uniform diffuse* Presence of intramyometrial diffuse areas of typical ultrasound features	*Focal, often isolated surrounded by normal myometrium*, presence of intramyometrial focal small areas of typical ultrasound features	*Focal, lobulated* presence in hyper-, iso-, hypoechogenic intramyometrial lobulated areas of typical ultrasound features
Vascularity	Translesional flow diffuse minimal or few vessels	Diffuse minimal sporadic vessels	Translesional flow diffuse vessels or circumferential flow
Endometrial rim	Irregular or ill-defined Distorted or imprinted	Often regular or imprinted by subendometrial focal lesion	Often regular or distorted by the lobulated lesion

Table 33.3 Ultrasound characteristics of adenomyosis that should be reported

Ultrasound description of adenomyosis	Ultrasound features
Type of features	Globally enlarged uterus Asymmetrically enlarged Inhomogeneous myometrial echotexture: Myometrial cystic areas Hyperechogenic islands Myometrial hypoechoic linear striations Junctional zone alterations: JZ hyperechogenic lines and buds Indistinct, poorly distinguishable endometrial-myometrial border "Irregular" and "interrupted" JZ
Location in the uterus	Anterior Posterior Lateral (left, right) Fundus Cervix
Type of the disease	Diffuse Focal Adenomyoma Mixed (both diffuse and focal)
Location in myometrial layers	Outer myometrium Inner myometrium or junctional zone
Size	Uterine wall maximum thickness Length of the affected JZ Max diameter of the focal lesion Max diameter of the adenomyoma
Extension of the disease	Mild Moderate Severe

33.3.1 TVS Types of Adenomyosis

The type of adenomyosis can be defined as diffuse, focal, and adenomyoma according to the TVS characteristics (Table 33.2; Figs. 33.2 and 33.6). Focal adenomyosis is identified when more than 25% of the lesion is surrounded by normal myometrium [48] (Fig. 33.6). When a focal lesion is completely surrounded by hypertrophic myometrium, this condition is named "adenomyoma." Furthermore, the same uterus can present with focal and diffuse lesions. In that case, the condition is called "mixed-type adenomyosis."

33.3.2 TVS Uterine Wall Location of Adenomyosis

Adenomyosis should be described in its location regarding uterine walls: anterior, posterior, lateral left, lateral right, or fundal and cervical. The affected uterine wall assessment could be important for surgical procedures on the adenomyosis itself or on deep endometriosis that can involve the uterus and the adenomyosis (Table 33.3).

33.3.3 TVS Myometrial Layer Location of Adenomyosis

The depth of myometrial infiltration is also variable, from cases limited to the more inner myometrium to those involving the whole myometrial thickness [1]. Adenomyosis may involve one or more of the uterine layers. If three uterine layers are considered, adenomyosis is defined as type 1 when only the JZ is involved, type 2 when the middle myometrium (the layer between the JZ and the vascular arcade) is involved, and type 3 if adenomyotic lesions are found in the outer myometrium [48]. Since the limitation between the middle and the outer myometrium is uncertain and difficult to perform at TVS, the differentiation in two layers inner and outer myometrium seems more practical considering also that these two layers are embryologically different (archimetrium and neometrium) and the middle layer belongs to the neometra. Diffuse and focal adenomyosis therefore can be subsequently divided for the outer myometrium and for the JZ (inner myometrium) (Figs. 33.2 and 33.3) [23] (Table 33.3).

33.3.4 TVS Size and Extension of Adenomyosis Inside the Uterus

The severity of adenomyosis is difficult to express in quantitative terms as the lesions are often poorly defined, and they may be disseminated throughout different parts of the myometrium. There are different attempts to describe by TVS the extension and the severity of the disease inside the uterus. The number of different morphological features in an individual woman has been proposed as an indirect semiquantitative measure of severity of adenomyosis [31–33].

The severity of adenomyosis may be classified according to MUSA [48] to the extent of the disease in terms of percentage of affected myometrium (mild <25%, moderate 25–50%, severe >50%). Another adenomyosis classification and reporting system proposed by us [16, 23] assesses the extension of each type of adenomyotic lesion (diffuse, focal, adenomyoma) in the external myometrium and in the junctional zone and is divided into four grades according to the parameters shown in Fig. 33.10. Measurements of the thickness of uterine affected wall, of the length and thickness of the infiltrated JZ, of the largest diameter of the focal lesions and of the adenomyoms should be taken and maximum diameters of the focal lesions and of the adenomyomas should be taken in order to determine the different grades. For diffuse adenomyosis of the outer myometrium, the degree is assigned according to the thickness of the uterine wall (> or <20 or 30 mm) and the number of the uterine walls affected (anterior, posterior, lateral left, lateral right). For the diffuse adenomyosis of the inner myometrium, the thickness of the JZ and the length of the infiltrated JZ tract were considered in four degrees. Focal adenomyosis of the inner and outer myometrium was assigned a degree according to the largest diameter of the focal lesion and the number of foci. Similarly, adenomyomas were divided into four degrees according to size (largest diameter 20, 30, 40 >40) and several adenomyomas. A score number of 1–4 was attributed to each degree of the disease considered. Then, the ultrasound extent of the disease was calculated through the sum of the

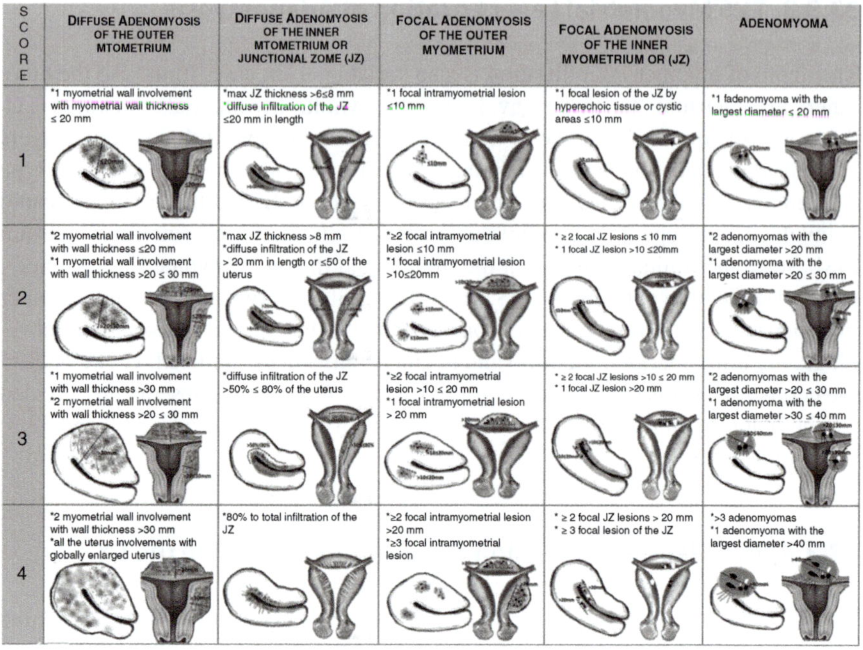

Fig. 33.10 Ultrasound score system for the evaluation and extension of adenomyosis inside the uterus

score numbers obtained and classified into three groups: mild (ranged between 1 and 3), moderate (4–6), and severe (>7) adenomyosis. In a recent paper [16], patients' characteristics, symptom severity, and uterine menstrual bleeding are correlated with the type of adenomyosis and score. Also the extent of adenomyosis, classified as mild, moderate, or severe, was correlated with symptom severity and uterine menstrual bleeding. Diffuse and severe disease occurs more in older patients with heavy menstrual bleeding and dysmenorrhea, whereas focal and mild disease is seen in younger patients and related more to infertility and recurrent miscarriage. The accuracy of the evaluation of localization, extent, and size of adenomyotic lesions, as well as the myometrial layer involved, should be tested in large series, in order to adequately define and differentiate focal versus diffuse forms. Furthermore, the relationship between the suggested US criteria and the clinical presentations of adenomyosis is still unknown and needs to be investigated, as well as the extent of adenomyotic lesions versus the severity of symptoms.

33.4 Ultrasound Diagnostic Accuracy of Adenomyosis Compared to Histology

Usually the diagnosis of adenomyosis is made on histological examination of a uterus following a hysterectomy. The histological frequency of adenomyosis ranges from 5% to 70% according to the series. This wide variation is affected by the histological criteria and the number of sections examined. The majority of previous studies reporting the accuracy of 2D TVS diagnosis of adenomyosis have assessed populations of women who underwent hysterectomy [3, 29, 54]. These included mainly women with severe symptoms who were more likely to have adenomyosis than the general population, and it is likely that the prevalence of adenomyosis in these studies is an overestimate. Furthermore, the 2D TVS findings are more likely to appear in advanced stage of disease. Reinhold et al. [40] reported that 2D ultrasound had a sensitivity of 80–86%, specificity of 50–96%, and overall accuracy of 68–86% for diagnosing diffuse adenomyosis. However, 2D ultrasound can yield equivocal results in case of focal adenomyosis and if there are coexistent fibroids [1, 54]. A meta-analysis of 14 trials and 1985 participants reported the sensitivity and specificity of ultrasound diagnosed adenomyosis to be as high as 82.5% and 84.6%, respectively [29]. Recent studies [52] reported a very high accuracy of 90% and specificity of 91%.

Targeted ultrasound-guided biopsies have been proposed in an attempt to correlate histological findings to ultrasound features of adenomyosis in those younger women who will not undergo hysterectomy [35, 51]. Nam and Lyu [35] performed abdominal ultrasound-guided transvaginal myometrial core needle biopsy in 1032 premenopausal women aged 22–53 years who had 2D ultrasound findings suggestive for adenomyosis. They reported a 92.26% of concordance rate between the transvaginal myometrial core needle biopsy and ultrasonographic diagnoses of adenomyosis.

Several studies have illustrated the sensitivity and specificity of 2D TVS in diagnosing adenomyosis, but 2D ultrasound findings generally described alterations of the outer myometrium and do not consider alterations of the JZ. JZ however forms the basis for MRI diagnosis of adenomyosis. The study of Kepkep et al. [19] was one of the first reports that included poor definition of the JZ as a diagnostic feature in assessment of the accuracy of various 2D transvaginal sonographic findings in adenomyosis. They found that poor definition of junctional zone had a high specificity (82%) but a low sensitivity (46%) in its diagnosis. Three-dimensional reconstruction of uterine anatomy in the coronal plane provides new view of the junctional zone [14, 34]. By comparing TVS features to histology of the uterus after hysterectomies, it was shown that junctional zone thickness $JZ_{max} \geq 6–8$ mm and $(JZ_{max}) - (JZ_{min}) \geq 4$ mm was significantly more associated with adenomyosis than other 2D features [14, 26]. Also the subjective evaluation of infiltration and disruption by endometrial tissue in the junctional zone is an accurate tool for the diagnosis of adenomyosis [9, 14, 26, 34, 37, 38]. Considering the hypothesis that adenomyosis is more likely to be caused by "invasion" of endometrial tissue across the junctional zone and into the myometrium [24], 3D evaluation of JZ may be able to detect early adenomyosis [15]. Alteration of JZ is correlated with adenomyosis and may be involved in the process that determines pelvic endometriosis [4, 20, 21, 24]. Therefore, the evaluation of junctional zone and its alterations by noninvasive imaging seems very important especially in patients with suspect of pelvic endometriosis and adenomyosis. Three-dimensional TVS seems to be more accurate than conventional 2D TVS to detect adenomyosis. Using 3D ultrasound JZ buds and striations as subendometrial adenomyotic cysts can now be detected in younger patients during their reproductive years and also in adolescents (Figs. 33.8 and 33.9) [27].

33.5 Ultrasound Diagnosis of Adenomyosis Compared to MRI Diagnosis

Multiple studies have measured the relative performance of TVS and MRI in diagnosing adenomyosis [1, 13, 39, 40, 44]. Three recent meta-analyses and systematic reviews demonstrated similar sensitivity for TVS (range: 72–79%) and MRI (range: 77–78%) [8, 25, 44]. However, MRI shows higher specificity (range: 88–93%) compared to TVS (range: 78–81%). The likelihood ratio for adenomyosis seems to be higher with MRI, but negative likelihood ratios were similar for both modalities. Overall, these results show that both TVS and MRI demonstrate high accuracy for the diagnosis of adenomyosis.

There are cost and patient outcome implications associated with the choice of imaging modality for the diagnosis of adenomyosis. The choice between US and MRI in the diagnosis of adenomyosis is contingent on several factors, including availability of the technology and imaging expertise, diagnostic performance, patient contraindications, and referring physician's preference. TVS is widely available and well tolerated by most patients. MRI scanners and expertise, while available to many patients, may not be an option in low-resource and geographically remote settings. The routine use of MRI where the resource is not readily available can lead to diagnostic and treatment delays [41]. TVS is more available in most of the gynecological offices and due to its reduced invasiveness could be carried out in all patients, including younger patients with fewer symptoms and a desire for pregnancy. Thus, ultimately, the choice of modality is left to the context of the individual patient's and care provider's preferences and defined by the locally available imaging resources and expertise of the practice setting [36].

33.6 Ultrasound Diagnosis of Adenomyosis and Association with Endometriosis

Adenomyosis diagnosed by TVS seems also to be associated with endometriosis [20, 22, 28, 31, 32]. Surely, both conditions share pathogenesis and symptoms such as *dysmenorrhea*, heavy menstrual bleeding, infertility, dyspareunia, and chronic pelvic pain. It has been reported that pelvic endometriosis, especially in advanced stages, is also strongly associated with JZ thickening due to adenomyosis [14, 21, 26].

Di Donato et al. [11] reported recently on a series of patients undergoing surgery for endometriosis a prevalence of adenomyosis diagnosed by ultrasound of 21.8%. This prevalence is slightly higher than the prevalence (20.9%) reported by Naftalin et al. [31, 32] who evaluated patients attending a general gynecological ultrasound unit who had only a TVS diagnosis of endometriosis. An interesting feature is also the strong association found between deep infiltrating endometriosis and adenomyosis reported in some recent studies [11, 22, 10]. Lazzeri confirmed the strong association between adenomyosis diagnosed by transvaginal ultrasound and deep endometriosis diagnosed and treated surgically. The incidence of adenomyosis in patients affected by deep infiltrating endometriosis was 48.7% [22]. It has been shown that the ultrasound "question mark sign" of the retroverted fixed uterus was strongly related to posterior deep infiltrating endometriosis (Fig. 33.5) [10, 11, 52]. It seems that this type of adenomyosis mostly of the outer myometrium is caused by external invasion of the deep endometriosis, whereas the adenomyosis that involved the JZ originates from the endometrium and extends outward to the myometrium toward the serosal uterine surface. Thus, it will appear contiguous with the junctional zone for adenomyosis. In contrast, deep infiltrating endometriosis, most commonly originating in the rectouterine pouch, invades from the serosal surface of the myometrium inward [9]. This type of adenomyosis will appear separate from the junctional zone – thereby supporting by imaging different theories for the pathogenesis of adenomyosis [9, 36, 53].

33.7 Ultrasound Diagnosis of Adenomyosis and Association with Symptoms

The association with symptoms could improve the diagnostic accuracy of ultrasound features for adenomyosis [2]. A number of factors encouraging the development of adenomyosis include history of spontaneous miscarriage, curettage, hysteroscopic resection of the endometrium, uterine myomectomy, caesarean section, and the use of tamoxifen [9, 45]. There are furthermore several studies that reported a correlation between ultrasound findings of adenomyosis, and symptoms like menorrhagia or dysmenorrhea, infertility, and recurrent miscarriages have been shown [2, 31–33, 49]. Recently, Zannoni et al. [52] reported that also the tenderness and pain caused by gentle pressure of the uterus with the transvaginal probe is associated with histologically proven adenomyosis. This study reported an accuracy rate of 90% in diagnosing adenomyosis by TVS with a high specificity of 96% and positive predictive value (PPV) of 91%.

Some authors suggest that the severity of symptoms and the clinical features correlate with the extent and depth of adenomyosis [16, 27, 30, 33]. There is a belief of a direct correlation between the extent of histopathological features and clinical manifestations with the consequent hypothesis of a causal relationship between the number and the depth of the adenomyotic foci and specific symptoms. Through TVS, it is possible to assess the characteristics of adenomyosis, the grades, the type, and its extension inside the uterus. Recently, the link between type and degree of adenomyosis scored by TVS and severity of clinical symptoms was evaluated [16]. It seems that ultrasound features of diffuse adenomyosis were more frequent in older women with heavy menstrual bleeding compared to those with focal disease. A higher percentage of infertility and miscarriage was observed in focal adenomyosis of the outer myometrium and the JZ, respectively (Figs. 33.6, 33.8, and 33.9). These findings could lead us to believe that different types and depth of adenomyosis (in terms of localization in the outer or inner myometrium) have an impact on symptoms and fertility. Severe diffuse adenomyosis is also correlated with severe dysmenorrhea and heavy menstrual bleeding (Fig. 33.1a, b). No other correlation to symptoms was observed when classifying the extension of the diseases inside the uterus in mild, moderate, and severe [16]. This is in contrast with the results previously reported by Naftalin et al., in which there was a correlation between ultrasound severity of adenomyosis, menstrual pain, and heavy bleeding [30, 33]. Nevertheless, in these studies, adenomyosis was not distinguished in types (focal and diffuse) or in regard to its extension inside the myometrial layers, but only according to the number of ultrasound features to evaluate the severity of the disease. Assessing the severity of adenomyosis based only on the number of sonographic characteristics could lead to false results: in some cases, a small focal lesion could show multiple ultrasound features of adenomyosis and vice versa.

The absence of a direct correlation between the ultrasound extension of adenomyosis within the uterus and the severity of symptoms could be partially explained by the presence of other coexisting conditions such as endometriosis, rather than the adenomyosis per se. Otherwise, it could be hypothesized that this condition is very similar to pelvic endometriosis, where often the severity of the disease is not related to the severity of symptoms. In fact, small endometriotic lesions may cause a lot of pain, whereas, sometimes, deep nodules are completely asymptomatic.

33.8 Conclusions

Two-dimensional transvaginal sonography has now achieved a high level of accuracy, and many authors have reported high agreement between ultrasound diagnosis of adenomyosis and histological findings. The TVS diagnosis of adenomyosis through specific features showed an accuracy up to 90%. TVS is a highly tolerable exam and due to its reduced invasiveness could be carried out in all patients, including younger patients with fewer symptoms. The use of TVS in the assessment of adenomyosis is a noninvasive test that allowed an accurate diagnosis, avoiding the need for histologic diagnosis, to assess also the correlation with the symptomatology. TVS is able to assess the type and severity of adenomyosis inside the uterus and may be helpful in selecting and evaluating the effectiveness of medical and surgical management, as well as the possible relationship between adenomyosis and infertility.

TVS should be the primary tool for the diagnosis of adenomyosis, with MRI being used where TVS is inconclusive or in the presence of large fibroids.

References

1. Bazot M, Cortez A, Darai E, Rouger J, Chopier J, Antoine JM, Uzan S. Ultrasonography compared with magnetic resonance imaging for the diagnosis of adenomyosis: correlation with histopathology. Hum Reprod. 2001;16:2427–33.
2. Bazot M, Darai E, Rouger J, Detchev R, Cortez A, Uzan S. Limitations of transvaginal sonography for the diagnosis of adenomyosis, with histopathological correlation. Ultrasound Obstet Gynecol. 2002;20:605–11.
3. Benagiano G, Brosens I. History of adenomyosis. Best Pract Res Clin Obstet Gynaecol. 2006;20:449–63.
4. Benagiano G, Habiba M, Brosens I. The pathophysiology of uterine adenomyosis: an update. Fertil Steril. 2012;98:572–9.
5. Bird CC, McElin TW, Manalo-Estrella P. The elusive adenomyosis of the uterus – revisited. Am J Obstet Gynecol. 1972;112:583–93.
6. Bromley B, Shipp TD, Benacerraf B. Adenomyosis: sonographic findings and diagnostic accuracy. J Ultrasound Med. 2000;19:529–34.
7. Brosens I, Derwig I, Brosens J, Fusi L, Benagiano G, Pijnenborg R. The enigmatic uterine junctional zone: the missing link between reproductive disorders and major obstetrical disorders? Hum Reprod. 2010;3:569–74.
8. Champaneria R, Abedin P, Daniels J, Balogun M, Khan KS. Ultrasound scan and magnetic resonance imaging for the diagnosis of adenomyosis: systematic review comparing test accuracy. Acta Obstet Gynecol Scand. 2010;89:1374–84.
9. Chapron C, S Vannuccini, Santulli P, Abrao MS, Carmona F, Fraser IS, Gordts S, Guo SW, Just PA, Noel JC Pistofidis G , Van den Bosch T and Petraglia F. Diagnosis of adenomyosis: an integrated clinical and imaging approach Hum Reprod Update 2020;26:392–411.
10. Di Donato N, Bertoldo V, Montanari G, Zannoni L, Caprara G, Seracchioli R. Question mark form of the uterus: a simple sonographic sign associated to the presence of adenomyosis. Ultrasound Obstet Gynecol. 2015;46:126–7.
11. Di Donato N, Montanari G, Benfenati A, Leonardi D, Bertoldo V, Monti G, Raimondo D, Seracchioli R. Prevalence of adenomyosis in women undergoing surgery for endometriosis. Eur J Obstet Gynecol Reprod Biol. 2014;181:289 93.
12. Dueholm M, Lundorf E, Hansen ES, Ledertoug S, Sorensen JS, Olesen F. Magnetic resonance imaging and transvaginal ultrasonography for diagnosis of adenomyosis. Fertil Steril. 2001;76:588–94.
13. Dueholm M, Lundorf E. Transvaginal ultrasound or MRI for diagnosis of adenomyosis. Curr Opin Obstet Gynecol. 2007;19:505–12.
14. Exacoustos C, Brienza L, Di Giovanni A, Szabolcs B, Romanini ME, Zupi E, Arduini D. Adenomyosis: three-dimensional sonographic findings of the junctional zone and correlation with histology. Ultrasound Obstet Gynecol. 2011;37:471–9.
15. Exacoustos C, Luciano D, Corbett B, De Felice G, Di Feliciantonio M, Luciano A, Zupi E. The uterine junctional zone: a 3-dimensional ultrasound study of patients with endometriosis. Am J Obstet Gynecol. 2013;209:248–55.
16. Exacoustos C, Morosetti G, Conway F, Camilli S, Martire FG, Lazzeri L, Piccione E, Zupi E. New sonographic classification of adenomyosis: do type and degree of adenomyosis correlate to severity of symptoms? J Minim Invasive Gynecol. 2020;27:1308–15.
17. Habiba M, Gordts S, Bazot M, Brosens I, Benagiano G. Exploring the challenges for a new classification of adenomyosis. Reprod Biomed Online. 2020;40:569–81.
18. Harmsen M, Van den Bosch T, de Leeuw A, Dueholm M, Exacoustos C, Valentin L, Hehenkamp W, Groenman F, de Bruyn C, Rasmussen C, Lazzeri L, Jokubkiene L Jurkovic D, Naftalin J, Tellum T, Bourne T, Timmerman D, Huirne JAF Applicability of Morphological Uterus Sonographic Assessment (MUSA) features associated with adenomyosis among experts and refinements of definitions. Ultrasound Obstet Gynecol. 2021; in press.

19. Kepkep K, Tuncay YA, Goynumer G, Tutal E. Transvaginal sonography in the diagnosis of adenomyosis: which findings are most accurate? Ultrasound Gynecol Obstet. 2007;30:341–5.
20. Kunz G, Beil D, Huppert P, Noe M, Kissler S, Leyendecker G. Adenomyosis in endometriosis-prevalence and impact on fertility. Evidence from magnetic resonance imaging. Hum Reprod. 2005;20:2309–16.
21. Larsen SB, Lundorf E, Forman A, Dueholm M. Adenomyosis and junctional zone changes in patients with endometriosis. Eur J Obstet Gynecol Reprod Biol. 2011;157:206–11.
22. Lazzeri L, Di Giovanni A, Exacoustos C, Tosti C, Pinzauti S, Malzoni M, Petraglia F, Zupi E. Preoperative and postoperative clinical and transvaginal ultrasound findings of adenomyosis in patients with deep infiltrating endometriosis. Reprod Sci. 2014;21:1027–33.
23. Lazzeri L, Morosetti G, Centini G, Monti G, Zupi E, Piccione E, Exacoustos C. A sonographic classification of adenomyosis: interobserver reproducibility in the evaluation of type and degree of the myometrial involvement. Fertil Steril. 2018;110:1154–61.
24. Leyendecker G, Wildt L, Mall G. The pathophysiology of endometriosis and adenomyosis: tissue injury and repair. Arch Gynecol Obstet. 2009;280:529–38.
25. Liu L, Wong L, Mol B, Condous G, Costa F, Leonardi M. Diagnostic accuracy of transvaginal ultrasound and magnetic resonance imaging for the diagnosis of adenomyosis: systematic review and meta-analysis. Ultrasound Med Biol. 2019;45:S54.
26. Luciano DE, Exacoustos C, Albrecht L, Lamonica R, Proffer A, Zupi E, Luciano AA. Three-dimensional ultrasound in diagnosis of adenomyosis: histologic correlation with ultrasound targeted biopsies of the uterus. J Minim Invasive Gynecol. 2013;20:803–10.
27. Martire FG, Lazzeri L, Conway F, Siciliano T, Pietropolli A, Piccione E, Solima E, Centini G, Zupi E, Exacoustos C. Adolescence and endometriosis: symptoms, ultrasound signs and early diagnosis. Fertil Steril. 2020;114:1049–57.
28. Maruyama S, Imanaka S, Nagayasu M, Kimura M, Kobayashi H. Relationship between adenomyosis and endometriosis; different phenotypes of a single disease? Eur J Obstet Gynecol Reprod Biol. 2020;253:191–7.
29. Meredith SM, Sanchez-Ramos L, Kaunitz AM. Diagnostic accuracy of transvaginal sonography for the diagnosis of adenomyosis: systematic review and meta analysis. Am J Obstet Gynecol. 2009;201:107.e1–107.
30. Naftalin J, Hoo W, Nunes N, Holland T, Mavrelos D, Jurkovic D. Association between ultrasound features of adenomyosis and severity of menstrual pain. Ultrasound Obstet Gynecol. 2016;47:779–8308.
31. Naftalin J, Hoo W, Nunes N, Mavrelos D, Nicks H, Jurkovic D. Inter- and intraobserver variability in three-dimensional ultrasound assessment of the endometrial-myometrial junction and factors affecting its visualization. Ultrasound Obstet Gynecol. 2012;39:587–91.
32. Naftalin J, Hoo W, Pateman K, Mavrelos D, Holland T, Jurkovic D. How common is adenomyosis? A prospective study of prevalence using transvaginal ultrasound in a gynaecology clinic. Hum Reprod. 2012;27:3432–9.
33. Naftalin J, Hoo W, Pateman K, Mavrelos D, Foo X, Jurkovic D. Is adenomyosis associated with menorrhagia? Hum Reprod. 2014;29:473–9.
34. Naftalin J, Jurkovic D. The endometrial-myometrial junction: a fresh look at a busy crossing. Ultrasound Obstet Gynecol. 2009;34:1–11.
35. Nam JH, Lyu GS. Abdominal ultrasound-guided transvaginal myometrial core needle biopsy for the definitive diagnosis of suspected adenomyosis in 1032 patients: a retrospective study. J Minim Invasive Gynecol. 2014;11:1553–650.
36. O'Shea A, Figueiredo G, Lee SI. Imaging diagnosis of adenomyosis. Semin Reprod Med. 2020;38:119–28.
37. Rasmussen CK, Hansen ES, Dueholm M. Inter-rater agreement in the diagnosis of adenomyosis by 2- and 3-dimensional trans- vaginal ultrasonography. J Ultrasound Med. 2019;38:657–66.
38. Rasmussen CK, Hansen ES, Ernst E, Dueholm M. Two- and three- dimensional transvaginal ultrasonography for diagnosis of adenomyosis of the inner myometrium. Reprod Biomed Online. 2019;38:750–60.
39. Reinhold C, McCarthy S, Bret PM, Mehio A, Atri M, Zakarian R, et al. Diffuse adenomyosis: comparison of endovaginal US and MR imaging with histopathologic correlation. Radiology. 1996;199:151–8.

40. Reinhold C, Tafazoli F, Mehio A, Wang L, Atri M, Siegelman ES, Rohoman L. Uterine adenomyosis: endovaginal US and MR imaging features with histopathologic correlation. Radiographics. 1999;19:S147–60.
41. Sam M, Raubenheimer M, Manolea F, et al. Accuracy of findings in the diagnosis of uterine adenomyosis on ultrasound. Abdom Radiol (NY). 2020;45:842–50.
42. Sammour A, Pirwany I, Usubutun A. Correlations between extent and spread of adenomyosis and clinical symptoms. Gynecol Obstet Investig. 2002;54:213e216.
43. Siegler AM, Camilien L. Adenomyosis. J Reprod Med. 1994;39:841e853.
44. Tellum T, Nygaard S, Lieng M. Noninvasive diagnosis of adenomyosis: a structured review and meta-analysis of diagnostic accuracy in imaging. J Minim Invasive Gynecol. 2020;27:408–18.
45. Tomassetti C, Mueleman C, Timmerman D, D'Hooghe T. Adenomyosis and subfertility: evidence of association and causation. Semin Reprod Med. 2013;31:101–8.
46. Van den Bosch T, Dueholm M, Leone FP, Valentin L, Rasmussen CK, Votino A, et al. Terms, definitions and measurements to describe sonographic features of the myometrium and uterine masses: a consensus opinion from the Morphological Uterus Sonographic Assessment (MUSA) group. Ultrasound Obstet Gynecol. 2015;46:284–29.
47. Van den Bosch T, Van Schoubroeck D, Alcazar JL, Guerriero S, Martins W. The importance of transient myometrial contractions in the diagnosis of adenomyosis and congenital uterine anomalies. Ultrasound Obstet Gynecol. 2021;57(4):651–653.
48. Van den Bosch T, de Bruijn AM, de Leeuw RA, Dueholm M, Exacoustos C, Valentin L, Bourne T, Timmerman D, Huirne JAF. Sonographic classification and reporting system for diagnosing adenomyosis. Ultrasound Obstet Gynecol. 2019;53:576–82.
49. Vercellini P, Consonni D, Dridi D, Bracco B, Frattaruolo MP, Somigliana E. Uterine adenomyosis and in vitro fertilization outcome: a systematic review and meta-analysis. Hum Reprod. 2014;29:964–7.
50. Vercellini P, Viganò P, Somigliana E, Daguati R, Abbiati A, Fedele L. Adenomyosis: epidemiological factors. Best Pract Res Clin Obstet Gynaecol. 2006;20:465–77.
51. Vercellini P, Cortesi I, De Giorgi O, Merlo D, Carinelli SG, Crosignani PG. Transvaginal ultrasonography versus uterine needle biopsy in the diagnosis of diffuse adenomyosis. Hum Reprod. 1998;13:2884–7.
52. Zannoni L, Ambrosio M, Raimondo D, Arena A, Del Forno S, Borghese G, Paradisi R, Seracchioli R. Question mark sign and transvaginal ultrasound uterine tenderness for the diagnosis of adenomyosis: a prospective validation. J Ultrasound Med. 2020;39:1405–12.
53. Zhai J, Vannuccini S, Petraglia F, Giudice LC. Adenomyosis: mechanisms and pathogenesis. Semin Reprod Med. 2020;38:129–43.
54. Dueholm M. Transvaginal ultrasound for diagnosis of adenomyosis: a review. Best Pract Res Clin Obstet Gynaecol. 2006;20:569–82.

Noninvasive Diagnosis of Adenomyosis: Magnetic Resonance Imaging (MRI)

34

Tina Tellum

Contents

34.1 Introduction

Magnetic resonance imaging (MRI) has been investigated for use in diagnosing adenomyosis since the 1980s. Interestingly, the observations from that time are largely still congruent with today's findings. However, higher resolution and new technology allow detecting very small foci of adenomyosis with MRI, and the diagnostic performance has since been improved.

34.1.1 The Role of MRI in Adenomyosis Diagnosis

In the last decades, not only MRI but also ultrasound technology underwent dramatic improvement. By today, the two modalities show the same diagnostic

T. Tellum (✉)
Department of Gynaecology, Oslo University Hospital, Oslo, Norway
e-mail: tina.tellum@ous-hf.no

E. Oral (ed.), *Endometriosis and Adenomyosis*,
https://doi.org/10.1007/978-3-030-97236-3_34

accuracy for the diagnosis of adenomyosis [1]. As it is more cost-effective and widely available, transvaginal ultrasound is an optimal first-line diagnostic modality to diagnose adenomyosis [2]. However, there are certain situations where ultrasound can fall short. An MRI can be required to discriminate fibroids from adenomyoma or when multiple large fibroids are present. An optimal visualization is especially relevant when uterus-sparing surgery is planned.

As MRI is costly and resource-intensive, there should be a clear clinical consequence resulting from the MRI that cannot be made based on an ultrasound examination alone. When MRI is considered, minimal technical requirements should be met. Also, the assessing radiologist needs to have expertise in gynecological imaging.

34.1.2 Overall Diagnostic Performance of MRI in Adenomyosis Diagnosis

In a structured review and meta-analysis [1], the overall diagnostic performance of MRI resulted in a positive likelihood ratio of 6.8 (95% CI 4.5–10), a negative likelihood ratio of 0.25 (95% CI 0.18–0.35), and an area under the curve (AUC) of 0.77, which is widely classified as a "good clinical test" [3]. The overall sensitivity of MRI for diagnosing adenomyosis was 78% (95% CI 70–84) and the specificity 88% (95% CI 83–92%) [1]. If the reader is not experienced in assessing MRI or adenomyosis, the diagnostic accuracy is likely to be lower. The described diagnostic performance might surprise many clinicians and be lower than expected. Even if the diagnostic qualities of MRI regarding diagnosing adenomyosis might be disappointing for some, one must bear in mind that adenomyosis is not a malignant condition, and therapeutic consequences should largely be determined by clinical factors and symptoms [2].

Also, it is not likely that minimal findings, such as single ectopic endometrial glands, play a significant clinical role [4]. Therefore, it is essential always to correlate clinical findings to imaging findings.

34.2 Uterine Zonal Anatomy in MRI and Adenomyosis

In MRI, a zonal anatomy of the uterus can be identified in T2W (Fig. 34.1) [5, 6]. The differentiation of three zones is relevant for the classification and reporting of adenomyosis [7]. The first and innermost layer is the central (eutopic) endometrium, located in the uterine cavity. It shows a high-intensity signal.

The second layer is a low-intensity signal band in the inner myometrial wall at the endometrial-myometrial junction. This layer is called the junctional zone (JZ), and it plays a central role in adenomyosis diagnosis and pathophysiology. The outer myometrium is the third zone, with an intermediate intensity signal. This outer zone is by some authors divided into the middle myometrium and outer myometrium, the

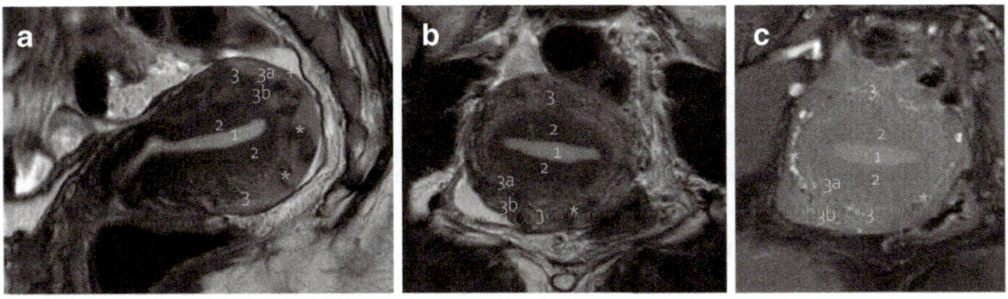

Fig. 34.1 Zonal anatomy of the uterus in MRI. T2W turbo spin echo (**a**, **b**), T1W with fat suppression (**c**), depicting a retroverted uterus of a 38-year-old woman. (**a**) Sagittal plane. (**b**, **c**) Coronal plane. (1) (Eutopic) endometrium, (2) junctional zone (JZ), (3) outer myometrium, (3a) middle myometrium, (3b) outer myometrium. *Arcuate veins. +Uterine serosa

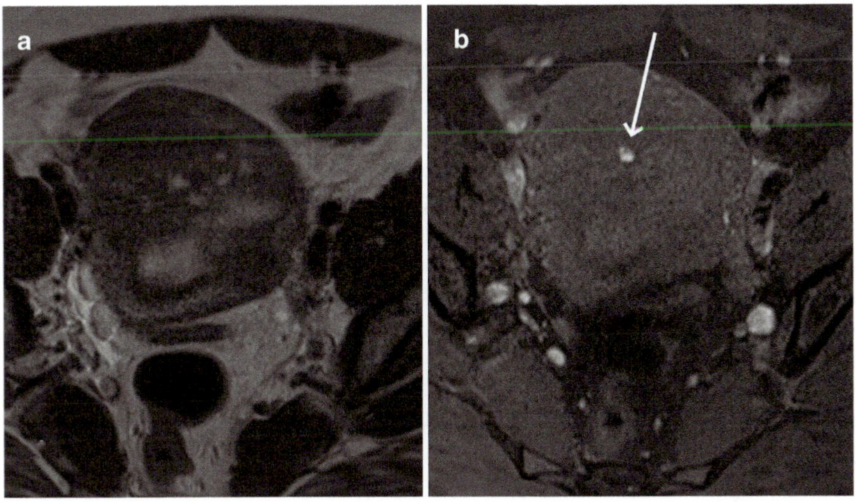

Fig. 34.2 Differences of T2W and T1W MRI in adenomyosis. Axial images of the same uterus in 42-year-old woman. (**a**) T2W sequence, showing several high-intensity signal islets. (**b**) T1W with fat suppression: only one of the ectopic areas as seen on **a** is hemorrhagic (arrow)

latter spanning from the arcuate arteries to the uterine serosa (Fig. 34.1). In T1W images, the zonal anatomy is not visible in the same way (Fig. 34.2). T1W images with fat suppression (FS) depict hemorrhagic content with a high-intensity signal (Fig. 34.2), resulting in a clear visualization of, for example, the arcuate uterine vessels (Fig. 34.1).

34.3 Diagnostic Signs of Adenomyosis in MRI

There are multiple diagnostic signs for adenomyosis. They can be divided into "direct" and "indirect" signs. Direct signs reflect the direct visualization of the ectopic endometrial glands in the myometrium and are pathognomonic for adenomyosis.

Indirect signs consist of morphological changes in the uterine shape and structure, caused by muscular hypertrophy secondarily to adenomyosis.

This division into direct and indirect signs is also used in ultrasound. As MRI depicts direct signs very well, indirect signs play a more subordinate role in diagnosing adenomyosis with MRI. Direct signs are highly specific, but they require a sufficient resolution to be detected. Indirect signs exempt less diagnostic accuracy as other conditions can cause them.

34.3.1 Direct Signs

Visualization of ectopic endometrial tissue is the main criterion for diagnosing adenomyosis on MRI. Ectopic endometrial glands can be displayed as tiny spots (1–3 mm in size), with a high signal on T2-weighted images and a low signal in T1W (Fig. 34.2) [8–11]. Those spots can be located in the junctional zone or disseminated throughout the myometrium. They are often found in ill-demarked areas of low-intensity signal (Figs. 34.3 and 34.5).

In contrast to "spots," larger high-intensity signal foci are either described as "cysts" or "islets." Those can vary in shape and size (Fig. 34.3) [7]. It is not clear if those phenotypes – spots, cysts, and islets – represent different variants of adenomyosis or if they are a continuum (smaller cysts developing to larger islets under certain stimuli). Various size cutoffs and nomenclatures have been suggested for those features. However, so far, there is no unanimous agreement for a precise terminology [12]. This can be the origin of confusion. For example, some authors describe only a phenotypical subtype with huge cysts as "cystic adenomyosis," while others use this term for larger islet as mentioned above [13, 14]. Those very large cysts are also called cystic adenomyoma. Those usually show hemorrhagic content (Fig. 34.4). The term "cystic juvenile adenomyosis" is also used in several publications; however, those might describe cases of accessory and cavitated uterine masses (ACUM) that resemble cystic adenomyosis [15]. ACUM are typically seen within the anterior lateral wall of the myometrium beneath the insertion of the round ligament and become symptomatic early on [16].

In older studies, small high-intensity signal foci were only detected in about half of the cases on T2W images [9, 17], but detection rates of 70% are described in more recent studies [10, 11]. The improvement of spatial resolution is most likely the main reason for this development and emphasizes the importance of technically satisfying image acquisition. An upgrade of MRI sequences and pelvic phased arrays can improve image quality and spatial resolution, namely, by 3D FSE T2W MRI [7].

Some foci of adenomyosis with functional endometrial deposits can contain blood. The iron within hemorrhage causes a shorter T1 and T2 relaxation, making them bright on T1W images and less bright on T2W images (Fig. 34.2).

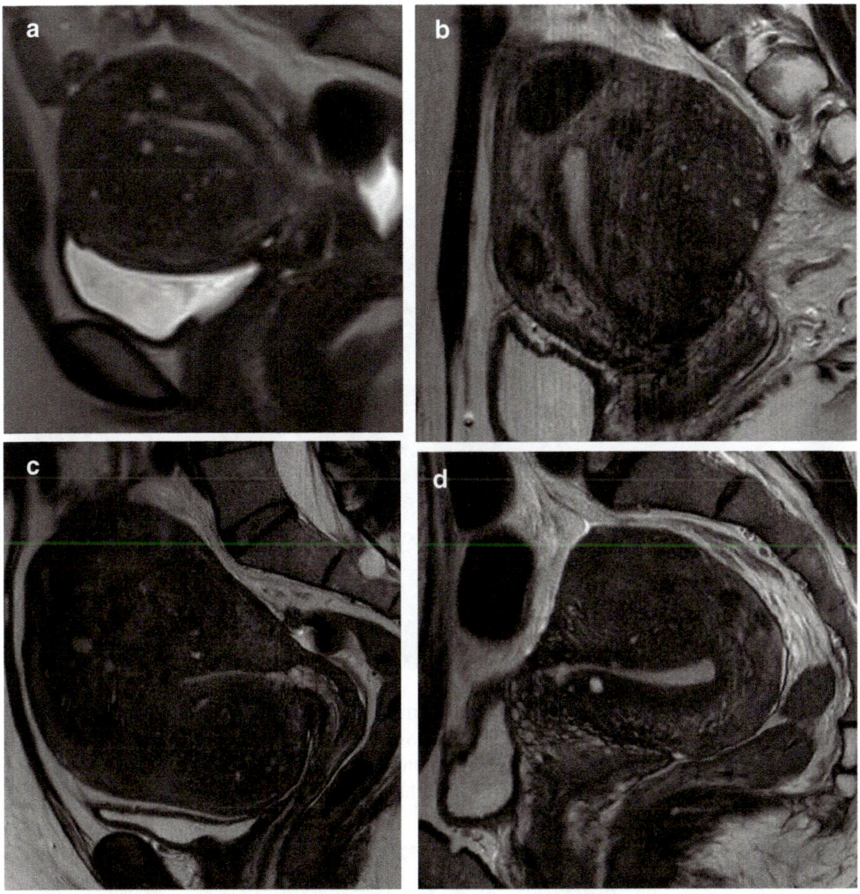

Fig. 34.3 Examples of typical adenomyosis features and adenomyoma. MRI of the uterus in sagittal view, all T2W turbo spin echo. All cases show diffusely demarcated low-intensity signal areas within the myometrium, containing high-intensity signal foci and/or islets. (**a**) Anteverted uterus with asymmetrical thickening of the anterior wall and globular shape. The junctional zone (JZ) is no more visible and almost completely invaded by adenomyosis. (**b**) Adenomyoma in the posterior wall. Several well-defined fibroids with a low signal are visible, which are in contrast to the ill-defined area affected by adenomyosis. Note that the JZ is thin and quite unaffected. (**c**) Grossly enlarged uterus containing no fibroids, only multiple adenomyoma and diffuse adenomyosis. (**d**) Retroverted uterus. A large adenomyoma distorts the anterior wall. The JZ is not thickened and shows smooth outer borders. However, several high signal cysts disrupt the JZ, which is highly suggestive of adenomyosis

34.3.2 Indirect Signs

Pathophysiological processes in adenomyosis can lead to myometrial hypertrophy of the uterus, usually seen as a low-intensity signal area in T2W sequences (Fig. 34.5) [18]. The signal intensity is not unlike some fibroids, but in contrast, adenomyosis lesions usually appear ill-demarked with diffuse borders (Figs. 34.3 and 34.5).

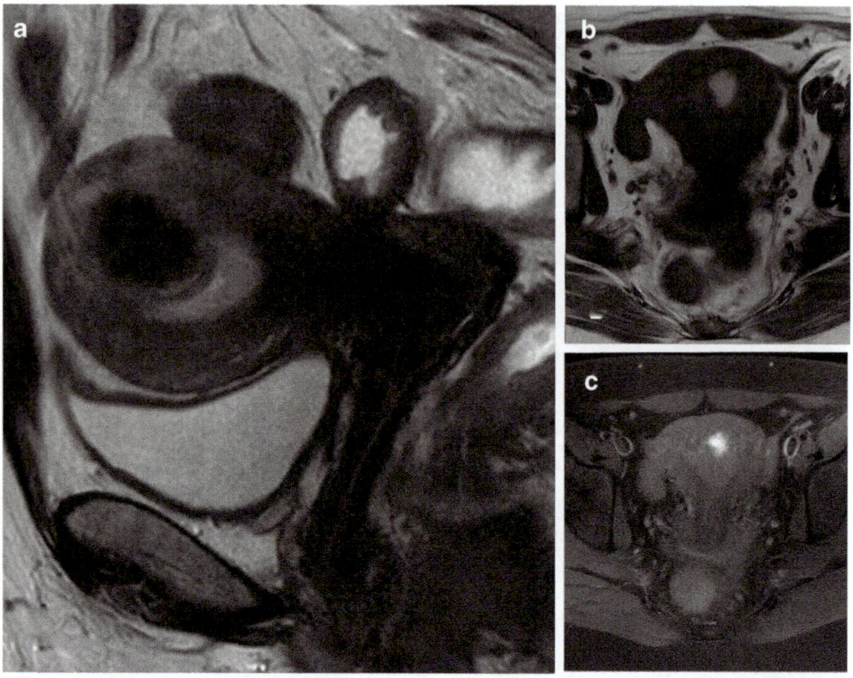

Fig. 34.4 A large cystic adenomyoma with hemorrhagic content. (**a**) T2W turbo spin echo (TSE), sagittal view. (**b**) T1W TSE, axial view. (**c**) T1W TSE with fat suppression. *Note:* small adenomyosis foci were found throughout the myometrium on histopathological examination after hysterectomy, explaining why removal of a cyst alone might not result in symptom relief

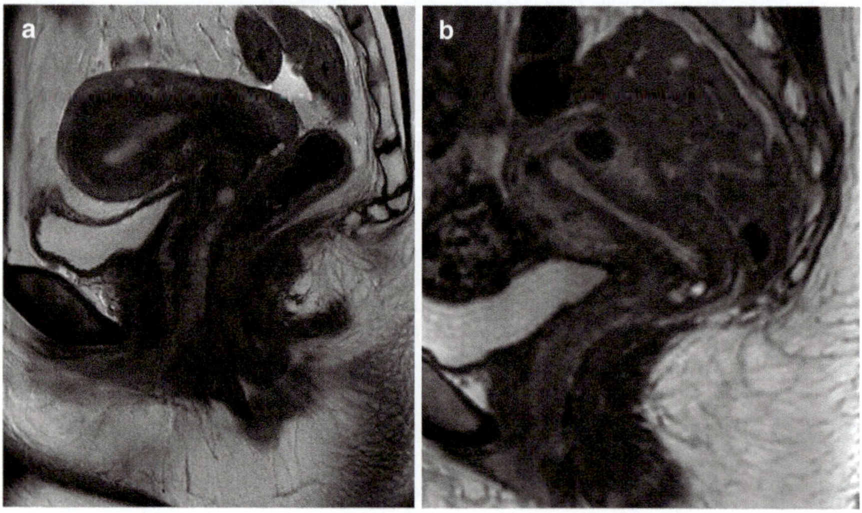

Fig. 34.5 Low-intensity signal areas in T2W images: adenomyosis vs fibroids. (**a**) Diffusely demarcated dark area of adenomyosis representing muscular hypertrophy in the posterior wall, not containing visible glandular structures. (**b**) Multiple, sharply demarcated fibroids throughout the myometrium

Other indirect signs demonstrating adenomyosis affecting the uterus are an enlarged and globular shape and asymmetrical thickening of the anterior and posterior walls (Fig. 34.3a) [10, 11]. Note that those shape changes do not always result in gross enlargement of the uterus (Fig. 34.5). However, indirect signs are more commonly used for the diagnosis by ultrasound and have a subordinate role in MRI as myometrial changes (direct and indirect) are usually more apparent in MRI, as demonstrated in the figures.

In the presence of multiple or large fibroids, indirect signs are usually not very well assessable. Also, there are no clearly defined cutoffs for myometrial thickness, ratios for myometrial asymmetry, or metric definition of globularity. Indirect signs have therefore to be assessed by subjective pattern recognition, requiring experience.

34.3.3 Alterations in the Junctional Zone

As described above, the JZ is depicted as a low-intensity signal band in T2W (Fig. 34.1). The JZ plays a central role in uterine function, for example, embryo implantation and transport and menstrual flow. Interestingly, it is not apparent what the JZ structurally represents, as it is not visible in formalin fixated specimen [19–21].

A JZ thickness measuring ≥12 mm has been used as a diagnostic marker for adenomyosis since it was first described in 1996 [22]. Also, various cutoffs for the ratio of JZ to wall thickness were described as diagnostic markers [10]. However, recent research has questioned if this is still valid with high-resolution MRI and a younger population [11]. While seemingly objective metric markers are very appealing to the investigating specialist, the JZ thickness cutoff of 12 mm has been developed on populations including a large proportion of postmenopausal women and women with endometrial cancer [9, 22]. When validated on a younger, premenopausal population, the correlation of JZ thickness with adenomyosis diagnosis could not be confirmed [11]. Therefore, caution is advised when diagnosing adenomyosis in younger women [7].

Rather than measuring the JZ thickness, it is advised to evaluate irregularities of the JZ indicating adenomyosis [7, 11]. Those can present themself in different shapes, for example, as high-intensity signal finger-like indentations at the endometrial-myometrial border in T2W (Figs. 34.1b and 34.3d) or as spots and cysts in the JZ [11]. Those findings represent the invasion of the endometrium into the myometrium and have a diagnostic specificity of 83% for adenomyosis [11].

Physiological thickening of the junctional zone can occur in line with uterine contractions and is also part of the menstrual cycle and represents a diagnostic pitfall [2, 7]. Also, hormonal treatment such as oral contraceptives, progestins, and gonadotropin-releasing hormone agonists can change the appearance of the junctional zone. A partial volume effect with the JZ not being depicted orthogonally to the cavity but tangentially can also mimic a focal thickening of the junctional zone. This pitfall can be avoided by proper angulation of the sequences.

On the other hand, adenomyosis only affecting the outer layers of the uterus, leaving the JZ intact, is also described. A normal junctional zone alone does, therefore, not confirm the absence of adenomyosis (Fig. 34.3).

In summary, a thickening of the JZ might be physiological or due to other pathologies. It is not suited to be used as a diagnostic sign alone, regardless of the thickness.

34.3.4 Adenomyoma

Especially when surgical removal is planned, the consequences of misdiagnosing adenomyoma as a fibroid can be fatal. Adenomyoma are myometrial masses that are hypointense on T2-weighted MRI (Fig. 34.3). They are usually more ill-defined than fibroids but can, in some cases, appear relatively circumscribed (Figs. 34.3b and 34.5). Adenomyoma virtually always contain high-intensity signal foci on T2W, which helps differentiate them from fibroids [23, 24]. Some authors use the terms adenomyoma and "focal adenomyosis" synonymously. Given the lack of a unanimous terminology for adenomyosis, it is essential to describe imaging findings in detail to avoid misunderstandings between the radiologist and the clinician.

34.4 Technical Requirements

Conventional 2D TSE-T2-weighted MR sequences in the sagittal and axial oblique plane, as well as T1W images with fat suppression, are the minimum requirements for diagnosing adenomyosis and are recommended by most authors [7]. When the slice thickness and intersection gap are set too wide, focal findings might be overlooked. As MRI should not be (mis)used as a diagnostic screening tool, a high image quality with a slice thickness of 1–2 mm should be considered when first utilizing this modality. Breath-hold T2-weighted sequences or 3D FSE T2-weighted MRI can optimize the image accuracy further [25].

The administration of spasmolytic agents is recommended to minimize bowel movement and prevent artifacts. Glucagon and butylscopolamine, commonly used spasmolytic substances, have different properties, but there is no evidence for the superiority of one agent to the other in diagnosing adenomyosis.

There is no reported benefit for the administration of gadolinium contrast or diffusion-weighted imaging in diagnosing adenomyosis [7, 26]. However, intravenous contrast might be beneficial when diagnosing endometriosis, a condition that frequently coexists with adenomyosis and, therefore, might be clinically relevant.

References

1. Tellum T, Nygaard S, Lieng M. Noninvasive diagnosis of adenomyosis: a structured review and meta-analysis of diagnostic accuracy in imaging. J Minim Invasive Gynecol. 2020;27(2):408–18.
2. Chapron C, Vannuccini S, Santulli P, Abrão MS, Carmona F, Fraser IS, et al. Diagnosing adenomyosis: an integrated clinical and imaging approach. Hum Reprod Update. 2020;26(3): 392–411.

3. McGee S. Simplifying likelihood ratios. J Gen Intern Med. 2002;17(8):646–9.
4. Naftalin J, Hoo W, Nunes N, Holland T, Mavrelos D, Jurkovic D. Association between ultrasound features of adenomyosis and severity of menstrual pain. Ultrasound Obstet Gynecol. 2016;47(6):779–83.
5. Mitchell DG, Schonholz L, Hilpert PL, Pennell RG, Blum L, Rifkin MD. Zones of the uterus: discrepancy between US and MR images. Radiology. 1990;174(3 Pt 1):827–31.
6. Turnbull LW, Manton DJ, Horsman A, Killick SR. Magnetic resonance imaging changes in uterine zonal anatomy during a conception cycle. Br J Obstet Gynaecol. 1995;102(4):330–1.
7. Bazot M, Darai E. Role of transvaginal sonography and magnetic resonance imaging in the diagnosis of uterine adenomyosis. Fertil Steril. 2018;109(3):389–97.
8. Tamai K, Togashi K, Ito T, Morisawa N, Fujiwara T, Koyama T. MR imaging findings of adenomyosis: correlation with histopathologic features and diagnostic pitfalls. Radiographics. 2005;25(1):21–40.
9. Bazot M, Cortez A, Darai E, Rouger J, Chopier J, Antoine JM, et al. Ultrasonography compared with magnetic resonance imaging for the diagnosis of adenomyosis: correlation with histopathology. Hum Reprod (Oxf, Engl). 2001;16(11):2427–33.
10. Dueholm M, Lundorf E, Hansen ES, Sorensen JS, Ledertoug S, Olesen F. Magnetic resonance imaging and transvaginal ultrasonography for the diagnosis of adenomyosis. Fertil Steril. 2001;76(3):588–94.
11. Tellum T, Matic GV, Dormagen JB, Nygaard S, Viktil E, Qvigstad E, et al. Diagnosing adenomyosis with MRI: a prospective study revisiting the junctional zone thickness cutoff of 12 mm as a diagnostic marker. Eur Radiol. 2019;29(12):6971–81.
12. Munro MG. Classification and reporting systems for adenomyosis. J Minim Invasive Gynecol. 2020;27(2):296–308.
13. Gordts S, Campo R, Brosens I. Hysteroscopic diagnosis and excision of myometrial cystic adenomyosis. Gynecol Surg. 2014;11(4):273–8.
14. Pontrelli G, Bounous VE, Scarperi S, Minelli L, Di Spiezio Sardo A, Florio P. Rare case of giant cystic adenomyoma mimicking a uterine malformation, diagnosed and treated by hysteroscopy. J Obstet Gynaecol Res. 2015;41(8):1300–4.
15. Brosens I, Gordts S, Habiba M, Benagiano G. Uterine cystic adenomyosis: a disease of younger women. J Pediatr Adolesc Gynecol. 2015;28(6):420–6.
16. Naftalin J, Bean E, Saridogan E, Barton-Smith P, Arora R, Jurkovic D. Imaging in gynecological disease: clinical and ultrasound characteristics of accessory cavitated uterine malformations. Ultrasound Obstet Gynecol. 2021;57(5):821–8.
17. Reinhold C, Tafazoli F, Mehio A, Wang L, Atri M, Siegelman ES, et al. Uterine adenomyosis: endovaginal US and MR imaging features with histopathologic correlation. Radiographics. 1999;19 Spec No:S147–60.
18. Tamai K, Koyama T, Umeoka S, Saga T, Fujii S, Togashi K. Spectrum of MR features in adenomyosis. Best Pract Res Clin Obstet Gynaecol. 2006;20(4):583–602.
19. Lee JK, Gersell DJ, Balfe DM, Worthington JL, Picus D, Gapp G. The uterus: in vitro MR-anatomic correlation of normal and abnormal specimens. Radiology. 1985;157(1):175–9.
20. Demas BE, Hricak H, Jaffe RB. Uterine MR imaging: effects of hormonal stimulation. Radiology. 1986;159(1):123–6.
21. Brown HK, Stoll BS, Nicosia SV, Fiorica JV, Hambley PS, Clarke LP, et al. Uterine junctional zone: correlation between histologic findings and MR imaging. Radiology. 1991;179(2):409–13.
22. Reinhold C, McCarthy S, Bret PM, Mehio A, Atri M, Zakarian R, et al. Diffuse adenomyosis: comparison of endovaginal US and MR imaging with histopathologic correlation. Radiology. 1996;199(1):151–8.
23. Byun JY, Kim SE, Choi BG, Ko GY, Jung SE, Choi KH. Diffuse and focal adenomyosis: MR imaging findings. Radiographics. 1999;19 Spec No:S161–70.
24. Song SE, Sung DJ, Park BJ, Kim MJ, Cho SB, Kim KA. MR imaging features of uterine adenomyomas. Abdom Imaging. 2011;36(4):483–8.

25. Bazot M, Darai E, Clement de Givry S, Boudghene F, Uzan S, Le Blanche AF. Fast breath-hold T2-weighted MR imaging reduces interobserver variability in the diagnosis of adenomyosis. AJR Am J Roentgenol. 2003;180(5):1291–6.
26. Agostinho L, Cruz R, Osorio F, Alves J, Setubal A, Guerra A. MRI for adenomyosis: a pictorial review. Insights Imaging. 2017;8(6):549–56.

Adenomyosis in Adolescence

35

Harald Krentel and Maribel Acien

Contents

A recently published retrospective population-based cohort study describes the age-related incidence of adenomyosis by analyzing ICD codes from 2006 to 2015 [1]. The study design presumes the correct diagnosis and recording of adenomyosis in the respective healthcare system. Although there is a growing awareness for adenomyosis, the disease still is underestimated as a possible cause for dysmenorrhea, dyspareunia, pelvic pain, and bleeding disorders, and the knowledge about adenomyosis in general is limited and minimal in the subgroup of female adolescents. Up to two-thirds of adolescent women report painful menstruation [2]. It is probable that a high number of unreported cases of adenomyosis in teen girls exist. The base for a plausible incidence rate of adenomyosis in fertile women and adolescents is a reliable diagnostic approach, which so far does not exist.

The original version of the chapter has been revised. A correction to this chapter can be found at https://doi.org/10.1007/978-3-030-97236-3_45

H. Krentel (✉)
Clinic of Gynecology, Obstetrics, Gynecological Oncology and Senology, Academic Teaching Hospital, Bethesda Hospital, Duisburg, Germany
e-mail: h.krentel@bethesda.de

M. Acien
Department of Obstetrics and Gynecology, San Juan University Hospital, Miguel Hernández University, Alicante, Spain

E. Oral (ed.), *Endometriosis and Adenomyosis*,
https://doi.org/10.1007/978-3-030-97236-3_35

35.1 Diagnosis of Adenomyosis in Adolescents

Currently, the diagnosis of adenomyosis is possible combining accurate anamnesis, gynecological examination, and transvaginal two-dimensional and three-dimensional ultrasound. MR imaging, power Doppler ultrasound, and sonographic elastography can be used as additional diagnostic tools [3]. In a 10-year meta-analysis, a pooled sensitivity of 83.8% and specificity of 63.9% of two-dimensional transvaginal ultrasound have been reported. The study described the ultrasound feature heterogeneous myometrium as the most sensitive sign and globular uterine enlargement as the most specific sign [4]. Similar studies reported comparable results regarding the overall accuracy of the method but showed a high variation of the typical relevant ultrasound features [5] in adenomyosis such as linear striation, question mark sign, myometrial cysts, or subendometrial microcysts (Fig. 35.1). The problem currently is that a score system on typical diagnostic features does not exist. And it is not yet known if the presence of special ultrasound features or the combination of those sonographic signs is more likely to predict adenomyosis. So far, the accuracy of the diagnosis adenomyosis completely depends on the experience of the sonographer and/or radiologist, the technical equipment, and the individual estimation of the diagnostic result. Usually, the suspicion of a disease diagnosed by imaging (e.g., breast tumor) can be proven by a biopsy of the suspicious lesion. In case of adenomyosis, a biopsy can be obtained by hysteroscopy [6], by laparoscopy [7], and by transvaginal or transcutaneous puncture [8]. Unfortunately, the sensitivity and specificity of these partly surgical techniques are not satisfying and therefore cannot be used as a standard. Recent guidelines do not recommend uterine biopsy in suspicion of adenomyosis [9]. A recent publication reports the detection of adenomyosis by transvaginal ultrasound in 5.2% of a group of 270 adolescent women examined in a university hospital setting. The overall detection rate of ultrasound signs of endometriosis was higher in patients with dysmenorrhea and dyspareunia compared to patients without symptoms [10]. However,

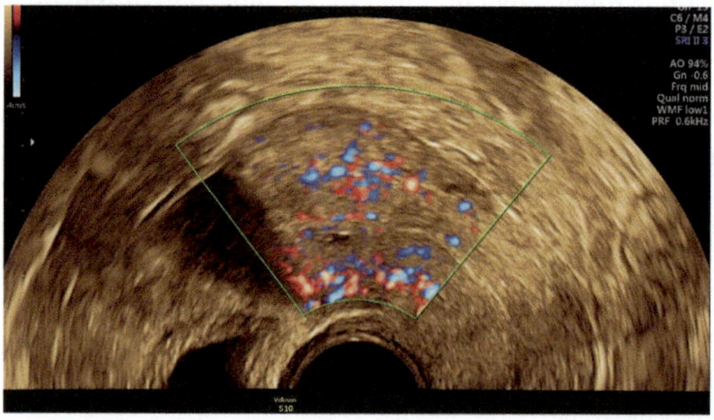

Fig. 35.1 Transvaginal ultrasound image of the uterus showing a subendometrial microcyst in adenomyosis. The additional colored Doppler sonography helps to distinguish blood vessels (*blue* and *red color*) from microcysts with no color signal. The shape and size of the uterus are normal. (With permission © H. Krentel, all rights reserved)

the detection rate of the typical ultrasound features of adenomyosis in adolescents might be more difficult compared to older fertile women. The diagnosis of adenomyosis by transvaginal ultrasound and the retrieval of a significant biopsy might be more challenging in adolescents.

The most important diagnostic sign in MR imaging seems to be the irregularity of the junctional zone. Other typical findings are low signal intensity areas in the myometrium and spots with high signal intensity in the T2-weighted technique [11, 12]. The accuracy of transvaginal ultrasound and MR imaging in the detection of adenomyosis has been described as comparable. The role of MR imaging in adolescents with assumed adenomyosis should be further investigated. Another clinical sign for the presence of adenomyosis in adolescents with dysmenorrhea and/or pelvic pain can be the persistence of symptoms after exclusion or excision of peritoneal endometriosis by laparoscopy.

35.2 Juvenile Cystic Adenomyomas

This entity, often reported as juvenile or isolated cystic adenomyomas in the literature, has been suggested to correspond to accessory and cavitated uterine masses (ACUM) with a functional endometrium [13]. Thus, a Müllerian anomaly possibly related to a dysfunction of the female gubernaculum [14].

An ACUM is a rare pathology, observed in young women (mostly under 30 years), who has significant clinical manifestations, particularly severe dysmenorrhea that has been progressive since menarche and recurrent pelvic pain that persists during the premenstrual and postmenstrual periods and does not respond to common analgesics. The differential diagnosis is broad including rudimentary and cavitated uterine horns, adenomyosis with cystic or degenerated areas, degenerated leiomyomas, and essential and primary dysmenorrhea. The criteria used to diagnose a case as an ACUM (Fig. 35.2) are (i) an isolated accessory cavitated mass or a couple, in the same lateral area of the uterus, typically located at the level of insertion of the round ligament; (ii) most likely a normal uterus with normal endometrial

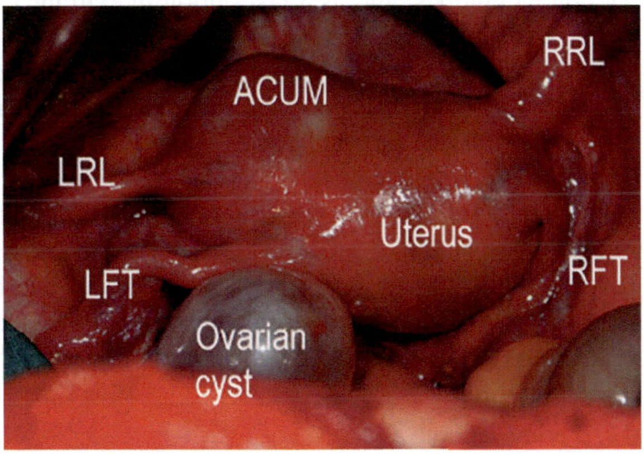

Fig. 35.2 Internal genitalia of the patient showing a left ACUM under the insertion of round ligament. ACUM accessory and cavitated uterine mass, LRL left round ligament, RRL right round ligament, LFT left fallopian tube, RFT right fallopian tube. (Taken from Acién et al. [15], with permission)

lumen, Fallopian tubes, and ovaries; (iii) an accessory cavity lined by endometrial epithelium with glands and stroma; (iv) a chocolate brown-colored fluid content; and (v) absence of adenomyosis or adenomyotic cysts in the remainder of the uterus, although there could be small foci of adenomyosis in the myometrium adjacent to the accessory cavity [15].

Adenomyomas and cystic adenomyosis are more characteristic of older women, who develop adenomyosis spread anywhere inside the uterine corpus, and the cysts frequently exhibit the absence of an internal epithelial lining. The diagnosis of an ACUM should be definitive once the mass has been excised and a pathological examination has been performed.

35.3 Surgical Treatment of Adenomyosis in Adolescents

The diagnosis of adenomyosis in adolescents is difficult, and the value of transvaginal ultrasound results and findings in MR imaging requires further investigation. But what would be the benefit of a safe diagnosis and histological proof of adenomyosis in adolescents? Would the early stage diagnosis change the treatment of teen girls with dysmenorrhea, dyspareunia, and/or pelvic pain? A standardized and evidence-based treatment of adenomyosis does not exist. Different medical and surgical treatment approaches are able to reduce symptoms and to increase fertility. The course of action depends on the family planning status of the patient.

Surgical treatment of adenomyosis is feasible in focal or cystic adenomyosis and can be an option in diffuse adenomyosis. The hysteroscopic and laparoscopic resection of cystic lesions has been reported in a variety of publications [16, 17]. In adolescents, juvenile cystic adenomyosis has been described including the surgical techniques of minimally invasive resection [18]. Endometrial lined myometrial cysts have been described as almost specific in adolescents and young women in a literature review [19]. However, these cases are very rare, and a surgical intervention requires a detailed informed consent and should be realized in a specialized center. Surgical resection of adenomyosis might be an option in symptomatic adolescent patients, patients with infertility despite assisted reproduction techniques, and as a last option in extreme cases (Fig. 35.3). The effect of surgery on fertility needs to be proven, so far surgery does not represent an evidence-based approach [20]. Especially in adolescents, risky surgical procedures should be avoided as they are related to a variety of complications and risks, like uterine rupture, intrauterine and intraperitoneal adhesions, and irregular placentation. High-intensity focused ultrasound (HIFU) and radiofrequency ablation may be possible alternatives for the treatment of adenomyosis in adolescents. Both techniques provide symptom relief and a low rate of complications. Recent studies describe a high conception and live birth rate after HIFU [21]. Both interventions seem to be an alternative in the treatment of small myometrial adenomyotic lesions. However, the feasibility and long-term outcome should be further investigated.

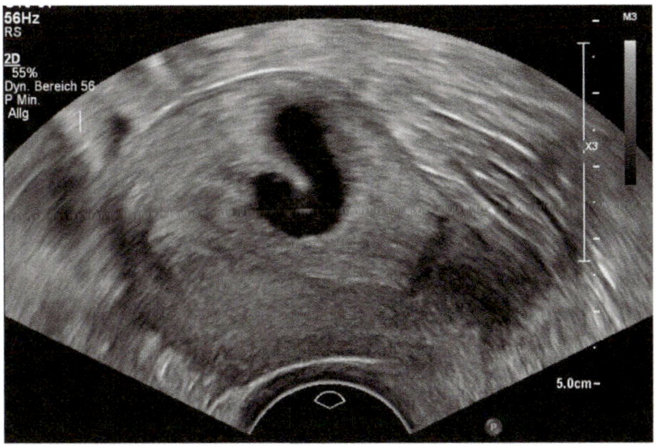

Fig. 35.3 Transvaginal ultrasound image of an intramural cystic adenomyosis in patient with ongoing family planning. (With permission © H. Krentel, all rights reserved)

35.4 Medical Treatment of Adenomyosis in Adolescents

All available suppressive hormonal treatments are able to reduce symptoms by reduction of adenomyosis. None of the medical treatment options is especially licensed for the specific treatment of adenomyosis. In adolescents, mostly oral contraceptives are used as treatment of first choice in case of painful menstruation. Combined oral contraceptives show a pain reduction but are related to bleeding disorders as main adverse effect. Progestins also can reduce pain but are related to dermatological side effects, libido reduction, and undesirable effects on body mass index. Dienogest is able to reduce adenomyosis-related dysmenorrhea and pain but is related with a risk of uterine bleeding in patients with adenomyosis [22]. This adverse effect has been reported in different publications [23, 24] and caused heavy bleedings in some cases [25]. The side effects cause a risk of treatment discontinuation especially in very young patients [26].

Another medical treatment option is the use of GnRH agonists or antagonists. The efficacy of GnRH agonists in adolescents with refractory chronic pelvic pain, failed therapy with combined oral contraceptives, and positive MR imaging has been recently reported. The treatment improved symptoms and caused regression of the lesions [27]. The efficacy of the treatment with levonorgestrel intrauterine device (LNG-IUD) in adenomyosis has also been shown in a variety of publications [28]. The use of LNG-IUD in adenomyosis represents a direct application of a hormonal treatment to the site of the disease. This treatment is able to reduce symptoms and menstrual blood loss. However, the spontaneous expulsion rate is higher in patients with adenomyosis and seems to be related to the insertion technique, the placement timing, and the type and size of the intrauterine device [29, 30]. The efficacy and safety of low-dose LNG-IUDs in the treatment of adolescent patients with adenomyosis need to be element of randomized trials.

The ideal medical treatment option in adolescents with adenomyosis guarantees a protective long-term effect with low complication rate. So far, the choice in daily practice needs to be individual and might be combined with interventional and surgical solutions. The detection of an abnormal menstrual pain by a regular assessment of adolescents' menstrual cycles should be the first diagnostic step [2]. Evidence-based treatment guidelines for adolescent patients with dysmenorrhea, dyspareunia, and pelvic pain and the suspicion of adenomyosis are needed in order to avoid overestimation or underestimation and overtreatment or undertreatment of the disease [31].

35.5 Conclusion

The meaning of an early diagnosis of the disease adenomyosis in adolescents is the preservation of the integrity of the uterus and the prevention of adenomyosis- and treatment-related harm of the central reproductive organ combined to an effective treatment of the symptoms. Prospective randomized trials are needed to describe the ideal combination of medical, interventional, and surgical treatment in order to reduce symptoms and maintain the uterine physiology in adolescent women.

References

1. Yu O, Schulze-Rath R, Grafton J, Hansen K, Scholes D, Reed SD. Adenomyosis incidence, prevalence and treatment: United States population-based study 2006–2015. Am J Obstet Gynecol. 2020;223(1):94.e1–10. https://doi.org/10.1016/j.ajog.2020.01.016. Epub 2020 Jan 15. PMID: 31954156.
2. Myszko O, Al-Husayni N, Talib HJ. Painful periods in the adolescent girl. Pediatr Ann. 2020;49(4):e176–82. https://doi.org/10.3928/19382359-20200318-01. PMID: 32275762.
3. Krentel H, Cezar C, Becker S, Di Spiezio Sardo A, Tanos V, Wallwiener M, De Wilde RL. From clinical symptoms to MR imaging: diagnostic steps in adenomyosis. Biomed Res Int. 2017;2017:1514029. https://doi.org/10.1155/2017/1514029. Epub 2017 Dec 4. PMID: 29349064; PMCID: PMC5733957.
4. Andres MP, Borrelli GM, Ribeiro J, Baracat EC, Abrão MS, Kho RM. Transvaginal ultrasound for the diagnosis of adenomyosis: systematic review and meta-analysis. J Minim Invasive Gynecol. 2018;25(2):257–64. https://doi.org/10.1016/j.jmig.2017.08.653. Epub 2017 Aug 30. PMID: 28864044.
5. Bazot M, Daraï E. Role of transvaginal sonography and magnetic resonance imaging in the diagnosis of uterine adenomyosis. Fertil Steril. 2018;109(3):389–97. https://doi.org/10.1016/j.fertnstert.2018.01.024. PMID: 29566851.
6. Dakhly DM, Abdel Moety GA, Saber W, Gad Allah SH, Hashem AT, Abdel Salam LO. Accuracy of hysteroscopic endomyometrial biopsy in diagnosis of adenomyosis. J Minim Invasive Gynecol. 2016;23(3):364–71. https://doi.org/10.1016/j.jmig.2015.11.004. Epub 2015 Nov 12. PMID: 26581187.
7. Jeng CJ, Huang SH, Shen J, Chou CS, Tzeng CR. Laparoscopy-guided myometrial biopsy in the definite diagnosis of diffuse adenomyosis. Hum Reprod. 2007;22(7):2016–9. https://doi.org/10.1093/humrep/dem084. Epub 2007 Apr 11. PMID: 17428879.
8. Movilla P, Morris S, Isaacson K. A systematic review of tissue sampling techniques for the diagnosis of adenomyosis. J Minim Invasive Gynecol. 2020;27(2):344–51. https://doi.org/10.1016/j.jmig.2019.09.001. Epub 2019 Sep 6. PMID: 31499191.
9. Burghaus S, Schäfer SD, Beckmann MW, Brandes I, Brünahl C, Chvatal R, Drahonovsky J, Dudek W, Ebert A, Fahlbusch C, Fehm T, Fehr PM, Hack CC, Häuser W, Hancke K, Heinecke V, Horn LC, Houbois C, Klapp C, Kramer H, Krentel H, Langrehr J, Matuschewski H, Mayer

I, Mechsner S, Müller A, Müller A, Müller M, Oppelt P, Papathemelis T, Renner SP, Schmidt D, Schüring A, Schweppe KW, Seeber B, Siedentopf F, Sirbu H, Soeffge D, Weidner K, Zraik I, Ulrich UA. Diagnostic and therapy of endometriosis. Guideline of the DGGG, SGGG and OEGGG (S2k-Level, AWMF-Registry Number 015/045, August 2020.
10. Martire FG, Lazzeri L, Conway F, Siciliano T, Pietropolli A, Piccione E, Solima E, Centini G, Zupi E, Exacoustos C. Adolescence and endometriosis: symptoms, ultrasound signs and early diagnosis. Fertil Steril. 2020;114(5):1049–57. https://doi.org/10.1016/j.fertnstert.2020.06.012. Epub 2020 Oct 6. PMID: 33036795.
11. Bazot M, Cortez A, Darai E, Rouger J, Chopier J, Antoine JM, Uzan S. Ultrasonography compared with magnetic resonance imaging for the diagnosis of adenomyosis: correlation with histopathology. Hum Reprod. 2001;16(11):2427–33. https://doi.org/10.1093/humrep/16.11.2427. PMID: 11679533.
12. Novellas S, Chassang M, Delotte J, Toullalan O, Chevallier A, Bouaziz J, Chevallier P. MRI characteristics of the uterine junctional zone: from normal to the diagnosis of adenomyosis. AJR Am J Roentgenol. 2011;196(5):1206–13. https://doi.org/10.2214/AJR.10.4877. PMID: 21512093.
13. Acién P, Acién M, Fernández F, José Mayol M, Aranda I. The cavitated accessory uterine mass: a Müllerian anomaly in women with an otherwise normal uterus. Obstet Gynecol. 2010;116(5):1101–9. https://doi.org/10.1097/AOG.0b013e3181f7e735. PMID: 20966695.
14. Acién P, Sánchez del Campo F, Mayol MJ, Acién M. The female gubernaculum: role in the embryology and development of the genital tract and in the possible genesis of malformations. Eur J Obstet Gynecol Reprod Biol. 2011;159(2):426–32. https://doi.org/10.1016/j.ejogrb.2011.07.040. PMID: 21831509.
15. Acién P, Bataller A, Fernández F, Acién M, Rodríguez JM, Mayol MJ. New cases of accessory and cavitated uterine masses (ACUM): a significant cause of severe dysmenorrhea and recurrent pelvic pain in young women. Hum Reprod. 2012;27(3):683–94. https://doi.org/10.1093/humrep/der471. PMID: 22252088.
16. Dueholm M. Minimally invasive treatment of adenomyosis. Best Pract Res Clin Obstet Gynaecol. 2018;51:119–37. https://doi.org/10.1016/j.bpobgyn.2018.01.016. Epub 2018 Feb 15. PMID: 29555380.
17. Gordts S, Campo R, Brosens I. Hysteroscopic diagnosis and excision of myometrial cystic adenomyosis. Gynecol Surg. 2014;11(4):273–8. https://doi.org/10.1007/s10397-014-0861-5. Epub 2014 Oct 3. PMID: 25419204; PMCID: PMC4237909.
18. Protopapas A, Kypriotis K, Chatzipapas I, Kathopoulis N, Sotiropoulou M, Michala L. Juvenile cystic adenomyoma vs blind uterine horn: challenges in the diagnosis and surgical management. J Pediatr Adolesc Gynecol. 2020;33(6):735–8. https://doi.org/10.1016/j.jpag.2020.08.010. Epub 2020 Aug 20. PMID: 32827760.
19. Brosens I, Gordts S, Habiba M, Benagiano G. Uterine cystic adenomyosis: a disease of younger women. J Pediatr Adolesc Gynecol. 2015;28(6):420–6. https://doi.org/10.1016/j.jpag.2014.05.008. Epub 2014 May 28. PMID: 26049940.
20. Dueholm M. Uterine adenomyosis and infertility, review of reproductive outcome after in vitro fertilization and surgery. Acta Obstet Gynecol Scand. 2017;96(6):715–26. https://doi.org/10.1111/aogs.13158. PMID: 28556124.
21. Zhang L, Rao F, Setzen R. High intensity focused ultrasound for the treatment of adenomyosis: selection criteria, efficacy, safety and fertility. Acta Obstet Gynecol Scand. 2017;96(6):707–14. https://doi.org/10.1111/aogs.13159. PMID: 28437003.
22. Osuga Y, Hayashi K, Kanda S. Long-term use of dienogest for the treatment of primary and secondary dysmenorrhea. J Obstet Gynaecol Res. 2020;46(4):606–17. https://doi.org/10.1111/jog.14209. Epub 2020 Feb 12. PMID: 32050307.
23. Nirgianakis K, Vaineau C, Agliati L, McKinnon B, Gasparri ML, Mueller MD. Risk factors for non-response and discontinuation of Dienogest in endometriosis patients: a cohort study. Acta Obstet Gynecol Scand. 2021;100(1):30–40. https://doi.org/10.1111/aogs.13969. Epub 2020 Sep 18. PMID: 32767677.

24. Matsubara S, Kawaguchi R, Akinishi M, Nagayasu M, Iwai K, Niiro E, Yamada Y, Tanase Y, Kobayashi H. Subtype I (intrinsic) adenomyosis is an independent risk factor for dienogest-related serious unpredictable bleeding in patients with symptomatic adenomyosis. Sci Rep. 2019;9(1):17654. https://doi.org/10.1038/s41598-019-54096-z. PMID: 31776404; PMCID: PMC6881344.
25. Nishino K, Hayashi K, Chaya J, Kato N, Yamamuro O. Effective salvage of acute massive uterine bleeding using intrauterine balloon tamponade in a uterine adenomyosis patient on dienogest. J Obstet Gynaecol Res. 2013;39(3):738–41. https://doi.org/10.1111/j.1447-0756.2012.02005.x. Epub 2012 Sep 25. PMID: 23003209.
26. Nagata C, Yanagida S, Okamoto A, Morikawa A, Sugimoto K, Okamoto S, Ochiai K, Tanaka T. Risk factors of treatment discontinuation due to uterine bleeding in adenomyosis patients treated with dienogest. J Obstet Gynaecol Res. 2012;38(4):639–44. https://doi.org/10.1111/j.1447-0756.2011.01778.x. Epub 2012 Mar 13. PMID: 22413833.
27. Mansouri R, Santos XM, Bercaw-Pratt JL, Dietrich JE. Regression of adenomyosis on magnetic resonance imaging after a course of hormonal suppression in adolescents: a case series. J Pediatr Adolesc Gynecol. 2015;28(6):437–40. https://doi.org/10.1016/j.jpag.2014.12.009. Epub 2014 Dec 29. PMID: 26233288.
28. Imai A, Matsunami K, Takagi H, Ichigo S. Levonorgestrel-releasing intrauterine device used for dysmenorrhea: five-year literature review. Clin Exp Obstet Gynecol. 2014;41(5):495–8. PMID: 25864246.
29. Park DS, Kim ML, Song T, Yun BS, Kim MK, Jun HS, Seong SJ. Clinical experiences of the levonorgestrel-releasing intrauterine system in patients with large symptomatic adenomyosis. Taiwan J Obstet Gynecol. 2015;54(4):412–5. https://doi.org/10.1016/j.tjog.2014.05.009. PMID: 26384061.
30. Youm J, Lee HJ, Kim SK, Kim H, Jee BC. Factors affecting the spontaneous expulsion of the levonorgestrel-releasing intrauterine system. Int J Gynaecol Obstet. 2014;126(2):165–9. https://doi.org/10.1016/j.ijgo.2014.02.017. Epub 2014 Apr 18. PMID: 24825498.
31. Hung YC, Westfal ML, Chang DC, Kelleher CM. Lack of data-driven treatment guidelines and wide variation in management of chronic pelvic pain in adolescents and young adults. J Pediatr Adolesc Gynecol. 2020;33(4):349–53.e1. https://doi.org/10.1016/j.jpag.2020.03.009. Epub 2020 Apr 4. PMID: 32259629.

Adenomyosis in Reproductive Years: Abnormal Uterine Bleeding and Pain

36

Yasushi Hirota and Yutaka Osuga

Contents

36.1 Introduction

Adenomyosis is defined as a disease in which endometrial-like glandular epithelium and stromal tissue develop in the myometrium. Although the pathological diagnosis according to the above definition requires surgical removal of the uterus or the lesions, recent advances in image diagnostic technology such as magnetic resonance imaging (MRI) and ultrasonography enable us to make accurate diagnosis of adenomyosis without surgery. Based on the improvement of image diagnosis in adenomyosis, there are accumulating evidence about the efficacy and adverse effects of medical treatment for the symptom of adenomyosis according to the condition of adenomyosis. Two major symptoms of adenomyosis are pain and

The original version of the chapter has been revised. A correction to this chapter can be found at https://doi.org/10.1007/978-3-030-97236-3_45

Y. Hirota (✉) · Y. Osuga
Department of Obstetrics and Gynecology, Graduate School of Medicine, The University of Tokyo, Tokyo, Japan

E. Oral (ed.), *Endometriosis and Adenomyosis*,
https://doi.org/10.1007/978-3-030-97236-3_36

Table 36.1 Major symptoms of adenomyosis

Symptom	Details
Pain	Dysmenorrhea, chronic pelvic pain, dyspareunia, and defecation pain
AUB	Heavy menstrual bleeding (HMB) and anemia, prolonged menstrual bleeding, and intermenstrual bleeding
Subfertility	Infertility, miscarriage, and preterm birth

abnormal uterine bleeding (AUB) (Table 36.1). In this chapter, we describe the points to deal with adenomyosis patients with pain and AUB at the reproductive age.

36.2 Symptoms of Pain and AUB

Typical symptoms of adenomyosis are pain, AUB, and subfertility. Adenomyosis is a disease affecting the women at reproductive age. According to the questionnaire survey in 2015 by the Japan Society of Obstetrics and Gynecology, the average age for the first diagnosis of adenomyosis was 38.2 years, and 79.0% of the cases diagnosed with adenomyosis had dysmenorrhea and/or heavy menstrual bleeding (HMB) [1]. A US survey using the ICD code reported that the prevalence of adenomyosis was highest in the early 40s [2]. Thus, the main age group receiving treatment for adenomyosis is in the late 30s to 40s, while some adenomyosis patients suffer from severe dysmenorrhea from menarche. Based on the patient background, especially age and desire of childbearing, the treatment plan needs to be determined, because recent studies have revealed that adenomyosis affects pregnancy outcomes.

Symptoms of AUB consist mainly of HMB, HMB-related anemia, and irregular uterine bleeding, and those of pain include dysmenorrhea, chronic pelvic pain, dyspareunia, and defecation pain (Table 36.1). Although adenomyosis does not necessarily result in infertility, recent meta-analysis studies have shown that in vitro fertilization (IVF) patients with adenomyosis tend to have a decrease in implantation rate and clinical pregnancy rate and an increase in miscarriage rate [3–5]. As symptomatic treatment, tranexamic acid and iron drug are used for menorrhagia, and nonsteroidal anti-inflammatory drugs (NSAIDs) are used for pain. NSAIDs have a temporary pain-relieving effect. Laxatives are used for constipation due to intestinal peristalsis associated with adenomyosis.

In 2011, the International Federation of Gynaecology and Obstetrics (FIGO) systems for nomenclature of symptoms of normal and AUB in the reproductive years (FIGO AUB System 1) and for classification of causes of AUB (FIGO AUB System 2; PALM-COEIN) were published [6–8]. In FIGO AUB System 2, PALM-COEIN (polyps, adenomyosis, leiomyoma, malignancy and hyperplasia, coagulopathy, ovulatory dysfunction, endometrial, iatrogenic, and not yet classified) is the acronym standing for disorders which cause AUB symptom. Adenomyosis is in the PALM categories which comprise disorders that are definable by imaging and/or histopathological evaluation. Thus, adenomyosis is recognized as the causative disorder of AUB.

36.3 Pain of Adenomyosis in Patients at Younger Reproductive Age

As for many of adenomyosis patients, their symptoms of pain and AUB first appear in the 30s and 40s and become worse. However, adenomyosis-related pain that occurs early after menarche is often caused by cystic adenomyosis which appears a hemorrhagic cyst with a diameter of 15–30 mm surrounded by the hypertrophic wall. Strong menorrhalgia characterizes juvenile-onset cystic adenomyosis and is sometimes hormonal treatment-resistant. The cause of juvenile cystic adenomyosis is suggested to be a congenital malformation caused by a defect in the developmental process of Müllerian ducts. The most common location of the lesion is the anterior wall of the uterus at the level of insertion of the round ligament. Figure 36.1 shows typical MRI findings of cystic adenomyosis. It has been reported that most of the uterine adenomyosis that led to surgery of the lesion removal in the early 10s to 20s was cystic adenomyosis [9–11]. As the initial choice of hormonal treatment of juvenile cystic adenomyosis, oral contraceptives/low-dose estrogen-progestins (OC/LEP) and a progestin dienogest (DNG) are used to control the symptoms as well as the progression of the disease. When cystic adenomyosis-related pain is resistant to hormonal treatment, surgical resection of the lesion should be considered, because cystic adenomyosis is relatively easy to distinguish the boundary between the lesion and the normal myometrium and the surgical removal of the lesion relieves pain markedly.

36.4 Pain and AUB of Adenomyosis in Patients at Elder Reproductive Age

The symptoms of women with adenomyosis emerge and worsen in the late 30s, which reduces their quality of life (QOL) and work performance. Therefore, both early diagnosis and proper therapeutic intervention are important in clinical

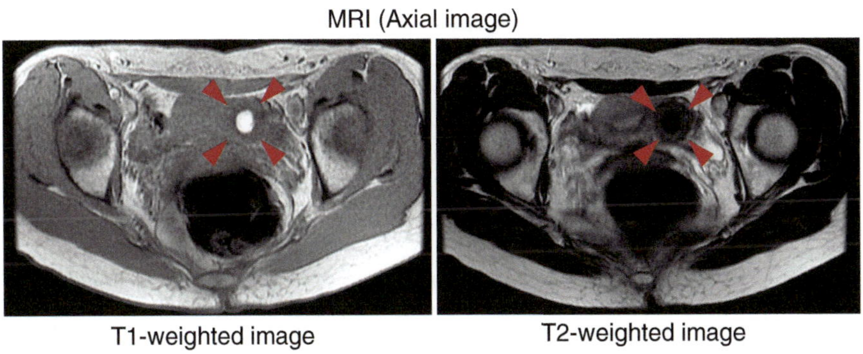

Fig. 36.1 *Magnetic resonance imaging (MRI) of cystic adenomyosis.* T1- and T2-weighted axial images were demonstrated. Arrowhead, cystic adenomyosis

practice. The presence of adenomyosis is associated with recurrent implantation failure, recurrent pregnancy loss, preterm birth, preeclampsia, and placenta previa [3, 4, 12–18]. To relieve pain in women with adenomyosis, may levonorgestrel-releasing intrauterine system (LNG-IUS), DNG, and OC/LEP are primarily selected [19–24]. To relieve HMB, LNG-IUS is primarily selected among progestins and OC/LEP [23–25]. An enlarged uterus is a major cause of LNG-IUS expulsion. Markedly enlarged uterus and HMB with severe anemia have increased risk of massive uterine bleeding during DNG treatment. It is speculated that venous thromboembolism (VTE) is a life-threatening event in adenomyosis patients with HMB accompanied by severe anemia, and OC/LEP may affect the increased risk of VTE in these patients. Once progestins and OC/LEP are effective in relieving the symptoms, they can suppress the disease progression for a long term (Fig. 36.2). When the patient has a desire to raise a baby at present, it is encouraged to attempt to conceive early after cancellation of the hormonal treatment (Fig. 36.2). Unless progestins and OC/LEP are effective, GnRH agonist and antagonist are chosen as alternative drugs [22, 25, 26]. GnRH agonist and antagonist alleviate the symptoms of adenomyosis most strongly but are not suitable for the long-term treatment

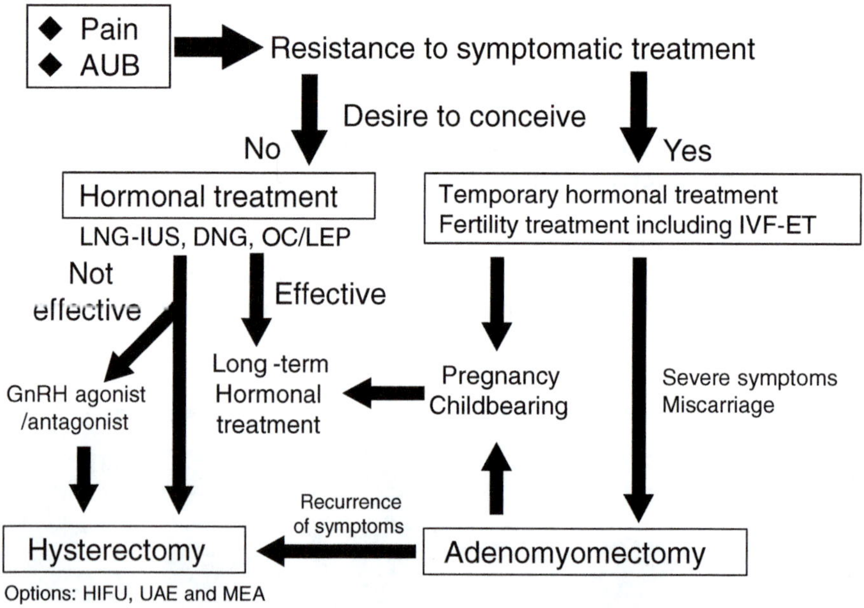

Fig. 36.2 *An example of the treatment strategy for adenomyosis patients with pain and abnormal uterine bleeding (AUB).* DNG, dienogest; LNG-IUS, levonorgestrel-releasing intrauterine system; OC/LEP, oral contraceptives and low-dose estrogen-progestin; HIFU, high-intensity focused ultrasound; UAE, uterine artery embolism; MEA, microwave endometrial ablation; IVF-ET, in vitro fertilization and embryo transfer

(Fig. 36.2) because of the adverse effects caused by strong inhibition of circulating estrogen levels.

Two major pathogenic theories of adenomyosis are considered [27]: (I) infiltration of endometriotic lesions from the uterine serosa to the myometrium and (II) infiltration of eutopic endometrium into the myometrium by way of the damaged interface between uterine endometrium and myometrium. Considering the theory in the pathogenesis of adenomyosis, hormonal therapy such as OC/LEP and DNG against endometriosis at the uterine serosa may help prevent the onset of adenomyosis, but further investigations are needed to elucidate this issue.

When the patient with adenomyosis does not have a desire to bear a child not only at present but in the future, hysterectomy is the best choice among the treatment of adenomyosis (Fig. 36.2). In hysterectomy, open, vaginal, and laparoscopic surgeries are selected according to the facility, taking into consideration factors such as the size of the uterus, history of pelvic surgery, and the presence or absence of endometriosis [28]. Microwave endometrial ablation (MEA), uterine artery embolization (UAE), and high-intensity focused ultrasound (HIFU) are the options of minimally invasive approaches (Fig. 36.2) [29–34]. For example, adenomyosis with a severe heart disease is a good indication for these treatments. MEA is selected when HMB is the main symptom of the patients who have no desire to raise children in the future [30]. Symptoms can be improved by cauterization of not only the endometrium but adenomyosis lesions close to the endometrium. When adenomyosis causes dilation or deformation of the uterine cavity, there is a high possibility of recurrence of symptoms after MEA due to the insufficient cauterization. Major complications of MEA are lower abdominal pain and uterine infection. UAE is also a treatment for symptomatic patients who do not want to conceive anymore [29, 32, 33]. UAE has adverse effects such as lower abdominal pain, uterine infection, and decreased ovarian function after the treatment. HIFU induces focal thermocoagulation of the adenomyotic lesions targeted by ultrasound or MRI. The coagulation necrosis obtained with HIFU is much less painful compared to the ischemic necrosis obtained by UAE. HIFU can only be recommended to women with symptomatic adenomyosis and no plans for future pregnancy, no suspect pelvic adhesions, no lower abdominal surgery, body weight < 100 kg, and abdominal wall thickness < 5 cm [29, 31, 34]. In contrast, when the patient with hormone treatment-resistant adenomyosis wants to conceive, adenomyomectomy, the uterus-sparing conservative surgery in adenomyosis, is an option to relieve the symptoms.

In 40s, the symptoms of adenomyosis become stronger, and the adenomyosis cases with resistance to hormonal therapy are increased. As the consequence, surgical intervention is more often required due to the severe symptoms, and it is often the case that hysterectomy should be considered in the end. Immediately before menopause, continuous treatment with GnRH agonist and antagonist is also an option of medical treatment. Recently, the number of adenomyosis patients in their 40s who wants to conceive is increasing, and early fertility treatment using assisted reproductive technology (ART) must be recommended for them, although their pregnancy rate and live birth rate are low even in the treatment with ART under the influence of aging. There is a lot of evidence about ovarian cancer derived from ovarian endometrioma [35]. Regarding adenomyosis, adenomyosis is often observed in the uterus with endometrial cancer. A recent study has demonstrated that patients with adenomyosis have an increased risk of endometrial and thyroid cancer [36]. In addition, several reports have demonstrated endometrial cancer that probably developed from adenomyosis [37–40], although it is difficult in many cases to pathologically certify whether endometrial cancer originates with adenomyosis. In our genomic analyses, 60% of adenomyosis lesions have some kinds of somatic mutations, and KRAS mutations were observed most frequently [41, 42], suggesting that gene mutation in adenomyosis is involved in the pathogenesis of adenomyosis-derived endometrial cancer.

36.5 The Efficacy of Adenomyomectomy for Symptomatic Adenomyosis

In the adenomyosis cases with infertility, it is difficult to determine whether adenomyosis is the cause of infertility, because uterine fibroid and endometriosis, which are often present together with adenomyosis, may cause infertility. Therefore, fertility treatment should be conducted primarily. In the ART program, freeze-all strategy, GnRH agonist treatment before embryo transfer, and thawed embryo transfer are recommended. When pain and HMB are too severe to continue fertility treatment, adenomyomectomy is considered. The presence of adenomyosis has been shown to increase miscarriage and preterm birth [3, 4, 12, 13, 15, 17, 18]. A history of miscarriage after 12 weeks or preterm birth less than 30 weeks can be an indication of adenomyomectomy. Adenomyomectomy is effective to improve AUB and pain regardless of the surgical procedure [43, 44]. Table 36.2 demonstrated that adenomyomectomy markedly improved severe pain and AUB in our facility. Although postoperative hormonal therapy is not always necessary, it should be considered according to the symptoms under the periodic postoperative observation. In principle, the mode of delivery in the pregnancy after adenomyomectomy is elective

Table 36.2 Pain and HMB are markedly improved by adenomyomectomy. The symptoms of 43 patients with symptomatic adenomyosis who underwent adenomyomectomy (open surgery) at the University of Tokyo Hospital from 2015 to 2017 were evaluated before and 3 months and 1 year after surgery. Dysmenorrhea, chronic pelvic pain, dyspareunia, and defecation pain were evaluated by visual analogue scale (VAS, 0–100). Menorrhagia was evaluated by menorrhagia multi-attribute scale (MMAS, 0–100). Of the 43 patients, the age at the surgery was 39.5 ± 3.9 years old, 36 patients (84%) were nulliparous, and 30 patients (70%) had endometriosis. *, $P < 0.05$ vs before surgery

			After surgery	
Symptom (mean ± SD)	Scale	Before surgery	3 months	1 year
Dysmenorrhea	VAS (0–100)	85 ± 17	18 ± 21*	14 ± 16*
Chronic pelvic pain	VAS (0–100)	41 ± 30	14 ± 21[a]	7 ± 13[a]
Dyspareunia	VAS (0–100)	33 ± 29	11 ± 18*	7 ± 12*
Defecation pain	VAS (0–100)	27 ± 27	11 ± 16*	7 ± 13*
Menorrhagia	MMAS (0–100)	24 ± 18	80 ± 20*	83 ± 17*

cesarean section [45]. In pregnancy after adenomyomectomy, the risks of uterine rupture and placenta accreta have been pointed out. According to a report on pregnancy cases after adenomyomectomy, uterine rupture was observed in 3.6% of postoperative pregnancies [46]. There is also a report of 6.3% for placenta accreta [47]. Therefore, the perinatal risk of pregnancy after adenomyomectomy is higher than that of other uterine surgeries, and pregnancy management at the intensive perinatal care facility is essential. Before conducting adenomyomectomy, this information about the perinatal complications needs to be fully understood by the patients who plan to undergo adenomyomectomy. A survey by the Japan Society of Obstetrics and Gynecology suggests that uterine adenomyomectomy is effective in preventing miscarriage for infertile women with focal adenomyosis [18, 48]. In 40 infertile patients with adenomyomectomy performed at the University of Tokyo Hospital, clinical pregnancy rate was 28% (11/40), and miscarriage rate was 9% (1/11). In addition, 91% of pregnant cases (10/11) were via ART, and 45% of pregnant women (5/11) were over 40 years old. These findings suggest that adenomyosis patients over 40 years old become increasingly like to be pregnant when they can obtain good-quality frozen embryos before surgery. Further accumulation of the evidence about the efficacy of adenomyomectomy on infertility is needed.

36.6 Conclusion

Pain and AUB in adenomyosis patients should be managed according to the severity of their symptoms, their ages, and their desires to conceive. Since the symptoms often worsen in the late 30s to early 40s, it is sometimes difficult to deal with adenomyosis-related infertility and recurrent miscarriage at that time. Hormonal therapy is usually conducted as the treatment for moderate and severe symptoms. However, regardless of the severity of the symptoms, it is acceptable to choose hormonal treatment for adenomyosis patients who want to bear children in their future, since hormonal therapy such as LNG-IUS and DNG has a potential to stop the progression of adenomyosis. Accumulation of new evidence will enable the optimization of the lifelong approaches to adenomyosis.

References

1. Sugino N, Kugu K, Kitawaki J, Narahara H, Minegishi T, Murakami T. Annual report of Reproductive Endocrinology Committee, Japan Society of Obstetrics and Gynecology, 2015. J Jpn Soc Obstet Gynecol (in Japanese). 2015;67:1493–511.
2. Yu O, Schulze-Rath R, Grafton J, Hansen K, Scholes D, Reed SD. Adenomyosis incidence, prevalence and treatment: United States population-based study 2006-2015. Am J Obstet Gynecol. 2020;223:94 e91–10.
3. Horton J, Sterrenburg M, Lane S, Maheshwari A, Li TC, Cheong Y. Reproductive, obstetric, and perinatal outcomes of women with adenomyosis and endometriosis: a systematic review and meta-analysis. Hum Reprod Update. 2019;25:592–632.

4. Nirgianakis K, Kalaitzopoulos DR, Schwartz ASK, Spaanderman M, Kramer BW, Mueller MD, Mueller M. Fertility, pregnancy and neonatal outcomes of patients with adenomyosis: a systematic review and meta-analysis. Reprod Biomed Online. 2021;42:185–206.
5. Vercellini P, Consonni D, Dridi D, Bracco B, Frattaruolo MP, Somigliana E. Uterine adenomyosis and in vitro fertilization outcome: a systematic review and meta-analysis. Hum Reprod. 2014;29:964–77.
6. Munro MG, Critchley HO, Broder MS, Fraser IS. FIGO classification system (PALM-COEIN) for causes of abnormal uterine bleeding in nongravid women of reproductive age. Int J Gynaecol Obstet. 2011;113:3–13.
7. Munro MG, Critchley HO, Fraser IS. The FIGO classification of causes of abnormal uterine bleeding in the reproductive years. Fertil Steril. 2011;95:2204–8, 2208 e2201–2203
8. Munro MG, Critchley HOD, Fraser IS. The two FIGO systems for normal and abnormal uterine bleeding symptoms and classification of causes of abnormal uterine bleeding in the reproductive years: 2018 revisions. Int J Gynaecol Obstet. 2018;143:393–408.
9. Brosens I, Gordts S, Habiba M, Benagiano G. Uterine cystic adenomyosis: a disease of younger women. J Pediatr Adolesc Gynecol. 2015;28:420–6.
10. Kriplani A, Mahey R, Agarwal N, Bhatla N, Yadav R, Singh MK. Laparoscopic management of juvenile cystic adenomyoma: four cases. J Minim Invasive Gynecol. 2011;18:343–8.
11. Takeuchi H, Kitade M, Kikuchi I, Kumakiri J, Kuroda K, Jinushi M. Diagnosis, laparoscopic management, and histopathologic findings of juvenile cystic adenomyoma: a review of nine cases. Fertil Steril. 2010;94:862–8.
12. Hashimoto A, Iriyama T, Sayama S, Nakayama T, Komatsu A, Miyauchi A, Nishii O, Nagamatsu T, Osuga Y, Fujii T. Adenomyosis and adverse perinatal outcomes: increased risk of second trimester miscarriage, preeclampsia, and placental malposition. J Matern Fetal Neonatal Med. 2018;31:364–9.
13. Juang CM, Chou P, Yen MS, Twu NF, Horng HC, Hsu WL. Adenomyosis and risk of preterm delivery. BJOG. 2007;114:165–9.
14. Kim SC, Lee NK, Yun KY, Joo JK, Suh DS, Kim KH. A rapidly growing adenomyosis associated with preterm delivery and postpartum abscess formation. Taiwan J Obstet Gynecol. 2016;55:620–2.
15. Mochimaru A, Aoki S, Oba MS, Kurasawa K, Takahashi T, Hirahara F. Adverse pregnancy outcomes associated with adenomyosis with uterine enlargement. J Obstet Gynaecol Res. 2015;41:529–33.
16. Razavi M, Maleki-Hajiagha A, Sepidarkish M, Rouholamin S, Almasi-Hashiani A, Rezaeinejad M. Systematic review and meta-analysis of adverse pregnancy outcomes after uterine adenomyosis. Int J Gynaecol Obstet. 2019;145:149–57.
17. Yamaguchi A, Kyozuka H, Fujimori K, Hosoya M, Yasumura S, Yokoyama T, Sato A, Hashimoto K. Risk of preterm birth, low birthweight and small-for-gestational-age infants in pregnancies with adenomyosis: a cohort study of the Japan Environment and Children's Study. Acta Obstet Gynecol Scand. 2019;98:359–64.
18. Tamura H, Kishi H, Kitade M, Asai-Sato M, Tanaka A, Murakami T, Minegishi T, Sugino N. Complications and outcomes of pregnant women with adenomyosis in Japan. Reprod Med Biol. 2017;16:330–6.
19. Osuga Y, Fujimoto-Okabe H, Hagino A. Evaluation of the efficacy and safety of dienogest in the treatment of painful symptoms in patients with adenomyosis: a randomized, double-blind, multicenter, placebo-controlled study. Fertil Steril. 2017;108:673–8.
20. Osuga Y, Hayashi K, Kanda S. Long-term use of dienogest for the treatment of primary and secondary dysmenorrhea. J Obstet Gynaecol Res. 2020;46:606–17.
21. Osuga Y, Watanabe M, Hagino A. Long-term use of dienogest in the treatment of painful symptoms in adenomyosis. J Obstet Gynaecol Res. 2017;43:1441–8.
22. Fawzy M, Mesbah Y. Comparison of dienogest versus triptorelin acetate in premenopausal women with adenomyosis: a prospective clinical trial. Arch Gynecol Obstet. 2015;292:1267–71.
23. Abbas AM, Samy A, Atwa K, Ghoneim HM, Lotfy M, Saber Mohammed H, Abdellah AM, El Bahie AM, Aboelroose AA, El Gedawy AM, Mostafa M, Elsenity MA, Samy M, Safwat

S, Abdelrahman RM, Salah El Din AS, Badran E, Abdelkader AM, Abdallah A. The role of levonorgestrel intra-uterine system in the management of adenomyosis: a systematic review and meta-analysis of prospective studies. Acta Obstet Gynecol Scand. 2020;99:571–81.
24. Vannuccini S, Luisi S, Tosti C, Sorbi F, Petraglia F. Role of medical therapy in the management of uterine adenomyosis. Fertil Steril. 2018;109:398–405.
25. Ozdegirmenci O, Kayikcioglu F, Akgul MA, Kaplan M, Karcaaltincaba M, Haberal A, Akyol M. Comparison of levonorgestrel intrauterine system versus hysterectomy on efficacy and quality of life in patients with adenomyosis. Fertil Steril. 2011;95:497–502.
26. Donnez O, Donnez J. Gonadotropin-releasing hormone antagonist (linzagolix): a new therapy for uterine adenomyosis. Fertil Steril. 2020;114:640–5.
27. Kishi Y, Suginami H, Kuramori R, Yabuta M, Suginami R, Taniguchi F. Four subtypes of adenomyosis assessed by magnetic resonance imaging and their specification. Am J Obstet Gynecol. 2012;207:114 e111–7.
28. Saito A, Hirata T, Koga K, Takamura M, Fukuda S, Neriishi K, Pastorfide G, Harada M, Hirota Y, Wada-Hiraike O, Fujii T, Osuga Y. Preoperative assessment of factors associated with difficulty in performing total laparoscopic hysterectomy. J Obstet Gynaecol Res. 2017;43:320–9.
29. Dueholm M. Minimally invasive treatment of adenomyosis. Best Pract Res Clin Obstet Gynaecol. 2018;51:119–37.
30. Nakamura K, Nakayama K, Ishikawa M, Katagiri H, Katagiri A, Ishibashi T, Sato E, Asakawa Y, Kyo S. Efficacy of multiple microwave endometrial ablation technique for menorrhagia resulting from adenomyosis. J Obstet Gynaecol Res. 2015;41:1769–72.
31. Cheung VY. Current status of high-intensity focused ultrasound for the management of uterine adenomyosis. Ultrasonography. 2017;36:95–102.
32. Liang E, Brown B, Rachinsky M. A clinical audit on the efficacy and safety of uterine artery embolisation for symptomatic adenomyosis: results in 117 women. Aust N Z J Obstet Gynaecol. 2018;58:454–9.
33. Wang S, Meng X, Dong Y. The evaluation of uterine artery embolization as a nonsurgical treatment option for adenomyosis. Int J Gynaecol Obstet. 2016;133:202–5.
34. Marques ALS, Andres MP, Kho RM, Abrao MS. Is high-intensity focused ultrasound effective for the treatment of adenomyosis? A systematic review and meta-analysis. J Minim Invasive Gynecol. 2020;27:332–43.
35. Kobayashi H, Sumimoto K, Moniwa N, Imai M, Takakura K, Kuromaki T, Morioka E, Arisawa K, Terao T. Risk of developing ovarian cancer among women with ovarian endometrioma: a cohort study in Shizuoka, Japan. Int J Gynecol Cancer. 2007;17:37–43.
36. Yeh CC, Su FH, Tzeng CR, Muo CH, Wang WC. Women with adenomyosis are at higher risks of endometrial and thyroid cancers: a population-based historical cohort study. PLoS One. 2018;13:e0194011.
37. Izumi Y, Yamamoto T, Matsunaga N, Ota T, Owaki Y, Shinohara K, Tsuzuki T, Suzuki K. Endometrial cancer arising from adenomyosis: case report and literature review of MRI findings. Radiol Case Rep. 2020;15:427–30.
38. Yanase T, Kikuchi A, Sasagawa M, Honma S. Two cases of endometrial cancer arising from adenomyosis during aromatase inhibitors therapy after mastectomy. J Obstet Gynaecol. 2017;37:952–4.
39. Marcus CC. Relationship of adenomyosis uteri to endometrial hyperplasia and endometrial carcinoma. Am J Obstet Gynecol. 1961;82:408–16.
40. Giammalvo JT, Kaplan K. The incidence of endometriosis interna in 120 cases of carcinoma of the endometrium. Am J Obstet Gynecol. 1958;75:161–6.
41. Inoue S, Hirota Y, Ueno T, Fukui Y, Yoshida E, Hayashi T, Kojima S, Takeyama R, Hashimoto T, Kiyono T, Ikemura M, Taguchi A, Tanaka T, Tanaka Y, Sakata S, Takeuchi K, Muraoka A, Osuka S, Saito T, Oda K, Osuga Y, Terao Y, Kawazu M, Mano H. Uterine adenomyosis is an oligoclonal disorder associated with KRAS mutations. Nat Commun. 2019;10:5785.
42. Inoue S, Yoshida E, Fukui Y, Ueno T, Kawazu M, Takeyama R, Ikemura M, Osuga Y, Terao Y, Hirota Y, Mano H. KRAS mutations in uterine endometrium are associated with gravidity and parity. Cell Death Dis. 2020;11:347.

43. Nishida M, Takano K, Arai Y, Ozone H, Ichikawa R. Conservative surgical management for diffuse uterine adenomyosis. Fertil Steril. 2010;94:715–9.
44. Osada H, Silber S, Kakinuma T, Nagaishi M, Kato K, Kato O. Surgical procedure to conserve the uterus for future pregnancy in patients suffering from massive adenomyosis. Reprod Biomed Online. 2011;22:94–9.
45. Grimbizis GF, Mikos T, Tarlatzis B. Uterus-sparing operative treatment for adenomyosis. Fertil Steril. 2014;101:472–87.
46. Osada H. Uterine adenomyosis and adenomyoma: the surgical approach. Fertil Steril. 2018;109:406–17.
47. Kishi Y, Yabuta M, Taniguchi F. Who will benefit from uterus-sparing surgery in adenomyosis-associated subfertility? Fertil Steril. 2014;102(802–807):e801.
48. Tamura H, Kishi H, Kitade M, Asai-Sato M, Tanaka A, Murakami T, Minegishi T, Sugino N. Clinical outcomes of infertility treatment for women with adenomyosis in Japan. Reprod Med Biol. 2017;16:276–82.

Adenomyosis in Reproductive Years: Fertility and ART in Adenomyosis

37

Jwal Banker, Manish Banker, and Juan Antonio Garcia-Velasco

Contents

37.1 Introduction

Adenomyosis is best defined by Bird in 1972 as "the benign invasion of endometrium into the myometrium, producing a diffusely enlarged uterus which microscopically exhibits ectopic non-neoplastic, endometrial glands and stroma

The original version of the chapter has been revised. A correction to this chapter can be found at https://doi.org/10.1007/978-3-030-97236-3_45

J. Banker (✉)
Nova IVF Fertility, Ahmedabad, India

IVI, Madrid, Spain

M. Banker
Nova IVF Fertility, Ahmedabad, India

J. A. Garcia-Velasco
IVI, Madrid, Spain

Rey Juan Carlos University, Madrid, Spain

E. Oral (ed.), *Endometriosis and Adenomyosis*,
https://doi.org/10.1007/978-3-030-97236-3_37

surrounded by the hypertrophic and hyperplastic myometrium" [1]. In the past, adenomyosis was thought to be present only in parous women. However, it is frequently encountered in nulliparous infertile patients also. Earlier, the only way for diagnosis was a retrospective histopathology after hysterectomy. Recently, adenomyosis is frequently diagnosed in infertile patients owing to better, accurate, and noninvasive diagnostic methods. Further, with the routine use of transvaginal ultrasound in infertility practice, the burden of adenomyosis in the infertile population has become more evident. Naftalin et al. and Puente et al. made it clearer for clinicians to uniformly diagnose and report the disease [2, 3]. In women undergoing assisted reproductive technologies (ARTs), studies show the prevalence to be about 25%, going up to 80% in the presence of endometriosis.

Given the broad and unclear spectrum of the disease and no clear guidelines from regional governing bodies on its types, the role of adenomyosis on fertility is not very clear. Generally, adenomyosis is divided into two types: diffuse, in which numerous foci of endometrial glands and stroma are dispersed within the myometrium, and focal (adenomyoma), in which circumscribed nodular aggregates are observed in the myometrium [also called focal adenomyosis of the outer myometrium (FAOM)]. A third type called cystic adenomyoma is also mentioned by some authors and is a rare variation of focal adenomyosis with additional compensatory hypertrophy of the surrounding myometrium [4]. FAOM is usually found in association with endometriosis, whereas diffuse type has not been found to have such a strong correlation.

Many theories have been proposed on the causal relation of adenomyosis and infertility, but its exact mechanism is still elusive. This difficulty can be due to the fact that a strong association exists between endometriosis and adenomyosis, which can be as high as 90%. This has led some authors to believe that the two represent the same underlying disease and the association with infertility has been explained in the same pathophysiological terms. Theories from abnormal uterine peristalsis to abnormal shape and composition of the endometrium have been postulated, but functional studies on the effects of adenomyosis on endometrial receptivity are still scarce.

The treatment options for such cases depend on the woman's age, reproductive status, and clinical symptoms. Many different medical and surgical methods are being offered, but there is still no drug specific for adenomyosis. Many medications are used off-label to manage pain and bleeding and sometimes even improve fertility outcome. The use of progestins like norethisterone acetate and dienogest is becoming popular due to its anti-proliferative and anti-inflammatory effects. Some minimally invasive surgical options like endometrial ablation, hysteroscopic adenomyoma resection, laparoscopic resection of adenomyosis, uterine artery embolization, and even high-intensity focused ultrasonography are offered. Laparoscopy for focal lesions and laparotomy for removal of the specimen in cases of larger diffuse lesions are other options. In spite of all these, there is no conclusive evidence of a "best" method, and proper randomized studies targeting impact on fertility are lacking.

37.2 Adenomyosis and Fertility Outcome

37.2.1 Proposed Theories for Factors Causing Infertility

Even though adenomyosis was first mentioned about 160 years ago, the disease is yet to be fully discovered [5]. It is hypothesized that adenomyosis might cause infertility by altering the normal myometrial architecture and function by affecting the uterine peristalsis and/or by interfering with sperm transport. In an interesting case control study on baboons, a clear correlation was found between adenomyosis and primary infertility [6]. Various mechanisms causing infertility are proposed by different authors, and any or a combination of many of these can lead to this dreadful condition.

It is known that specific uterine peristalsis that directs the sperm transport toward the peritoneal opening of the fallopian tubes especially on the side of dominant follicle is crucial in the early reproductive process. This characteristic depends on the myometrial architecture. In adenomyosis, this normal architecture is disturbed, and this results in abnormal peristalsis with increased intrauterine pressure [7]. It seems reasonable to assume that this may affect fertility in these women.

A rapid sperm transport from the cervix to the tubes is observed and is essential in humans for effective reproduction. The dynamics involved in this transport were described by Kunz et al. who used technetium-labeled albumin macrospheres of the size of sperms at the external os and followed these using serial scintigrams. Their analysis revealed that the progress of these spheres increased with advancement of the follicular phase. Lyons et al. observed that uterine peristaltic contractions had maximum frequency during the preovulatory period and were of cervico-fundal pattern [7, 8]. Hence, dysperistalsis caused due to adenomyosis might affect this effective sperm transport and cause problems in conceiving.

Besides causing abnormal uterine peristalsis, adenomyosis can interfere in reproduction by altering the shape of the uterine cavity itself. Using ultrasound, Puente et al. analyzed the coronal sections of the uterine cavity in patients with adenomyosis and found that 22.6% women had moderate alterations, while 10.1% had severe modifications showing a pseudo T-shaped uterine cavity [2]. This modification has an impact on implantation in natural as well as assisted reproduction pregnancies.

Many authors have suggested changes at a cellular level that can hinder endometrial receptivity and implantation. P450 (P450arom) protein and mRNA expression was found to be present in patients with adenomyosis and not in controls [9]. Clinical pregnancy rates were found to be statistically lower in patients with high endometrial P450arom mRNA levels, and Brosens et al. proposed this could be an important reason even in IVF [10]. Research also suggests alteration of estrogen and progesterone receptors in these women which can reduce the β-3 integrin secretion and hinder receptivity. It has also been found that leukemia inhibitory factor (LIF) is an essential molecule for successful implantation during human reproduction. Dysregulation of LIF in women with adenomyosis, especially during the window of implantation, can cause difficulty in implantation [11]. Furthermore, abnormal expression levels of many implantation-related factors (HOXA10, LIF, IL-6, cytochrome P450) in the eutopic endometrium of adenomyotic women have been found to result in impaired implantation of even good-quality embryos [12]. Having said that, it is also found that the genes involved in the timing of the window of implantation or the endometrial receptiveness are not dysregulated in this disease, which means that there is mainly a defect with the functional aspect of implantation [13]. All these factors, either alone or in combination, can cause problems in achieving a successful pregnancy, and some of these changes are an intriguing target for future investigation.

37.2.2 Effect on Pregnancy Outcomes

It has become quite evident in recent times that adenomyosis can have a negative impact in the fertile life of a woman. In this matter, Puente et al. performed a cross-sectional study of more than 1000 patients prior to reproductive treatment. They found that the prevalence of adenomyosis was 24.4% and 22% in women aged ≥40 years and ≤40 years, respectively. This was found to be higher in women with recurrent pregnancy loss (38.2%) and previous ART failure (34.7%) when compared with the rest. Interestingly, they also found that four out of five patients had the diagnosis missed in earlier transvaginal ultrasonography [2]. Given this, at what stage adenomyosis will affect the pregnancy is not clearly understood, but this can occur at various stages.

Given the fact that adenomyosis causes abnormal uterine shape, vascularity, and peristalsis, it has been thought that this can affect the implantation of the embryo. Various studies addressing this have had inconclusive varied results. In a classic study by Martinez-Conejero et al., the authors evaluated the role of the disease in women undergoing ovum donation cycles where the embryo quality was good and endometrial hormonal milieu was similarly managed by exogenous hormones. They found that implantation rates were similar in women with and without the disease. Moreover, the gene expression profile of the endometrial samples during the window of implantation did not differ between the groups [13]. However, a recent meta-analysis found that implantation was significantly lower in women with adenomyosis undergoing ART [14]. This variation begs the question whether adenomyosis directly affects implantation or whether it is due to other confounding factors, and further research is still necessary.

Based on the above speculations, it is also thought that adenomyosis can affect the clinical pregnancy rate (CPR) in ART cycles. Due to the different definitions of CPR used in various studies, this information is difficult to obtain. Younes et al. evaluated 12 different studies and found significantly reduced CPR per cycle. An earlier meta-analysis also showed that women with adenomyosis had a 28% reduction of CPR in IVF/ICSI cycles as compared to controls [14, 15]. This makes it quite evident that these women have a reduced chance of a clinical pregnancy; however, randomized studies using similar definitions for CPR will be more helpful.

Adenomyosis causes changes in the myometrial architecture and thus affects the vascularity by distorting the spiral arteries. This vascular change is assumed to cause increased miscarriages in these women. While some studies have found a similar miscarriage rate, most others have not. In the study performed using donor oocytes on women with and without adenomyosis with similar age and reason for infertility, there was a significant increase in miscarriage rates in the affected women (13.1% vs. 7.2%) [13]. Similar results were obtained in the two meta-analyses showing that adenomyotic women had a significantly higher miscarriage rate as compared to controls [14, 15]. Despite the fact that the exact cause leading to abortions is not clear, we do know that adenomyosis has a negative impact and it causes increased miscarriage rates.

The most important indicator of whether the disease has an impact on the overall fertility of the woman is the live birth rate. By reducing the CPR and increasing the abortions, it is safe to assume that the overall live birth rate (LBR) will also drop. Very few studies have followed up these women up to their delivery and calculated the live births. While many studies found that there was a fall in the LBR, the drop was not found to be significant in some. To address this, Younes et al. made it quite evident in their meta-analysis that there is a 41% drop in LBR in patients with adenomyosis compared to healthy women, and more recent studies also agree to that [14, 15]. Hence, to put in simple terms, adenomyosis dose affect the fertility and that is reflected by the reduced live birth rates.

It is assumed that adenomyosis can affect the pregnancy outcome due to its various effects on the myometrial architecture and blood supply. To date, there are only one or two meta-analysis on establishing a relationship between the disease and perinatal complication. In a very recent systemic review, such outcomes were analyzed according to the mode of conception and adjusted to age when possible. It was found that for risk factors like preterm delivery, preeclampsia, small for gestational age, low birth weight, and postpartum hemorrhage, adenomyosis was a significant risk factor independent of the mode of conception [16]. Even after such strong calculations, data on this aspect is still inadequate, and more studies are needed.

In spite of this evidence, there is still a lack of information on exactly which type of adenomyosis is more relevant in view of the reproductive life of the woman. Studies on animals have already found an association of adenomyosis with primary infertility. A very recent and thought-provoking study by Bourdon et al., which had a database spanning more than 10 years and consisted of women who had adenomyosis diagnosed exclusively by MRI by experienced radiologists, has found that focal adenomyosis is associated with primary infertility. Even though the focal phenotype was frequently associated with severe forms of endometriosis, deeper analysis suggested that it had an independent association [17]. To summarize, adenomyosis does affect fertility by increasing miscarriages and reducing clinical pregnancies and the live births and also that the focal variant might be of more significance.

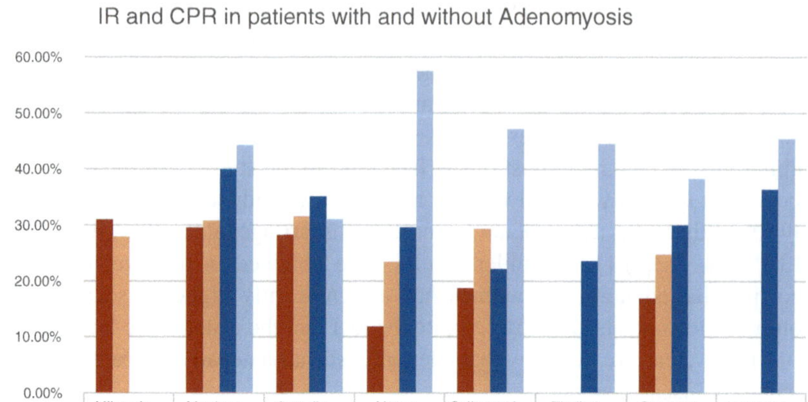

	Mijatovic et al. 2010	Martinez et al. 2011	Costello et al. 2011	Youm et al. 2011	Salim et al. 2012	Thalluri et al. 2012	Camargo et al. 2012	Yan et al. 2014
IR (A)	31.00%	29.60%	28.30%	11.86%	18.80%		16.90%	
IR (H)	28.00%	30.80%	31.60%	23.50%	29.40%		24.80%	
CPR (A)		40.00%	35.10%	29.60%	22.20%	23.60%	30.00%	36.40%
CPR (H)		44.40%	31.10%	57.50%	47.20%	44.60%	38.30%	45.50%

(IR)–Implantation Rate, (CPR) –Clinical Pregnancy Rate; (A) -with Adenomyosis; (H) –Healthy, without Adenomyosis

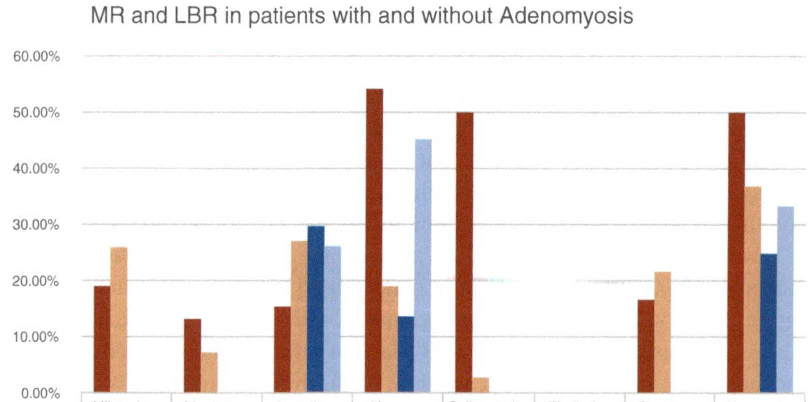

	Mijatovic et al. 2010	Martinez et al. 2011	Costello et al. 2011	Youm et al. 2011	Salim et al. 2012	Thalluri et al. 2012	Camargo et al. 2012	Yan et al. 2014
MR (A)	19.00%	13.10%	15.40%	54.20%	50.00%		16.70%	50.00%
MR (H)	26.00%	7.20%	27.10%	19.00%	2.80%		21.70%	36.90%
LBR (A)			29.70%	13.60%				24.80% *
LBR (H)			26.10%	45.20%				33.30% *

(MR) –MiscarriageRate, (LBR) –Live Birth Rate; (A) -with Adenomyosis; (H) –Healthy, without Adenomyosis
**-Delivery rate*

37.3 Management

37.3.1 Medical Management of Adenomyosis-Related Infertility

It is believed that endometrial cells invade the myometrium at sites in the junctional zone that are weakened, either from genetic predisposition or from uterine auto-traumatization and induced hypoxia. This causes neoangiogenesis and leads to a vicious cycle. Like endometriosis, adenomyosis is an estrogen-dependent condition that usually responds to medical treatment. Medical management in adenomyosis is focused on breaking this cycle and trying to achieve a hypoestrogenic environment which in turn causes reduction in the size of the lesion and normalize the uterus. These various treatment modalities are being tried before and after IVF procedures and are scrutinized.

Most of the literature is focused mainly on medical management for adenomyosis-associated dysmenorrhea, abnormal uterine bleeding, and pelvic pain, with less focus on associated subfertility. It is still assumed that by reducing the volume of the uterus and the defect, it will help improve fertility outcomes. Treatment options include GnRH-a, oral contraceptives (OCs), progestins, danazol, and, more recently, selective estrogen receptor modulators (SERMs), selective progesterone receptor modulators (SPRMs), and aromatase inhibitors (AIs) along with some other experimental drugs.

Adenomyotic tissue contains estrogen, progesterone, and androgen receptors and also aromatase and sulfatase enzymes which catalyze the conversion of androgens to estrogens. Together with circulating hormones, locally produced estrogens also stimulate the growth of this estrogen-dependent tissue. Physiology suggests that if we reverse this process, we can obtain good results. The most widely used drug for this purpose is a GnRH agonist. Along with causing a hypoestrogenic state, these agents also reduce the expression of aromatase cytochrome P450 in the eutopic endometrium. To assess this on IVF outcomes, Xiaoni Hou et al. recently compared outcomes using long agonist protocols with and without prior suppression by GnRH agonist depots. They found that the suppressed patients needed a significantly longer and higher dose of gonadotropins for stimulation and a number of oocytes retrieved were also less. But, on the other hand, these women had a significantly higher implantation and live birth rate [18]. On the other hand, another study found CLBR to be higher in the non-pretreatment group, and this was attributed to the fact that the hyperestrogenic environment during ovarian stimulation negates the effect of the suppression [19]. In another older study, the authors used agonist suppression before frozen embryo transfer cycles and found a significantly higher implantation and clinical pregnancy rate [20]. Based on existing literature, we can assume that agonist pretreatment can have a beneficial effect on implantation and live birth rates, but with a negative effect of longer and increased stimulation and lower oocyte retrieval [14]. More prospective trials and meta-analyses are still needed for a definitive answer.

Besides the use of GnRH agonists, various other drugs are used in patients with adenomyosis. These are mainly focused on relieving other ill effects like pain or AUB, but many also help in reducing the overall uterine volume. A very recent study has demonstrated a correlation between the uterine volume and pregnancy outcome in these women by analyzing frozen embryo transfer cycles [21]. Medications like COCs, danazol, and LNG-IUD have been found to help in reducing the uterine volume, but the time required to achieve this extended to more than 2 years. This is not desired in women wishing pregnancy. In another randomized trial, Badawy A et al. found that aromatase inhibitors, specially letrozole, was as effective as agonists in reducing the adenomyoma size (adenomyoma volume reduction by 8.6% and 29.7% vs. 5.7% and 34.6% after 4 and 8 weeks of treatment) [22]. There is also new evidence to suggest a role of antiplatelet therapy in treating adenomyotic lesions by suggesting that these undergo repeated tissue injury and repair (ReTIAR), and platelets induce epithelial-mesenchymal transition (EMT) and fibroblast-to-myofibroblast transdifferentiation (FMT), leading ultimately to fibrosis. Studies on mice have demonstrated beneficial effects, but clinical use cannot be advocated yet without further studies. Hence, either due to the lack of studies or due to an increased "time to pregnancy" effect of these medications, medical management prior to fertility treatment is not a popular choice while dealing with adenomyosis-related infertility.

Along with the drugs, many newer nonsurgical techniques are in the process of evaluation. These procedures include uterine artery embolization (UAE) and high-intensity focused ultrasound (HIFU). Though UAE has been found to help in relieving the symptoms by decreasing the vascularity, it is associated with complications like infarctions and hence seldom used. Its role in preserving and enhancing fertility is not studied. On the other hand, HIFU is a noninvasive local thermal ablation technique which has been used in the treatment of both focal and diffuse adenomyoses and has been found beneficial. In a review article, many studies were included which evaluated the safety profile and fertility outcomes in women undergoing HIFU. In one study, out of 68 patients who had HIFU procedure, 54 conceived and 21 had a live birth [23]. This can be an attractive treatment option in the future, but its use should be based on strict selection criteria, and its efficacy, safety, and long term side effects need to be validated by randomized trials.

Overall, it seems that all these factors work by reducing the size of the lesion and the uterus and ultimately creating a favorable environment. This can then help improve pregnancy and live birth rates. The most commonly used and studied drug is GnRH agonist, but as it has negative effects in IVF cycles, it can be used after ovarian stimulation and before a frozen embryo transfer. It also seems that long agonist protocols can offer some benefit and can be used in these women. Newer drugs and techniques need proper validation and approvals from regional governing bodies before implementing in daily practice.

37.3.2 Surgical Management of Adenomyosis-Related Infertility

The surgical management of women with associated subfertility is highly controversial, and there remains an overall lack of consensus regarding the value of conservative surgery with or without medical management to improve reproductive outcomes. Surgery for adenomyosis is a less popular but yet a valid option. While it is assumed that by removing the pathology one can improve fertility outcomes, it is still invasive and hence carries its own risks. Various techniques like adenomyomectomy with or without myometrial reduction, electrocoagulation of adenomyoma, and myometrial excision have been used, but no method has been proven to be superior. Laparoscopy, hysteroscopy, or laparotomy is being used, but laparotomy is usually preferred, as meticulous identification, excision, and proper closure of the defect are mandatory to prevent uterine rupture. Factors like the method of removal of adenomyotic tissue, the degree of residual adenomyosis, the method of reconstructing the uterine wall, postoperative complications, and the interval between the procedure and conception are of immense importance. The role of surgery in improving fertility outcomes is still questionable and requires further research.

Since 1990, various kinds of surgeries have been demonstrated. From excision of adenomyotic tissue after longitudinal incision of the uterus to the wedge resection and using.

Classical V-shaped resection technique, multiple newer techniques have been experimented, including a uterine "muscle flap" method that stresses fertility preservation. This procedure was described by Osada et al. in 113 women. Of these women, 81.4% demonstrated normal blood flow in that area after 6 months, and a significant number of women conceived and delivered. No cases of uterine rupture were reported. Similarly, a study including 102 women in search of pregnancy who underwent a laparoscopic adenomyomectomy observed a 31.4% clinical pregnancy rate post-surgery; however, two cases of placenta accreta which required a postpartum hysterectomy were reported. The evidence suggests that the triple-flap technique, when performed by surgical experts, seems beneficial in women who fail to achieve a live birth after all efforts.

Another approach using hysteroscopy can be useful in cases with cavity modifications. Regarding such cavity abnormalities induced by adenomyosis, a prospective study evaluating the role of hysteroscopic enlargement metroplasty in women with a T-shaped uterus and infertility demonstrated better live birth and reduced miscarriage rates after the procedure [24]. Surgical procedures which were initially done for a focal lesion are now also being done for diffuse adenomyosis. Studies have wide heterogenicity and hence all methods are not comparable. In a systemic review and meta-analysis, it was found that these procedures can be helpful in reducing the uterine volume and getting superior reproductive outcomes but proper care must be taken to avoid complications [25]. All cases must be evaluated on a case-to-case basis, and decisions should be made accordingly after careful evaluation.

37.4 Conclusion

Adenomyosis still continues to mystify patients and gynecologists. As we are eventually learning more about the disease, we realize that it is quite prevalent in the infertile population. Due to its frequent association with endometriosis, the disease in the uterus is often overlooked, which according to many can be the primary source of these estrogen-dependent conditions. A lack of standardization in diagnoses makes this disease challenging to study. Although pain and bleeding problems are common symptoms, sometimes subfertility or even infertility is the only sign of this uterine disease. Advances in science and technology have provided us with quite new information regarding the immunological and vascular defects causing infertility in these women, and this can help in developing new and targeted treatment options in the future. Existing literature suggests early IVF and embryo culture with or without the use of suppression using GnRH agonists or even aromatase inhibitors prior to embryo transfer can give good and early results. Surgical management, in spite of being helpful in some instances, is still not recommended for all, and patient selection guidelines are pending. Guidelines from regional governing bodies, when available, will be helpful. All cases must be evaluated individually, and a personalized treatment plan must be suggested depending on the patients' need and the extent of the disease.

References

1. Bird CC, McElin TW, Manalo-Estrella P. The elusive adenomyosis of the uterus-revisited. Am J Obstet Gynecol. 1972;112:583–93.
2. Puente JM, Fabris A, Patel J, Patel A, Cerrillo M, Requena A, et al. Adenomyosis in infertile women: prevalence and the role of 3D ultrasound as a marker of severity of the disease. Reprod Biol Endocrinol. 2016;14:60.
3. Naftalin J, Hoo W, Pateman K, Mavrelos D, Holland T, Jurkovic D. How common is adenomyosis? A prospective study of prevalence using transvaginal ultrasound in a gynaecology clinic. Hum Reprod. 2012;27:3432–9.
4. Marcellin L, Santulli P, Bourdon M, Maignien C, Campin L, Lafay-Pillet MC, et al. Focal adenomyosis of the outer myometrium and deep infiltrating endometriosis severity. Fertil Steril. 2020;114:818–27.
5. Benagiano G, Brosens I. History of adenomyosis. In: Best practice and research: clinical obstetrics and gynaecology, vol. 20. Baillière Tindall; 2006. p. 449–63.
6. Barrier BF, Malinowski MJ, Dick EJ, Hubbard GB, Bates GW. Adenomyosis in the baboon is associated with primary infertility. Fertil Steril. 2004;82:1091–4.
7. Lyons EA, Taylor PJ, Zheng XH, Ballard G, Levi CS, Kredentser J, v. Characterization of subendometrial myometrial contractions throughout the menstrual cycle in normal fertile women. Fertil Steril. 1991;55:771–4.
8. Kunz B, Beil D, Huppert P, Leyendecker G. Structural abnormalities of the uterine wall in women with endometriosis and infertility visualized by vaginal sonography and magnetic resonance imaging. Hum Reprod. 2000;15:76–82.
9. Kitawaki J, Noguchi T, Amatsu T, Maeda K, Tsukamoto K, Yamamoto T, et al. Expression of aromatase cytochrome P450 protein and messenger ribonucleic acid in human endometriotic and adenomyotic tissues but not in normal endometrium. Biol Reprod. 1997;57:514–9.

10. Brosens J, Verhoeven H, Campo R, Gianaroli L, Gordts S, Hazekamp J, et al. High endometrial aromatase P450 mRNA expression is associated with poor IVF outcome. Hum Reprod. 2004;19:352–6.
11. Xiao Y, Sun X, Yang X, Zhang J, Xue Q, Cai B, et al. Leukemia inhibitory factor is dysregulated in the endometrium and uterine flushing fluid of patients with adenomyosis during implantation window. Fertil Steril. 2010;94:85–9.
12. Wang J, Huang C, Jiang R, Du Y, Zhou J, Jiang Y, Yan Q, Xing J, Hou X, Zhou J, Sun H. Decreased endometrial IL-10 impairs endometrial receptivity by downregulating HOXA10 expression in women with adenomyosis. Biomed Res Int. 2018;2018
13. Martínez-Conejero JA, Morgan M, Montesinos M, Fortuño S, Meseguer M, Simón C, et al. Adenomyosis does not affect implantation, but is associated with miscarriage in patients undergoing oocyte donation. Fertil Steril. 2011;96:943–950.e1.
14. Younes G, Tulandi T. Effects of adenomyosis on in vitro fertilization treatment outcomes: a meta-analysis. Fertil Steril. 2017;108:483–490.e3.
15. Vercellini P, Consonni D, Dridi D, Bracco B, Frattaruolo MP, Somigliana E. Uterine adenomyosis and in vitro fertilization outcome: a systematic review and meta-analysis. Hum Reprod. 2014;29:964–77.
16. Nirgianakis K, Kalaitzopoulos DR, Schwartz AS, Spaanderman M, Kramer BW, Mueller MD, Mueller M. Fertility, pregnancy and neonatal outcomes of patients with adenomyosis: a systematic review and meta-analysis. Reprod Biomed Online. 2020;42:185–206.
17. Bourdon M, Santulli P, Oliveira J, Marcellin L, Maignien C, Melka L, et al. Focal adenomyosis is associated with primary infertility. Fertil Steril. 2020;114:1271–7.
18. Hou X, Xing J, Shan H, Mei J, Sun Y, Yan G, et al. The effect of adenomyosis on IVF after long or ultra-long GnRH agonist treatment. Reprod Biomed Online. 2020;41:845–53.
19. Chen M, Luo L, Wang Q, Gao J, Chen Y, Zhang Y, et al. Impact of gonadotropin-releasing hormone agonist pre-treatment on the cumulative live birth rate in infertile women with Adenomyosis treated with IVF/ICSI: a retrospective cohort study. Front Endocrinol. 2020;11:318.
20. Niu Z, Chen Q, Sun Y, Feng Y. Long-term pituitary downregulation before frozen embryo transfer could improve pregnancy outcomes in women with adenomyosis. Gynecol Endocrinol. 2013;29:1026–30.
21. Li X, Pan N, Zhang W, Wang Y, Ge Y, Wei H, et al. Association between uterine volume and pregnancy outcomes in adenomyosis patients undergoing frozen-thawed embryo transfer. Reprod Biomed Online. 2021;42:384–9.
22. Badawy AM, Elnashar AM, Mosbah AA. Aromatase inhibitors or gonadotropin-releasing hormone agonists for the management of uterine adenomyosis: a randomized controlled trial. Acta Obstet Gynecol Scand. 2012;91:489–95.
23. Zhang L, Rao F, Setzen R. High intensity focused ultrasound for the treatment of adenomyosis: selection criteria, efficacy, safety and fertility. Acta Obstet Gynecol Scand. 2017;96:707–14.
24. Alonso Pacheco L, Laganà AS, Garzon S, Pérez Garrido A, Flores Gornés A, Ghezzi F. Hysteroscopic outpatient metroplasty for T-shaped uterus in women with reproductive failure: results from a large prospective cohort study. Eur J Obstet Gynecol Reprod Biol. 2019;243:173–8.
25. Mikos T, Lioupis M, Anthoulakis C, Grimbizis GF. The outcome of fertility-sparing and nonfertility-sparing surgery for the treatment of adenomyosis. A Systematic Review and Meta-analysis. J Minim Invasive Gynecol. 2020;27:309–31.

Pregnancy and Obstetric Outcomes in Adenomyosis

38

Michael D. Mueller, Konstantinos Nirgianakis, and U. Leone Roberti Maggiore

Contents

38.1 Introduction

Adenomyosis, characterized by the presence of endometrial epithelial and stromal cells within the myometrium, is an enigmatic gynecological disorder with an estimated prevalence of 20–35% [1, 2]. It is a significantly heterogeneous disease, both in phenotype and clinical outcomes varying from normally sized to much enlarged uterus and from heavy dysmenorrhea and hypermenorrhea to no symptom [3]. Several studies demonstrated a negative impact of adenomyosis on fertility, pregnancy, and neonatal outcomes [4].

M. D. Mueller (✉) · K. Nirgianakis
Department of Gynecology and Gynecological Oncology, Inselspital, Bern University Hospital, Bern, Switzerland
e-mail: michel.mueller@insel.ch

U. L. R. Maggiore
Gynecologic Oncology Unit, Fondazione IRCCS, Istituto Nazionale dei Tumori, Milano, Italy

E. Oral (ed.), *Endometriosis and Adenomyosis*,
https://doi.org/10.1007/978-3-030-97236-3_38

38.1.1 Fertility Outcomes after ART

Adenomyosis is associated with a significantly lower clinical pregnancy rate and higher miscarriage rate after ART especially when a short downregulation protocol is administered for ovarian stimulation. Indeed, the protocol for ovarian stimulation may be crucial for the fertility outcome in patients with adenomyosis [5]. Long GnRHa protocols produce a period of estrogen deficiency that may temporarily inactivate adenomyosis, reduce the uterine volume, and normalize some of the distorted endometrial functions. This period of potentially therapeutic estrogen deficiency does not occur in GnRH antagonist or short GnRHa cycles.

The positive effect of the long GnRHa pretreatment before ART in patients with adenomyosis is supported by two retrospective controlled studies comparing GnRHa pretreatment versus no treatment before fresh embryo [6] and frozen embryo transfer [7]. Currently, two RCT studies are ongoing to conclusively elucidate this issue [8, 9]. Finally, it is currently unknown if alternative treatments with less side effects such as progestins could be beneficial prior to ART.

As mentioned above, adenomyosis is a very heterogenic disorder with varying extent of lesions, ranging from multiple lesions with diffuse myometrial hypertrophy to more discrete focal lesions [10]. It is plausible that the impact of adenomyosis on the reproductive course is not always the same rather than dependent on the degree of the uterus involvement.

Two studies compared the effects of focal versus diffuse adenomyosis on clinical pregnancy rate after ART [6, 11]. The pooled results gave a statistically nonsignificant OR of 1.36 favoring focal adenomyosis (CI: 0.67–2.75) [12]. In another prospective study, 152 women had MRI prior to in vitro fertilization [13]. The pregnancy rate in the group with maximum JZ thickness < 10 vs. >10 mm was 63 vs. 14%. Implantation failure rate was 96% in patients with an average JZ thickness > 7 mm and a maximal JZ >10 mm, compared with 38% in other patient groups. This study indicates an increase in adverse implantation outcome in relation to the JZ thickness.

In a study which included only patients with adenomyosis receiving donated oocytes, it has been demonstrated that despite having no difference in the pregnancy rate, a higher risk of miscarriage was reported in the adenomyosis group, indicating a detrimental effect of adenomyosis on the reproductive outcome irrespective of the embryo quality [14]. A large Chinese retrospective cohort study aimed to investigate the effect of ultrasound-diagnosed adenomyosis on assisted pregnancy outcomes. This study included 18,568 women undergoing in vitro fertilization and confirmed that despite there was no statistical difference in the embryo implantation rate, clinical pregnancy rate, or multiple pregnancy rate between two groups, early miscarriage rate in the adenomyosis group was significantly higher than that in the control group. Furthermore, the live birth rate was 22.8% in women with adenomyosis and was observed to be significantly lower than 33.3% in the control group ($P = 0.026$) [15].

38.1.2 Pregnancy Outcomes

Most of the studies that evaluated pregnancy outcomes in patients with adenomyosis included a much higher number of ART pregnancies in the case group than in the control group. Since ART pregnancies are anyway at a higher risk of adverse pregnancy outcomes such as preterm birth and low birth weight [16], it is uncertain if the observed adverse outcomes can be attributed to adenomyosis or are just the effect of the ART conception. However, in a recent study, all outcomes measured were analyzed according to the mode of conception and adjusted to age when possible [4]. Interestingly, the increased risk of preeclampsia, SGA, preterm delivery (<37 weeks), low birth weight, and PPH in patients with adenomyosis persisted. It seems that at least for these pregnancy complications adenomyosis represents a significant risk factor independently of the mode of conception. A retrospective study aimed to explore if fetal and maternal outcomes, in particular the incidence of a SGA infant, are different in pregnant women with endometriosis only from those with the concomitant presence of diffuse or focal adenomyosis. Patients with diffuse adenomyosis compared with those with endometriosis only had significantly lower pregnancy-associated plasma protein A, higher mean uterine artery pulsatility index in the first and second trimesters of pregnancy, and higher incidence of SGA [17].

Although the risk of preterm delivery, adjusted for endometriosis, is higher in patients with adenomyosis (OR 2.49; 95% CI 1.81, 3.41) [28], a meta-analysis showed no significant difference in severe preterm delivery (<32 weeks) [4].

38.1.3 Obstetrical Outcomes

Women with adenomyosis have a higher risk of fetal malpresentation (OR 2.84; 95% CI 1.60, 5.81) and C-section delivery (OR 4.44; CI 2.64, 7.47) than women without adenomyosis [4]. Operative vaginal deliveries are not more frequent in women with adenomyosis [18].

The reported increased risk of C-section in patients with endometriosis has to be interpreted with caution as the biggest study on the topic was based on a patient-reported questionnaire collected during the pregnancy for the diagnosis of adenomyosis, while a significant difference in age, primiparity, and sterility treatment between groups was described [19]. Nevertheless, a sensitivity analysis, which included only two studies with balanced groups for age and mode of conception showed also an increased risk for C-section [4]. The significantly increased risk of fetal malpresentation indicates an independent association with adenomyosis since no other factor could be demonstrated as the reason for fetal malpresentation in the concerned studies. Consequently, the increased risk of elective C-section in patients with adenomyosis could be partially attributed to the adenomyosis-dependent increased risk of fetal malpresentation. If patients with adenomyosis are also at an increased risk of failed vaginal delivery and secondary C-section is unclear.

An increased risk of severe PPH in women with adenomyosis has been described in an older study, supported by a prevalence of 17.2% histologically confirmed adenomyosis cases found in women who needed a cesarean hysterectomy [20]. The higher rate of placental malpresentation could also contribute to the increased blood loss [21].

Women with adenomyosis have also a significantly higher risk of placental malposition (OR 4.94; 95% 1.70, 14.34) and of PPH than women without adenomyosis (OR 2.90; 1.39, 6.05) [4].

38.1.4 Neonatal Outcomes

A meta-analysis of four studies [7, 8, 22, 28] showed a significantly higher risk for small for gestational age (SGA) infants in women with adenomyosis (OR 2.86, 95% CI 1.68, 4.88) [4]. Studies matched for endometriosis showed that the risk of SGA remained significantly higher in patients with endometriosis (2 studies, OR 2.10; 95% CI 1.17, 3.77) [4]. Two studies including both natural and ART pregnancies showed also a higher risk of birth weight < 2500 g and < 1500 g in the adenomyosis group [23, 28]. Shin et al. examined the risk of low birth weight (<2500gr) separately in pregnancies after ART and natural conception. In ART pregnancies, a significantly higher risk in the adenomyosis group was shown (25 vs. 187 women; OR 7.69; 95% CI 2.56, 35.34). However, in natural conception pregnancies, no significant difference between groups was found.

No statistical difference has been demonstrated for intrauterine growth restriction or intrauterine fetal death in patients with adenomyosis when compared to patients without adenomyosis.

38.2 Conclusion

Due to the large variety of criteria used to diagnose adenomyosis, the inadequate characterization and classification of adenomyosis in most of the published studies, a comparison between women with adenomyosis and women without adenomyosis is often difficult. Certain diagnostic criteria for adenomyosis have been proposed [24], and we strongly suggest that these are systematically used in future studies in order to investigate which adenomyosis characteristics, if any, are the most significant for the reproductive course. A recent article proposed that seven items should be assessed when examining and describing a uterus with adenomyosis by ultrasound: presence, location, differentiation (focal/diffuse), appearance (cystic/non-cystic), uterine layer involvement, extent, and size of lesion [25]. A similar MRI-based classification distinguishing between internal adenomyosis, external adenomyosis, and structural-related adenomyoma subtypes with a potential relation for therapeutic strategy has been proposed [26].

The frequent coexistence of adenomyosis with other gynecologic disorders such as endometriosis and uterine fibroids is well known [27, 28]. As both endometriosis and uterine fibroids correlate with adverse pregnancy outcomes [29–32], future studies have to consider the existence of endometriosis and uterine fibroids.

Meanwhile, as a negative association between adenomyosis and fertility outcome has been reported in several studies after short protocol downregulation in ART, a mixed or ultralong GnRHa protocol should be followed as this association is less significant in ART following these regimens. Adenomyosis also correlates with adverse pregnancy outcomes such as preterm delivery, preeclampsia, C-section, fetal malpresentation, SGA, low birth weight, and PPH. Gynecologists should be aware of these risks to indicate proper pregnancy controls enabling an early diagnosis and treatment of pregnancy complications. Matched controlled studies with proper adenomyosis classification extending from fertility desire to postpartum period are needed to investigate the role of specific adenomyosis subtypes and their treatment in every aspect of the reproductive course.

References

1. Abbott JA. Adenomyosis and Abnormal Uterine Bleeding (AUB-A)-Pathogenesis, diagnosis, and management. Best Pract Res Clin Obstet Gynaecol. 2017;40:68–81.
2. Vercellini P, Vigano P, Somigliana E, Daguati R, Abbiati A, Fedele L. Adenomyosis: epidemiological factors. Best Pract Res Clin Obstet Gynaecol. 2006;20:465–77.
3. Chapron C, Vannuccini S, Santulli P, Abrao MS, Carmona F, Fraser IS, et al. Diagnosing adenomyosis: an integrated clinical and imaging approach. Hum Reprod Update. 2020;26:392–411.
4. Nirgianakis K, Kalaitzopoulos DR, Schwartz ASK, Spaanderman M, Kramer BW, Mueller MD, Mueller M. Fertility, pregnancy and neonatal outcomes of patients with adenomyosis: a systematic review and meta-analysis. Reprod Biomed Online. 2021;42(1):185–206.
5. Thalluri V, Tremellen KP. Ultrasound diagnosed adenomyosis has a negative impact on successful implantation following GnRH antagonist IVF treatment. Hum Reprod. 2012;27:3487–92.
6. Park CW, Choi MH, Yang KM, Song IO. Pregnancy rate in women with adenomyosis undergoing fresh or frozen embryo transfer cycles following gonadotropin-releasing hormone agonist treatment. Clin Exp Reprod Med. 2016;43:169–73.
7. Niu Z, Chen Q, Sun Y, Feng Y. Long-term pituitary downregulation before frozen embryo transfer could improve pregnancy outcomes in women with adenomyosis. Gynecol Endocrinol. 2013;29:1026–30.
8. Impact of Ultra-long Versus Long Down-regulation Protocol on IVF/ICSI in Adenomyosis. clinicaltrials.gov
9. Modified Downregulation for Women With Adenomyosis of the Uterus Prior to Frozen-thawed Embryo Transfer. clinicaltrials.gov
10. Chapron C, Tosti C, Marcellin L, Bourdon M, Lafay-Pillet MC, Millischer AE, et al. Relationship between the magnetic resonance imaging appearance of adenomyosis and endometriosis phenotypes. Hum Reprod. 2017;32:1393–401.
11. Benaglia L, Cardellicchio L, Leonardi M, Faulisi S, Vercellini P, Paffoni A, et al. Asymptomatic adenomyosis and embryo implantation in IVF cycles. Reprod Biomed Online. 2014;29:606–11.
12. Younes G, Tulandi T. Effects of adenomyosis on in vitro fertilization treatment outcomes: a meta-analysis. Fertil Steril. 2017;108:483–90.e3.
13. Maubon A, Faury A, Kapella M, Pouquet M, Piver P. Uterine junctional zone at magnetic resonance imaging: a predictor of in vitro fertilization implantation failure. J Obstet Gynaecol Res. 2010;36:611–8.
14. Martínez-Conejero JA, Morgan M, Montesinos M, Fortuño S, Meseguer M, Simón C, et al. Adenomyosis does not affect implantation, but is associated with miscarriage in patients undergoing oocyte donation. Fertil Steril. 2011;96:943–50.e1.
15. Zhang XP, Zhang YF, Shi R, Zhang YJ, Zhang XL, Hu XM, Hu XY, Hu YJ. Pregnancy outcomes of infertile women with ultrasound-diagnosed adenomyosis for in vitro fertilization

and frozen-thawed embryo transfer. Arch Gynecol Obstet. 2021;304(4):1089–96. https://doi.org/10.1007/s00404-021-06011.
16. Qin JB, Sheng XQ, Wu D, Gao SY, You YP, Yang TB, et al. Worldwide prevalence of adverse pregnancy outcomes among singleton pregnancies after in vitro fertilization/intracytoplasmic sperm injection: a systematic review and meta-analysis. Arch Gynecol Obstet. 2017;295:285–301.
17. Scala C, Leone Roberti Maggiore U, Racca A, Barra F, Vellone VG, Venturini PL, Ferrero S. Influence of adenomyosis on pregnancy and perinatal outcomes in women with endometriosis. Ultrasound Obstet Gynecol. 2018;52(5):666–71.
18. Mochimaru A, Aoki S, Oba MS, Kurasawa K, Takahashi T, Hirahara F. Adverse pregnancy outcomes associated with adenomyosis with uterine enlargement. J Obstet Gynaecol Res. 2015;41:529–33.
19. Yamaguchi A, Kyozuka H, Fujimori K, Hosoya M, Yasumura S, Yokoyama T, et al. Risk of preterm birth, low birthweight and small-for-gestational-age infants in pregnancies with adenomyosis: a cohort study of the Japan environment and Children's study. Acta Obstet Gynecol Scand. 2019;98:359–64.
20. Sandberg EC, Cohn F. Adenomyosis in the gravid uterus at term. Am J Obstet Gynecol. 1962;84:1457–65.
21. Hashimoto A, Iriyama T, Sayama S, Nakayama T, Komatsu A, Miyauchi A, et al. Adenomyosis and adverse perinatal outcomes: increased risk of second trimester miscarriage, preeclampsia, and placental malposition. J Matern Fetal Neonatal Med. 2018;31:364–9.
22. Scala C, Leone Roberti Maggiore U, Racca A, Barra F, Vellone VG, Venturini PL, et al. Influence of adenomyosis on pregnancy and perinatal outcomes in women with endometriosis. Ultrasound Obstet Gynecol. 2018;52:666–71.
23. Shin YJ, Kwak DW, Chung JH, Kim MY, Lee SW, Han YJ. The risk of preterm births among pregnant women with adenomyosis. J Ultrasound Med. 2018;37:1937–43.
24. Gordts S, Grimbizis G, Campo R. Symptoms and classification of uterine adenomyosis, including the place of hysteroscopy in diagnosis. Fertil Steril. 2018;109(380–8):e1.
25. Van den Bosch T, de Bruijn AM, de Leeuw RA, Dueholm M, Exacoustos C, Valentin L, et al. Sonographic classification and reporting system for diagnosing adenomyosis. Ultrasound Obstet Gynecol. 2019;53:576–82.
26. Bazot M, Darai E. Role of transvaginal sonography and magnetic resonance imaging in the diagnosis of uterine adenomyosis. Fertil Steril. 2018;109:389–97.
27. Eisenberg VH, Arbib N, Schiff E, Goldenberg M, Seidman DS, Soriano D. Sonographic signs of adenomyosis are prevalent in women undergoing surgery for endometriosis and may suggest a higher risk of infertility. Biomed Res Int. 2017;2017:8967803.
28. Lazzeri L, Di Giovanni A, Exacoustos C, Tosti C, Pinzauti S, Malzoni M, et al. Preoperative and postoperative clinical and transvaginal ultrasound findings of adenomyosis in patients with deep infiltrating endometriosis. Reprod Sci. 2014;21:1027–33.
29. Zullo F, Spagnolo E, Saccone G, Acunzo M, Xodo S, Ceccaroni M, et al. Endometriosis and obstetrics complications: a systematic review and meta-analysis. Fertil Steril. 2017;108:667–72.e5.
30. Karlsen K, Schioler Kesmodel U, Mogensen O, Humaidan P, Ravn P. Relationship between a uterine fibroid diagnosis and the risk of adverse obstetrical outcomes: a cohort study. BMJ Open. 2020;10:e032104.
31. Klatsky PC, Tran ND, Caughey AB, Fujimoto VY. Fibroids and reproductive outcomes: a systematic literature review from conception to delivery. Am J Obstet Gynecol. 2008;198:357–66.
32. Lam S-J, Best S, Kumar S. The impact of fibroid characteristics on pregnancy outcome. Am J Obstet Gynecol. 2014;211:395.e1.

Does Adenomyosis Increase Cancer Risk?

39

Harald Krentel and Ioannis Vlachodimitris

Contents

39.1 Introduction

A review and meta-analysis of 8 retrospective cohort studies assessing 5573 patients with endometrial cancer by Raffone et al. recently attempted to answer the question if cancer risk is increased in patients with adenomyosis. The authors concluded that the supposed association between adenomyosis and endometrial cancer appears unsupported. The prevalence of adenomyosis in patients with endometrial cancer was not different from that reported for other gynecological disorders [1]. The co-occurrence of adenomyosis and endometrial cancer might be due to the high incidence of adenomyosis in perimenopausal and postmenopausal women [2]. However, even if adenomyosis does not increase the risk of endometrial cancer, the presence of adenomyosis still seems to be related to the following questions: Is adenomyosis

The original version of the chapter has been revised. A correction to this chapter can be found at https://doi.org/10.1007/978-3-030-97236-3_45

H. Krentel (✉) · I. Vlachodimitris
Clinic of Gynecology, Obstetrics, Gynecological Oncology and Senology, Academic Teaching Hospital, Bethesda Hospital, Duisburg, Germany
e-mail: h.krentel@bethesda.de

E. Oral (ed.), *Endometriosis and Adenomyosis*,
https://doi.org/10.1007/978-3-030-97236-3_39

a confounder in the diagnosis and staging of endometrial cancer? Does endometrial cancer arise from adenomyosis? Is there a malignant transformation or do the entities coexist? Is there a special risk for endometrial cancer in patients with adenomyosis using hormone replacement therapy or patients with breast cancer and related endocrine treatment and adenomyosis?

39.2 Malignant Transformation of Adenomyosis

Adenomyosis is one of the most common benign histological findings in hysterectomy specimens in patients with endometrial cancer. In the current literature, several case reports describe endometrial cancer arising from adenomyosis and differentiate this entity from endometrial cancer coexisting with adenomyosis [3–5]. Kucera et al. described a rate of 6.8% of malignant changes of adenomyosis in a total of 219 patients with endometrial cancer. The authors identified benign glandular hyperplasia or atypical complex hyperplasia simultaneously in all cases of cancer-positive adenomyosis [6]. Machida et al. compared cases with endometrial cancer arising in adenomyosis (EC-AIA) ($n = 46$) to 350 cases of coexisting endometrial cancer and adenomyosis (EC-A) and described the clinical differences between both entities [7]. EC-AIA can be defined by the following histopathological characteristics: endometrial cancer should not be present in the eutopic endometrium and must arise from the epithelium of adenomyotic foci, and endometrial stromal cells have to surround the ectopic endometrial glands as a feature of adenomyosis [1] (Figs. 39.1 and 39.2). At present, the mechanism of malignant transformation of adenomyosis is not completely understood due to its low incidence, missing clinical trials and the heterogeneity of the current research [8]. So far, the effect of hormone replacement therapy and endocrine treatment in patients with breast cancer on adenomyotic lesions is not fully understood [9, 10].

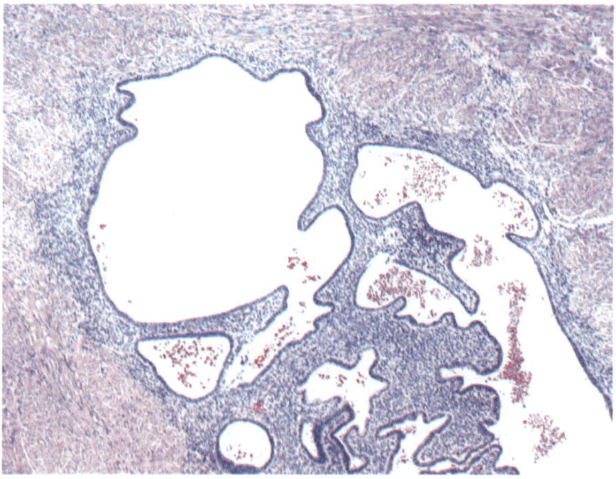

Fig. 39.1 Adenomyosis within the uterine myometrium. Endometrial glands surrounded by myometrial cells. Hematoxylin-eosin stain. (Photograph by H. Krentel)

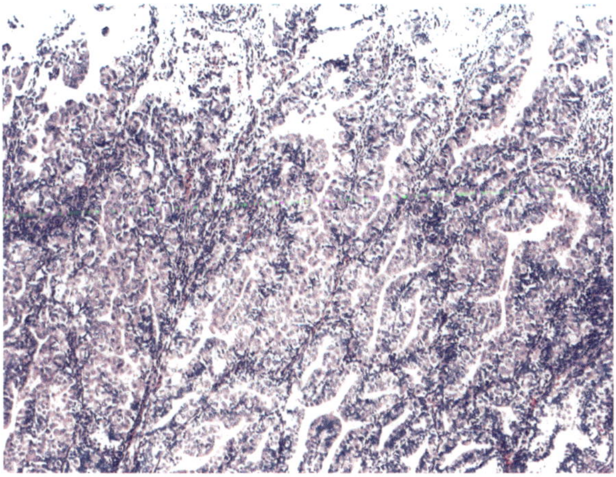

Fig. 39.2 Endometrial cancer within adenomyosis. Hematoxylin-eosin stain. (Photograph by H. Krentel)

39.3 Diagnosis and Staging of Endometrial Cancer in Patients with Adenomyosis

The differentiation between adenomyosis, EC-A, and EC-AIA is challenging. The classical first sign of a beginning endometrial cancer, a postmenopausal bleeding, might be missing or be delayed in patients with endometrial cancer within the myometrium. Usually endometrial lesions can be detected by transvaginal ultrasound. The endometrium might be thickened or irregular. Additionally, intracavitary tumors can be visualized by hydrosonography. Diagnostic hysteroscopy with intrauterine biopsy and abrasion is the next step in the diagnosis of suspicious endometrial lesions. The histopathological examination of the uterus reveals malignant lesions and allows a clear differentiation. In patients with endometrial cancer arising in adenomyotic lesions, the diagnosis by transvaginal ultrasound might be hindered as a reliable differentiation between adenomyosis and endometrial cancer within adenomyosis lesions is not possible. Transvaginal Doppler sonography might detect irregular vascularization as a sign of malignancy. However, in patients with endometrial cancer arising from adenomyosis, the tumor can be found within the myometrium without intracavitary extension in 50–67% of the cases [7, 11]. Thus, these lesions cannot be visualized by hysteroscopy, and it turns out to be difficult to obtain a reliable biopsy. A hysteroresectoscopic approach is an additional option in the hands of the skilled hysteroscopic surgeon [12]. However, a uterine perforation with possible spillage of cancer cells to the peritoneal cavity should be avoided. A possible imaging alternative in the differentiation of endometrial carcinoma and uterine benign lesions is the use of 3D amide proton transfer-weighted MR imaging [13].

In cases of endometrial cancer within adenomyotic lesions, the initial localization of the malignant lesion also represents a challenge for staging and classification of endometrial cancer [14]. The definition of depth of malignant infiltration of the uterine wall and thus the oncological classification can be difficult. This can also affect the subsequent decisions regarding lymphadenectomy and adjuvant therapy. Compared to endometrial cancer coexisting with adenomyosis, endometrial cancer arising in adenomyotic lesions is associated with a deep myometrial tumor invasion [7, 15, 16]. Matsuo and co-authors associated EC-AIA with a decreased disease-free survival and a worse survival outcome [7, 11]. Other authors reported a less deep myometrial invasion in EC-A compared to patients with endometrial cancer without adenomyosis [17]. This might be related to the simple fact of an increased diameter of the uterine wall in patients with coexisting adenomyosis. The results regarding the prognosis of adenomyosis-related endometrial cancer remain controversial. EC-A seems to be associated with favorable tumor characteristics, while EC-AIA could be related to a poorer prognosis [2, 17–20]. A comparison of the results appears to be difficult as some authors did not differ between EC without adenomyosis, EC-A, and EC-AIA.

39.4 Conclusion

The recent literature shows that adenomyosis does not increase the risk of endometrial cancer. The presence of adenomyosis can be a confounder in the accurate diagnosis and staging of uterine malignancies. Endometrial cancer arising in adenomyotic lesions is rare and has to be differentiated from endometrial cancer coexisting with adenomyosis. EC-AIA seems to be related to a deep myometrial tumor invasion. Its impact on the oncological outcome requires further investigations. The possible correlation between endometrial cancer and adenomyosis should be considered, especially in perimenopausal and postmenopausal patients and patients using hormone replacement therapy.

References

1. Raffone A, Seracchioli R, Raimondo D, Maletta M, Travaglino A, Raimondo I, Giaquinto I, Orsini B, Insabato L, Pellicano M, Zullo F. Prevalence of adenomyosis in endometrial cancer patients: a systematic review and meta-analysis. Arch Gynecol Obstet. 2020. https://doi.org/10.1007/s00404-020-05840-8. Epub ahead of print. PMID: 33098006.
2. Habiba M, Pluchino N, Petignat P, Bianchi P, Brosens IA, Benagiano G. Adenomyosis and endometrial cancer: literature review. Gynecol Obstet Investig. 2018;83(4):313–28. https://doi.org/10.1159/000487320. Epub 2018 Jun 6. PMID: 29874641.
3. Rubod C, Narducci F, Delattre C, Decocq J, Verbert A, Delahousse G. Adénocarcinome endométrioïde résultant de foyers d'adénomyose: à propos d'un cas et revue de la littérature [Endometrioid adenocarcinoma arising from adenomyosis. A case report and literature review]. J Gynecol Obstet Biol Reprod (Paris). 2004;33(2):140–4. https://doi.org/10.1016/s0368-2315(04)96413-7. French. PMID: 15052180.
4. Kazandi M, Zeybek B, Terek MC, Zekioglu O, Ozdemir N, Oztekin K. Grade 2 endometrioid adenocarcinoma arising from adenomyosis of the uterus: report of a case. Eur J Gynaecol Oncol. 2010;31(6):719–21. PMID: 21319528.

5. Boes AS, Tousseyn T, Vandenput I, Timmerman D, Vergote I, Moerman P, Amant F. Pitfall in the diagnosis of endometrial cancer: case report of an endometrioid adenocarcinoma arising from uterine adenomyosis. Eur J Gynaecol Oncol. 2011;32(4):431–4. PMID: 21941970.
6. Kucera E, Hejda V, Dankovcik R, Valha P, Dudas M, Feyereisl J. Malignant changes in adenomyosis in patients with endometrioid adenocarcinoma. Eur J Gynaecol Oncol. 2011;32(2):182–4. PMID: 21614909.
7. Machida H, Maeda M, Cahoon SS, Scannell CA, Garcia-Sayre J, Roman LD, Matsuo K. Endometrial cancer arising in adenomyosis versus endometrial cancer coexisting with adenomyosis: are these two different entities? Arch Gynecol Obstet. 2017;295(6):1459–68. https://doi.org/10.1007/s00404-017-4375-z. Epub 2017 Apr 25
8. Yuan H, Zhang S. Malignant transformation of adenomyosis: literature review and meta-analysis. Arch Gynecol Obstet. 2019;299(1):47–53. https://doi.org/10.1007/s00404-018-4991-2. Epub 2018 Dec 5. PMID: 30519753.
9. Kossaï M, Penault-Llorca F. Role of hormones in common benign uterine lesions: endometrial polyps, leiomyomas, and adenomyosis. Adv Exp Med Biol. 2020;1242:37–58. https://doi.org/10.1007/978-3-030-38474-6_3. PMID: 32406027.
10. Benagiano G, Brosens I, Habiba M. Adenomyosis: a life-cycle approach. Reprod Biomed Online. 2015;30(3):220–32. https://doi.org/10.1016/j.rbmo.2014.11.005. Epub 2014 Nov 20. PMID: 25599903.
11. Matsuo K, Moeini A, Machida H, Scannell CA, Casabar JK, Kakuda M, Adachi S, Garcia-Sayre J, Ueda Y, Roman LD. Tumor characteristics and survival outcome of endometrial cancer arising in adenomyosis: an exploratory analysis. Ann Surg Oncol. 2016;23(3):959–67. https://doi.org/10.1245/s10434-015-4952-y. Epub 2015 Nov 5. PMID: 26542589; PMCID: PMC7521605.
12. Honda M, Tsuchiya A, Isono W, Takahashi M, Fujimoto A, Kawamoto M, Nishii O. Endophytic-type endometrial cancer with adenomyosis successfully diagnosed with hysteroscopic endometrial biopsy using an 8.3-mm operative resectoscope: a case report. Case Rep Oncol. 2018;11(2):311–7. https://doi.org/10.1159/000489084. PMID: 29928209; PMCID: PMC6006659.
13. Li Y, Lin CY, Qi YF, Wang XQ, Chen B, Zhou HL, Ren J, Yang JJ, Xiang Y, He YL, Xue HD, Jin ZY. Non-invasive differentiation of endometrial adenocarcinoma from benign lesions in the uterus by utilization of amide proton transfer-weighted MRI. Mol Imaging Biol. 2021;23(3):446–55. https://doi.org/10.1007/s11307-020-01565-x. Epub 2020 Nov 13. PMID: 33185840.
14. Khalifa MA, Atri M, Klein ME, Ghatak S, Murugan P. Adenomyosis as a confounder to accurate endometrial cancer staging. Semin Ultrasound CT MR. 2019;40(4):358–63. https://doi.org/10.1053/j.sult.2019.04.004. Epub 2019 Apr 18. PMID: 31375175.
15. Taneichi A, Fujiwara H, Takahashi Y, Takei Y, Machida S, Saga Y, Takahashi S, Suzuki M. Influences of uterine adenomyosis on muscle invasion and prognosis of endometrioid adenocarcinoma. Int J Gynecol Cancer. 2014;24(8):1429–33. https://doi.org/10.1097/IGC.0000000000000243. PMID: 25188882.
16. Ismiil N, Rasty G, Ghorab Z, Nofech-Mozes S, Bernardini M, Ackerman I, Thomas G, Covens A, Khalifa MA. Adenomyosis involved by endometrial adenocarcinoma is a significant risk factor for deep myometrial invasion. Ann Diagn Pathol. 2007;11(4):252–7. https://doi.org/10.1016/j.anndiagpath.2006.08.011. PMID: 17630108.
17. Aslan K, Sarı ME, Yalçın HR, Yalçın İ, Cüylan ZF, Özdal B. Coexistence of uterine adenomyosis is not associated with a better prognosis in endometrioid-type endometrial cancer. Ir J Med Sci. 2020;189(3):835–42. https://doi.org/10.1007/s11845-020-02172-z. Epub 2020 Jan 23. PMID: 31970616.
18. Chao X, Wu M, Ma S, Tan X, Zhong S, Bi Y, Wu H, Lang J, Li L. The clinicopathological characteristics and survival outcomes of endometrial carcinoma coexisting with or arising in adenomyosis: a pilot study. Sci Rep. 2020;10(1):5984. https://doi.org/10.1038/s41598-020-63065-w. PMID: 32249826; PMCID: PMC7136226.

19. Erkilinç S, Taylan E, Gülseren V, Erkilinç G, Karadeniz T, Bağci M, Temel O, Solmaz U, Gökçü M, Sanci M. The effect of adenomyosis in myometrial invasion and overall survival in endometrial cancer. Int J Gynecol Cancer. 2018;28(1):145–51. https://doi.org/10.1097/IGC.0000000000001137. PMID: 29040186.
20. An M, Duan H, Zhang Y. Prognostic significance of co-existent adenomyosis on outcomes and tumor characteristics of endometrial cancer: a meta-analysis. J Obstet Gynaecol Res. 2020;46(9):1851–63. https://doi.org/10.1111/jog.14371. Epub 2020 Jul 19. PMID: 32686169.

Part V

Clinical Pharmaceutical Features of Drugs Used in Endometriosis and Adenomyosis Treatment and Guidelines

Hormonal Therapy in Endometriosis and Adenomyosis: Oral Contraceptives

40

Hiroaki Komatsu, Fuminori Taniguchi, and Tasuku Harada

Contents

40.1 Treatment of Endometriosis

The most commonly laparoscopic removal of endometriosis lesions can improve pain; however, the procedure is associated with complications and a high recurrence rate [1, 2]. A more radical surgery including cystectomy has also constant recurrence rates [3]. In cases of deep infiltrating endometriosis, resection of the nodule with part of the bowel may resolve symptoms without affecting fertility. However, it associates with serious complications, and postoperative follow-up alone is insufficient to prevent recurrence; therefore, drug therapy is necessary to reduce the recurrence rate. Koga et al. reported that regular and prolonged medication until the patient wishes to conceive is highly recommended to prevent postoperative recurrence of endometriosis [4, 5]. Hence, an alternative to surgery is the use of long-term hormonal therapies. Several therapies have been thoroughly investigated or approved for treating endometriosis [6]. Gonadotropin-releasing hormone agonists have been widely used; however, their duration of use is limited because of unwanted symptoms and loss of

The original version of the chapter has been revised. A correction to this chapter can be found at https://doi.org/10.1007/978-3-030-97236-3_45

H. Komatsu · F. Taniguchi · T. Harada (✉)
Obstetrics and Gynecology, Tottori University, Yonago, Japan
e-mail: tasuku@tottori-u.ac.jp

E. Oral (ed.), *Endometriosis and Adenomyosis*,
https://doi.org/10.1007/978-3-030-97236-3_40

bone mineral density associated with low estrogen (E) status. Progestins have recently been more commonly used, and oral contraceptives (OC), such as, low-dose estrogen plus progestin (LEP), are used as off-label first-line treatments [7, 8].

The most commonly used LEP products are administered on a 28-day (21 + 7 placebo) cyclic regimen. Although the 28-day cycle mimics the length of a natural menstrual cycle, there is no scientific/medical rationale for this approach [9, 10]. Treatment guidelines from the American College of Obstetricians and Gynecologists recommend extended-cycle combined oral contraceptives as initial treatment [11]. Extended LEP regimens may involve 12 weeks of administration rather than 3 weeks of active tablets, followed by 1 week of placebo tablets, thereby reducing the number of withdrawal bleeds. Moreover, several additional studies on the continuous use of LEP had been conducted [12–14]. Extended LEP regimens suppress ovarian function more reliably than 28-day cyclic regimens, with greater improvement of symptoms associated with menstruation [13–15].

Hormone withdrawal symptoms experienced with 28-day LEP products are common during drug-free intervals. Dysmenorrhea is often a typical symptom of endometriosis-related pain. Therefore, extended LEP products, which reduce the frequency of menstrual periods, may be particularly beneficial in patients with endometriosis [16]. However, patients receiving fixed extended LEP products frequently experience irregular bleeding/spotting while taking active tablets [17].

Recently, a placebo-controlled, double-blind, randomized trial is conducted to evaluate the efficacy and safety of 28-day cyclic and 84-day extended regimens of ethinylestradiol 0.02 mg plus levonorgestrel 0.09 mg (NPC-16) in patients with dysmenorrhea in Japan. The cyclic and extended regimens of NPC-16 significantly reduced dysmenorrhea severity compared to placebo. The extended regimen was superior to cyclic regimen in reducing the dysmenorrhea [18].

A more recent development is a flexible extended LEP product comprising 20 μg of ethinylestradiol/3 mg of drospirenone (DRSP) [19]. The flexible regimen consists of a repeat cycle of 120 consecutive days of an active tablet followed by a 4-day tablet-free interval, either after 120 days or after ≥3 consecutive days of bleeding and/or spotting between days 25 and 120 [20]. Studies on flexible regimens have shown that extending the established 28-day cyclic regimen to a flexible extended regimen does not change the steady-state pharmacokinetics of ethinylestradiol or DRSP and have confirmed the efficacy and tolerability of flexible regimens for contraception and dysmenorrhea. Therefore, a flexible regimen could provide a valuable additional treatment choice for women with endometriosis and adenomyosis. Due to coagulation and reactivation of the fibrinolytic system during menstruation in adenomyosis, the use of LEP should be avoided in patients at risk for thrombosis, such as those who are obese, those who smoke, and those aged [21].

40.2 Treatment of Adenomyosis

No randomized controlled trials have shown the efficacy of LEP for adenomyosis. However, LEP is expected to decrease menstrual bleeding and relieve pain in patients with adenomyosis by causing endometrial desquamation and atrophy.

However, it is well known that LEP treatment may not be enough to control pain symptoms of adenomyosis. Dienogest may be beneficial in cases of pelvic pain due to adenomyosis and unresponsive to LEP [22]. Dienogest is an anti-androgenic drug with high selectivity for progesterone receptors. It suppresses ovulation and ovarian function and has a direct effect on endometriosis lesions and is highly effective in the treatment of chronic pelvic pain with endometriosis [23]. In particular, it is an effective treatment for perimenopausal or obese patients in whom LEP use is unfavorable. Irregular uterine bleeding is a problem; however, its frequency can be reduced with continuous administration.

40.3 Mechanism of LEP

LEP acts on the hypothalamus and pituitary gland, suppressing ovulation and resulting in the loss of cyclic fluctuations in estrogen secretion. As a result, the proliferation of the endometrium is suppressed, and the amount of menstrual blood decreases. Since prostaglandin (PG) levels are lowest in the early follicular phase, it suppresses excessive PG production from the endometrium, which is seen in patients with dysmenorrhea, and reduces the size of endometrioma [24]. Patients with endometriosis have higher intrauterine pressure and more frequent contractions. Inhibition of PG production reduces excessive uterine contractions, which is the main cause of dysmenorrhea [25]. In addition, basic data on LEP exists. A study by Meresman et al. showed that the ectopic endometria of endometriotic patients had higher proliferative capacities and a lower number of apoptotic cells than the endometrium of women without endometriosis; however, the number was comparable after LEP administration [26]. Moreover, the number of nerve fibers in the endometriosis tissue was exhibited to decrease after LEP administration [27].

40.4 Endometriosis in Adolescents

Recently, the need for dysmenorrhea and endometriosis management in adolescent women has been increasingly discussed, and early intervention in young women is crucial. The American College of Obstetricians and Gynecologists developed the following recommendations and conclusions [28]: First, most adolescents experiencing dysmenorrhea have primary dysmenorrhea, which is defined as painful menstruation in the absence of pelvic pathology. Primary dysmenorrhea usually begins when adolescents reach ovulatory cycles, usually within 6–12 months of menarche. Second, secondary dysmenorrhea refers to painful menses due to pelvic pathology or a recognized pathological medical condition. Furthermore, Martin et al. reported that the prevalence of endometriosis among adolescents with pelvic pain is high but treatable and prompt identification helps ensure that adolescents are referred earlier to appropriate specialists [29]. Thus, the management of adolescents with endometriosis should be consistent with best practice guidelines. Furthermore, based on a recent report, we believe that there is an overwhelming preference for initiating hormone treatments in young women.

The long-term maintenance therapy of OC is expected to alleviate symptoms and shrink the lesions. The Practice Committee of the American Society for Reproductive Medicine (ASRM) in 2014 mentioned that endometriosis should be viewed as a chronic disease that requires a lifelong management plan with the goal of maximizing the use of medical treatment and avoiding repeated surgical procedures [30]. The timing of the onset of symptoms, the desire to have a baby, and the beginning of the decline in fertility are different individually, and it is often difficult to find a best solution. To maintain the quality of life of women at each stage of life, it is important to select the most effective treatment method, taking into account the implementation of reproductive medicine, including assisted reproductive technology.

References

1. Guo SW. Recurrence of endometriosis and its control. Hum Reprod Update. 2009;15:441–61.
2. Vercellini P, Crosignani P, Somigliana E, et al. 'Waiting for Godot': a commonsense approach to the medical treatment of endometriosis. Hum Reprod. 2011;26:3–13.
3. Shakiba K, Bena JF, McGill KM, et al. Surgical treatment of endometriosis: a 7-year follow-up on the requirement for further surgery. Obstet Gynecol. 2008;11:1285–92.
4. Kaori K, Masashi T, Tomoyuki F, et al. Prevention of the recurrence of symptom and lesions after conservative surgery for endometriosis. Fertil Steril. 2015;104:793–801.
5. Koga K, Osuga Y, Takemura Y, et al. Recurrence of endometrioma after laparoscopic excision and its prevention by medical management. Front Biosci (Elite Ed). 2013;5:676–83.
6. Dunselman GA, Vermeulen N, Becker C, et al. ESHRE guideline: management of women with endometriosis. Hum Reprod. 2014;29:400–12.
7. Harada T, Momoeda M, Taketani Y, et al. Low-dose oral contraceptive pill for dysmenorrhea associated with endometriosis: a placebo-controlled, double-blind, randomized trial. Fertil Steril. 2014;90:1583–8.
8. Guideline on the management of women with endometriosis. European Society of Human Reproduction and Embryology. 2014;29(3):400–12. file:///C:/Users/komat/Downloads/ESHRE%20guideline%20on%20endometriosis%202013.pdf.
9. Kaunitz AM. Menstruation: choosing whether…and when. Contraception. 2000;62:277–84.
10. Thomas SL, Ellertson C. Nuisance or natural and healthy: should monthly menstruation be optional for women? Lancet. 2000;355:922–4.
11. Armstrong C. ACOG updates guideline on diagnosis and treatment of endometriosis. Am Fam Physician. 2011;83:84–5.
12. Archer DF. Menstrual-cycle-related symptoms: a review of the rationale for continuous use of oral contraceptives. Contraception. 2006;74:359–66.
13. Sulak PJ. Continuous oral contraception: changing times. Best Pract Res Clin Obstet Gynaecol. 2008;22:355–74.
14. Wiegratz I, Kuhl H. Long-cycle treatment with oral contraceptives. Drugs. 2004;6:2447–62.
15. Birtch RL, Olatunbosun OA, Pierson RA. Ovarian follicular dynamics during conventional vs. continuous oral contraceptive use. Contraception. 2006;73:235–43.
16. Vercellini P, Frontino G, De Giorgi O, et al. Continuous use of an oral contraceptive for endometriosis-associated recurrent dysmenorrhea that does not respond to a cyclic pill regimen. Fertil Steril. 2003;80:560–3.
17. Anderson FD, Hait H. A multicenter, randomized study of an extended cycle oral contraceptive. Contraception. 2003;68:89–96.

18. Harada T, Momoeda M. Efficacy of cyclic and extended regimens of ethinylestradiol 0.02 mg -levonorgestrel 0.09 mg for dysmenorrhea: a placebo-controlled, double-blind, randomized trial. Reprod Med Biol. 2021;20(2):215–23.
19. Harada T, Kosaka S, Elliesen J, et al. Ethinylestradiol 20 μg/drospirenone 3 mg in a flexible extended regimen for the management of endometriosis-associated pelvic pain: a randomized controlled trial. Fertil Steril. 2017;108:798–805.
20. Klipping C, Duijkers I, Fortier MP, et al. Contraceptive efficacy and tolerability of ethinylestradiol 20 mug/drospirenone 3 mg in a flexible extended regimen: an open-label, multicentre, randomised, controlled study. J Fam Plann Reprod Health Care. 2012;38:73–83.
21. Osuga Y, Fujimoto-Okabe H, Hagino A. Evaluation of the efficacy and safety of dienogest in the treatment of painful symptoms in patients with adenomyosis: a randomized, double-blind, multicenter, placebo-controlled study. Fertil Steril. 2017;108:673–8.
22. Osuga Y, Hayashi K, Kanda S, et al. Long-term use of dienogest for the treatment of primary and secondary dysmenorrhea. J Obstet Gynaecol Res. 2020;46:606–17.
23. Harada T, Momoeda M, Taketani Y, et al. Low-dose oral contraceptive pill for dysmenorrhea associated with endometriosis: a placebo-controlled, double-blind, randomized trial. Fertil Steril. 2008;90:1583–8.
24. Harada T, Momoeda M, Taketani Y, et al. Dienogest is as effective as intranasal buserelin acetate for the relief of pain symptoms associated with endometriosis--a randomized, double-blind, multicenter, controlled trial. Fertil Steril. 2009;91(3):675–81.
25. Bulletti C, De Ziegler D, Polli V, et al. Characteristics of uterine contractility during menses in women with mild to moderate endometriosis. Fertil Steril. 2002;77:1156–61.
26. Meresman GF, Augé L, Barañao RI, et al. Oral contraceptives suppress cell proliferation and enhance apoptosis of eutopic endometrial tissue from patients with endometriosis. Fertil Steril. 2002;77:1141–7.
27. Tokushige N, Markham R, Russell P, et al. Effect of progestogens and combined oral contraceptives on nerve fibers in peritoneal endometriosis. Fertil Steril. 2009;92:1234–9.
28. ACOG Committee Opinion No. 760: dysmenorrhea and endometriosis in the adolescent. Obstet Gynecol. 2001;132(6):e249–58.
29. Martin H, Rima D, Alfred S, et al. The prevalence of endometriosis in adolescents with pelvic pain: a systematic review. J Pediatr Adolesc Gynecol. 2020;33:623–30.
30. Practice Committee of the American Society for Reproductive M. Treatment of pelvic pain associated with endometriosis: a committee opinion. Fertil Steril. 2014;101(4):927–35.

Hormonal Therapy in Endometriosis and Adenomyosis: Progestins

41

Ezgi Darici and Engin Oral

Contents

41.1 Introduction

Endometriosis is defined as "the presence of viable, estrogen-sensitive, endometrial-like glands and stroma associated with inflammatory response outside the uterus" [1]. Endometriosis affects 6–10% of women of reproductive age, and it has been reported to be found in women between 12 and 80 years old [2]. The average

E. Darici (✉)
Department of Obstetrics Gynecology, İznik State Hospital, Bursa, Turkey

E. Oral
Department of Obstetrics and Gynecology, Bezmialem Vakif University Medical Faculty, Istanbul, Turkey

E. Oral (ed.), *Endometriosis and Adenomyosis*,
https://doi.org/10.1007/978-3-030-97236-3_41

diagnosis is approximately 28 years old [3]. It is reported in 21–47% of women with subfertility and 71–87% of women with chronic pelvic pain [4, 5]. Pain symptoms such as dysmenorrhea, deep dyspareunia, nonmenstrual pelvic pain, and dyschezia are the major symptoms in endometriosis which was reported in 92% of the patients [1]. Typically, the pain precedes the onset of menses and lasts for the duration of the cycle. Less commonly patients also present with cyclical pain at other sites, relating to endometriosis at extrapelvic sites. Endometriosis has a multifactorial etiology [1]. The theories on the disease include retrograde menstruation and refluxed endometrial tissue implanting on pelvic structures, metaplasia of the coelomic pluripotent mesothelial cells in the peritoneum, and implantation of cells via hematogenous or lymphatic embolization. The discovery of the molecular mechanisms associated with endometriosis improved the understanding of traditional theories. Recently discovered features of endometriosis are chronic inflammation with increased cyclooxygenase activity and increased local aromatase activity, increased number of activated macrophages, and proinflammatory cytokines. Concomitant immune dysfunction impairs the clearance of the refluxed endometrial tissue and promotes the progression of the disease by aiding adherence and invasion, angiogenesis, and sensory (sympathetic and parasympathetic) innervations [1]. Treatment of endometriosis is very challenging, and commonly preferred methods are medical therapy and surgical interventions. The surgical intervention provides a treatment that is directly correlated to patient symptoms with long-term pain relief and is associated with improved quality of life. Hence, it remains a necessary part of the management algorithm [6]; however, it may be associated with complications. Moreover, the recurrence rate of pain symptoms after surgery is not negligible [7], so medical treatment strategies play a pivotal role in endometriosis treatment and appears as the first choice in the case of pain, deep endometriosis, extragenital endometriosis, adenomyosis, and infertility (before IVF). Prevention recurrence after surgery, in patients not desiring surgery, empiric treatment, recurrence after a complete excision in the first surgery, and medical therapy with surgical therapy are the other indications to consider medical therapy. The most important issue about medical treatment of endometriosis is that alternate treatments are all effective, but the symptoms tend to recur after the discontinuation of the treatments [1]. Whatever treatment is chosen, often long-term or repeated medication is necessary. Therefore, not only the efficacy but also the tolerability and costs of a drug are relevant. First-line medical treatment should focus on the drugs that can be used for a long term with minimal adverse effect profile (Table 41.1).

NSAIDs may be utilized to control the pain due to endometriosis. On the failure of NSAID treatment, suppressive treatment should be initiated. Estradiol (E2) has the highest importance in the maintenance of endometriosis; hence, the medical therapies used to treat endometriosis-related pain primarily acts by suppressing ovulation, and the main principle is to induce amenorrhea [9].

The first-line treatment choices are combined oral contraceptives (COCs) and oral progestins. The GnRH analogs follow these drugs. Current guidelines recommend an accurate diagnostic workup of women with endometriosis prior to administering second-line hormonal treatments, which include gonadotropin-releasing

Table 41.1 Criteria for the ideal medication for endometriosis [8]

Curative rather than suppressive
Treats pain and fertility at the same time
Acceptable side-effect profile
Long-term use should be safe and affordable
Noncontraceptive nature
No interference with spontaneous ovulations and normal implantation
Enhances spontaneous conception
No teratogenic potential and safe to use periconceptionally
Inhibits the growth of already existing lesions
Aborts the development of new lesions
Efficacious for all endometriosis phenotypes including superficial disease, endometriomas, deep-infiltrating endometriosis, and extrapelvic endometriosis and adenomyosis

hormone analogs (GnRH-as) or aromatase inhibitors (AIs) [2]. Danazol has been shown to be effective in controlling endometriosis-related pain. Levonorgestrel-containing intrauterine system can be used for the endometriosis-related pain so as antiprogesterone gestrinone and aromatase inhibitors such as letrozole and anastrozole (Table 41.2). Norethisterone acetate (NETA), depot medroxyprogesterone acetate (DMPA), GnRH analogs/antagonists, and danazol are FDA-approved drugs in the treatment of endometriosis.

41.2 Progestins in the Treatment of Endometriosis

Progesterone is a steroid hormone and the main source of production is in the ovaries, adrenal glands, and placenta. During the menstrual cycle, with the effect of estrogen endometrium proliferates and following ovulation, secretion of progesterone from the corpus luteum inhibits proliferation of the endometrium, and it enters into the secretory phase in which tissue remodeling is stimulated until the pregnancy or the menstrual shedding. Progestins are synthetic compounds that mimic the effects of progesterone. The progestins differ concerning their profile and potency of action on the hypothalamic-pituitary axis, metabolic processes, breast, and genital organs. Progestins decrease the frequency and increase the amplitude of pulsatile gonadotropin-releasing hormone (GnRH) release in the hypothalamus. This effect decreases the release of follicle-stimulating hormone and luteinizing hormone. Continuous exposure to progestins suppresses ovarian steroidogenesis causing anovulation with decreased ovarian sex steroids production. The hypoestrogenic status caused by the drugs induces the decidualization both in the eutopic and ectopic endometrial tissues. Another suggested mechanism might be the direct anti-inflammatory effect of progestin therapy since the association between changes in cytokine mRNA expression and nuclear receptors protein expression has previously been shown by Grandi et al. [11].

When compared with COCs, progestins pose a reduced risk for thrombosis, myocardial infarction, and stroke and can be administered to patients with migraine with aura and patients of less than 35 years of age with migraine without aura [12].

Table 41.2 Medical treatment alternatives for endometriosis-associated pelvic pain [10]

Medical treatment	Indication	Priority	Adverse effects and complications	Comment
NSAID	Dysmenorrhea	First	Nausea, vomiting, GI irritation, vertigo, headache	Only symptomatic
Combined oral contraceptives				
Cyclic	Dysmenorrhea	First	Nausea, weight gain, water retention, depression, intercyclic bleeding, breast tenderness, headache, decrease in menstrual bleeding	
Continuous	Dysmenorrhea noncyclic chronic pelvic pain	First	Nausea, weight gain, water retention, depression, intercyclic bleeding, breast tenderness, headache, amenorrhea	
Progestins				
MPA, NETA, CPA, DNG, DYD	Dysmenorrhea noncyclic chronic pelvic pain	First	Nausea, weight gain, water retention, depression, intercyclic bleeding, breast tenderness, headache, amenorrhea, delay in regulation of menstrual pattern	NETA and MPA are approved for endometriosis treatment by FDA
LNG-IUS	Dysmenorrhea dyspareunia	Second or third	Bloating, weight gain, headache, breast tenderness	Effective in symptomatic rectovaginal endometriosis, not approved for endometriosis by US FDA
GnRH agonists	Dysmenorrhea dyspareunia	Second or third	Hypoestrogenism (vasomotor symptoms, vaginal dryness, decrease in libido, irritability, decrease in bone mineral density)	Approved for endometriosis by FDA
GnRH antagonists	Dysmenorrhea dyspareunia Chronic pelvic pain	Second or third	Vasomotor symptoms, decrease in bone mineral density, headache, nausea, difficulty sleeping, absence of periods, anxiety, joint pain, depression, and mood changes	Approved for endometriosis treatment by FDA
Aromatase inhibitors	Dysmenorrhea noncyclic chronic pelvic pain	Third	Hypoestrogenism ovulation induction	Should be combined with COC or GNRHa; not approved for endometriosis by FDA

Table 41.2 (continued)

Medical treatment	Indication	Priority	Adverse effects and complications	Comment
Danazol	Dysmenorrhea noncyclic chronic pelvic pain	Second or third	Hyperandrogenism (acne, edema, decrease in breast size)	Approved for endometriosis treatment by FDA

Modified from the study, Gezer and Oral [10]
CPA cyproterone acetate, *DNG* dienogest, *FDA* Food and Drug Administration, *GI* gastrointestinal, *GnRH* gonadotropin-releasing hormone, *IUS* intrauterine system, *LNG* levonorgestrel, *MPA* medroxyprogesterone acetate, *NETA* norethisterone acetate

Table 41.3 Classification of progestogens [16]

Progestogens			
Progesterone and structurally related compounds		Compounds structurally related to testosterone	
Progesterone	Retroprogesterone	19-nortestosterone derivatives	
Progesterone	Dydrogesterone	Estrane	Gonanes
		Norethisterone	Oesogestrel
17-OH-progesterone derivatives	19-norprogesterone derivatives	Estrane/pregnane	Gestodene
		Dienogest	Norgestimate
Chlormadinone acetate	Nomegestrol acetate		Norgestrel
Medroxyprogesterone acetate	Promegestone	Spironolactone derivative	
	Nestorone	Drospirenone	
Cyproterone acetate	Trimegestone		
Megestrol acetate			

Generally, progestins have good long-term tolerability. The potential disadvantages might be in women desiring contraception since few options are approved as contraceptives (desogestrel, the etonogestrel-releasing subdermal implant, and the levonorgestrel intrauterine device) [13].

41.2.1 Classification

Progestins can be classified according to their chemical structure in 17-hydroxyprogesterone derivatives and 19-nortestosterone derivatives [2, 9]. Different forms of the C-21 progesterone (medroxyprogesterone acetate and dydrogesterone) or C-19 nortestosterone (norethisterone, lynestrenol, desogestrel, and dienogest) have been widely utilized in the treatment of endometriosis [14] (Table 41.3). Several progestins are available for the treatment including norethisterone acetate (NETA), cyproterone acetate (CPA), medroxyprogesterone acetate (MPA), desogestrel (DSG), etonogestrel (ETG), levonorgestrel (LNG), and dienogest (DNG). Currently, only depot MPA and NETA as monotherapies are approved by the FDA for the treatment of endometriosis [15].

41.2.2 Mechanism of Action

The exact mechanism of action of progestins in controlling endometriosis-related pain is still unknown since the basic mechanism of the endometriosis-related pain is unexplained. There are three main mechanisms suggested for the pain in endometriosis:

- The effect of active bleeding from the endometriotic lesions
- The overexpression of the growth factors and proinflammatory cytokines in the ectopic endometrium
- The irritation or direct invasion of pelvic nerves

The progestins stimulate atrophy or regression of endometrial lesions. The effectiveness of progestins for treating endometriosis is not just related to its growth inhibiting actions, but also to its induction of anovulation, inhibition of blood vessel growth, and anti-inflammatory actions [17]. The common characteristic of progestins is the secretory transformation of estrogen-primed uterine endometrium, but the doses required to achieve this effect differ among the different derivatives [17]. Progestins also reduce the frequency and increase the amplitude of pulsatile gonadotropin-releasing hormone (GnRH) release, resulting in a reduction in follicle-stimulating hormone (FSH) and luteinizing hormone (LH) secretion. As a result of this effect, continuous application of progestins leads to the suppression of ovarian steroidogenesis with anovulation and low serum levels of ovarian steroids [17]. The long-standing hypoestrogenic and hypergestagenic state causes decidual transformation of the eutopic endometrium, and to some degree, the same effect is observed in ectopic lesions. In order to induce decidual transformation with resultant necrosis and resorption of the implant, however, concomitant estrogen action is required. As continuous progestin therapy results in low serum estradiol levels, breakthrough bleeding is a common occurrence.

There is a portion of patients with endometriosis who does not respond to medical therapy with progestins. In a very recent review, Donnez et al. found that OCPs and progestogens are effective in two-thirds of women suffering from endometriosis. However, other options are required in case of failure, and in one-third of women it is due to progesterone resistance [18].

Bulun et al. explained this theory owing to reduced levels of progesterone receptors and lack of PR isoform named progesterone receptor B. Progesterone induces secretion of paracrine factors on stromal cells, and neighboring epithelial cells induce the expression of 17-hydroxysteroid dehydrogenase type 2. 17-hydroxysteroid dehydrogenase type 2 is responsible for metabolizing the estradiol (E2) to estrone (E1). The inability of endometriotic stromal cells to produce progesterone-induced paracrine factors may be due to the lack of PR-B and very low levels of progesterone receptor A [19]. Furthermore, there are also underlying dysregulated signaling factors in endometriosis and decreased progesterone signaling pathways leading to progesterone resistance [20].

41.2.3 Molecular Effects on Target Tissue

The mode of action of the progestins on the endometriotic implant is still an unsettled issue. Earlier studies postulated activity via the steroid receptor mechanism that secretory changes in ectopic lesions were followed by decidual transformation and atrophy. Later studies did not confirm this hypothesis. Endometriotic foci either contain progesterone receptors in very low concentrations or do not contain progesterone receptors (mainly PR-β is undetectable and PR-α is markedly reduced), and the function of the enzyme systems differs widely between eutopic and ectopic endometrial tissues [21]. As a contradiction, progestins cause the downregulation of their effects by reducing the synthesis of the receptors, and as a result of all these alterations, sensitivity of the implants to progesterone decreases during long-term treatment. Endometriosis has different patterns of action: some implants remain unchanged at the end of long-term progestin treatment; in some implants, an arrest of growth is observed and some have secretory changes, but the expected decidual reaction and necrosis could not be revealed [22]. On the comparison of ultrastructural changes between eutopic and ectopic endometrium, endometriotic foci are found to remain proliferative in the luteal phase [23]. This insensitivity to the effect of progestins (progesterone blockage) may be as a result of alterations in enzyme or reduced receptor concentrations systems in the ectopic endometriotic implants [23]. In ectopic endometrium, 17-β-hydroxysteroiddehydrogenase type 2 is defective and cannot be activated by progestins, resulting in increased proliferation, as estradiol is not inactivated [23]. Furthermore, aromatase in ectopic implants has been found to have a pathologic activity [23]. It is known that the endometriotic foci produce more estradiol, converting androgens to estrogens. A new mechanism of controlling the growth of endometriosis by progesterone and progestins was proposed recently, which postulates progestins were found to reduce TNF-α-induced NF-κB which in turn inhibits the proliferation of endometriotic stromal cells [24]. Moreover, progestins suppress the matrix metalloproteinases, which enable the implantation and progression of ectopic endometriotic implants [24]. In a rat endometrial autograft model, it was demonstrated that progestins (dienogest) inhibited the process of angiogenesis in the ectopic endometrium that reduced the development and progression of endometriotic implants. In addition, progestins were found to inhibit the proliferation of endometrial stromal cells in vitro due the arrest of cells in the G0/G1 phase of the cell cycle [25]. Another mechanism of action could be progestins' direct effect on nerve fibers. Progestins and COCs were found to reduce nerve fiber density and nerve growth factor and nerve growth factor receptor p75 expression in peritoneal endometriotic lesions [26].

The suggested mechanisms of progestins in resolving endometriosis-related pain are summarized as follows [14, 17]:

- Ovarian suppression
- Effects on endometrial morphology (desidualization, atrophy, and alteration in steroid receptor ligand binding)

- Local modulation of immune response (suppression of IL-8 production, increase of nitric oxide production, reduction of TNF-α-induced nuclear factor-χ-β)
- Effects on angiogenesis (suppression of transcription of bFGF, suppression of VEGF and cysteine-rich angiogenic inducer [CYR61])
- Progesterone receptor expression and progesterone resistance
- Direct effect on nerve fiber intensity

41.2.4 Route of Administration

Progestins can be administered as oral preparations, injections, subdermal implants, and intrauterine systems (Table 41.4).

41.2.4.1 Oral Route

41.2.4.1.1 Dienogest

Dienogest (DNG) is a C-19-nortestosterone progestogen derivative and is a fourth-generation selective progestin with anti-inflammatory properties [27]. DNG has a strong progestational effect as dydrogesterone but differs from it with its moderate antagonist action on the androgen receptors and moderate antigonadotrophic effects [28]. It has no androgenic, glucocorticoid, mineralocorticoid activity, or estrogenic

Table 41.4 Available forms of progestins in the treatment of endometriosis [10]

Route of administration	Generic name	Dosage
Oral route	Dienogest	2 mg a day
	Medroxyprogesterone acetate	Usually 30 mg a day, but may be up to 60 mg a day if necessary
	Norethisterone	Usually 2.5–5 mg a day
	Dydrogesterone	10–30 mg a day
	Cyproterone acetate	10–12.5 mg a day
	Progestogen only pill	75 mcg a day
	Desogestrel	4 mg a day
	Drospirenone	
Depot injection	Depot medroxyprogesterone acetate	One 50 mg injection each week, or one 100 mg injection every 2 weeks, or one 150 mg injection every 2–3 months. Injected into muscle
Subdermal implant	Etonogestrel	In single rod, 68 mg with a life span of 3 s
Intrauterine system	Levonorgestrel intrauterine system	This device contains 52 mg of levonorgestrel, which is slowly released into the uterus over a period of up to 3 years. The device has two strings attached that protrude through the cervix into the vagina. Regularly check that the strings are still present, as the device may be expelled unnoticed. Heavier bleeding may be a sign that the device has been expelled

Modified from the study, Gezer and Oral [10]

activity. Like the other 19-norprogestins, it enables the suppression of the endometrium in low doses, having a short half-life and high bioavailability. Dienogest is bound to albumin and does not accumulate in oral doses of 2 mg/day. It has been shown to be effective with good tolerability with doses 2–4 mg daily in continuous administration for 3–24 months in patients with endometriosis [29–31]. DNG has been compared with GnRH agonists (buserelin acetate and leuprolide acetate) [30] and has been found to have a lower adverse effect profile. The main side effects were the bleeding problems that were observed in 80% of patients within the first 3 months of treatment, which later on were reduced [30]. It has a good safety and efficacy profile, with a progressive decrease in adverse effects and bleeding irregularities, and the decrease in pain for at least 6 months after cessation of the treatment [31]. Prospective randomized studies that evaluated dienogest 2 mg daily against placebo or versus leuprorelin depot showed a significant improvement in endometriosis-related symptoms with comparable effectiveness to GnRH agonist treatment [28, 32].

A potential adverse effect of the DNG treatment is decreased bone mineral density. Seo et al. conducted a study to evaluate the effect of long-term postoperative dienogest use for the treatment of endometriosis on bone mineral density. The results of the study suggested that long-term postoperative DNG treatment might have an adverse effect on BMD in reproductive-aged women, a bone loss occurring mostly during the first 6 months of treatment [33]. The results of a very recent retrospective study were in line with the previous literature. Kim et al. searched the changing pattern of bone mineral density levels after 3 years of dienogest use post endometrioma surgery and investigated the possible predictive factors for BMD reduction. The results showed that the treatment was associated with a significant and gradual decrease in BMD, and no predictive factors for BMD reduction during the first year of treatment with dienogest were found [34]. In 2017, Ebert et al. conducted a 52-week, open-label, single-arm study named "The VISanne Study to Assess Safety in ADOlescents-VISADO" including 21 centers among six European countries to evaluate the safety and efficacy of dienogest 2 mg in adolescents between 12 and 18 years with suspected endometriosis. In adolescents, dienogest 2 mg for 52 weeks was associated with a decrease in lumbar BMD, followed by partial recovery after treatment discontinuation. The authors concluded that a tailored approach is needed in this population to decrease the risk of osteoporosis [33].

41.2.4.1.2 Norethisterone (Norethindrone) Acetate

NETA is a C-91-nortestesterone derivative. It has been approved for the treatment of endometriosis (2.5 mg daily continuous administration) by FDA. In randomized controlled trials, NETA has been shown to be effective in endometriosis-related pelvic pain [15, 35]. The advantages of NETA are control of uterine bleeding, positive effect on calcium metabolism, and lack of negative effect on lipoprotein profile [35]. There is also increasing data on the effective use of NETA in rectovaginal endometriosis [15, 17].

41.2.4.1.3 Dydrogesterone

Dydrogesterone was first reported to be effective in endometriosis treatment in the 1960s [36]. It is manufactured by treating progesterone with ultraviolet light. A daily dose of 10–30 mg is used for the treatment of endometriosis. It has good oral bioavailability and is very similar to natural progesterone structurally as it binds the receptor 50% more than progesterone [37]. Several studies used dydrogesterone at doses of between 10 and 60 mg/day, for various numbers of days per cycle for periods of 3–9 months showed that the majority of the patients reported a reduction in their symptom severity or being symptom-free after taking the medication [38–44]. Cyclical usage of the drug was also studied and shown to be effective in reduced blood loss and shortened bleeding times with satisfying symptom relief among women with dysmenorrhea [43, 44]. In a Cochrane review published in 2012 to determine the effectiveness of both the progestagens and anti-progestagens in the treatment of painful symptoms of endometriosis, Brown et al. found that only one RCT out of 13 was on dydrogesterone and concluded that there was no evidence of a difference in objective efficacy at 6 months between dydrogesterone and placebo (OR 0.53, 95% CI 0.14–1.94) [45]. Dydrogesterone is a good treatment of choice especially in patients with a desire for fertility since the drug does not inhibit ovulation and can be used in the treatment of pain, bleeding, and cycle control.

41.2.4.1.4 Medroxyprogesterone Acetate

Medroxyprogesterone acetate (MPA) is a C-21-progestogen derivative. It has been studied comparing placebo to GnRH agonist (Nafarelin) in 15–50 mg doses daily in continuous administration [46]. MPA has been shown to have greater efficacy at alleviating the pain and improving the quality of life against placebo, but the effectiveness was found to be equivalent to GnRH agonist [46]. MPA causes breakthrough bleeding in long-term use.

41.2.4.1.5 Cyproterone Acetate

Cyproterone acetate (CPA) is a C-21-progestogen derivative. It is mainly an anti-androgen with weak progestational activity. CPA in 10–12.5 mg daily in continuous administration has been studied comparing to oral contraceptives (desogestrel and ethinyl estradiol) for treatment of endometriosis [47]. Both study groups have been found equally improved due to pain, sexual satisfaction, and quality of life after 6 months of treatment. The side effects of CPA are the main drawback of its generalized use. It is associated with depression, decreased libido, hot flushes, and vaginal dryness.

41.2.4.2 Other Routes of Application

41.2.4.2.1 Depot Injections

Depot injections of MPA are very effective in suppressing endometriosis-related complaints. Depot MPA (DMPA) has been studied in doses 150 mg intramuscularly or 104 mg subcutaneously in 3 months. It was compared with combination of oral contraceptive with danazol and GnRH agonist (leuprolide acetate) [48, 49]. No differences were observed in the reduction of pain symptoms, but demineralization of bone and hypoestrogenism side effects were found in the GnRH agonist group and bleeding problems were frequent in the MPA group. DMPA achieved good pain relief and minimal side effects (bloating and spotting). The optimum interval for administration should be every 3 months. In long-term use of DMPA, prolonged delay of resumption of ovulation is a major concern in women desiring pregnancy. Therefore, this type of application is recommended only in elderly patients, who do not desire pregnancy. Breakthrough bleeding is an important side effect that interferes with the quality of life. Furthermore, bone demineralization due to hypoestrogenism may be detrimental for the long-term use.

41.2.4.2.2 Subdermal Implants

A new approach to improve the use of progestins in endometriosis is the development of subcutaneous implants. Subdermal implants (etonogestrel contraceptive implant/Implanon-68 mg in single rod with a life span of 3 years) have been found to be equally effective compared with DMPA in pain relief in 12 months use [50]. It is a safe, well-tolerated alternative for the treatment of endometriosis and achieving long-term contraception. A study aimed to investigate the efficacy of etonogestrel (ENG)-releasing implant in treating patients with rectovaginal endometriosis showed that the treatment quickly improved the intensity of nonmenstrual pelvic pain, deep dyspareunia, dysmenorrhea, and dyschezia. At the 6-month follow-up, there were improvements in all domains of the Endometriosis Health Profile (EHP-30) compared with baseline. At the 6-month follow-up, volume of the rectovaginal nodules was significantly lower compared with baseline [51].

41.2.4.2.3 Intrauterine Systems

To reduce the adverse side effects of medical treatments, a new aspect is the intrauterine administration of progestins, which can be an effective treatment of symptomatic endometriosis. The precise mechanism of action of levonorgestrel intrauterine system (LNG-IUS/Mirena-releasing 0.02 mg levonorgestrel/day with a lifespan of 5 years) in the treatment of endometriosis is unclear. However, the patients with pelvic pain due to endometriosis have been shown to be improved after LNG-IUS administration, and antiproliferative effects in the ectopic endometrium have been shown [52]. LNG-IUS was compared with depot GnRH agonist and has been shown to have similar efficacy to control the pain-related symptoms [53]. It has also been suggested to be effective against the pain in rectovaginal endometriosis [52]. LNG-IUS has been found to be effective in the treatment of adenomyosis [54]. Main advantages of LNG-IUS are lack of necessity for repeated administrations, institution of highly effective contraception, and minimal hypoestrogenic side effects. As the disadvantages, the cost and the probability of unexpected bleeding should be noted. Irregular bleeding during the initial months of application is frequent side effect of the device, but 70% of the women will be amenorrheic in 6 months.

41.2.5 Side Effects

The main side effects of progestins can be listed as follows:

- The disturbances of lipid and carbohydrate metabolism and the clotting system, observed more with C-19-derivatives
- Negative influences on mood swings and depression, experienced more with C-17-derivatives

The individual reactions to the progestins differ depending on the type and dosage of the progestin [55–57]. Levonorgestrel is the cause of spotting, breakthrough bleeding, bloating, weight gain, and headache in up to a third of the patients.

41.3 Results for Treatment for Pain

Progestins in treating the pain associated with endometriosis have shown to be efficient [28, 47, 58]. Symptom improvement was reported between 60% and 94% [14, 17]. The results, in general, were similar to the results obtained with continuous use of oral contraceptives (estrogen-progestin combination therapy). Furthermore, progestins were also effective in gastrointestinal symptoms in patients with colorectal endometriosis [59], as well as urinary symptoms [60] and ovarian endometriomas [60]. The advantages of progestins are related to the escaping of estrogen-based side effects. The disadvantages are the bleeding problems such as spotting, which can be managed with increasing dosages, adding estrogen, or discontinuing the progestin for 5–7 days [17].

Several RCTs have investigated the efficacy of DNG in treating endometriosis. In a randomized, double-blind trial, the efficacy of dienogest 2 mg for providing pain relief was compared with placebo in 12 weeks among 198 women with endometriosis, dienogest significantly reduced the mean VAS score representing a statistically significant difference in favor of dienogest [27]. A systematic review by Andres et al. reported that DNG (2 mg/day) is superior to placebo and as effective as GnRH analogs in reducing pelvic pain and growth of endometriotic lesions. They also found that extended therapy with DNG (2 mg/day) showed an improvement in pelvic pain after 24–52 weeks with tolerable side effects [61]. Two years later, Pinto et al. reported that DNG is an effective medication to control symptoms of pain related to DIE, even without reducing the volume of DIE nodules. A literature review conducted by Murji et al. was in line with the previous literature reporting that dienogest offers an effective and tolerable alternative or adjunct to surgery and provides many advantages over combined hormonal contraceptives for the treatment of endometriosis [62]. In a recent RCT comparing the effects of dienogest and a combined oral contraceptive pill (COCP) after laparoscopic surgery on pain and quality of life in women with severe endometriosis, Kashi et al. found that postoperative administration of dienogest or COCP reduced endometriosis-associated pain and improved quality of life in women with severe endometriosis; however, no significant difference was registered between the two intervention group regarding the pelvic pain scores [63].

NETA is one of the most frequently studied progestogens in literature with DNG. Both drugs are associated with safety drawbacks as NETA may modify serum cholesterol lipoprotein distribution, whereas DNG may deplete bone mineral content [58, 64]. Among the literature, NETA was also found to be an effective treatment option in endometriosis-associated pain. In a study conducted by Muneyyirci-Delale and Karacan, NETA seemed to be a cost-effective alternative with relatively mild side effects in the treatment of symptomatic endometriosis. Dysmenorrhea and noncyclic pelvic pain were relieved in 48/52 (92.3%) and 25/28 (89.2%) of patients, respectively [65]. Vercellini et al. compared the patient satisfaction with NETA versus DNG, the implementation of dienogest was not associated with statistically significant amelioration in overall pain relief, psychological status, sexual functioning, or health-related quality of life [66]. In a retrospective study conducted by Forno et al. in 2019, colleagues compared the effects of dienogest and norethindrone acetate in symptomatic women with ovarian endometriomas, analyzing the efficacy in reducing endometrioma size and symptom relief. Progestin therapy was effective in both groups in reducing the size of endometriomas and related symptoms, but dienogest had a greater effect on symptoms relief and higher drug tolerability [67].

In a very recent meta-analysis, Peng et al. investigated the effect of dydrogesterone for the treatment of endometriosis and found that with limited evidence, dydrogesterone may have some advantages over gestrinone, GnRH agonists, and other therapeutic interventions in treating endometriosis [68]. In the ORCHIDEA study, Sukhikh et al. compared the effectiveness of two different treatment regimens of dydrogesterone in the management of endometriosis-related chronic pelvic pain (10 mg 2 or 3 times daily, either between the 5th and 25th days of the menstrual cycle or continuously) and found that both regimens demonstrated a pronounced and similar reduction in the severity of chronic pelvic pain and dysmenorrhea and led to marked improvements in all study parameters related to the quality of life and sexual well-being [69].

In a prospective, randomized trial with MPA, the regression rate of ectopic implants was reported as 50% and the partial regression rate as 13% in the treatment group which was 12% and 6%, respectively, in the placebo group. Pain reduction with MPA was found as effective as danazol [70].

Gonadotropin-releasing hormone agonists are second-line medical therapies in the treatment of endometriosis. The prospective randomized studies in the literature comparing GnRH analogs with low-dose progestins are limited. Vercellini et al. used a monthly combination of ethinyl estradiol 0.02 mg and desogestrel 0.15 mg versus goserelin 3.6 mg, while Regidor et al. compared daily lynestrenol 5 mg versus monthly leuprorelin 3.7 mg and Strowitzki et al. studied dienogest 2 mg daily versus leuprorelin depot monthly injections [30, 71, 72]. In a double-blind study, a significant reduction of pain was found during and 1 year after treatment, but there were no differences between the medications used. In the aforementioned study, Vercellini et al. found a significant reduction of deep dyspareunia and cyclic pain in both groups, with goserelin superior to the oral contraceptive [72]. Nonmenstrual pain was diminished in all of the treatments [72]. Utilizing the repeat laparoscopy, Regidor et al. observed a significant reduction of endometriotic implants in the leuprorelin group (r-American Fertility Society scores were reduced from 21.8 to 11.5 points with leuprorelin and from 27.2 to 25.5 points with lynestrenol; $p < 0.000014$ Wilcoxon test). There was no significant improvement in symptoms such as chronic pelvic pain and dyspareunia [71].

In a recent Cochrane review in which 11 RCTs were included, the authors concluded that both continuous progestins (especially continuous high-dose progestin (in the form of MPA)) and the antiprogestin, gestrinone, are effective therapies for the treatment of painful symptoms associated with endometriosis, but there had been no evidence of progestin use, either in oral or depot form, being superior to other types of treatment in endometriosis-related pain symptoms [45]. This conclusion should be treated with caution particularly in light of the absence of suitable placebo-controlled trials.

In conclusion, pain relief established by utilizing acceptable dosages of progestins is indistinguishable from the results of danazol or GnRH analogs. Systematic investigations of various progestins in altered dosages are lacking, and there are no conclusive data from prospective randomized placebo-controlled trials up to date. Studies comparing DNG with GnRH analogs and DNG with NETA have found both drugs to be equally effective [66, 73].

41.4 Patients with Rectovaginal Endometriosis

In deep-infiltrating rectovaginal endometriosis, the guidelines recommend complete excision, but treatment symptomatically with progestin is also possible [14]. In a prospective randomized controlled trial comparing NETA versus a combination of estrogen and CPA, the symptom reduction was proved to be feasible [58]. In both treatment groups, dyschezia, pelvic pain, deep dyspareunia, and dysmenorrhea were reduced significantly [58]. A study comparing NETA alone versus NETA combined with an aromatase inhibitor in symptomatic pain relief has confirmed NETA's effects [74]. The positive effect of CPA was also observed in a prospective randomized controlled trial comparing CPA for 6 months versus an oral contraceptive; the quality of life and psychiatric profile improved significantly in the treatment group [47]. Another study conducted by Morotti et al. evaluated patient satisfaction at 6-month dienogest treatment in women with symptomatic rectovaginal endometriosis who had pain persistence after 6 months of norethisterone acetate therapy. The results of this 24-week pilot open-label prospective study showed that DNG was superior to NETA in improving pain and quality of life, and DNG may be an alternative to surgery for the patients resistant to other progestins [75]. LNG-IUS was also proposed to be effective in rectovaginal endometriosis in observational studies [52].

41.5 Patients with Infertility

The reported rates of pregnancy following progestin treatment (MPA, lynestrenol, or norethisterone acetate) vary from 5% to 90% depending on the stage of endometriosis. Lynestrenol 5–10 mg daily was reported with 60% subjective improvement and a 5% pregnancy rate. On the contrary, 40% failure and the recurrence rate were observed [76].

Progestins are also a treatment of choice before fertility treatments. In a prospective study, Iwami et al. analyzed a new controlled ovarian hyperstimulation (COH) regimen: progestin-primed ovarian stimulation (PPOS) in patients with endometriosis and compared DNG with dydrogesterone (DYG) to show the appropriate progestin for PPOS. The results show that a smaller number of oocytes were retrieved in the DNG group than in the DYG group; however, the rate of mature oocytes was significantly higher in the DNG group than in the DYG group. The fertilization rate was comparable between the two groups, and the authors concluded that the patients taking DNG for PPOS can continue endometriosis treatment and obtain good-quality embryos during COH [77].

A prolonged course of hormonal therapy before IVF treatment for suppression of the disease is acclaimed to play an important role in endometriosis-related infertility. The use of progestins in this regard was studied by Mueller et el., among infertile women of reproductive age, who planned to undergo IVF after the laparoscopic resection of ovarian endometriomas. They divided patients into three groups as dienogest group, the GnRH analog group, and patients without any hormonal therapy within 6 months preceding IVF. The results show that dienogest be a possibly more efficient treatment option for this kind of patient as the clinical pregnancy rate was 2.5 times (44.7% vs. 16.7%, $p = .012$) and delivery rate was three times higher (36.8% vs. 11.1%, $p = .013$) in dienogest pretreatment group when compared with no intervention group. In a study conducted in 2019 by Tamure et al., authors investigated the benefit of dienogest (DNG) treatment just before IVF-embryo transfer and found that DNG treatment did not provide any benefits to improve the clinical outcomes for infertile women with endometriosis [78]. A year later, Barra et al. evaluated the administration of DNG before IVF in women with endometriosis who had previously failed one IVF cycle and hypothesized that the anti-inflammatory and anti-angiogenic activity of DNG may theoretically improve IVF outcomes in women with endometriosis. The results show that the cumulative implantation, clinical pregnancy, and live birth rates were significantly higher in the DNG-treated group (39.7%, 33.3%, and 28.6%) than in the nontreated group (23.9%, 18.2%, and 14.8%; $p = 0.049$, 0.037, and 0.043, respectively). They also found that the largest diameter of endometriomas significantly decreased after DNG pretreatment and the use of DNG increased significantly the number of oocytes retrieved [79]. The results of a very recent RCT, comparing DNG pretreatment for endometriosis suppression with gonadotropin-releasing hormone agonist in patients with endometriosis pursuing IVF treatment, showed that there was no statistically significant difference between both groups regarding ovarian stimulation, response parameters, and pregnancy outcomes, but the DNG group had a lower cost of treatment, lower side effects, higher FertiQoL treatment scores, and higher tolerability scores indicating that DNG is a suitable and safe substitute for GnRHa pretreatment in endometriosis patients [80].

MPA was suggested as another treatment of choice in women with ovarian endometriosis undergoing controlled ovarian hyperstimulation for IVF. A study investigated the use of medroxyprogesterone acetate or a short protocol for controlled ovarian hyperstimulation in patients with advanced endometriosis who have normal ovarian function showed higher rates of the mature oocyte, D3 high quality embryo, and hMG dose in the study groups using MPA compared with the short protocol. The number of >10–14 mm follicles on the trigger day, D3 top-quality embryos, viable embryos, rates of cancellation, fertilization, implantation, and pregnancy outcomes were similar among the groups. Authors suggested that MPA COH could be effective for women with ovarian advanced endometriosis who has a normal ovarian function [81].

41.6 Postoperative Hormonal Suppression

"Adjuvant" medical therapy following endometriosis surgery to prevent the recurrence of the disease was a suggested treatment of choice from the point that the existence of microscopic lesions after the surgery may lead to proceeding symptoms. According to clinical data available, the length of the postsurgical medical suppression is the key point for reducing the symptoms.

In a Cochrane meta-analysis in 2004, updated in 2011, authors investigated the effectiveness of medical therapies (GnRHas, danazol, progestogens, gestrinone, or COCs) for hormonal suppression after surgery for improving painful symptoms, reducing disease recurrence, and increasing pregnancy rates and found that there was no evidence of benefit associated with postsurgical medical therapy [82]. However, in most of the included studies, the patients' outcomes were examined at 3 months. In another RCT including 450 women testing the benefits of a 3 month course of medical therapy after surgery confirmed the previous findings [83]. In contrast with the previous findings, Muzii et al. found that lower recurrence rates for dysmenorrhea were obtained with a continuous COC schedule [84]. In line with the previous paper, Grandi et al. reported in a systematic review that some COCs decreased the risk of disease recurrence after conservative surgery, but progestin-only contraceptives did not [85]. In a recent review, Zakhari et al. reported that when hormonal suppression (CHC, progestin, LNG-IUS, GnRH agonist) is initiated within 6 weeks of endometriosis surgery, there is a significant reduction in endometriosis recurrence and pain scores at up to 1 year postoperatively [86].

In conclusion, with the current data available, short course of suppressive therapy may not be beneficial, and longer periods are needed to prevent disease recurrence, and also more RCTs are needed to analyze the effect of progestins on disease recurrence after surgery.

41.7 Progestins in Adenomyosis

Hysterectomy is a "gold standard" and definitive therapy for uterine adenomyosis; however, conservative treatment is required in a group of patients who have a desire for fertility and deny surgical management. Available literature on the medical treatment of adenomyosis is limited. According to the fact that both endometriosis and adenomyosis share similar origins regarding estrogen dependency, medical treatment strategies follow the same principles which aim to reduce endogenous estrogen production or inducing endometrial differentiation with progestins [87]. Although there are merging data on the efficacy of medical treatment in patients with adenomyosis, no drug is currently labeled for adenomyosis.

The first study investigating the effect of DNG treatment for up to 24 weeks on symptomatic adenomyosis showed that DNG is an effective and well-tolerated therapy for symptomatic adenomyosis although some patients experienced reported worsening menorrhagia [88]. In a double-blind, placebo-controlled trial conducted in 2017, Osuga et al. investigated 67 patients randomly assigned to receive DNG (2 mg/day, orally) or placebo for 16 weeks with adenomyosis. After 16 weeks of treatment with DNG, the results showed that DNG was effective and well tolerated as a treatment for painful symptoms in patients with adenomyosis, not complicated by a severe uterine enlargement or severe anemia [89]. The comparison between DNG and GnRH analogs found both drugs to be effective for the pain symptoms, while GnRH analogs were more effective on abnormal bleeding and uterine volume reduction with 4 months of treatment [90].

A study conducted by Muneyyirci-Delale showed that treatment with a low dose (5 mg/day) of NETA for the treatment of adenomyosis in women with pelvic pain, dysmenorrhea, and abnormal uterine bleeding showed significant improvement in both dysmenorrhea and bleeding [91].

LNG-IUD is the most promising treatment option for the medical treatment of adenomyosis. In a study, overall satisfaction was 72% among women treated with LNG-IUD for 3 years, and a significant decrease in dysmenorrhea and uterine volume was observed compared to baseline [54]. In line with the previous reports, a prospective longitudinal study conducted among 1100 women with adenomyosis who received the LNG -IUD were followed up over 60 months showed that 25.9% of the patients had amenorrhea and 21.9% had shortened periods. The incidence of adverse events was <10%; hence, long-term use of LNG-IUD was reported as effective and acceptable for the treatment of symptomatic adenomyosis [92]. Moreover, LNG-IUD seems to be the best optimal treatment in women with the moderate enlarged uterus [93]. Regarding the increased expulsion rates with the increased uterine volume [93], combining GnRHa and LNG-IUD treatment may be efficacious in patients with adenomyosis and enlarged uterus [94]. When compared with COCs, LNG-IUD seems to be more effective and has a better effect on quality of life when compared with hysterectomy [95].

In a study, Liang et al. investigated the effect of pretreatment with the levonorgestrel-releasing intrauterine system on IVF outcomes in women with adenomyosis, and differences were found in implantation rates (32.1% vs. 22.1%, $p = 0.005$) and clinical pregnancy rates (44% vs. 33.5%, $p = 0.045$) between the LNG-IUD group and control group [96].

41.8 Recent Guidelines on Hormonal Therapy with Progestins in Endometriosis

European Society of Human Reproduction and Embryology (ESHRE) [97]
Endometriosis - Guideline of European Society of Human Reproduction and Embryology (2022)
Progestogens (including progestogen-only contraceptives)

- It is recommended to prescribe women progestogens to reduce endometriosis-associated pain (strong recommendation).
- The GDG recommends that clinicians take the different side effect profiles of progestogens into account when prescribing them (GPP).
- It is recommended to prescribe women a levonorgestrel-releasing intrauterine system or an etonogestrel-releasing subdermal implant to reduce endometriosis-associated pain (strong recommendation).

American College of Obstetricians and Gynecologists (ACOG) [98]
Committee Opinion on Dysmenorrhea and Endometriosis in the Adolescent (2018)

- First-line therapy for adolescents with either surgically diagnosed and destroyed endometriosis or presumed endometriosis includes suppressive hormonal therapy using a continuous combined hormonal contraceptive, a progestin-only agent, or 52 mg of LNG-IUD.

National Institute for Health and Care Excellence (NICE) [99]
Endometriosis: Diagnosis and Management (2017)

Hormonal Treatments

- Offer hormonal treatment (e.g., the combined oral contraceptive pill or a progestogen) to women with suspected, confirmed, or recurrent endometriosis.

European Society of Human Reproduction and Embryology (ESHRE) [100]
Guideline on the Management of Women with Endometriosis (2013)

Empirical Treatment of Pain

- The GDG recommends clinicians to counsel women with symptoms presumed to be due to endometriosis thoroughly, and to empirically treat them with adequate analgesia, combined hormonal contraceptives, or progestagens—GPP.

Hormonal Therapies for Treatment of Endometriosis-Associated Pain

- Clinicians are recommended to prescribe hormonal treatment [hormonal contraceptives (level B), progestagens (level A), antiprogestagens (level A), or GnRH agonists (level A)] as one of the options, as it reduces endometriosis-associated pain.

Progestagens and Antiprogestagens

- Clinicians are recommended to use progestagens (medroxyprogesterone acetate [oral or depot], dienogest, cyproterone acetate, norethisterone acetate, or danazol) or antiprogestagens (gestrinone) as one of the options, to reduce endometriosis-associated pain—A.

- The GDG recommends that clinicians take the different side-effect profiles of progestagens and antiprogestagens into account when prescribing these drugs, especially irreversible side effects (e.g., thrombosis, androgenic side effects)—GPP.
- Clinicians can consider prescribing a levonorgestrel-releasing intrauterine system as one of the options to reduce endometriosis-associated pain—B.

World Endometriosis Society (WES) [101]

Consensus on Current Management of endometriosis (2013)

Empirical Medical Treatment

- Well-tolerated, low-cost, easily accessible options such as nonsteroidal anti-inflammatory drugs (NSAIDs), other analgesics, combined OCP, and progestins should be considered for use as first-line empirical medical treatment (strong).
- In some circumstances, second-line medical treatment with gonadotrophin-releasing hormone agonists (GnRH-a) with add-back HRT, or the LNG-IUS may be considered for use as empirical medical treatment for women who are not optimally treated with first-line empirical therapy prior to surgical diagnosis and treatment, while awaiting laparoscopic surgery (weak).

Medical Therapy for Women with Symptomatic Endometriosis

- Well-tolerated, low-cost, easily accessible options such as nonsteroidal anti-inflammatory drugs (NSAIDs), other analgesics, combined OCP, and progestins should be considered for first-line medical treatment of laparoscopically diagnosed endometriosis (strong).
- Second-line medical treatments could include gonadotrophin-releasing hormone agonists (GnRH-a, which should be used with add-back HRT, routinely), the LNG-IUS and depot progestins (weak).

Society of Obstetricians and Gynaecologists of Canada (SOGC) [102]
Clinical Practice Guideline on Endometriosis—Diagnosis and Management (2010)

Medical Management of Pain Associated with Endometriosis

- Administration of progestin alone—orally, intramuscularly, or subcutaneously—may also be considered as first-line therapy (I-A).

American College of Obstetricians and Gynecologists (ACOG) [103]
Practice Bulletin for Management of Endometriosis (2010)

- In patients with known endometriosis and dysmenorrhea, OCs and oral norethindrone or DMPA are effective compared with placebo and are equivalent to other more costly regimens—B.

American Society of Reproductive Medicine (ASRM) [104]
Treatment of Pelvic Pain Associated with Endometriosis—A Committee Opinion (2014)

Medical Therapies for Endometriosis

- Progestogens most commonly used for the treatment of endometriosis include medroxyprogesterone acetate (MPA) and 19-nortestosterone derivatives (e.g., levonorgestrel, norethindrone acetate, and dienogest). As with OCs, their proposed mechanism of action involves decidualization and subsequent atrophy of endometrial tissue. Another more recently proposed mechanism involves progestogen-induced suppression of matrix metalloproteinases, a class of enzymes important in the growth and implantation of ectopic endometrium. Inhibition of angiogenesis has also been proposed as a mechanism to explain the effectiveness of progestins in the treatment of endometriosis. In observational studies involving treatment with MPA, dydrogesterone, or norethindrone acetate, pain has been reduced by 70–100%. A meta-analysis of four randomized, controlled trials comparing MPA to danazol alone, danazol and combined OCs, or a GnRH-a (goserelin acetate) concluded that MPA was as effective as the other treatments (odds ratio [OR] 1.1; 95% CI 0.4–3.1). Randomized studies concluded that dienogest was significantly better than placebo and as effective as the GnRH-a buserelin, LA, or triptorelin in reducing pain symptoms with diminished side effects of hot flushes and bone mineral density loss. The levonorgestrel-releasing intrauterine system (LNGIUD) represents another approach to the medical treatment of endometriosis. A randomized, controlled trial comparing the LNG-IUD to expectant management after laparoscopic surgical treatment for symptomatic endometriosis found that the LNG-IUD was more effective than no treatment in reducing symptoms of dysmenorrhea. Other studies have demonstrated improved symptoms associated with rectovaginal endometriosis and a significant decrease in the extent of disease observed at second-look laparoscopy after 6 months of treatment with the LNG-IUD. Relief of endometriosis pain with the LNG-IUD is similar to GnRH-a.

41.9 Conclusion

New effective substances have been introduced for the medical treatment of endometriosis in the last 50 years. Although there have been few studies with a limited number of subjects on progestin use in endometriosis, the beneficial effect of progestins for the treatment of endometriosis-related complaints was confirmed. Progestins are accepted to be one of the major treatment choices in the management of pain and other symptoms related to endometriosis. They are exceptionally useful especially when long-term treatment is indicated and repeated courses of treatment are necessary. Medical treatment is also one of the mainstays of adenomyosis treatment. Although hysterectomy is a "gold standard" and definitive therapy for uterine adenomyosis, conservative treatment is required in a group of patients who have a desire for fertility and denies surgical management. LNG-IUD is the most promising treatment option for the medical treatment of adenomyosis.

References

1. Falcone T, Lebovic DI. Clinical management of endometriosis. Obstet Gynecol. 2011;118(3):691–705.
2. Giudice LC, Kao LC. Endometriosis. Lancet. 2004;364(9447):1789–99.
3. Rawson JM. Prevalence of endometriosis in asymptomatic women. J Reprod Med. 1991;36(7):513–5.
4. Balasch J, Creus M, Fábregues F, Carmona F, Ordi J, Martinez-Román S, et al. Visible and non-visible endometriosis at laparoscopy in fertile and infertile women and in patients with chronic pelvic pain: a prospective study. Hum Reprod. 1996;11(2):387–91.
5. Carter JE. Combined hysteroscopic and laparoscopic findings in patients with chronic pelvic pain. J Am Assoc Gynecol Laparosc. 1994;2(1):43–7.
6. Duffy JM, Arambage K, Correa FJ, Olive D, Farquhar C, Garry R, et al. Laparoscopic surgery for endometriosis. Cochrane Database Syst Rev. 2014;(4):Cd011031.
7. Shakiba K, Bena J, McGill KM, Minger J, Falcone T. Surgical treatment of endometriosis: a 7-year follow-up on the requirement for further surgery. Obstet Gynecol. 2008;111:1285–92.
8. Bedaiwy MA, Alfaraj S, Yong P, Casper R. New developments in the medical treatment of endometriosis. Fertil Steril. 2017;107(3):555–65.
9. Tafi E, Leone Roberti Maggiore U, Alessandri F, Bogliolo S, Gardella B, Vellone VG, et al. Advances in pharmacotherapy for treating endometriosis. Expert Opin Pharmacother. 2015;16(16):2465–83.
10. Gezer A, Oral E. Progestin therapy in endometriosis. Womens Health. 2015;11(5):643–52.
11. Grandi G, Mueller MD, Bersinger NA, Facchinetti F, McKinnon BD. The association between progestins, nuclear receptors expression and inflammation in endometrial stromal cells from women with endometriosis. Gynecol Endocrinol. 2017;33(9):712–5.
12. Morotti M, Remorgida V, Venturini PL, Ferrero S. Progestogen-only contraceptive pill compared with combined oral contraceptive in the treatment of pain symptoms caused by endometriosis in patients with migraine without aura. Eur J Obstet Gynecol Reprod Biol. 2014;179:63–8.
13. Berlanda N, Somigliana E, Viganò P, Vercellini P. Safety of medical treatments for endometriosis. Expert Opin Drug Saf. 2016;15(1):21–30.
14. Schweppe KW. Current place of progestins in the treatment of endometriosis-related complaints. Gynecol Endocrinol. 2001;15(Suppl 6):22–8.
15. Barra F, Scala C, Ferrero S. Current understanding on pharmacokinetics, clinical efficacy and safety of progestins for treating pain associated to endometriosis. Expert Opin Drug Metab Toxicol. 2018;14(4):399–415.
16. Schindler AE, Campagnoli C, Druckmann R, Huber J, Pasqualini JR, Schweppe KW, et al. Classification and pharmacology of progestins. Maturitas. 2008;61(1–2):171–80.
17. Horne A, Critchley HOD. Medical therapies: progestins. In: Endometriosis: Science and Practice. Giudice LC, Evers JLH, Healy DL (Eds). Blackwell Publishing Ltd, UK. 2012. p. 351–6.
18. Donnez J, Dolmans M-M. Endometriosis and medical therapy: from progestogens to progesterone resistance to GnRH antagonists: a review. J Clin Med. 2021;10(5):1085.
19. Bulun SE, Cheng YH, Yin P, Imir G, Utsunomiya H, Attar E, et al. Progesterone resistance in endometriosis: link to failure to metabolize estradiol. Mol Cell Endocrinol. 2006;248(1–2):94–103.
20. Marquardt RM, Kim TH, Shin JH, Jeong JW. Progesterone and estrogen signaling in the endometrium: what goes wrong in endometriosis? Int J Mol Sci. 2019;20(15):3822.
21. Vierikko P, Kauppila A, Rönnberg L, Vihko R. Steroidal regulation of endometriosis tissue: lack of induction of 17 beta-hydroxysteroid dehydrogenase activity by progesterone, medroxyprogesterone acetate, or danazol. Fertil Steril. 1985;43(2):218–24.

22. Zeitoun K, Takayama K, Sasano H, Suzuki T, Moghrabi N, Andersson S, et al. Deficient 17beta-hydroxysteroid dehydrogenase type 2 expression in endometriosis: failure to metabolize 17beta-estradiol. J Clin Endocrinol Metab. 1998;83(12):4474–80.
23. Attar E, Bulun SE. Aromatase and other steroidogenic genes in endometriosis: translational aspects. Hum Reprod Update. 2006;12(1):49–56.
24. Horie S, Harada T, Mitsunari M, Taniguchi F, Iwabe T, Terakawa N. Progesterone and progestational compounds attenuate tumor necrosis factor alpha-induced interleukin-8 production via nuclear factor kappa B inactivation in endometriotic stromal cells. Fertil Steril. 2005;83(5):1530–5.
25. Fu L, Osuga Y, Morimoto C, Hirata T, Hirota Y, Yano T, et al. Dienogest inhibits BrdU uptake with G0/G1 arrest in cultured endometriotic stromal cells. Fertil Steril. 2008;89(5 Suppl):1344–7.
26. Zhang X, Lu B, Huang X, Xu H, Zhou C, Lin J. Endometrial nerve fibers in women with endometriosis, adenomyosis, and uterine fibroids. Fertil Steril. 2009;92(5):1799–801.
27. Harada T, Taniguchi F. Dienogest: a new therapeutic agent for the treatment of endometriosis. Womens Health (Lond). 2010;6(1):27–35.
28. Strowitzki T, Faustmann T, Gerlinger C, Seitz C. Dienogest in the treatment of endometriosis-associated pelvic pain: a 12-week, randomized, double-blind, placebo-controlled study. Eur J Obstet Gynecol Reprod Biol. 2010;151(2):193–8.
29. Cosson M, Querleu D, Donnez J, Madelenat P, Konincks P, Audebert A, et al. Dienogest is as effective as triptorelin in the treatment of endometriosis after laparoscopic surgery: results of a prospective, multicenter, randomized study. Fertil Steril. 2002;77(4):684–92.
30. Strowitzki T, Marr J, Gerlinger C, Faustmann T, Seitz C. Detailed analysis of a randomized, multicenter, comparative trial of dienogest versus leuprolide acetate in endometriosis. Int J Gynaecol Obstet. 2012;117(3):228–33.
31. Petraglia F, Hornung D, Seitz C, Faustmann T, Gerlinger C, Luisi S, et al. Reduced pelvic pain in women with endometriosis: efficacy of long-term dienogest treatment. Arch Gynecol Obstet. 2012;285(1):167–73.
32. Strowitzki T, Marr J, Gerlinger C, Faustmann T, Seitz C. Dienogest is as effective as leuprolide acetate in treating the painful symptoms of endometriosis: a 24-week, randomized, multicentre, open-label trial. Hum Reprod. 2010;25(3):633–41.
33. Ebert AD, Dong L, Merz M, Kirsch B, Francuski M, Böttcher B, et al. Dienogest 2 mg daily in the treatment of adolescents with clinically suspected endometriosis: the VISanne study to assess safety in ADOlescents. J Pediatr Adolesc Gynecol. 2017;30(5):560–7.
34. Kim SE, Lim HH, Lee DY, Choi D. The long-term effect of dienogest on bone mineral density after surgical treatment of endometrioma. Reprod Sci. 2021;28(5):1556–62.
35. Bergqvist A, Theorell T. Changes in quality of life after hormonal treatment of endometriosis. Acta Obstet Gynecol Scand. 2001;80(7):628–37.
36. Backer MH Jr. Isopregnenone (Duphaston): a new progestational agent. Obstet Gynecol. 1962;19:724–9.
37. King RJ, Whitehead MI. Assessment of the potency of orally administered progestins in women. Fertil Steril. 1986;46(6):1062–6.
38. WIH J. Dydrogesterone and endometriosis. BJOG Int J Obstet Gynaecol. 1976;83(1):77–80.
39. Overton CE, Lindsay PC, Johal B, Collins SA, Siddle NC, Shaw RW, et al. A randomized, double-blind, placebo-controlled study of luteal phase dydrogesterone (Duphaston) in women with minimal to mild endometriosis. Fertil Steril. 1994;62(4):701–7.
40. Tumasian KP, Bespoiasnaia VV, Voronovskaia IV. Treatment of endometriosis in female infertility. Lik Sprava. 2001;3:103–5.
41. Makhmudova GM, Nazhmutdinova DK, Gafarova D, Lukmanova ID. Efficacy of duphaston treatment in women with endometriosis after reconstructive surgery. Akush Ginekol (Sofiia). 2003;42(4):42–6.
42. Trivedi P, Selvaraj K, Mahapatra PD, Srivastava S, Malik S. Effective post-laparoscopic treatment of endometriosis with dydrogesterone. Gynecol Endocrinol. 2007;23(Suppl 1):73–6.

43. Bishop PM. A new oral progestogen in the treatment of dysmenorrhoea. Proc R Soc Med. 1961;54(9):752–4.
44. Fairweather DV. Duphaston in dysmenorrhoea; the results of a double blind clinical trial. J Obstet Gynaecol Br Commonw. 1965;72:193–5.
45. Brown J, Kives S, Akhtar M. Progestagens and anti-progestagens for pain associated with endometriosis. Cochrane Database Syst Rev. 2012;2012(3):Cd002122.
46. Harrison RF, Barry-Kinsella C. Efficacy of medroxyprogesterone treatment in infertile women with endometriosis: a prospective, randomized, placebo-controlled study. Fertil Steril. 2000;74(1):24–30.
47. Vercellini P, De Giorgi O, Mosconi P, Stellato G, Vicentini S, Crosignani PG. Cyproterone acetate versus a continuous monophasic oral contraceptive in the treatment of recurrent pelvic pain after conservative surgery for symptomatic endometriosis. Fertil Steril. 2002;77(1):52–61.
48. Crosignani PG, Luciano A, Ray A, Bergqvist A. Subcutaneous depot medroxyprogesterone acetate versus leuprolide acetate in the treatment of endometriosis-associated pain. Hum Reprod. 2006;21(1):248–56.
49. Simon MA, Shulman LP. Subcutaneous versus intramuscular depot methoxyprogesterone acetate: a comparative review. Womens Health (Lond). 2006;2(2):191–7.
50. Walch K, Unfried G, Huber J, Kurz C, van Trotsenburg M, Pernicka E, et al. Implanon versus medroxyprogesterone acetate: effects on pain scores in patients with symptomatic endometriosis--a pilot study. Contraception. 2009;79(1):29–34.
51. Ferrero S, Scala C, Ciccarelli S, Vellone VG, Barra F. Treatment of rectovaginal endometriosis with the etonogestrel-releasing contraceptive implant. Gynecol Endocrinol. 2020;36(6):540–4.
52. Vercellini P, Viganò P, Somigliana E. The role of the levonorgestrel-releasing intrauterine device in the management of symptomatic endometriosis. Curr Opin Obstet Gynecol. 2005;17(4):359–65.
53. Petta CA, Ferriani RA, Abrao MS, Hassan D, Rosa ESJC, Podgaec S, et al. Randomized clinical trial of a levonorgestrel-releasing intrauterine system and a depot GnRH analogue for the treatment of chronic pelvic pain in women with endometriosis. Hum Reprod. 2005;20(7):1993–8.
54. Sheng J, Zhang WY, Zhang JP, Lu D. The LNG-IUS study on adenomyosis: a 3-year follow-up study on the efficacy and side effects of the use of levonorgestrel intrauterine system for the treatment of dysmenorrhea associated with adenomyosis. Contraception. 2009;79(3):189–93.
55. Vercellini P, Aimi G, Panazza S, De Giorgi O, Pesole A, Crosignani PG. A levonorgestrel-releasing intrauterine system for the treatment of dysmenorrhea associated with endometriosis: a pilot study. Fertil Steril. 1999;72(3):505–8.
56. Vercellini P, De Giorgi O, Oldani S, Cortesi I, Panazza S, Crosignani PG. Depot medroxyprogesterone acetate versus an oral contraceptive combined with very-low-dose danazol for long-term treatment of pelvic pain associated with endometriosis. Am J Obstet Gynecol. 1996;175(2):396–401.
57. Moore C, Kohler G, Muller A. The treatment of endometriosis with dienogest. Drugs Today (Barcelona, Spain: 1998). 1999;35(Suppl. C):41–52.
58. Vercellini P, Pietropaolo G, De Giorgi O, Pasin R, Chiodini A, Crosignani PG. Treatment of symptomatic rectovaginal endometriosis with an estrogen-progestogen combination versus low-dose norethindrone acetate. Fertil Steril. 2005;84(5):1375–87.
59. Ferrero S, Camerini G, Ragni N, Venturini PL, Biscaldi E, Seracchioli R, et al. Letrozole and norethisterone acetate in colorectal endometriosis. Eur J Obstet Gynecol Reprod Biol. 2010;150(2):199–202.
60. Angioni S, Nappi L, Pontis A, Sedda F, Luisi S, Mais V, et al. Dienogest. A possible conservative approach in bladder endometriosis. Results of a pilot study. Gynecol Endocrinol. 2015;31(5):406–8.
61. Andres Mde P, Lopes LA, Baracat EC, Podgaec S. Dienogest in the treatment of endometriosis: systematic review. Arch Gynecol Obstet. 2015;292(3):523–9.

62. Murji A, Biberoğlu K, Leng J, Mueller MD, Römer T, Vignali M, et al. Use of dienogest in endometriosis: a narrative literature review and expert commentary. Curr Med Res Opin. 2020;36(5):895–907.
63. Mehdizadeh Kashi A, Niakan G, Ebrahimpour M, Allahqoli L, Hassanlouei B, Gitas G, et al. A randomized, double-blind, placebo-controlled pilot study of the comparative effects of dienogest and the combined oral contraceptive pill in women with endometriosis. Int J Gynaecol Obstet. 2022;156(1):124–32.
64. Chwalisz K, Surrey E, Stanczyk FZ. The hormonal profile of norethindrone acetate: rationale for add-back therapy with gonadotropin-releasing hormone agonists in women with endometriosis. Reprod Sci. 2012;19(6):563–71.
65. Muneyyirci-Delale O, Karacan M. Effect of norethindrone acetate in the treatment of symptomatic endometriosis. Int J Fertil Womens Med. 1998;43(1):24–7.
66. Vercellini P, Bracco B, Mosconi P, Roberto A, Alberico D, Dhouha D, et al. Norethindrone acetate or dienogest for the treatment of symptomatic endometriosis: a before and after study. Fertil Steril. 2016;105(3):734–43.e3.
67. Del Forno S, Mabrouk M, Arena A, Mattioli G, Giaquinto I, Paradisi R, et al. Dienogest or Norethindrone acetate for the treatment of ovarian endometriomas: can we avoid surgery? Eur J Obstet Gynecol Reprod Biol. 2019;238:120–4.
68. Peng C, Huang Y, Zhou Y. Dydrogesterone in the treatment of endometriosis: evidence mapping and meta-analysis. Arch Gynecol Obstet. 2021;304(1):231–52.
69. Sukhikh GT, Adamyan LV, Dubrovina SO, Baranov II, Bezhenar VF, Kozachenko AV, et al. Prolonged cyclical and continuous regimens of dydrogesterone are effective for reducing chronic pelvic pain in women with endometriosis: results of the ORCHIDEA study. Fertil Steril. 2021;116(6):1568–77.
70. Telimaa S, Rönnberg L, Kauppila A. Placebo-controlled comparison of danazol and high-dose medroxyprogesterone acetate in the treatment of endometriosis after conservative surgery. Gynecol Endocrinol. 1987;1(4):363–71.
71. Regidor PA, Regidor M, Schmidt M, Ruwe B, Lübben G, Förtig P, et al. Prospective randomized study comparing the GnRH-agonist leuprorelin acetate and the gestagen lynestrenol in the treatment of severe endometriosis. Gynecol Endocrinol. 2001;15(3):202–9.
72. Vercellini P, Trespidi L, Colombo A, Vendola N, Marchini M, Crosignani PG. A gonadotropin-releasing hormone agonist versus a low-dose oral contraceptive for pelvic pain associated with endometriosis. Fertil Steril. 1993;60(1):75–9.
73. Ceccaroni M, Clarizia R, Liverani S, Donati A, Ceccarello M, Manzone M, et al. Dienogest vs GnRH agonists as postoperative therapy after laparoscopic eradication of deep infiltrating endometriosis with bowel and parametrial surgery: a randomized controlled trial. Gynecol Endocrinol. 2021;37(10):930–3.
74. Ferrero S, Camerini G, Seracchioli R, Ragni N, Venturini PL, Remorgida V. Letrozole combined with norethisterone acetate compared with norethisterone acetate alone in the treatment of pain symptoms caused by endometriosis. Hum Reprod. 2009;24(12):3033–41.
75. Morotti M, Sozzi F, Remorgida V, Venturini PL, Ferrero S. Dienogest in women with persistent endometriosis-related pelvic pain during norethisterone acetate treatment. Eur J Obstet Gynecol Reprod Biol. 2014;183:188–92.
76. Timonen S, Johansson CJ. Endometriosis treated with lynestrenol. Ann Chir Gynaecol Fenn. 1968;57(2):144–7.
77. Iwami N, Kawamata M, Ozawa N, Yamamoto T, Watanabe E, Mizuuchi M, et al. New treatment strategy for endometriosis using progestin-primed ovarian stimulation with dienogest: a prospective cohort study, comparison of dienogest versus dydrogesterone. Reprod Biol. 2021;21(1):100470.

78. Tamura H, Yoshida H, Kikuchi H, Josaki M, Mihara Y, Shirafuta Y, et al. The clinical outcome of Dienogest treatment followed by in vitro fertilization and embryo transfer in infertile women with endometriosis. J Ovarian Res. 2019;12(1):123.
79. Barra F, Laganà AS, Scala C, Garzon S, Ghezzi F, Ferrero S. Pretreatment with dienogest in women with endometriosis undergoing IVF after a previous failed cycle. Reprod Biomed Online. 2020;41(5):859–68.
80. Khalifa E, Mohammad H, Abdullah A, Abdel-Rasheed M, Khairy M, Hosni M. Role of suppression of endometriosis with progestins before IVF-ET: a non-inferiority randomized controlled trial. BMC Pregnancy Childbirth. 2021;21(1):264.
81. Guo H, Wang Y, Chen Q, Chai W, Sun L, Ai A, et al. Use of medroxyprogesterone acetate in women with ovarian endometriosis undergoing controlled ovarian hyperstimulation for in vitro fertilization. Sci Rep. 2017;7(1):11927.
82. Yap C, Furness S, Farquhar C. Pre and post operative medical therapy for endometriosis surgery. Cochrane Database Syst Rev. 2004;2004(3):CD003678.
83. Mettler L, Ruprai R, Alkatout I. Impact of medical and surgical treatment of endometriosis on the cure of endometriosis and pain. Biomed Res Int. 2014;2014:264653.
84. Muzii L, Di Tucci C, Achilli C, Di Donato V, Musella A, Palaia I, et al. Continuous versus cyclic oral contraceptives after laparoscopic excision of ovarian endometriomas: a systematic review and metaanalysis. Am J Obstet Gynecol. 2016;214(2):203–11.
85. Grandi G, Barra F, Ferrero S, Sileo FG, Bertucci E, Napolitano A, et al. Hormonal contraception in women with endometriosis: a systematic review. Eur J Contracept Reprod Health Care. 2019;24(1):61–70.
86. Zakhari A, Delpero E, McKeown S, Tomlinson G, Bougie O, Murji A. Endometriosis recurrence following post-operative hormonal suppression: a systematic review and meta-analysis. Hum Reprod Update. 2021;27(1):96–107.
87. Tsui KH, Lee WL, Chen CY, Sheu BC, Yen MS, Chang TC, et al. Medical treatment for adenomyosis and/or adenomyoma. Taiwan J Obstet Gynecol. 2014;53(4):459–65.
88. Hirata T, Izumi G, Takamura M, Saito A, Nakazawa A, Harada M, et al. Efficacy of dienogest in the treatment of symptomatic adenomyosis: a pilot study. Gynecol Endocrinol. 2014;30(10):726–9.
89. Osuga Y, Fujimoto-Okabe H, Hagino A. Evaluation of the efficacy and safety of dienogest in the treatment of painful symptoms in patients with adenomyosis: a randomized, double-blind, multicenter, placebo-controlled study. Fertil Steril. 2017;108(4):673–8.
90. Fawzy M, Mesbah Y. Comparison of dienogest versus triptorelin acetate in premenopausal women with adenomyosis: a prospective clinical trial. Arch Gynecol Obstet. 2015;292(6):1267–71.
91. Muneyyirci-Delale O, Chandrareddy A, Mankame S, Osei-Tutu N, Hv G. Norethindrone acetate in the medical management of adenomyosis. Pharmaceuticals (Basel). 2012;5(10):1120–7.
92. Li L, Leng J, Jia S, Lang J. Treatment of symptomatic adenomyosis with the levonorgestrel-releasing intrauterine system. Int J Gynaecol Obstet. 2019;146(3):357–63.
93. Lee KH, Kim JK, Lee MA, Ko YB, Yang JB, Kang BH, et al. Relationship between uterine volume and discontinuation of treatment with levonorgestrel-releasing intrauterine devices in patients with adenomyosis. Arch Gynecol Obstet. 2016;294(3):561–6.
94. Zhang P, Song K, Li L, Yukuwa K, Kong B. Efficacy of combined levonorgestrel-releasing intrauterine system with gonadotropin-releasing hormone analog for the treatment of adenomyosis. Med Princ Pract. 2013;22(5):480–3.
95. Dueholm M. Minimally invasive treatment of adenomyosis. Best Pract Res Clin Obstet Gynaecol. 2018;51:119–37.

96. Liang Z, Yin M, Ma M, Wang Y, Kuang Y. Effect of pretreatment with a levonorgestrel-releasing intrauterine system on IVF and vitrified-warmed embryo transfer outcomes in women with adenomyosis. Reprod Biomed Online. 2019;39(1):111–8.
97. Group TmotEGC, Becker CM, Bokor A, Heikinheimo O, Horne A, Jansen F, et al. ESHRE guideline: endometriosis. Human Reprod Open. 2022;2022:hoac009.
98. ACOG Committee Opinion No. 760: dysmenorrhea and endometriosis in the adolescent. Obstet Gynecol. 2018;132(6):e249–58.
99. National Guideline A. National Institute for Health and Care Excellence: clinical guidelines. Endometriosis: diagnosis and management. London: National Institute for Health and Care Excellence (UK) © nice; 2017.
100. Dunselman GA, Vermeulen N, Becker C, Calhaz-Jorge C, D'Hooghe T, De Bie B, et al. ESHRE guideline: management of women with endometriosis. Hum Reprod. 2014;29(3):400–12.
101. Johnson NP, Hummelshoj L, Abrao MS, Adamson GD, Allaire C, Consortium ftWESM, et al. Consensus on current management of endometriosis. Hum Reprod. 2013;28(6):1552–68.
102. Leyland N, Casper R, Laberge P, Singh SS. Endometriosis: diagnosis and management. J Obstet Gynaecol Can. 2010;32(7 Suppl 2):S1–32.
103. Practice bulletin no. 114: management of endometriosis. Obstet Gynecol. 2010;116(1):223–36.
104. Practice Committee of the American Society for Reproductive Medicine. Treatment of pelvic pain associated with endometriosis: a committee opinion. Fertil Steril. 2014;101(4):927–35.

Hormonal Therapy in Endometriosis and Adenomyosis: Danazol, Aromatase Inhibitors

42

Simone Ferrero and Fabio Barra

Contents

42.1 Introduction

Although endometriosis and adenomyosis are different diseases, they both grow and regress in an estrogen-dependent fashion. Both endometriotic and adenomyotic lesions express steroid receptors and enzyme aromatase [1]. Circulating estrogens produced by the ovaries and locally produced estrogens stimulate the growth of endometriotic and adenomyotic tissue. Both danazol and aromatase inhibitors have been used to treat endometriosis and adenomyosis because they have hypoestrogenic effects.

The original version of the chapter has been revised. A correction to this chapter can be found at https://doi.org/10.1007/978-3-030-97236-3_45

S. Ferrero (✉) · F. Barra
Academic Unit of Obstetrics and Gynecology, IRCCS Ospedale Policlinico San Martino, Genoa, Italy

Department of Neurosciences, Rehabilitation, Ophthalmology, Genetics, Maternal and Child Health (DiNOGMI), University of Genoa, Genoa, Italy

E. Oral (ed.), *Endometriosis and Adenomyosis*,
https://doi.org/10.1007/978-3-030-97236-3_42

Danazol is an isoxazole derivative of 17 alpha-ethinyl testosterone, which is characterized by anti-gonadotropic, hypoestrogenic, and hyperandrogenic properties. It lowers the mid-cycle luteinizing hormone surge and increases serum free testosterone levels. In vitro, danazol has direct inhibitory activity on endometrial or endometriotic cells [2–4], which can alleviate endometriosis-related pain. Also, danazol competitively inhibits aromatase activity in endometriosis-derived stromal cells supporting its local application to treat endometriotic lesions [5]. It was also demonstrated that danazol diminishes the expression of aromatase cytochrome P450 in the eutopic endometrium of women with adenomyosis [6].

The aromatase P450 is a crucial enzyme for estrogen biosynthesis because it catalyzes the conversion of androstenedione and testosterone to estrone and estradiol via hydroxylation. The aromatase P450 is aberrantly expressed in the eutopic and ectopic endometrium of women with endometriosis. Estrogen stimulates the production of cyclooxygenase type 2 enzyme, resulting in elevated levels of prostaglandin E_2, which is a potent stimulator of aromatase P450 activity [7]. Based on this biological background, aromatase inhibitors (AIs) have been used to treat endometriosis and adenomyosis.

42.2 Endometriosis

42.2.1 Danazol

Danazol was very popular for the treatment of endometriosis during the 1970s and 1980s. However, due to the severe androgenic side effects and to the marketing of other drugs, the use of danazol significantly declined in the last 20 years [8, 9].

Several randomized controlled trials (RCTs) demonstrated the efficacy of danazol in treating endometriosis-related pain. A double-blind, placebo-controlled RCT compared the efficacy and tolerability of danazol and medroxyprogesterone acetate (MPA) in the treatment of mild-moderate endometriosis [10]. After diagnostic laparoscopy, 59 patients randomly received danazol (200 mg three times daily; 18 women), medroxyprogesterone acetate (MPA; 100 mg/day; 16 women), or placebo (17 women) for 6 months. A second laparoscopy was performed 6 months after the discontinuation of the hormonal therapy, demonstrating full or partial resolution of peritoneal implants in 60% of the patients receiving danazol and in 63% of those receiving MPA. In contrast, in the placebo group, the resolution was observed in 18%, and the implant size was increased in 23% of the patients. Pelvic pain, lower back pain, and dyschezia significantly improved in patients treated with danazol and MPA compared with placebo, but they did not differ from each other in these actions. Another RCT investigated the efficacy of postsurgical treatment with danazol in women with American Fertility Society (AFS) stage III or IV endometriosis [11]. Women were assigned either to treatment with oral danazol (600 mg/day; 36 women) for 3 months or no therapy (41 women). At 6-month follow-up, 23% of patients on danazol and 31% of those without any treatment had moderate/severe pelvic pain recurrence; the respective cumulative pain recurrence rates at

12 months were 26% and 34% in the two study groups. Fedele et al. compared cyproterone acetate (CPA; 27 mg plus ethinyl estradiol 0.035 mg/day; 11 women) and danazol (600 mg/day; 12 women) for 6 months in patients with laparoscopically diagnosed endometriosis [12]. A second laparoscopy was performed at the end of treatment in some patients, showing a partial regression of endometriotic lesions in both groups, with no significant differences between them. Dysmenorrhea disappeared in all patients during treatment. At 6-month follow-up after treatment discontinuation, dysmenorrhea recurred in 66% of the patients treated with CPA and in 58% of those treated with danazol; at 12-month follow-up, the recurrence rates were 89% and 92%, respectively. Noncyclic pelvic pain improved during treatment in both groups; 6 months after treatment interruption, it recurred in four patients both in the CPA and in the danazol group; after 12 months, just one woman in the danazol group did not have this symptom. Deep dyspareunia was less affected by both treatments, and after 12 months, it recurred in all women. An RCT including infertile patients with a laparoscopic diagnosis of endometriosis compared a 6-month treatment of oral gestrinone (2.5 mg twice weekly; 20 women) with oral danazol (600 mg/day; 19 women) [13]. Women were followed for at least 12 months after the end of the treatment. During both treatments, there was a significant decrease in the severity of pain. Symptoms recurred during the follow-up in 57% of the patients treated with gestrinone and 53% of those treated with danazol. Twenty-seven studies included in a Cochrane review evaluated the use of danazol versus gonadotrophin-releasing hormone (GnRH) agonists in patients with endometriosis showing no significant difference between the two treatments in improving dysmenorrhea, deep dyspareunia, and noncyclic pelvic pain [14]. In 1988, a large RCT compared a 6-month treatment with oral danazol (800 mg per day; 80 women) or intranasal nafarelin (400 or 800 μg/day; 77 and 79 women, respectively) in 213 patients with laparoscopically confirmed endometriosis [15]. More than 80% of the women in each treatment group had a decrease in the extent of disease. Also, the rate of patients who experienced severe pain symptoms decreased from about 40% to 5–10%, while the percentage with no or minimal discomfort grew from 25% to 70%. Wheeler et al. conducted a double-blind, multicenter RCT, including 270 patients [11]. Patients were randomized to a 24-week treatment with leuprolide acetate (3.75 mg every month; 128 women) or oral danazol (800 mg/day; 125 women). At baseline, there was no difference in dysmenorrhea, dyspareunia, and pelvic pain between the study groups. After 6 months of treatment, pain symptoms similarly improved in both groups: a complete resolution of dysmenorrhea and pelvic pain was reported by 99% and 55% of patients on leuprolide and 96% and 60% of patients on danazol, respectively. At the same follow-up, patients treated with danazol had greater improvement of dyspareunia than those treated with leuprolide. An open-label RCT compared oral danazol efficacy (200 mg three times daily; 20 women) and intramuscular triptorelin (3.75 mg every 6 weeks; 20 women) for 6 months in the management of moderate and severe endometriosis. Both pain control and the revised AFS score at second-look laparoscopy did not show a significant difference between the two medications [16]. An open-label, parallel-group RCT compared a combined oral contraceptive (COC; ethinylestradiol 0.02 mg and

desogestrel 0.15 mg) plus oral danazol (50 mg/day for 21 days of each 28-day cycle; 40 women) versus intramuscular depot MPA (150 mg every 3 months; 40 women) [17]. At 1-year follow-up, symptoms significantly improved in both study groups; dysmenorrhea was greater in women allocated to COC plus danazol because of the virtual absence of regular flow in patients receiving depot MAP.

Vaginally administered danazol can be used in combination with other therapies. A prospective pilot study (15 women) demonstrated the effectiveness of treatment with vaginal danazol (100 mg per day) in improving the pain symptoms caused by rectovaginal endometriosis that persist after insertion of a levonorgestrel-releasing intrauterine device. Adverse effects of the treatment were minimal and well tolerated [18].

In conclusion, several randomized controlled trials demonstrated that danazol effectively treats endometriosis-associated pain symptoms (Table 42.1). However, its use is limited by the occurrence of androgenic side effects (Table 42.2) and the availability of other efficacious and better-tolerated drugs.

42.2.2 Aromatase Inhibitors

Over the last 15 years, several studies documented the efficacy of AIs in treating endometriosis-related pain symptoms. An open-label RCT compared the effectiveness of letrozole (LTZ, 2.5 mg/day) combined with either norethindrone acetate (NETA; 2.5 mg/day; 17 women) or triptorelin (11.25 mg/day every 3 months; 18 women) for 6 months in treating pain symptoms caused by rectovaginal endometriosis [19]. The severity of both nonmenstrual pelvic pain and deep dyspareunia significantly decreased during treatment in both study groups, although no statistical difference between the two groups was reported. A recent RCT compared the efficacy and tolerability of continuous COC (one tablet of 20 mg ethinyl estradiol/0.1 mg levonorgestrel) versus continuous COC combined with LTZ (2.5 mg/day) in treating pain in patients with a surgical diagnosis of endometriosis [20]. Eight hundred twenty patients were included in the study, and they received the treatment for 6 months. The intensity of chronic pelvic pain and deep dyspareunia significantly decreased at 1-month after treatment in both study groups; chronic pelvic pain continued to decline during treatment. Similarly, the intensity of deep dyspareunia significantly decreased at 6-month follow-up in both study groups. The intensity of chronic pelvic pain and deep dyspareunia was significantly lower in patients receiving LTZ and COC than in those receiving COC alone. Pain scores continued to decrease throughout the trial. In all patients, menstrual cycles resumed within 8 weeks after the discontinuation of the treatment. At 6-month follow-up after completing therapy, the intensity of dysmenorrhea, deep dyspareunia, and chronic pelvic pain was significantly decreased compared with baseline values in both study groups. At 12-month follow-up, no significant difference was observed in the intensity of dysmenorrhea symptoms between the two study groups.

Several studies documented the efficacy of AIs in treating pain caused by deep-infiltrating endometriosis. A prospective open-label nonrandomized trial compared

Table 42.1 Most important randomized controlled trials investigating the efficacy of danazol in treating endometriosis-related pain

First author, year published	Study location	No. of partici-pants	Age (y), mean (± SD)	Treatment group	Dosage	Treatment duration (weeks)	Pain score/ symptoms scale	Changes in pain symptoms	Stage of disease	Main results
Telimaa, 1987 [10]	Finland	18	31.4 ± 5.2	Danazol	600 mg/day	24	NA	NA	AFS (I-II)	Pelvic pain, lower back pain, and defecation pain significantly decreased both with danazol and MPA compared with placebo, but they did not differ from each other in these actions
		16	32.2 ± 5.4	MPA	100 mg/day					
		17	32.4 ± 5.7	Placebo	–					
Henzl, 1988 [48]	United States	79	NA	Nafarelin	800 µg/day	24	NA	NA	AFS	Nafarelin given by nasal spray is as effective in treating endometriosis as the established therapy with danazol
		77	NA	Nafarelin	400 µg/day					
		80	NA	Danazol	800 mg/day					
Fedele, 1989 [12]	Italy	11	25.5 ± 7.2	CPA/EE	27 mg + 0.035 mg/day	24	Andersh & Milson questionnaires and VAS	NA	r-AFS	Dysmenorrhea disappeared in all patients during treatment, noncyclic pelvic pain significantly improved during treatment in both groups; deep dyspareunia was less affected by both treatments. After 12 months, it recurred in all women
		12	27.2 ± 3.9	Danazol	600 mg/day			NA		

(continued)

Table 42.1 (continued)

First author, year published	Study location	No. of partici-pants	Age (y), mean (± SD)	Treatment group	Dosage	Treatment duration (weeks)	Pain score/ symptoms scale	Changes in pain symptoms	Stage of disease	Main results
Fedele, 1989 [13]	Italy	20	29.7 ± 3.9	Gestrinone	2.5 mg twice weekly	24	NA	NA	Stage I to IV (r-AFS)	Significant improvement of pain symptoms during the treatment was reported in both groups without significant differences between the two compounds
		19	29.1 ± 4.5	Danazol	600 mg/day					
Dmowsky, 1989 [49]	United States	10	30.8 ± 0.6	Buserelin (intranasal)	1200 μg/day	24	Pelvic pain score (0–3 point scale)	Pre-treatment 2.7 ± 0.5; post-treatment 0.7 ± 0.2	r-AFS	Pelvic pain scores decreased significantly during treatment in all the study groups
		9		Buserelin (subcutaneous)	200 μg/day					
		10		Danazol	800 mg/day			Pre-treatment 3.3 ± 0.5; post-treatment 0.4 ± 0.2		
Wheeler, 1992 [11]	United States	128	31.0	Leuprolide acetate	3.75 mg monthly	24	B & B	NA	r-AFS	After 6 months of treatment, pain symptoms similarly improved in both groups: a complete resolution of dysmenorrhea and pelvic pain was reported by 99% and 55% of patients on leuprolide and 96% and 60% of patients on danazol, respectively
		125	29.8	Danazol	800 mg/day			NA		

Adamson, 1994 [50]	United States	45	NA	Nafarelin acetate	800 μg/day	24	Pain reports %	Dysmenorrhea: PR % at baseline 100; PR % at 6 months 0. Dyspareunia: PR % at baseline 100; PR % at 6 months 31. Pelvic pain PR % at baseline 100; PR % at 6 months 35	NA	Nafarelin at both high and low doses and danazol provided significant relief of several types of pain associated with endometriosis during 6 months of daily treatment
		45	NA	Nafarelin acetate	400 μg/day			Dysmenorrhea: PR % at baseline 100; PR % at 6 months 0. Dyspareunia: PR % at baseline 100; PR % at 6 months 32. Pelvic pain PR % at baseline 100; PR % at 6 months 43		
		34	NA	Danazol	800 mg/day			Dysmenorrhea: PR % at baseline 100; PR % at 6 months 6. Dyspareunia: PR % at baseline 100; PR % at 6 months 17. Pelvic pain PR % at baseline 100; PR % at 6 months 36		

(continued)

Table 42.1 (continued)

First author, year published	Study location	No. of partici-pants	Age (y), mean (± SD)	Treatment group	Dosage	Treatment duration (weeks)	Pain score/ symptoms scale	Changes in pain symptoms	Stage of disease	Main results
Bromham, 1995 [51]	UK	132	NA	Gestrinone	2.5 mg twice weekly	24	NA	NA	AFS	A significant reduction in the severity of dysmenorrhea by the third month in the danazol group and at 6 months in both groups
		137	NA	Danazol	400 mg/day					
Vercellini, 1996 [17]	Italy	40	NA	MPA (intramuscular)	150 mg once every 3 months	48	Modified B & B and VAS	Dysmenorrhea at baseline: 7; at 6 and 12 months: 0. Dyspareunia at baseline: 4; at 6 and 12 months: 0. Nonmenstrual pain at baseline: 4; at 6 and 12 months: 0	r-AFS	
		40	NA	EE/DSG + Danazol (oral)	0.02 mg + 0.15 mg + 50 mg/day for 21/28 days			Dysmenorrhea at baseline: 6.5; at 6 months: 2; at 12 months: 0.5. Dyspareunia at baseline: 3.5; at 6 and 12 months: 0. Nonmenstrual pain at baseline: 4; at 6 and 12 months 0		More impact on BMD, less bleeding

B & B Biberoglu & Behrman, *BMD* bone mineral density, *CPA* cyproterone acetate, *DSG* desogestrel, *EE* ethinylestradiol, *MPA* medroxyprogesterone acetate, *VAS* visual analog scale

Table 42.2 Adverse effects reported in randomized controlled trials investigating the efficacy of danazol in patients with endometriosis

First author, year published	Dosage of danazol	Side effects
Telimaa, 1987 [10]	600 mg/day	Weight increase in 6 months from (59.3 ± 1.2 kg) to (62.7 ± 2.6 kg); acne frequency after 1 month (30%), after 6 months (63%). Edema frequency (65%) after 1 month, (47%) after 6 months. Muscle cramps frequency after 6 months (32%). Spotting after 1 month (55%), after 6 months (26%)
Henzl, 1988 [48]	800 mg/day	Hot flushes (68%). Weight increase, edema, and myalgia (statistically significantly greater than the nafarelin group)
Fedele, 1989 [12]	600 mg/day	Weight increase (2.8 ± 1.1 kg). Hot flushes. Breast pain-tension. Acne. Seborrhea. Nausea. Hirsutism. Liver enzymes increase
Fedele, 1989 [13]	600 mg/day	Weight increase (68%). Hot flushes (31%). Decreased breast size (26%). Vaginal dryness (11%). Acne (31%). Seborrhea (21%). Nausea (16%). Muscle cramps (26%). Deepening of voice (5%). Hirsutism (11%). Increase of liver transaminases (11%)
Dmowsky, 1989 [49]	800 mg/day	Headaches (60%). Fatigue (40%). Irritability (40%). Depression (50%). Sleep disturbances (30%). Vaginal dryness (30%). Vasomotor symptoms (60%). Acne (60%). Weight increase (3.9 kg).
Bromham, 1995 [51]	400 mg/day	Headache (4.4%). Skin rush (1.5%). Hirsutism (2.2%). Nausea (3.7%). Vomiting (1.5%). Voice change (3.7%). Tiredness (1.5%). Muscle cramps (2.2%). Depression (2.9%). Shaking (1.5%). Acne (0.73%). Dizziness (1.5%). Faintness (0.73%). Increase of liver transaminases (1.5%)

the effectiveness of NETA or a combination of LTZ and NETA in treating pain symptoms caused by rectovaginal endometriosis [21]. The study included 82 patients, and the treatment was administered for 6 months. Both treatments improved the intensity of chronic pelvic pain and deep dyspareunia. However, the intensity of the symptoms was significantly better in patients receiving the combined therapy than in those treated with NETA alone. Pain symptoms recurred after the discontinuation of treatment in both study groups. A prospective study including six women with colorectal endometriosis demonstrated that LTZ and NETA administration improves pain and dyschezia, symptoms mimicking diarrhea-predominant irritable bowel syndrome, intestinal cramping, abdominal bloating, and passage of mucus in the stools [22]. The same authors showed that the combined treatment with LTZ and NETA quickly improves pain and urinary symptoms of patients with bladder endometriosis [23].

Some studies investigated the impact of aromatase inhibitors on ovarian endometriomas. As expected, all the studies proved that aromatase inhibitors decrease the size of ovarian endometrioma. However, contradictory results have been reported that aromatase inhibitors cause the complete disappearance of ovarian endometriotic cysts. Lall Seal et al. treated five patients with recurrent ovarian endometrioma with LTZ, desogestrel, and ethinylestradiol for 6 months [24]. In all patients, the size of the ovarian endometriomas decreased within 3 months of initiation of treatment. One patient had complete regression of cyst within 3 months of initiation of treatment; the remaining patients had complete regression of cysts at the end of the 6-month treatment. Subsequent follow-up showed no recurrence of the endometriotic ovarian cyst (maximum up to 2 years). All the patients reported improvement in the intensity of pain within 1 month of treatment initiation; the intensity of pain continued to decrease throughout treatment. A prospective study investigated the impact of 3-month treatment with LTZ (5 mg/day) combined with NETA (5 mg/day) on ovarian endometrioma size [25]. Eight women with 14 endometriomas were enrolled in the study. The mean endometrioma diameter decreased 50% (from 4.6 ± 1.6 cm to 2.3 ± 1.6 cm, $p < 0.01$). This change in diameter corresponds to a mean endometrioma volume reduction of 75%. Dysmenorrhea, dyspareunia, and nonmenstrual pelvic pain also improved with treatment. More recently, an Italian patient-preference study including 40 women compared the efficacy of NETA or NETA combined with LTZ in treating ovarian endometriotic cysts [26]. After 6 months of treatment, the endometriomas volume significantly decreased compared with baseline in both study groups; it was significantly smaller in patients receiving the combined treatment than in those treated with NETA alone. However, in none of the 40 patients included in the study did the endometriomas disappear. Furthermore, in both study groups, at 6 months after the discontinuation of treatment, the volume of the endometriotic cysts was comparable to baseline. Therefore, the author concluded that aromatase inhibitors' efficacy should be balanced with the need to administer long-term treatment.

AIs have also been used to prevent the recurrence of endometriosis after surgery. In an RCT, Soysal et al. compared 6-month treatment of anastrozole (1 mg/day) plus subcutaneous goserelin (3.6 mg every month; 40 women) with subcutaneous goserelin alone (3.6 mg every month; 40 women) in patients who underwent conservative surgery for severe endometriosis [27]. The combination of anastrozole and goserelin was better in improving pain than goserelin alone. Furthermore, patients treated with goserelin plus anastrozole, compared to those treated with goserelin alone, had a longer symptom recurrence period (>24 vs. 17 months). At 24-month follow-up, symptoms recurred in three women (7.5%) treated with goserelin plus anastrozole, while recurrence was observed in 14 women (35%) treated with goserelin-only. A prospective Iranian RCT including 144 infertile patients with endometriosis compared the following three postoperative treatments: LTZ (2.5 mg/day for 2 months; 47 women; group 1), triptorelin (3.75 mg every month for 2 months; 40 patients; group 2), and no medication (57 women; group 3) [28]. At baseline, there was no difference in the prevalence of pain symptoms among the three groups. After 1 year of follow-up, the rate of symptom recurrence was similar in the three study groups: 6.4% in patients treated with LTZ, 5% in those treated with triptorelin, and 5.3% in those who did not receive postoperative hormonal therapy. The pregnancy rate was 23.4% in patients treated with LTZ, 27.5% in those treated with triptorelin, and 28.1% in those who did not receive postoperative treatment.

Theoretically, the vaginal administration or aromatase inhibitors may guarantee the efficacy in improving pain symptoms, and it may minimize the adverse effects. A cynomolgus monkey study showed that anastrozole could be administered by a vaginal polymer-based drug delivery system [29]. Subsequently, a phase 1, randomized, multicenter, parallel-group, three-arm, open-label study investigated the doses, pharmacokinetics, pharmacodynamics, and safety/tolerability of anastrozole and the levonorgestrel delivered to the systemic circulation by an intravaginal ring [30]. In addition, a phase 2 trial showed that there is no interaction of anastrozole on levonorgestrel [31].

42.3 Adenomyosis

42.3.1 Danazol

Limited data are available on the systemic treatment of adenomyosis with danazol due to the high incidence of androgenic adverse effects.

Igarashi used an intrauterine device containing 175 mg of danazol to treat patients affected by adenomyosis [32]. The treatment effectively reduced the size of the uterus, and pregnancy was achieved in 66.6% of the patients. In another study, an intrauterine device containing 300–400 mg of danazol was employed for the treatment of 14 women with adenomyosis [33]. During treatment, there was complete remission of dysmenorrhea in 9, reduction in 4, and no change in 1 patient, respectively; additionally, there was complete remission of hypermenorrhea in 12 and no change in 2 patients, respectively. A decrease in dysmenorrhea and hypermenorrhea was observed at the first menstruation following the initiation of treatment and persisted after removing the danazol IUD. With the danazol-IUD therapy, in 9 out of 14 patients a reduction in the myometrium's maximum thickness (from the surface of the uterus to the border between the myometrium and the endometrium) as measured by MRI was observed. During the treatment, blood danazol levels were undetectable, ovulation was not inhibited, and no side effects were reported. The same device loaded with danazol was used in a murine model of adenomyosis. In this preclinical study, it was reported that the adenomyotic nodule number decreased as the danazol dose increased, with a low and stable plasma drug concentration [34]. Another study published in the abstract form confirmed the efficacy of the danazol-loaded intrauterine device in the treatment of adenomyosis [35]. The device was inserted in 50 patients resistant to previous oral danazol therapy or GnRH analog treatment. The therapy improved dysmenorrhea and hypermenorrhea. There were no systemic side effects because serum danazol concentration was not detectable. Ovulation and menstruation were the same as in pre-treatment cycles.

Cervical injections of danazol at 2-week intervals for 12 weeks have also been successfully used for treating adenomyosis, showing a 60% improvement in bleeding, pain, and dyspareunia, and a decrease in uterine size [36].

A prospective noncomparative study including 21 symptomatic women with adenomyosis found that the danazol-loaded intrauterine device was responsible for complete relief of dysmenorrhea in 17 (81%) and improvement of menstrual bleeding in 16 (76%) patients after 6 months of treatment. The treatment caused no systemic side effects. The only disadvantage of the danazol-loaded intrauterine device in this series was uterine spotting and spontaneous expulsion [37].

A prospective Italian study investigated the efficacy of vaginally administered danazol (200 mg/day) in treating young women with menorrhagia [38]. The treatment was administered every day at night and continued for 6 months. The severity of blood loss was significantly reduced in all of the women after 2 months of treatment. After 6 months of treatment, there was a decrease in bleeding duration and the total number of pads and/or tampons used. Uterine volume was significantly reduced, and hematocrit, hemoglobin, and red blood cell count increased. The medical treatment did not affect hormonal parameters, and the menstrual cycle remained unaffected; few local vaginal adverse effects (such as vaginal irritation) were recorded. After 6 months of treatment, 80% of women were very satisfied with their treatment, 16% were satisfied, 4% were uncertain, and none were dissatisfied. Dysmenorrhea, dyspareunia, and pelvic pain significantly decreased after 3 months of treatment, with a persistent effect of 6 months. A subsequent retrospective study investigated the clinical efficacy of long-term vaginal danazol treatment in patients with adenomyosis [39]. Women were treated with a daily low-dose vaginal danazol (200 mg) for 6 months, followed by two different schedules: continuous treatment for further 18 months ($n = 30$) or intermittent cyclic treatment with 3 months' therapy followed by 3 months' interval for further 18 months. Both protocols improved dysmenorrhea, dyspareunia, and menstrual bleeding at 6, 12, and 24 months of treatment.

A study published only in the abstract form compared low-dose dienogest with low-dose danazol for the long-term treatment, and of adenomyosis [40]. The daily dose of dienogest could be decreased from 2.0 to 1.5 or 1.0 mg. The daily dose of danazol could be reduced from 200 to 50 or 33 mg. Both therapies were effective in the treatment of adenomyosis. Still, some patients in the low-dose danazol treatment group developed polycythemia as an adverse effect, and the administration of the drug was therefore discontinued. There was no significant difference in the values of serum hormones, tumor markers, or lipid metabolism between both groups.

42.3.2 Aromatase Inhibitors

A non-blind RCT compared the efficacy of GnRH-a and aromatase inhibitors in treating adenomyosis [41]. Thirty-two patients were allocated to receive oral LTZ (2.5 mg/day) or subcutaneous goserelin (3.6 mg) for 12 weeks. There were no significant differences between the post-treatment adenomyoma volume of the two groups. Goserelin was more efficacious than LTZ in improving chronic pelvic pain, dysmenorrhea, menorrhagia, metrorrhagia, and dyspareunia, although the difference did not reach statistical significance. Hot flashes were significantly more frequent in patients treated with GnRH-a than in those treated with LTZ.

A case report described the use of an aromatase inhibitor combined with a GnRH-a in a 34-year-old woman wishing to preserve fertility [42]. The patient suffered severe menorrhagia and hypermenorrhea. The patient failed previous treatments with buserelin acetate, goserelin acetate, E2 and medroxyprogesterone acetate, and oral danazol. The patient was thus treated with oral anastrozole (1 mg/day) and goserelin acetate. The combined therapy caused a rapid decrease in the uterine volume; a small amount of bleeding continued for 30 days and ultimately stopped. Forty-five days after the initiation of this treatment, the uterine size was reduced by 60%, with no further reduction after that. The dosage of anastrozole was increased to 2 mg/day at 65 days after treatment initiation. After 120 days of combined treatment, the patient continued the therapy with goserelin alone. After 6 months, there was no increase in the uterine size.

A prospective study published only in the abstract form investigated the changes in the sonographically detectable alterations of the myometrium caused by adenomyosis after treatment with aromatase inhibitor [43]. Overall, 34 patients received oral LTZ (2.5 mg/day) for 6 months; 4 patients (11.8%) discontinued the therapy because of adverse effects. After 3-month treatment, there was a significant decrease in uterine volume; a further decrease was observed after 6 months of treatment. The treatment caused a significant decrease in the size of the anechoic area, the thickness of the uterine wall, the larger diameter of localized adenomyomas, and the total adenomyoma volume. Also, the treatment improved pain symptoms.

42.4 Conclusion

Several RTCs performed between 1980 and 1990 documented the efficacy of danazol in treating endometriosis-related pain (Table 42.1). However, as it is now well accepted that patients with endometriosis require long-term treatment, the high incidence of androgenic adverse effects (Table 42.2) has significantly decreased the use of this drug [8, 9, 44]. Several studies documented the efficacy of AIs in treating different forms of endometriosis, including ovarian endometrioma and deep-infiltrating endometriosis (Table 42.3). However, AIs cause significant adverse effects and, therefore, they are not suitable for the long-term treatment of endometriosis [45, 46]. The use of AIs can be considered in patients with severe pain that is not responsive to other hormonal therapies and in which surgery may be associated with potentially relevant complications.

Limited data are available on the use of danazol for the treatment of adenomyosis. Some studies showed that a danazol-load intrauterine device might improve symptoms of patients with adenomyosis [33, 35, 47]. However, this device has never been introduced in the market. Vaginally administered danazol may decrease the menstrual blood loss in premenopausal women with adenomyosis [38, 39]. An RCT demonstrated that AIs might improve the symptoms caused by adenomyosis [41]; however, these results were not confirmed by other studies. Therefore, AIs should not be routinely used for the treatment of adenomyosis.

Table 42.3 Studies investigating the use of aromatase inhibitors to treat endometriosis

Authors	Study design	n	Treatment	Length of treatment (months)	Findings
Ailawadi, 2004 [52]	Phase 2, open-label, nonrandomized proof-of-concept study	10	LTZ (2.5 mg/day) and NETA (2.5 mg/day)	6	Improved ASRM score and symptoms Stable BMD
Soysal, 2004 [27]	RCT	40 vs. 40	ANZ (1 mg/day) + goserelin (3.6 mg/4 weeks) Placebo + goserelin (3.6 mg/4 weeks)	6	Higher time to recurrence after surgery in the ANZ group (> 24 months vs. 17 months) After 24 months: recurrence in 3/40 in the combined treatment vs. 14/40 in patients treated with goserelin alone Higher BMD loss in patients treated with the combined therapy
Amsterdam, 2005 [53]	Prospective open-label phase 2 trial	18	ANZ (1 mg/day) + ethinyl estradiol (20 mcg/day) and levonorgestrel (0.1 mg/day)	6	Improved pain symptoms Stable BMD
Hefler, 2005 [54]	Nonrandomized pilot study	10	LTZ (0.25 mg) in 2 g vaginal suppository	6	Improved dysmenorrhea and QoL Stable dyspareunia and CPP Stable BMD
Remorgida, 2006 [55]	Open-label prospective study	12	LTZ (2.5 mg/day) + NETA (2.5 mg/day)	6	Improved pain symptoms and QoL Stable BMD
Remorgida, 2007 [56]	Open-label prospective study	12	LTZ (2.5 mg/day) + desogestrel 75mcg/day	6	Interrupted for functional ovarian cysts

Table 42.3 (continued)

Authors	Study design	n	Treatment	Length of treatment (months)	Findings
Ferrero, 2009 [21]	Prospective, open-label, nonrandomized trial	41 vs. 41	LTZ (2.5 mg/day) + NETA (2.5 mg/day) NETA 2.5 mg/day	6	Comparable pain symptoms and QoL improvement—lower dyspareunia and CPP after 3- and 6-month treatment with LTZ Stable and comparable BMD
Loss, 2009 [57]	Prospective pilot study	20	ANZ (1 mg/day) + goserelin (3.6 mg/4 week)	3	15/20 reduction of endometrioma volume Ca-125 reduced by 61%
Ferrero, 2010 [22]	Prospective study	6	LTZ (2.5 mg/day) + NETA (2.5 mg/day)	6	Improved pain and gastrointestinal symptoms Stable BMD
Roghaei, 2010 [58]	RCT	38 vs. 37 vs. 31	LTZ (2.5 mg/day) Danazol (600 mg/day) No hormonal therapy	6	Comparable pain symptoms improvement in LTZ and danazol groups after surgery; return to baseline for the placebo group
Alborzi, 2011 [28]	RCT	47 vs. 40 vs. 57	LTZ (2.5 mg/day) Triptorelin (3.75 mg/4 weeks) Control	2	Comparable pain symptoms recurrence and reproductive outcomes Ovarian functional cysts in 24.3% LTZ and 2.5% triptorelin groups

(continued)

Table 42.3 (continued)

Authors	Study design	n	Treatment	Length of treatment (months)	Findings
Ferrero, 2011 [19]	RCT	17 vs. 18	LTZ (2.5 mg/day) + NETA (2.5 mg/day) LTZ (2.5 mg/day) + triptorelin 11.25 mg/3 months	6	Comparable pain symptoms improvement Higher reduction of rectovaginal nodule in triptorelin group Higher adverse effects in the triptorelin group Reduced BMD in the triptorelin group and stable in NETA groups
Ferrero, 2013 [59]	Prospective, nonrandomized, self-controlled study	8	LTZ (2.5 mg/day) + NETA (2.5 mg/day)	12	Significant and comparable reduction in the volume of rectovaginal nodules after 6 and 12 months for all the treatment options
Ferrero, 2014 [26]	Patient-preference study	20 vs 20	LTZ (2.5 mg/day) + NETA (2.5 mg/day) NETA (2.5 mg/day)	6	Comparable pain symptoms improvement Higher reduction in endometrioma volume in LTZ group Return to baseline in both groups after 6 months of follow-up Stable and comparable BMD
Agarwal, 2015 [25]	Prospective cohort study	8	LTZ (5 mg/day) + NETA (5 mg/day)	3	Pain symptoms improvement Reduction in endometrioma volume

ANZ anastrozole, *ASRM* American Society for Reproductive Medicine, *BMD* bone mineral density, *CPP* chronic pelvic pain, *LTZ* letrozole, *QoL* quality of life, *RCT* randomized controlled trial

References

1. Kitawaki J, Noguchi T, Amatsu T, Maeda K, Tsukamoto K, Yamamoto T, et al. Expression of aromatase cytochrome P450 protein and messenger ribonucleic acid in human endometriotic and adenomyotic tissues but not in normal endometrium. Biol Reprod. 1997;57(3):514–9.
2. Chamness GC, Asch RH, Pauerstein CJ. Danazol binding and translocation of steroid receptors. Am J Obstet Gynecol. 1980;136(4):426–9.
3. Surrey ES, Halme J. Direct effects of medroxyprogesterone acetate, danazol, and leuprolide acetate on endometrial stromal cell proliferation in vitro. Fertil Steril. 1992;58(2):273–8.
4. Braun DP, Gebel H, Dmowski WP. Effect of danazol in vitro and in vivo on monocyte-mediated enhancement of endometrial cell proliferation in women with endometriosis. Fertil Steril. 1994;62(1):89–95.
5. Murakami K, Nomura K, Shinohara K, Kasai T, Shozu M, Inoue M. Danazol inhibits aromatase activity of endometriosis-derived stromal cells by a competitive mechanism. Fertil Steril. 2006;86(2):291–7.
6. Ishihara H, Kitawaki J, Kado N, Koshiba H, Fushiki S, Honjo H. Gonadotropin-releasing hormone agonist and danazol normalize aromatase cytochrome P450 expression in eutopic endometrium from women with endometriosis, adenomyosis, or leiomyomas. Fertil Steril. 2003;79(Suppl 1):735–42.
7. Zeitoun KM, Bulun SE. Aromatase: a key molecule in the pathophysiology of endometriosis and a therapeutic target. Fertil Steril. 1999;72(6):961–9.
8. Ferrero S, Evangelisti G, Barra F. Current and emerging treatment options for endometriosis. Expert Opin Pharmacother. 2018;19(10):1109–25.
9. Ferrero S, Barra F, Leone Roberti Maggiore U. Current and emerging therapeutics for the management of endometriosis. Drugs. 2018;78(10):995–1012.
10. Telimaa S, Puolakka J, Ronnberg L, Kauppila A. Placebo-controlled comparison of danazol and high-dose medroxyprogesterone acetate in the treatment of endometriosis. Gynecol Endocrinol. 1987;1(1):13–23.
11. Wheeler JM, Knittle JD, Miller JD. Depot leuprolide versus danazol in treatment of women with symptomatic endometriosis. I. Efficacy results. Am J Obstet Gynecol. 1992;167(5):1367–71.
12. Fedele L, Arcaini L, Bianchi S, Baglioni A, Vercellini P. Comparison of cyproterone acetate and danazol in the treatment of pelvic pain associated with endometriosis. Obstet Gynecol. 1989;73(6):1000–4.
13. Fedele L, Bianchi S, Viezzoli T, Arcaini L, Candiani GB. Gestrinone versus danazol in the treatment of endometriosis. Fertil Steril. 1989;51(5):781–5.
14. Brown J, Pan A, Hart RJ. Gonadotrophin-releasing hormone analogues for pain associated with endometriosis. Cochrane Database Syst Rev. 2010;(12):CD008475.
15. Agarwal SK, Hamrang C, Henzl MR, Judd HL. Nafarelin vs. leuprolide acetate depot for endometriosis. Changes in bone mineral density and vasomotor symptoms. Nafarelin Study Group. J Reprod Med. 1997;42(7):413–23.
16. Wong AY, Tang L. An open and randomized study comparing the efficacy of standard danazol and modified triptorelin regimens for postoperative disease management of moderate to severe endometriosis. Fertil Steril. 2004;81(6):1522–7.
17. Vercellini P, De Giorgi O, Oldani S, Cortesi I, Panazza S, Crosignani PG. Depot medroxyprogesterone acetate versus an oral contraceptive combined with very-low-dose danazol for long-term treatment of pelvic pain associated with endometriosis. Am J Obstet Gynecol. 1996;175(2):396–401.
18. Ferrero S, Tramalloni D, Venturini PL, Remorgida V. Vaginal danazol for women with rectovaginal endometriosis and pain symptoms persisting after insertion of a levonorgestrel-releasing intrauterine device. Int J Gynaecol Obstet. 2011;113(2):116–9.
19. Ferrero S, Venturini PL, Gillott DJ, Remorgida V. Letrozole and norethisterone acetate versus letrozole and triptorelin in the treatment of endometriosis related pain symptoms: a randomized controlled trial. Reprod Biol Endocrinol. 2011;9:88.
20. Zhao Y, Luan X, Wang Y. Letrozole combined with oral contraceptives versus oral contraceptives alone in the treatment of endometriosis-related pain symptoms: a pilot study. Gynecol Endocrinol. 2021;37(1):51–5.

21. Ferrero S, Camerini G, Seracchioli R, Ragni N, Venturini PL, Remorgida V. Letrozole combined with norethisterone acetate compared with norethisterone acetate alone in the treatment of pain symptoms caused by endometriosis. Hum Reprod. 2009;24(12):3033–41.
22. Ferrero S, Camerini G, Ragni N, Venturini PL, Biscaldi E, Seracchioli R, et al. Letrozole and norethisterone acetate in colorectal endometriosis. Eur J Obstet Gynecol Reprod Biol. 2010;150(2):199–202.
23. Ferrero S, Biscaldi E, Luigi Venturini P, Remorgida V. Aromatase inhibitors in the treatment of bladder endometriosis. Gynecol Endocrinol. 2011;27(5):337–40.
24. Lall Seal S, Kamilya G, Mukherji J, De A, Ghosh D, Majhi AK. Aromatase inhibitors in recurrent ovarian endometriomas: report of five cases with literature review. Fertil Steril. 2011;95(1):291 e15–8.
25. Agarwal SK, Foster WG. Reduction in endometrioma size with three months of aromatase inhibition and progestin add-back. Biomed Res Int. 2015;2015:878517.
26. Ferrero S, Remorgida V, Venturini PL, Leone Roberti Maggiore U. Norethisterone acetate versus norethisterone acetate combined with letrozole for the treatment of ovarian endometriotic cysts: a patient preference study. Eur J Obstet Gynecol Reprod Biol. 2014;174: 117–22.
27. Soysal S, Soysal ME, Ozer S, Gul N, Gezgin T. The effects of post-surgical administration of goserelin plus anastrozole compared to goserelin alone in patients with severe endometriosis: a prospective randomized trial. Hum Reprod. 2004;19(1):160–7.
28. Alborzi S, Hamedi B, Omidvar A, Dehbashi S, Alborzi S, Alborzi M. A comparison of the effect of short-term aromatase inhibitor (letrozole) and GnRH agonist (triptorelin) versus case control on pregnancy rate and symptom and sign recurrence after laparoscopic treatment of endometriosis. Arch Gynecol Obstet. 2011;284(1):105–10.
29. Rotgeri A, Korolainen H, Sundholm O, Schmitz H, Fuhrmann U, Prelle K, et al. Characterization of anastrozole effects, delivered by an intravaginal ring in cynomolgus monkeys. Hum Reprod. 2015;30(2):308–14.
30. Schultze-Mosgau MH, Waellnitz K, Nave R, Klein S, Kraetzschmar J, Rautenberg T, et al. Pharmacokinetics, pharmacodynamics, safety and tolerability of an intravaginal ring releasing anastrozole and levonorgestrel in healthy premenopausal women: a phase 1 randomized controlled trial. Hum Reprod. 2016;31(8):1713–22.
31. Nave R, Mellinger U, Klein S, Hochel J, Schmitz H. Absence of drug-drug interaction of anastrozole on levonorgestrel delivered simultaneously by an intravaginal ring: results of a phase 2 trial. J Clin Pharmacol. 2019;59(7):1022–8.
32. Igarashi M. A new therapy for pelvic endometriosis and uterine adenomyosis: local effect of vaginal and intrauterine danazol application. Asia Oceania J Obstet Gynaecol. 1990;16(1):1–12.
33. Igarashi M, Abe Y, Fukuda M, Ando A, Miyasaka M, Yoshida M, et al. Novel conservative medical therapy for uterine adenomyosis with a danazol-loaded intrauterine device. Fertil Steril. 2000;74(2):412–3.
34. Zhang X, Yuan H, Deng L, Hu F, Ma J, Lin J. Evaluation of the efficacy of a danazol-loaded intrauterine contraceptive device on adenomyosis in an ICR mouse model. Hum Reprod. 2008;23(9):2024–30.
35. Igarashi M. Further studies on danazol-loaded IUD in uterine adenomyosis. Fertil Steril. 2002;77:S25.
36. Takebayashi T, Fujino Y, Umesaki N, Ogita S. Danazol suspension injected into the uterine cervix of patients with adenomyosis and myoma. Preliminary study. Gynecol Obstet Invest. 1995;39(3):207–11.
37. Shawki OA. Danazol loaded intrauterine device (D-IUD): a novel conservative management for uterine adenomyosis. Middle East Fertil Soc J. 2002;7:214–20.
38. Luisi S, Razzi S, Lazzeri L, Bocchi C, Severi FM, Petraglia F. Efficacy of vaginal danazol treatment in women with menorrhagia during fertile age. Fertil Steril. 2009;92(4): 1351–4.
39. Tosti C, Vannuccini S, Troia L, Luisi S, Centini G, Lazzeri L, et al. Long-term vaginal danazol treatment in fertile age women with adenomyosis. J Endometr Pelvic Pain Disord. 2017;9(1):39–43.

40. Sasa H, Imai K, Suzuki A, Kiguna S, Makimura N, Kenichi F. Comparison of low-dose dienogest with low-dose danazol for long-term treatment of adenomyosis. Obstet Gynecol. 2014;123:97S–8S.
41. Badawy AM, Elnashar AM, Mosbah AA. Aromatase inhibitors or gonadotropin-releasing hormone agonists for the management of uterine adenomyosis: a randomized controlled trial. Acta Obstet Gynecol Scand. 2012;91(4):489–95.
42. Kimura F, Takahashi K, Takebayashi K, Fujiwara M, Kita N, Noda Y, et al. Concomitant treatment of severe uterine adenomyosis in a premenopausal woman with an aromatase inhibitor and a gonadotropin-releasing hormone agonist. Fertil Steril. 2007;87(6):1468 e9–12.
43. Ferrero S, Leone Roberti Maggiore U, Scala C, Biscaldi E, Venturini P, Remorgida V. Changes in sonographic findings of adenomyosis after treatment with aromatase inhibitor. Ultrasound Obstet Gynecol. 2014;44(S1):125.
44. Ferrero S, Remorgida V, Venturini PL. Current pharmacotherapy for endometriosis. Expert Opin Pharmacother. 2010;11(7):1123–34.
45. Ferrero S, Venturini PL, Ragni N, Camerini G, Remorgida V. Pharmacological treatment of endometriosis: experience with aromatase inhibitors. Drugs. 2009;69(8):943–52.
46. Garzon S, Lagana AS, Barra F, Casarin J, Cromi A, Raffaelli R, et al. Aromatase inhibitors for the treatment of endometriosis: a systematic review about efficacy, safety and early clinical development. Expert Opin Investig Drugs. 2020;29(12):1377–88.
47. Cobellis L, Razzi S, Fava A, Severi FM, Igarashi M, Petraglia F. A danazol-loaded intrauterine device decreases dysmenorrhea, pelvic pain, and dyspareunia associated with endometriosis. Fertil Steril. 2004;82(1):239–40.
48. Henzl MR, Corson SL, Moghissi K, Buttram VC, Berqvist C, Jacobson J. Administration of nasal nafarelin as compared with oral danazol for endometriosis. A multicenter double-blind comparative clinical trial. N Engl J Med. 1988;318(8):485–9.
49. Dmowski WP, Radwanska E, Binor Z, Tummon I, Pepping P. Ovarian suppression induced with Buserelin or danazol in the management of endometriosis: a randomized, comparative study. Fertil Steril. 1989;51(3):395–400.
50. Adamson GD, Kwei L, Edgren RA. Pain of endometriosis: effects of nafarelin and danazol therapy. Int J Fertil Menopausal Stud. 1994;39(4):215–7.
51. Bromham DR, Booker MW, Rose GL, Wardle PG, Newton JR. Updating the clinical experience in endometriosis--the European perspective. Br J Obstet Gynaecol. 1995;102(Suppl 12):12–6.
52. Ailawadi RK, Jobanputra S, Kataria M, Gurates B, Bulun SE. Treatment of endometriosis and chronic pelvic pain with letrozole and norethindrone acetate: a pilot study. Fertil Steril. 2004;81(2):290–6.
53. Amsterdam LL, Gentry W, Jobanputra S, Wolf M, Rubin SD, Bulun SE. Anastrazole and oral contraceptives: a novel treatment for endometriosis. Fertil Steril. 2005;84(2):300–4.
54. Hefler LA, Grimm C, van Trotsenburg M, Nagele F. Role of the vaginally administered aromatase inhibitor anastrozole in women with rectovaginal endometriosis: a pilot study. Fertil Steril. 2005;84(4):1033–6.
55. Remorgida V, Abbamonte HL, Ragni N, Fulcheri E, Ferrero S. Letrozole and norethisterone acetate in rectovaginal endometriosis. Fertil Steril. 2007;88(3):724–6.
56. Remorgida V, Abbamonte LH, Ragni N, Fulcheri E, Ferrero S. Letrozole and desogestrel-only contraceptive pill for the treatment of stage IV endometriosis. Aust N Z J Obstet Gynaecol. 2007;47(3):222–5.
57. Lossl K, Loft A, Freiesleben NL, Bangsboll S, Andersen CY, Pedersen AT, et al. Combined down-regulation by aromatase inhibitor and GnRH-agonist in IVF patients with endometriomas-a pilot study. Eur J Obstet Gynecol Reprod Biol. 2009;144(1):48–53.
58. Roghaei MA, Tehrany HG, Taherian A, Koleini N. Effects of letrozole compared with danazol on patients with confirmed endometriosis: a randomized clinical trial. Int J Fertil Steril. 2010;4(2):67–72.
59. Ferrero S, Leone Roberti Maggiore U, Scala C, Di Luca M, Venturini PL, Remorgida V. Changes in the size of rectovaginal endometriotic nodules infiltrating the rectum during hormonal therapies. Arch Gynecol Obstet. 2013;287(3):447–53.

GnRH Agonists and Antagonists in Endometriosis and Adenomyosis Therapy

43

H. Paige Anglin, Warren G. Foster, and Sanjay K. Agarwal

Contents

The original version of the chapter has been revised. A correction to this chapter can be found at https://doi.org/10.1007/978-3-030-97236-3_45

H. P. Anglin
Department of Obstetrics, Gynecology & Reproductive Sciences, UC San Diego, La Jolla, CA, USA

W. G. Foster
Department of Obstetrics and Gynecology and the School of Biomedical Engineering, McMaster University, Hamilton, ON, Canada

S. K. Agarwal (✉)
Fertility Services & Center for Endometriosis Research and Treatment, Department of Obstetrics, Gynecology & Reproductive Sciences, UC San Diego, La Jolla, CA, USA
e-mail: skagarwal@health.ucsd.edu

E. Oral (ed.), *Endometriosis and Adenomyosis*,
https://doi.org/10.1007/978-3-030-97236-3_43

43.1 GnRH Physiology

GnRH is a decapeptide released in a pulsatile fashion from the hypothalamus. It acts on the pituitary plasma membrane receptor, which has a characteristic seven transmembrane configuration, leading to the release of follicle stimulating hormone (FSH) and luteinizing hormone (LH) from the anterior pituitary. This further leads to stimulation of the end organ, the ovary, with the production of sex steroids. The pulsatile nature of GnRH release is critical to its function and when administered continuously leads to an initial stimulation of FSH/LH release followed by down regulation of receptors responsible for the release of gonadotropins [1]. The desensitization and down regulation of these gonadotropin receptors ultimately leads to reduction in ovarian sex steroid production.

Knobil's groundbreaking work in which rhesus monkeys with lesions were given pulsatile synthetic GnRH hourly to restore the release of gonadotropins from the pituitary [1] was pivotal in our understanding of the HPO axis. When synthetic GnRH was administered continuously, gonadotropin release was inhibited and it was discovered that the pattern of GnRH delivery had a critical impact on its downstream effects. The finding that pulsatile GnRH release is critical to HPO function, together with the realization that treatment with exogenous continuous GnRH agonist/analogue would lead to blockage of gonadotropin and thus ovarian sex steroid release, was key in our understanding of this complex physiologic phenomenon. Ultimately, this work has led to the clinical use of GnRH agonists to suppress the gonadotropin secretions by the hypothalamus and ovarian estradiol production for multiple clinical applications.

43.2 Clinical Uses

The work of Knobil and others has led to the use of GnRH agonists to suppress the HPO for the purposes of treating a wide variety of conditions including endometriosis, uterine fibroids, dysmenorrhea, adenomyosis, dysfunctional uterine bleeding, and for fertility preservation [1]. In addition, GnRH analogues are also widely used in the world of assisted reproductive technology to chemically shut down the HPO axis in a reversible manner, thereby allowing for the blockage of ovulation. Conversely, one of the early uses of GnRH agonists was in a pulsatile manner to induce ovulation in patients with PCOS or with hypothalamic hypogonadism.

43.3 Impact of GnRH Agonist Amino Acid Substitution on Clinical Effect

The 1977 Nobel Prize in Physiology and Medicine was awarded jointly to Drs. Roger Guillemin and Andrew Schally for the discovery of brain peptide production including the sequencing of GnRH [2, 3]. Since that time, amino acid substitutions have been made to the synthetic decapeptide in order to increase biological stability and enhance potency resulting in chemical hypophysectomy. The half-life of endogenous GnRH and gonadorelin, its synthetic analog, is just 2–4 min [4]. Renal clearance and degradation by peptidases are the key reasons for the short half-life. The fast clearance is key to its ability to act in a pulsatile manner. In order to limit degradation and lead to a longer duration of action together with a higher potency at suppressing the HPO axis, synthetic analogs have to be structurally altered by substituting amino acids. For example, by substituting more hydrophobic amino acids at the 6th and 10th positions of the decapeptide (see Fig. 43.1), the molecule's vulnerability to degradation by peptidases, which cleave at these sites, is markedly decreased. This leads to a longer half-life for the synthetic analogue and a more potent physiologic effect. As an example of their protection from elimination and degradation, the synthetic analogs nafarelin and leuprolide have half-lives of about 3 h [5].

In addition to amino acid sequence, the route and frequency of GnRH agonist administration may also be important determinants of clinical effect. GnRH agonists can be administered in several forms for the treatment of endometriosis. For example, nafarelin acetate is a nasal spray, that is administered twice daily. In addition, a short acting leuprolide acetate formulation can also be injected subcutaneously on a daily basis. Alternative options for long acting forms are depot leuprolide acetate or goserelin acetate, whose properties allow administration in a monthly or quarterly dosing regimen [6]. Efficacy in suppressing ovarian function has enabled GnRH agonists to become important medications in the management of endometriosis and adenomyosis. However, although effective, these medications are sub-optimal owing to their side-effects and thus alternative approaches

Amino Acid Configurations of GnRH Agonists

	Peptide position									
AGENT	1	2	3	4	5	6	7	8	9	10
GnRH	Pyrog	His	Trp	Ser	Tyr	Gly	Leu	Arg	Pro	Gly
Gonadorelin	Pyrog	His	Trp	Ser	Tyr	Gly	Leu	Arg	Pro	Gly
Leuprolide*	Pyrog	His	Trp	Ser	Tyr	**Leu**	Leu	Arg	Pro	**Ethylamide**
Nafarelin*	Pyrog	His	Trp	Ser	Tyr	**Nap**	Leu	Arg	Pro	Gly
Goserelin*	Pyrog	His	Trp	Ser	Tyr	**Ser**	Leu	Arg	Pro	**AzaGly**
Deslorelin	Pyrog	His	Trp	Ser	Tyr	**Trp**	Leu	Arg	Pro	**Ethylamide**
Buserelin	Pyrog	His	Trp	Ser	Tyr	**Ser**	Leu	Arg	Pro	**Ethylamide**
Tryptorelin	Pyrog	His	Trp	Ser	Tyr	**Trp**	Leu	Arg	Pro	Gly

Major sites of cleavage

Fig. 43.1 Amino acid configurations of GnRH agonists. *FDA approved for the treatment of endometriosis. (Adapted from [5])

to achieving ovarian suppression without complete loss of circulating estrogens have been sought.

43.4 Adenomyosis

Adenomyosis is the growth of endometrial glands and stroma within the myometrium. Challenges in studying adenomyosis treatment include inconsistent diagnosis without hysterectomy and the overlap in presence of endometriosis. The first report of the efficacy of GnRH agonist for treatment of adenomyosis, which had been confirmed pathologically, was in 1991. A uterus had a 64% reduction in uterine volume along with clinical improvement of dysmenorrhea and pelvic pain. However, on discontinuation of GnRH agonist, the symptoms quickly returned [7]. The data on adenomyosis treatment with GnRH agonists and antagonists is limited to mostly case reports. However, preliminary empiric treatment with these agents for suspected adenomyosis related pain results in relief of pelvic pain and dysmenorrhea [8].

43.5 Endometriosis

Endometriosis, which is the presence of endometrial glandular tissue and stroma outside the uterine cavity, occurs in approximately 6–10% of reproductively aged women. Many women with endometriosis experience severe dysmenorrhea, dyspareunia, and non-menstrual pelvic pain; others remain asymptomatic [6]. The traditional diagnosis of endometriosis is made when endometriotic implants are visualized in the surgical field and confirmed by pathologic evaluation of tissue biopsy [6].

As may be expected with other chronic pain syndromes, the physical and emotional burden perpetrated by endometriosis can lead to a significant reduction in the quality of life and reductions in household and workplace productivity [9]. The endometrial-like tissue can be present anywhere in the pelvis or abdomen and responds to estrogen in the same manner as the endometrium. Circulating estradiol levels stimulate endometriosis growth and can cause the significant pain associated with this disease. Although comprehensive multidisciplinary programs have been proposed and established [10], the primary treatment options for endometriosis are surgical excision and/or ablation of the ectopic endometrium, hormonal manipulation, or a combination. Many patients only experience relief from a lifetime of pain when they enter menopause at which point circulating estradiol levels are low, and usually lead to regression of the endometriosis. By decreasing circulating estradiol levels pharmacologically, the goal is to maintain a level of estradiol high enough to prevent unnecessary bone loss, but lower than premenopausal physiologic levels resulting in atrophy of endometriotic implants. This goal has proven challenging with single medications.

43.6 GnRH Agonists for the Treatment of Endometriosis

Given that endometriosis is an estrogen dependent disorder, GnRH agonist induced suppression of estradiol has been a cornerstone in the medical management of endometriosis. Several early studies demonstrated agonists to be as effective as previously FDA approved danazol in the treatment of endometriosis but without the androgenic side effects [11–13]. However, hypoestrogenemia induced impact on bone limited FDA approval to 6 months. Three FDA approved GnRH Agonists are currently used for the treatment of endometriosis: leuprolide acetate (Lupron), goserelin acetate (Zoladex), and nafarelin acetate (Synarel). Lupron and Zoladex are depot injections. Lupron has a one month 3.75 mg form as well as with dosing of 11.25 mg subcutaneous every 3 months. Zoladex, also a depot preparation, is administered 3.6 mg subcutaneously every 28 days. Intranasal nafarelin dosing is either 400 or 800 ug daily.

An important weakness with the above treatments is recurrence of endometriosis symptoms following discontinuation of medical therapy. The recurrence rate following cessation of GnRH therapy within 5 years is between 53 and 74%. The recurrence rate is higher in patients with advanced disease (73%) when compared with minimal disease (37%); however, the overall median recurrence rate was 53% over 5 years [14]. Hence the search for improved agonists for the management of endometriosis continues. Currently, orally administered GnRH agonists are being evaluated for the treatment of endometriosis including relugolix and linzagolix. As yet, neither is FDA approved for this indication.

43.7 Impact on GnRH Agonists on Bone

The major adverse effects associated with GnRH agonists and antagonists are related to the hypoestrogenemia that occurs as a result of their mechanisms of action. These commonly include vaginal dryness, vasomotor symptoms, decreased libido, mood changes, irregular bleeding/amenorrhea, and a reversible reduction in bone mineral density. Prolonged use results in the increased loss of bone mineral density, which led to restrictions on the approved duration of therapy with these drugs. Six months of agonist use can lead to around 6–12% BMD loss [15]. Although the pain relief experienced by patients using these drugs is significant, this side effect profile is a deterrent to their use.

43.8 Add-Back Therapy as a Strategy to Protect Bone and Extend GnRH Agonist Use

Use of add-back is the recommended strategy to maintain efficacy of the GnRH agonist, while at the same time reducing unwanted hypoestrogenic side effects. Add-back relies on the realization that agonists may suppress the HPO axis beyond that necessary for an endometriosis therapeutic effect. Therefore, sex-steroids are prescribed in conjunction with the agonist (add-back) to reduce unwanted hypoestrogenic effects without compromising efficacy.

Much of the initial work on add-back was conducted at UCLA by Drs. Judd and Surrey who evaluated norethindrone as add-back [16, 17]. They demonstrated that hypoestrogenic side effects could be reduced with add-back without compromising efficacy [17]. Since those foundational studies, many hormonal and non-hormonal such as etidronate add-backs have been evaluated. For example, high dose medroxyprogesterone acetate (MPA) supplementation at 100 mg/day diminishes the hypoestrogenic side effects of goserelin acetate 3.6 mg daily without changing its efficacy in endometriosis [18]. As an alternative, 0.3 mg/day or 0.635 mg/day conjugated estradiol + MPA (Provera) 5 mg/d, administered in conjunction with 3.6 mg monthly goserelin was as effective as goserelin alone in improving pelvic symptoms of endometriosis but reduced both the vasomotor symptoms/vaginal dryness and loss of bone mineral density (BMD) associated with goserelin therapy alone administered over 6 months [19]. Similarly, use of either goserelin alone or together with 17-beta estradiol (2 mg/d) plus 1 mg/d norethisterone acetate were equally effective in treatment of endometriosis of 88 women randomly assigned to one of the two treatment groups; however, the menopausal symptoms were significantly reduced in the patients whose treatment included hormone replacement therapy (HRT) compared to goserelin alone plus placebo [20].

In 1998, one of the largest studies of its kind showed that add-back hormone therapy resulted in relief of endometriosis symptoms in addition to protection of bone mineral density at 1 year of treatment with Leuprolide acetate depot. Bone density was maintained in all three treatment arms, which included either: norethindrone acetate 5 mg daily alone, norethindrone acetate 5 mg and conjugated equine estrogens 0.625 mg daily, or norethindrone acetate 5 mg and conjugated equine estrogens 1.25 mg daily. Add-back therapy with 5 mg norethindrone acetate alone maintained the efficacy of the leuprolide while providing bone protection leading to FDA approval for this use [21]. Norethindrone acetate 5 mg remains the only FDA approved add back therapy at this time. However, some patients do not tolerate the side effects of this high dose progestin only add-back and would prefer the hypoestrogenic side effects over the side effects of norethindrone acetate. An additional alternative to progestin alone add-back involved the use of testosterone, which is also bone protecting [22]. Further, tibolone is a synthetic steroid with weak progesterone, estrogen, and androgen activity, used in the treatment of menopausal symptoms has been explored as an alternative for add-back therapy and to mitigate unwanted side-effects. A prospective, randomized placebo controlled double-blind study of 29 women with moderate to severe endometriosis observed that vasomotor symptoms associated with GnRH agonist treatment were significantly reduced with the addition of Tibolone 2.5 mg/day. Although BMD was not one of the study outcomes, a decrease in the urinary calcium to creatinine ratio, which is a clinical indicator of the metabolic effects hypoestrogenism has on bone, was observed in the treatment group when compared to the placebo group which received only Goserelin and iron supplementation [23]. Agarwal et al. showed that 6 months treatment with daily intranasal GnRH agonist deslorelin along with low estradiol +/− testosterone add-back resulted in reduction in endometriosis symptoms without significant hypoestrogenic side effects. Women were randomized to receive one of three add-back regimens with the deslorelin. They received either 50 mcg/d transdermal estradiol via a patch, 300 mcg/d intranasal estradiol spray or the estradiol spray along with 275 mcg/d testosterone spray. Importantly, even in the two estradiol alone add-back groups, there were no cases of endometrial hyperplasia. In each of these three groups, changes in BMD after 6 months of treatment was negligible when compared to baseline [24]. This pilot study was the first to report the use of unopposed estradiol or estradiol plus testosterone as add-back and demonstrated a good safety profile and supports the concept that complete ablation of ovarian function may not be necessary to achieve beneficial effects on endometriosis symptoms.

43.9 Estrogen Threshold Hypothesis and the Suggestion of an Alternative Strategy

Problems with add-back are that it adds a degree of complexity and expense. An alternative concept to add-back for the reduction of unwanted GnRH induced hypoestrogenic effects on bone was proposed by Barbieri in 1992 [25]. His estrogen threshold hypothesis (ETH) pertains to the concept that a range of estradiol concentrations approximately between 30–50 pg/ml are sufficient for bone calcium metabolism to minimize bone loss while maximizing the therapeutic effects of estrogen suppression on endometriosis. Therefore, there is a key therapeutic estradiol range of 30–50 pg/ml at which bone turnover by osteoclasts is minimized, yet the endometriotic implants are adequately deprived of the stimulatory effects of estradiol, to block the growth of endometriosis (Fig. 43.2) [25].

Support for the ETH is derived from a randomized placebo-controlled study comparing nafarelin 400 mcg daily and leuprolide 3.75 mg monthly in terms of efficacy and adverse effects. Patients were treated with either drug for 6 months, and then followed for an additional 6 months. Both treatment arms of the study showed improvement in dysmenorrhea, pelvic pain, and dyspareunia to equal degrees; however, the side effect profile differed significantly between the two groups. The leuprolide had a significantly larger reduction in bone mineral density ($P = 0.002$), and increased frequency of vasomotor symptoms [26].

The other key differences between the two were circulating estradiol levels. In the nafarelin group, estradiol levels remained higher (around 30 pg/ml) than in the leuprolide arm (around 15 pg/ml), indicating a lesser degree of hypothalamic suppression. Since both therapies were equally effective at improving endometriosis pelvic pain, the differences observed between the two groups could be explained by the ETH [15] and reinforced the concept that complete suppression of the HPO function was not necessary for clinical benefit and maintenance of vasomotor function and bone mineral density.

A second pilot study from Japan compared conventional dose nafarelin to half dose after the first month and found comparable efficacy in both groups but with much less of a negative impact on bone mineral density in the low dose group

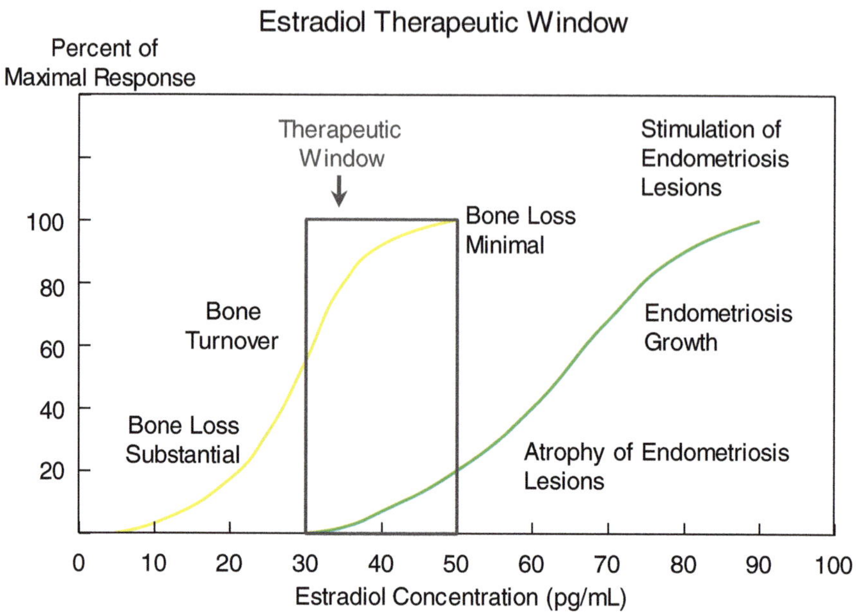

Fig. 43.2 Estrogen threshold therapeutic window. (Adapted from [25])

(5.56% versus 1.38%). This further supported the concept of low dose agonist use or variable suppression of the HPO axis [27].

43.10 Empiric Use of GnRH Agonists

In a study by Ling et al., 100 women were randomized to receive placebo or depot leuprolide 7.5 mg/month over 3 months for suspected endometriosis based on moderate to severe pelvic pain. Women in the intervention group had significantly more improvement in all pelvic pain measures when compared to placebo. Following the study, all subjects had laparoscopy to confirm suspected endometriosis and 78% and 87% of women had surgically confirmed disease in the leuprolide and placebo groups, respectively. These results lead to the conclusion that empiric therapy with leuprolide can be started when endometriosis is suspected, leading to avoidance of the requirement that surgical intervention for diagnosis [28]. As a result, since 1999, ACOG sanctioned the empiric use of GnRH agonists prior to surgical confirmation of disease.

43.11 Post-Operative Use of GnRH Agonists

Another special clinical situation for the use of GnRH agonists is immediately following conservative surgery. Endometriosis recurrence rates vary greatly between studies depending on diagnostic and follow up criteria. However, the overall recurrence rates range between 6 to 67% [29]. Some studies have evaluated the use of biomarkers for surveillance following treatment of endometriosis in an attempt to diagnose and tailor treatment accordingly. Although a high priority research area in women's health that has seen important recent advances with novel clinical markers such as differential expression of microRNA and exosomes in women with endometriosis compared to controls, none have proven adequate or been validated for use in the diagnosis of endometriosis [29–33].

Postoperative treatment of endometriosis is important to prolong the pain-free interval after surgery. This may be particularly important when residual disease that could not be surgically addressed has clearly been left in the pelvis (ACOG Practice Bulletin: Endometriosis 2010). A large RCT with 109 women, who had undergone laparoscopy to confirm and treat endometriosis, received either Nafarelin 200 mg twice daily or placebo for 6 months following surgery. They were followed long term to determine if the length of time required to initiate alternative medical treatment was different between the two groups. The patients in the Nafarelin group had a >2 year period requiring no alternative therapy versus not even 1 year (11.7 months) in the placebo group. In addition, the treatment group had significantly improved pelvic pain scores following the 6 months of treatment. This study led to the conclusion that medical management with GnRH agonists significantly prolongs the recurrence of symptoms following surgical management [34]. In a further study to assess the value of postoperative agonist therapy [35], conservative (uteriovarian sparing) surgery was performed on 269 women with mild to moderate disease and then randomized postoperatively to receive either goserelin depot injections or placebo for 6 months. Patients were followed for 2 years with monitoring of dysmenorrhea, deep dyspareunia, non-menstrual pelvic pain, and general discomfort. Both symptom severity and time to recurrence were significantly less in the treatment arm when compared to placebo at both the one and two year follow ups (Fig. 43.3). This study further supports the use of postoperative treatment with goserelin following conservative surgery for endometriosis to prolong the symptom free period following surgery.

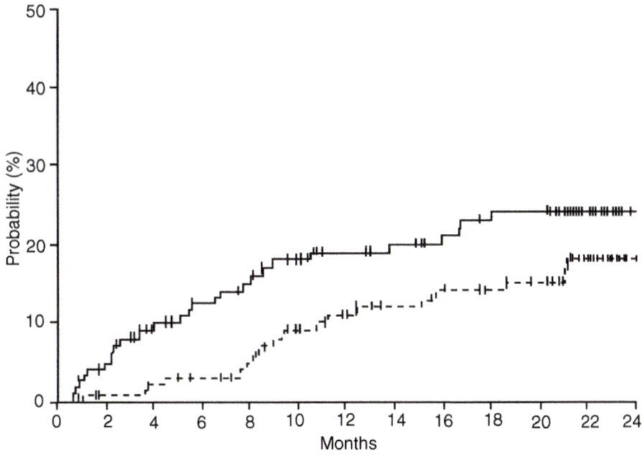

Fig. 43.3 24 months probability of recurrence following conservative surgery with expectant management (solid line) versus Goserelin therapy x 6 months (dotted line) [35]

Recurrence rate following surgical treatment of endometriosis is upwards of 40% [36]. The recurrence rate of endometriosis following excisional surgery is high (up to 53% at 5 years), especially in young patients who have uterine and ovarian sparing procedures when compared with hysterectomy or hysterectomy with ovaries removed [37].

Hysterectomy with bilateral salpingo-oophorectomy reduces risk of recurrence sixfold when compared with hysterectomy alone; further supporting the theory that the growth of endometrial implants is driven by the presence of estrogen. However, in young premenopausal women, conservation of at least one ovary is recommended [36]. The complex nature of these excisional procedures may lead to incomplete removal of endometrial implants for treatment of pelvic pain, due to either extensiveness of the disease complicating the excision process or the microscopic nature, resulting in missed lesions even with high resolution laparoscopic surgeries. Much work with ultrasound and other technologies is being conducted to better define extent of disease and lesion margins both pre- and intra-operatively [38–40] with a view to either avoiding diagnostic surgery or more complete surgical excision of disease during surgery. These strategies have yet to be used on a widespread basis and hence, for the time being, surgical limitations further contribute to medical management being used first line to treat this disease.

43.12 GnRH Antagonists for the Treatment of Endometriosis

Pituitary gonadotropins and sex steroid production from the ovary are blocked by continuous stimulation of the GnRH receptor by an agonist or blockage by an antagonist. Agonist therapy had been utilized for a number of years, prior to the availability of a competitive antagonist. By binding competitively to the GnRH receptor, they also block the GnRH receptor expression, leading to a fast, dose dependent suppression of gonadotropin release [41]. Although the initial flare with GnRH agonists may be utilized in the setting of an "agonist trigger" in modern ART protocols, this can be detrimental in the treatment of endometriosis, where an early rise in gonadotropins and estradiol prior to desensitization of GnRH receptors can lead to an exacerbation of pelvic pain. In a large randomized controlled trial of 120 women treated with a GnRH agonist, patients were found to have a statistically significant increase in pelvic pain accompanied by a decrease in quality of life temporarily when compared to placebo alone [42]. A major benefit of antagonist therapy is rapid suppression of the HPO without the initial "flare" that is observed with GnRH agonists.

Elagolix is the first GnRH antagonist approved for the treatment of endometriosis. It is a small, non-peptide molecule that is a potent antagonist of the GnRH receptor. Because of its non-peptide structure, it can be taken orally. This is in contrast to GnRH agonists which are peptides and are subject to GI degradation [43]. Elagolix is FDA approved for the treatment of endometriosis, with limitations for its length of treatment due to bone loss resulting from the therapeutic hypoestrogenemia. The half-life of elagolix is a mere 4–6 h, requiring daily dosing. An RCT of

45 premenopausal women showed that FSH, LH, and estradiol concentrations dropped in a dose dependent manner within 1 day of taking the oral elagolix with 200 mg twice daily causing maximal estradiol suppression. At concentrations of 100 mg twice daily, cessation of ovulation occurred with undetectable progesterone levels throughout the 21 day course of treatment [44]. Elaris Endometriosis I and II were two Phase 3, double blind RCTs which compared low (150 mg daily) and high (200 mg twice daily) dose elagolix in 872 women with surgically diagnosed endometriosis accompanied by moderate to severe pelvic pain. When compared to the placebo groups, both doses had significantly improved symptoms of dysmenorrhea and non-menstrual pelvic pain (Fig. 43.4). Patients in the higher dose group had significantly better results, including reduced analgesic use and reduction of dyspareunia [45]. Both doses in the phase 3 clinical trials led to adverse effects, notably a reversible reduction in bone mineral density (Fig. 43.5) and elevated serum lipids at the end of the 6 month treatment period [45] which were not observed in the 3 month Phase 2 trial.

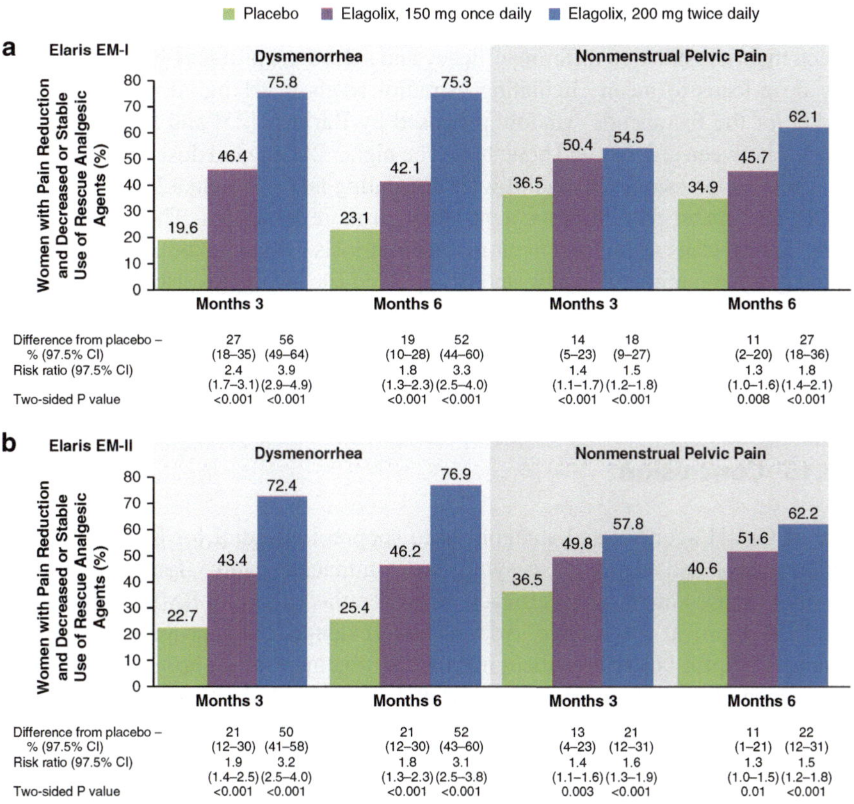

Fig. 43.4 Reduction in dysmenorrhea and non-menstrual pelvic pain with Elagolix in two large Phase 3 studies. Two 6-month phase 3 trials were completed (**a**). Elaris Endometriosis I (EM-1) and (**b**). Elaris Endometriosis II (EM-II) (From Taylor et al. NEJM 2017)

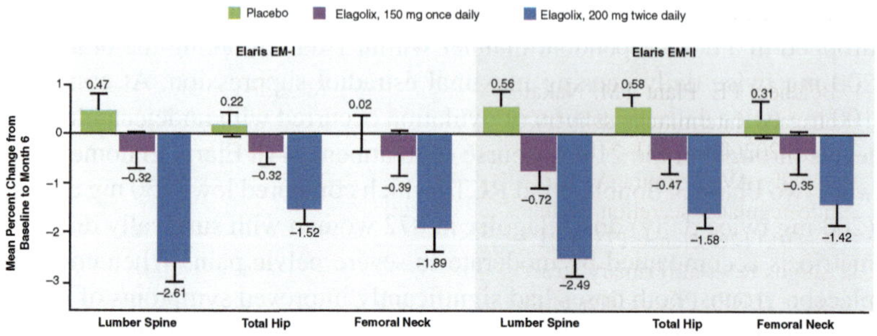

	Lumber Spine (EM-I)			Total Hip (EM-I)			Femoral Neck (EM-I)			Lumber Spine (EM-II)			Total Hip (EM-II)			Femoral Neck (EM-II)		
		**	***		**	***		NS	***		***	***		***	***		*	***
Difference from placebo (%)		−0.79	−3.08		−0.54	−1.74		−0.41	−1.91		−1.28	−3.04		−1.05	−2.16		−0.66	−1.73
95% CI, lower boundary		−1.29	−3.58		−0.93	−2.13		−1.02	−2.53		−1.75	−3.51		−1.46	−2.57		−1.23	−2.28
95% CI, upper boundary		−0.30	−2.59		−0.15	−1.35		0.20	−1.29		−0.80	−2.58		−0.64	−1.76		−0.10	−1.17
No. of women	282	186	182	280	185	182	280	185	182	271	174	183	271	172	182	271	172	182

Fig. 43.5 Mean percent change from baseline to month 6 in bone mineral density with Elagolix. (From Taylor et al. NEJM 2017)

In the 12 month extended phase 3 studies, the two now FDA approved dosages of elagolix resulted in dose-dependent magnitudes of serum estradiol suppression, which in turn resulted in differing efficacy and side effect profiles [46]. The 150 mg/day dose leads to mean circulating estradiol levels of 41 pg/ml which is in the middle of the therapeutic window proposed by Barbieri [25] and leads to a good balance between efficacy and bone loss. The higher 200 mg bid dose leads to a more profound suppression of estradiol with circulating levels around 12 pg/ml and as a result has greater pain improvement but with more bone loss. The 150 mg once daily dosing leads to improvement in endometriosis symptoms without substantial impact on bone mineral density and is approved for 24 months. However, because of the more profound suppression of estradiol with the higher 200 mg bid dosing, a greater negative impact on BMD occurred with approval being limited to 6 months of use.

43.13 Conclusion

Use of GnRH agonists and antagonists to suppress estradiol for the treatment of endometriosis and adenomyosis symptoms continues to evolve. Early studies with agonists focused on ensuring efficacy. However, the impact on BMD lead to a limited FDA approval of 6 months. Add-back has extended the approval to 12 months, which is helpful but still challenging for the treatment of a chronic disease. The acceptance of variable ovarian suppression together with the availability of an oral GnRH antagonist have been notable advances. However, even with low dose elagolix and because of bone concerns, approval is limited to 24 months use. Future work will hopefully help better define mechanisms of bone loss and endometriosis pain suppression and will need to address the disjoin between duration of approval and chronic nature of the disease. The use of low dose addback in conjunction with variable and incomplete ovarian suppression may well lead to therapeutic options that are both efficacious and safe for long-term use.

References

1. Belchetz PE, Plant TM, Nakai Y, Keogh EJ, Knobil E. Hypophysial responses to continuous and intermittent delivery of hypothalamic gonadotropin-releasing hormone. Science. 1978;202(4368):631–3. https://doi.org/10.1126/science.100883.
2. Schally AV, Arimura A, Kastin AJ, et al. Gonadotropinreleasing hormone: one polypeptide regulates secretion of luteinizing and follicle-stimulating hormones. 1971. https://doi.org/10.1126/science.173.4001.1036.
3. Burgus R, et al. Primary structure of the ovine hypothalamic luteinizing hormone-releasing factor (LRF). Proceedings of the National Academy of Sciences. 1972;69(1):278–82.
4. Kumar P, Sharma A. Gonadotropin-releasing hormone analogs: understanding advantages and limitations. J Human Reproduct Sci. 2014;7(3):170–174. Medknow Publications. https://doi.org/10.4103/0974-1208.142476
5. Agarwal SK. Differential effects of GnRH agonist therapies: implications regarding the Estrogen Threshold Hypothesis. In: Lemay A, Maheux R, editors. Understanding and managing endometriosis: advances in research and practice (proceedings of the VIth world congress on endometriosis). Parthenon Publishing; 1999. p. 199–204.
6. Practice Committee of the American Society for Reproductive Medicine, T. Treatment of pelvic pain associated with endometriosis: a committee opinion. Fertil Steril. 2014;101(4):927–35. https://doi.org/10.1016/j.fertnstert.2014.02.012.
7. Nelson JR, Corson SL. Long-term management of adenomyosis with a gonadotropin-releasing hormone agonist: a case report. Fertil Steril. 1993;59(2):441–3. https://doi.org/10.1016/s0015-0282(16)55704-5.
8. Pontis A, et al. Adenomyosis: a systematic review of medical treatment. Gynecological endocrinology: the official journal of the International Society of Gynecological Endocrinology. 2016;32(9):696–700. https://doi.org/10.1080/09513590.2016.1197200.
9. Surrey ES, Soliman AM, Palac HL, Agarwal SK. Impact of Elagolix on workplace and household productivity among women with moderate to severe pain associated with endometriosis: a pooled analysis of two phase III trials. Patient. 2019;12(6):651–60. https://doi.org/10.1007/s40271-019-00394-7.
10. Agarwal SK et al. Clinical diagnosis of endometriosis: a call to action. Am J Obstet Gynecol. 2019;220(4):354.e1–354.e12. https://doi.org/10.1016/j.ajog.2018.12.039.
11. Becker CM, Gattrell WT, Gude K, Singh SS. Reevaluating response and failure of medical treatment of endometriosis: a systematic review. Fertil Steril. 2017;108(1):125–36. https://doi.org/10.1016/j.fertnstert.2017.05.004.
12. Ishihara H, Kitawaki J, Kado N, Koshiba H, Fushiki S, Honjo H. Gonadotropin-releasing hormone agonist and danazol normalize aromatase cytochrome P450 expression in eutopic endometrium from women with endometriosis, adenomyosis, or leiomyomas. Fertil Steril. 2003;79(Suppl 1):735–42. https://doi.org/10.1016/s0015-0282(02)04813-6. PMID: 12620485
13. Strowitzki T, Marr J, Gerlinger C, Faustmann T, Seitz C. Detailed analysis of a randomized, multicenter, comparative trial of dienogest versus leuprolide acetate in endometriosis. Int J Gynecol Obstet. 2012;117(3):228–33. https://doi.org/10.1016/j.ijgo.2012.01.009.
14. Waller KG, Shaw RW. Gonadotropin-releasing hormone analogues for the treatment of endometriosis: long-term follow-up. Fertil Steril. 1993;59(3):511–5. https://doi.org/10.1016/S0015-0282(16)55791-4.
15. Agarwal SK. Comparative effects of GnRH agonist therapy. Review of clinical studies and their implications. J Reprod Med. 1998;43(3 Suppl):293–8.
16. Surrey ES, Gambone JC, Lu JK, Judd HL. The effects of combining norethindrone with a gonadotropin-releasing hormone agonist in the treatment of symptomatic endometriosis. Fertil Steril. 1990;53(4):620–6. PMID: 2108056
17. Surrey ES, Judd HL. Reduction of vasomotor symptoms and bone mineral density loss with combined norethindrone and long-acting gonadotropin-releasing hormone agonist therapy of symptomatic endometriosis: a prospective randomized trial. J Clin Endocrinol Metab. 1992;75(2):558–63. https://doi.org/10.1210/jcem.75.2.1386374. PMID: 1386374

18. Makarainen L, Ronnberg L, Kauppila A. Medroxyprogesterone acetate supplementation diminishes the hypoestrogenic side effects of gonadotropin-releasing hormone agonist without changing its efficacy in endometriosis. Fertil Steril. 1996;65(1):29–34. https://doi.org/10.1016/S0015-0282(16)58023-6.
19. Moghissi KS, Schlaff WD, Olive DL, Skinner MA, Yin H. Goserelin acetate (Zoladex) with or without hormone replacement therapy for the treatment of endometriosis. Fertil Steril. 1998;69(6):1056–62. https://doi.org/10.1016/S0015-0282(98)00086-7.
20. Kiilholma P, Tuimala R, Kivinen S, Korhonen M, Hagman E. Comparison of the gonadotropin-releasing hormone agonist goserelin acetate alone versus goserelin combined with estrogen-progestogen add-back therapy in the treatment of endometriosis. Fertil Steril. 1995;64(5):903–8. https://doi.org/10.1016/S0015-0282(16)57900-X.
21. Hornstein MD, Surrey ES, Weisberg GW, Casino LA. Leuprolide acetate depot and hormonal add-back in endometriosis: a 12- month study. Obstet Gynecol. 1998;91(1):16–24. https://doi.org/10.1016/S0029-7844(97)00620-0.
22. Behre HM, Kliesch S, Leifke E, Link TM, Nieschlag E. Long-term effect of testosterone therapy on bone mineral density in Hypogonadal men. J Clin Endocrinol Metabol. 1997;82(8):2386–90. https://doi.org/10.1210/jcem.82.8.4163.
23. Taskin O, Yalcinoglu AI, Kucuk S, Uryan I, Buhur A, Burak F. Effectiveness of tibolone on hypoestrogenic symptoms induced by goserelin treatment in patients with endometriosis. Fertil Steril. 1997;67(1):40–5. https://doi.org/10.1016/S0015-0282(97)81853-5.
24. Agarwal SK, Daniels A, Drosman SR, Udoff L, Foster WG, Pike MC, Spicer DV, Daniels JR. Treatment of endometriosis with the GnRHa deslorelin and add-back estradiol and supplementary testosterone. Biomed Res Int. 2015;2015 https://doi.org/10.1155/2015/934164.
25. Barbieri RL. Hormone treatment of endometriosis: the estrogen threshold hypothesis. Am J Obstet Gynecol. 1992;166(2):740–5. https://doi.org/10.1016/0002-9378(92)91706-G.
26. Agarwal SK, Hamrang C, Henzl MR, Judd HL. Nafarelin vs. leuprolide acetate depot for endometriosis. Changes in bone mineral density and vasomotor symptoms. Nafarelin Study Group. J Reprod Med. 1997;42(7):413–23. PMID: 9252932
27. Tahara M, Matsuoka T, Yokoi T, Tasaka K, Kurachi H, Murata Y. Treatment of endometriosis with a decreasing dosage of a gonadotropin-releasing hormone agonist (nafarelin): a pilot study with low-dose agonist therapy ("draw-back" therapy). Fertil Steril. 2000;73(4):799–804. https://doi.org/10.1016/s0015-0282(99)00636-6. PMID: 10731543
28. Ling FW. Randomized controlled trial of depot leuprolide in patients with chronic pelvic pain and clinically suspected endometriosis. Obstet Gynecol. 1999;93(1):51–8. https://doi.org/10.1016/S0029-7844(98)00341-X.
29. Selçuk I, Bozdağ G. Recurrence of endometriosis; risk factors, mechanisms and biomarkers; review of the literature. J Turkish German Gynecol Assoc. 2013;14(2):98–103. AVES. https://doi.org/10.5152/jtgga.2013.52385
30. Papari E, et al. Identification of candidate microRNA markers of endometriosis with the use of next-generation sequencing and quantitative real-time polymerase chain reaction. Fertil Steril. 2020;113(6):1232–41. https://doi.org/10.1016/j.fertnstert.2020.01.026.
31. Vanhie A, et al. Peritoneal fluid exosomes as potential biomarkers for endometriosis: mind and bridge the gap between innovation and validation/development into benefit for patients. Fertil Steril. 2020;113(2):326–7. https://doi.org/10.1016/j.fertnstert.2019.12.031.
32. Nisenblat V, et al. Imaging modalities for the non-invasive diagnosis of endometriosis. The Cochrane database of systematic reviews. 2016;2(2):CD009591. https://doi.org/10.1002/14651858.CD009591.pub2.
33. Cosar E, et al. Serum microRNAs as diagnostic markers of endometriosis: a comprehensive array-based analysis. Fertil Steril vol. 2016;106(2):402–9. https://doi.org/10.1016/j.fertnstert.2016.04.013.
34. Hornstein MD, Hemmings R, Yuzpe AA, Leroy Heinrichs W. Use of nafarelin versus placebo after reductive laparoscopic surgery for endometriosis. Fertil Steriliw. 1997;68:Issue 6.
35. Vercellini P, Crosignani PG, Fadini R, Radici E, Belloni C, Sismondi P. A gonadotrophin-releasing hormone agonist compared with expectant management after conservative surgery

for symptomatic endometriosis. BJOG Int J Obstetr Gynaecol. 1999;106(7):672–7. https://doi.org/10.1111/j.1471-0528.1999.tb08366.x.
36. Vercellini P, Barbara G, Abbiati A, Somigliana E, Viganò P, Fedele L. Repetitive surgery for recurrent symptomatic endometriosis: what to do? Eur J Obstet Gynecol Reprod Biol. n.d.; https://doi.org/10.1016/j.ejogrb.2009.05.007.
37. Falcone T, Shakiba K, Bena JF, McGill KM, Minger J. Surgical treatment of endometriosis: a 7-year follow-up on the requirement for further surgery. Obstet Gynecol. 2008;111(6):1285–92. https://doi.org/10.1097/AOG.0b013e3181758ec6.
38. Bar-Shavit Y, Jaillet L, Chauvet P, Canis M, Bourdel N. Use of indocyanine green in endometriosis surgery. Fertil Steril. 2018;109(6):1136–7. https://doi.org/10.1016/j.fertnstert.2018.02.113.
39. Leonardi M, Martin E, Reid S, Blanchette G, Condous G. Deep endometriosis transvaginal ultrasound in the workup of patients with signs and symptoms of endometriosis: a cost analysis. BJOG. 2019;126(12):1499–506. https://doi.org/10.1111/1471-0528.15917. Epub 2019 Sep 18
40. Leonardi M, Robledo KP, Goldstein SR, Benacerraf BR, Condous G. International survey finds majority of gynecologists are not aware of and do not utilize ultrasound techniques to diagnose and map endometriosis. Ultrasound Obstet Gynecol. 2020;56(3):324–8. https://doi.org/10.1002/uog.21996.
41. Heber D, Dodson R, Swerdloff RS, Channabasavaiah K, Stewart JM. Pituitary receptor site blockade by a gonadotropin-releasing hormone antagonist in vivo: mechanism of action. Science. 1982;216(4544):420–1. https://doi.org/10.1126/science.6280278.
42. Miller JD. Quantification of endometriosis-associated pain and quality of life during the stimulatory phase of gonadotropin-releasing hormone agonist therapy: a double-blind, randomized, placebo-controlled trial. Am J Obstet Gynecol. 2000;182(6):1483–8. https://doi.org/10.1067/mob.2000.106846.
43. Chen C, Wu D, Guo Z, Xie Q, Reinhart GJ, Madan A, Wen J, Chen T, Huang CQ, Chen M, Chen Y, Tucci FC, Rowbottom M, Pontillo J, Zhu YF, Wade W, Saunders J, Bozigian H, Struthers RS. Discovery of sodium R-(+)-4-{2-[5-(2-Fluoro-3-methoxyphenyl)-3-(2-fluoro-6- [trifluoromethyl]-benzyl)-4-methyl-2,6-dioxo-3,6-dihydro-2H-pyrimidin-1-yl] -1-phenylethylamino}butyrate (elagolix), a potent and orally available nonpeptide antagonist of the human gonadotropin-releasing hormone receptor. J Med Chem. 2008;51(23):7478–85. https://doi.org/10.1021/jm8006454.
44. Ng J, Chwalisz K, Carter DC, Klein CE. Dose-dependent suppression of gonadotropins and ovarian hormones by Elagolix in healthy premenopausal women. J Clin Endocrinol Metab. 2017;102:1683–91. https://doi.org/10.1210/jc.2016-3845.
45. Taylor HS, Giudice LC, Lessey BA, Abrao MS, Kotarski J, Archer DF, Diamond MP, Surrey E, Johnson NP, Watts NB, Gallagher JC, Simon JA, Carr BR, Dmowski WP, Leyland N, Rowan JP, Duan WR, Ng J, Schwefel B, et al. Treatment of endometriosis-associated pain with Elagolix, an Oral GnRH antagonist. N Engl J Med. 2017;377(1):28–40. https://doi.org/10.1056/NEJMoa1700089.
46. Surrey E, et al. Longt-term outcomes of elagolix in women with endometriosis: results from two extension studies. Obstet Gynecol. 2018;132(1):147–60. https://doi.org/10.1097/AOG.0000000000002675.

Recent Guidelines on Endometriosis and Adenomyosis

44

Ertan Sarıdoğan and Nura Fitnat Topbas Selcuki

Contents

44.1 Introduction

Guidelines for clinical practice are systematically developed statements to assist care providers and patient decisions about appropriate health care for specific clinical circumstances [1]. Their purpose is to improve patient care by informing clinical practice, to reduce unwarranted variability and to expedite implementation of effective intervention. A number of national and international guidelines have been published on the diagnosis and management of endometriosis in the last two decades

The original version of the chapter has been revised. A correction to this chapter can be found at https://doi.org/10.1007/978-3-030-97236-3_45

E. Sarıdoğan (✉)
Institute for Women's Health, University College London, University College London Hospital, London, UK
e-mail: ertan.saridogan@nhs.net

N. F. Topbas Selcuki
Department of Obstetrics and Gynecology, University of Health Sciences Turkey, Istanbul Sisli Hamidiye Etfal Training and Research Hospital, Istanbul, Turkey

E. Oral (ed.), *Endometriosis and Adenomyosis*,
https://doi.org/10.1007/978-3-030-97236-3_44

([2, 3], ACOG 2010 [4], [5], ACCEPT 2012 [6], ASRM 2012 [7], [8, 9]). Although there are some differences, many aspects in these guidelines are in agreement with each other. This is not surprising as most guidelines use a similar methodology, some more robust than others, and look at the same published evidence. This usually results in agreement in most areas. However, there are many knowledge gaps in certain areas, and this usually requires development of recommendations based on opinion which probably accounts for the variability between different guidelines. A list of the major international guidelines is given in Table 44.1 and national

Table 44.1 List of some of the available international guidelines on endometriosis*

European Society of Human Reproduction and Embryology (ESHRE) guideline, management of women with endometriosis, 2013 [8]
WES (World Endometriosis Society) consensus on current management of endometriosis, 2013 [10]
European Society of Urogenital Radiology (ESUR) guidelines: MR imaging of pelvic endometriosis [11]
Systematic approach to sonographic evaluation of the pelvis in women with suspected endometriosis, including terms, definitions and measurements: a consensus opinion from the International Deep Endometriosis Analysis (IDEA) group [12]
ACCEPT (Australasian Certificate of Reproductive Endocrinology and Infertility Consensus Expert Panel on Trial Evidence 2012 Endometriosis and infertility [6]
ACOG 2010 Practice Bulletin: management of endometriosis [4]

*ESHRE Guidelines have been recently updated and the new full guidelines are available at https://www.eshre.eu/Guidelines-and-Legal/Guidelines/Endometriosis-guideline.aspx

Table 44.2 List of some of the available national guidelines on endometriosis

National Institute for Health and Care Excellence Guideline, Endometriosis: diagnosis and management [13]
Obstetrical and Gynaecological Society of Malaysia, Clinical Guidelines for the Management of Endometriosis, [14]
CNGOF (College National des Gynecologues et Obstetriciens Francais) Guidelines for the Management of Endometriosis, [9]
Turkish Society of Endometriosis and Adenomyosis Guidelines, Diagnosis and Management of Endometriosis, [15]
National German Guideline (S2k), Diagnosis and treatment of endometriosis, [16]
SOGC (Society of Obstetricians and Gynaecologists of Canada), Endometriosis: Diagnosis and Management, [5]
Federation of Obstetrics and Gynaecological Societies of India, Good clinical practice recommendations on endometriosis, [17]
Endometriosis – new clinical guidelines for better and equal care in Sweden [18]
Clinical practice guidelines for the treatment of extragenital endometriosis in Japan, 2018 [19]
Clinical evaluation and management of endometriosis: guideline for Korean patients from the Korean Society of Endometriosis [20]
Guideline for the diagnosis and treatment of endometriosis (Cooperative Group of Endometriosis, Chinese Society of Obstetrics and Gynecology, Chinese Medical Association) [21]
Federacion Mexicana de Colegios de Obstetricia y Ginecologia, Diagnosis and treatment of endometriosis, [22]
The statement of Polish Society's Experts Group concerning diagnostics and methods of endometriosis treatment [23]
Diagnosis and Management of Endometriosis in New Zealand, [24]
South African guideline for treatment of endometriosis [25]

guidelines in Table 44.2. Some guidelines cover management of endometriosis-associated infertility (ASRM [7], ACCEPT [6]) or diagnosis only (ESUR [11] and IDEA group guidelines [12]), whereas others cover all aspects of endometriosis including diagnosis, medical or surgical treatment and management of endometriosis-associated infertility (ESHRE, ACOG, CNGOF, National German, Turkish, Indian, Malaysian and Korean). Although all of the international and most of the national guidelines are published in English language, Swedish, Chinese, Mexican and Polish guidelines are only available in their national languages.

There have been fewer guidelines on adenomyosis, and this may reflect the fact that the knowledge gap on this condition is much bigger compared to endometriosis.

Endometriosis is quite often described as an enigmatic disease. Its aetiology, pathogenesis and even diagnosis are poorly understood. Similarly, there are many unknowns about its management; hence, both clinicians and patients resort to guidelines prepared by experts from respected societies.

44.2 Methodology

Guideline development methodology varies considerably between various examples. Some organizations have well-established methodology for guideline development in line with internationally agreed standards. For example, ESHRE has developed a manual in 2007 for its guideline development groups, and this has been updated in 2019 in line with Guidelines for Research and Evaluation in Europe (AGREE) instrument [1]. In contrast, some other organizations have developed documents based on consensus agreed by 'experts' depending on their personal experience, their opinion and their knowledge of the published literature (WES Consensus document, [10]). Older guidelines are written more in line with a 'narrative review' style (ASRM, Endometriosis and infertility: a committee opinion).

After deciding on a topic, development of guidelines usually starts with the formation of the 'guideline development group (GDG)' which may include experts in the field, non-expert clinicians, patient representative(s), relevant allied health-care professionals and research specialists who are experienced in systematic literature searches. However, most guidelines have been developed by 'expert clinicians' only; only the ESHRE GDG includes all individuals listed above.

The GDG determines the 'scope' of the guidelines and may determine the 'key questions' that would need to be covered within the guideline. The questions are quite often formed in a standard format to include 'population', 'intervention', 'comparison' and 'outcome' (PICO). This then helps preparing the search terms that will be used for the systematic literature search. ASRM and ACCEPT guidelines cover fertility aspects of endometriosis, whereas other guidelines cover both pain and infertility.

The evidence available in the published literature is usually graded on the basis of its strength. There are a number of grading systems, but in general these classify the published evidence under a number of groups:

1. Systematic review and meta-analysis of randomized controlled trials (RCTs)
2. Well-designed controlled studies without randomization or quasi-experimental studies
3. Well-designed descriptive studies, comparative/correlation studies, case series
4. Expert committee opinions or reports

The quality of evidence may be upgraded in the presence of large effect or dose response but would be downgraded for the risk of bias, inconsistency, indirectness, imprecision and publication bias [26]. Once the evidence is gathered and summarized, 'recommendations' are written and make condensed statements on the use/usefulness of a particular approach, supported by summary evidence.

44.3 Diagnosis of Endometriosis

Recommendations on the diagnosis of endometriosis vary amongst the guidelines and cover statements on the significance of symptoms, examination, imaging such as ultrasound and magnetic resonance imaging (MRI), biomarkers, laparoscopy and histopathological examination. There is low-quality evidence on the usefulness of symptoms and clinical examination; however, some guidelines make recommendations on these tools in diagnosing endometriosis. For example, ESHRE guidelines recommend considering endometriosis in women with dysmenorrhea, non-cyclical pelvic pain, deep dyspareunia, infertility, fatigue and cyclical nongynaecological symptoms such as dyschezia, dysuria, rectal bleeding and shoulder pain (ESHRE). Similarly, NICE, CNGOF and SOGC recommend using symptoms in the diagnosis, but most other guidelines do not make specific recommendations.

Similarly, the recommendations on the place of clinical examination in the diagnosis of endometriosis are based on low-quality evidence or expert opinion. CNOF, ESHRE, NICE and SOGC make specific recommendations on pelvic, abdominal or rectal examination.

Most guidelines advise against the use of biomarkers such as CA-125 in the diagnosis of endometriosis. In contrast, there is overall agreement that transvaginal ultrasound examination is useful in diagnosing ovarian endometriomas and deep endometriosis based on good-quality evidence. In order to standardize the reporting of ultrasonographic findings, the International Deep Endometriosis Analysis (IDEA) group developed a consensus statement to implement terms and definitions to describe the anatomical structures and locations when diagnosing endometriosis [12]. With such standardization, they aim to minimize the terminology used between endometriosis centres and allow comparison of data.

The opinion on the use of MRI for diagnosis is divided, whilst ESHRE guidelines state that the place of MRI is not well established, NICE and Turkish guidelines advise against the use of MRI, and CNGOF guideline suggests MRI can be used for the diagnosis of endometriosis. The European Society of Urogenital

Radiology (ESUR) developed a guideline to establish protocols on the indications, technical requirements, patient preparation and reporting of the findings for the diagnosis of pelvic endometriosis on MRI [11].

Visualization of endometriosis with or without histological confirmation at laparoscopy (or at laparotomy) is recommended for the diagnosis of endometriosis in CNGOF, ESHRE, NICE and Turkish guidelines, but there are no specific recommendations on the place of laparoscopy in other guidelines.

44.4 Medical Treatment for Endometriosis-Associated Pain

The CNGOF guidelines recommend histological or surgical confirmation of endometriosis before instituting long-term medical treatment, as far as possible. However, ESHRE, NICE, Malaysian, Korean, Indian and Turkish guidelines recommend empirical treatment with combined oral contraceptives (COC) or progestins for the treatment of pain due to presumed endometriosis. ACOG guidelines also recommend that gonadotropin-releasing hormone analogues or agonists (GnRHa) can be used for 3 months for empirical treatment.

There is overall agreement that medical treatment using combined hormonal contraceptives, progestins and GnRHa can be used for the treatment of pain associated with endometriosis. It is suggested that efficacy, patient preference, cost, availability and side-effect profile will need to be taken into account when deciding on the medical treatment option. Danazol is mentioned in some guidelines (CNGOF, Korean, Indian and Turkish guidelines) without clearly endorsing its use due to its side-effect profile, but others do not make a recommendation on it (e.g. ESHRE and NICE guidelines). ESHRE, Turkish and Malaysian guidelines state that aromatase inhibitors have a limited place in the treatment of pain related to endometriosis.

44.5 Surgical Treatment for Endometriosis-Associated Pain

There is overall consensus that surgical treatment of endometriosis is recommended for the treatment of endometriosis-associated pain based on high-quality evidence, although ACOG guidelines state that this may be the case in the short term. There is again overall agreement that excision of endometrioma is a preferred surgical approach over drainage and coagulation in all guidelines. German guidelines recommend removal of peritoneal endometriosis, whereas ESHRE, Indian and South African guidelines suggest that both excisional ablative approaches can be utilized. ESHRE and Turkish guidelines state that deep endometriosis can be surgically treated by excising it but that this treatment should take place in a centre of expertise by a multidisciplinary team. Hysterectomy with or without oophorectomy has been recommended in guidelines which address the subject of endometriosis-associated pain. CNGOF, ESHRE, Korean and Turkish guidelines specifically recommend hysterectomy with bilateral salpingo-oophorectomy together with removal of endometriotic lesions in women who do not have a desire to have further pregnancies, whereas ACOG guidelines indicate that the ovaries should be conserved in women with normal ovaries.

44.6 Management of Endometriosis-Associated Infertility

All published guidelines recommend against the use of hormonal therapies to improve fertility in women with endometriosis-associated infertility. The CNGOF, ESHRE, German, Indian, Korean, South African and Turkish guidelines recommend surgical treatment of endometriosis, particularly for early endometriosis, to improve spontaneous pregnancy rates. However, the ASRM guidelines state that there is insufficient evidence to recommend surgical treatment and that ACOG guidelines suggest that surgery does improve pregnancy rates, but the magnitude of improvement is unclear. Overall, there is agreement amongst the guidelines that excision of endometrioma is superior to drainage and coagulation in improving spontaneous pregnancy rates when the subject of endometrioma is specifically addressed. ESHRE guidelines highlight the detrimental impact of endometrioma surgery on ovarian function, particularly in those who had previous surgery. Some guidelines indicate that the benefits of surgery to improve fertility in women with deep endometriosis are not well established (CNGOF, ESHRE) or are not recommended due to limited/weak evidence of benefit and higher risk of complications (Turkish guidelines). There is overall agreement that in infertile women who had previous surgery, assisted reproductive technologies (ART) are better than repeat surgery.

ASRM, ESHRE and Turkish guidelines recommend intrauterine insemination with superovulation (or controlled ovarian stimulation) in women with early stage (ASRM stage I/II) endometriosis. ART is recommended when other treatments have failed or when there is additional male factor or severe tubal damage. Some guidelines (ACCEPT, ESHRE, Turkish guidelines) highlight the issue that women with endometriosis tend to have lower pregnancy rates following ART. Most guidelines advise against surgical treatment of endometriomas prior to ART to improve pregnancy rates.

44.7 Adenomyosis

Adenomyosis has been included in CNGOF, German, Turkish and Indian guidelines as a separate section. These guidelines identify MRI as the most reliable method of diagnosis, although transvaginal ultrasound is deemed to be sufficiently reliable. Levonorgestrel intrauterine system is identified as an effective treatment for adenomyosis-associated heavy menstrual bleeding and pain. These guidelines state that hysterectomy is the preferred surgical treatment in women who no longer desire pregnancy. Turkish guidelines also cover the impact of adenomyosis on fertility and emphasize there is some evidence that adenomyosis may compromise fertility and have a detrimental impact on the outcome of IVF treatment. Limited evidence on the potential benefit of uterus-sparing surgery for adenomyosis in women who wish to preserve uterus/fertility has been summarized in the Turkish guidelines.

44.8 Conclusion

A number of national and international guidelines have been available since the publication of the first ESHRE Guidelines on the Management of Women with Endometriosis in 2005 [2]. These have gradually evolved, and revised or updated versions have been published (ESHRE, CNGOF Guidelines). There are significant differences between the scope and focus of these guidelines; whilst some cover all aspects of endometriosis, others solely address endometriosis-associated infertility. The majority of recommendations are in agreement with each other, although there are subtle differences between different guidelines.

References

1. Vermeulen N, Le Clef N, Mcheik S, D'Angelo A, Tilleman K, Veleva Z, Nelen W. Manual for ESHRE guideline development, 2019. https://www.eshre.eu/.../Guidelines/Guidelines/Manual-guidelines.pdf
2. Kennedy S, Bergqvist A, Chapron C, D'Hooghe T, Dunselman G, Greb R, Hummelshoj L, Prentice A, Saridogan E, ESHRE Special Interest Group for Endometriosis and Endometrium Guideline Development Group. ESHRE guideline for the diagnosis and treatment of endometriosis. Hum Reprod. 2005;20(10):2698–704. https://doi.org/10.1093/humrep/dei135. Epub 2005 Jun 24. PMID: 15980014.
3. RCOG Green-Top Guidelines. Endometriosis, Investigation and Management, 2007, Endometriosis, Investigation and Management (Green-top Guideline No. 24) (rcog.org.uk).
4. Practice bulletin no. 114: management of endometriosis. Obstet Gynecol 2010;116(1):223–236. doi: https://doi.org/10.1097/AOG.0b013e3181e8b073. PMID: 20567196.
5. Leyland N, Casper R, Laberge P, Singh SS, SOGC. Endometriosis: diagnosis and management. J Obstet Gynaecol Can. 2010;32(7 Suppl 2):S1–32. PMID: 21545757.
6. Koch J, Rowan K, Rombauts L, Yazdani A, Chapman M, Johnson N. Endometriosis and infertility – a consensus statement from ACCEPT (Australasian CREI consensus expert panel on trial evidence). Aust N Z J Obstet Gynaecol. 2012;52(6):513–22. https://doi.org/10.1111/j.1479-828X.2012.01480.x. Epub 2012 Sep 27. PMID: 23016798.
7. ASRM2012: Practice Committee of the American Society for Reproductive Medicine. Endometriosis and infertility: a committee opinion. Fertil Steril. 2012;98(3):591–8. https://doi.org/10.1016/j.fertnstert.2012.05.031.
8. Dunselman GA, Vermeulen N, Becker C, Calhaz-Jorge C, D'Hooghe T, De Bie B, Heikinheimo O, Horne AW, Kiesel L, Nap A, Prentice A, Saridogan E, Soriano D, Nelen W, European Society of Human Reproduction and Embryology. ESHRE guideline: management of women with endometriosis. Hum Reprod. 2014;29(3):400–12. https://doi.org/10.1093/humrep/det457. Epub 2014 Jan 15. PMID: 24435778.
9. College National des Gynecologues et Obstetriciens Francais. Management of endometriosis CNGOF/HAS clinical practice guidelines, 2018. http://www.cngof.fr/pratiques-cliniques/

guidelines/apercu?path=RPC_CNGOF-HAS_Endometriose_Recommandations_2017-VA.pdf&i=20535
10. Johnson NP, Hummelshoj L, World Endometriosis Society Montpellier Consortium. Consensus on current management of endometriosis. Hum Reprod. 2013;28(6):1552–68. https://doi.org/10.1093/humrep/det050. Epub 2013 Mar 25. PMID: 23528916.
11. Bazot M, Bharwani N, Huchon C, et al. European society of urogenital radiology (ESUR) guidelines: MR imaging of pelvic endometriosis. Eur Radiol. 2017;27:2765–75. https://doi.org/10.1007/s00330-016-4673-z.
12. Guerriero S, Condous G, van den Bosch T, Valentin L, Leone FPG, Van Schoubroeck D, Exacoustos C, Installé AJF, Martins WP, Abrao MS, Hudelist G, Bazot M, Alcazar JL, Gonçalves MO, Pascual MA, Ajossa S, Savelli L, Dunham R, Reid S, Menakaya U, Bourne T, Ferrero S, Leon M, Bignardi T, Holland T, Jurkovic D, Benacerraf B, Osuga Y, Somigliana E, Timmerman D. Systematic approach to sonographic evaluation of the pelvis in women with suspected endometriosis, including terms, definitions and measurements: a consensus opinion from the International Deep Endometriosis Analysis (IDEA) group. Ultrasound Obstet Gynecol. 2016;48:318–32. https://doi.org/10.1002/uog.15955.
13. National institute for health and care excellence guideline, endometriosis: diagnosis and management, 2017. Overview | Endometriosis: diagnosis and management | Guidance | NICE
14. Obstetrics and Gynaecological Society of Malaysia, Clinical Guidelines for the Management of Endometriosis, 2016. https://www.ogsm.org.my/docs/Endometriosis-guideline.pdf
15. Turkish Endometriosis and Adenomyosis Society Guidelines, Diagnosis and management of endometriosis, 2014. Microsoft Word - Guideline english final.docx (endometriozis-dernegi.org).
16. Ulrich U, Buchweitz O, Greb R, Keckstein J, von Leffern I, Oppelt P, Renner SP, Sillem M, Stummvoll W, De Wilde RL, Schweppe KW, German and Austrian Societies for Obstetrics and Gynecology. National German guideline (S2k): guideline for the diagnosis and treatment of endometriosis: long version – AWMF Registry No. 015-045. Geburtshilfe Frauenheilkd. 2014;74(12):1104–18. https://doi.org/10.1055/s-0034-1383187. PMID: 26157194; PMCID: PMC4470398.
17. Federation of Obstetrics & Gynecological Societies of India, Good Clinial Practice Recommendations on Endometriosis, 2016. https://www.fogsi.org/wp-content/uploads/2017/01/GCRP-2017-final.pdf
18. Björk E, Gustavsson M, Palmstierna M, Valentin A, Olovsson M, Melin AS. Nationellt vårdprogram för bättre och jämlik vård vid endometrios [Endometriosis - new clinical guidelines for better and equal care in Sweden]. Lakartidningen. 2020;117:19231. Swedish. PMID: 32542617
19. Hirata T, Koga K, Kai K, Katabuchi H, Kitade M, Kitawaki J, Kurihara M, Takazawa N, Tanaka T, Taniguchi F, Nakajima J, Narahara H, Harada T, Horie S, Honda R, Murono K, Yoshimura K, Osuga Y. Clinical practice guidelines for the treatment of extragenital endometriosis in Japan, 2018. J Obstet Gynaecol Res. 2020;46:2474–87. https://doi.org/10.1111/jog.14522.
20. Hwang H, Chung YJ, Lee SR, Park HT, Song JY, Kim H, Lee DY, Lee EJ, Kim MR, Oh ST. Clinical evaluation and management of endometriosis: guideline for Korean patients from Korean Society of Endometriosis. Obstet Gynecol Sci. 2018;61(5):553–64. https://doi.org/10.5468/ogs.2018.61.5.553. Epub 2018 Sep 7. PMID: 30254991; PMCID: PMC6137012.
21. Cooperative Group of Endometriosis, Chinese Society of Obstetrics and Gynecology, Chinese Medical Association. [Guideline for the diagnosis and treatment of endometriosis]. Zhonghua Fu Chan Ke Za Zhi. 2015;50(3):161–169. Chinese. PMID: 26268404.
22. Federación Mexicana de Colegios de Obstetricia y Ginecología. Diagnóstico y tratamiento de endometriosis [Diagnosis and treatment of endometriosis]. Ginecol Obstet Mex. 2011;79(11):697–710. Spanish. PMID: 22168117.
23. Basta A, Brucka A, Górski J, Kotarski J, Kulig B, Oszukowski P, Poreba R, Radowicki S, Radwan J, Sikora J, Skret A, Skrzypczak J, Szyłło K, Polish Gynocologic Society Experts Group. Stanowisko Zespołu Ekspertów Polskiego Towarzystwa Ginekologicznego dotyczace

diagnostyki i metod leczenia endometriozy [The statement of Polish Society's Experts Group concerning diagnostics and methods of endometriosis treatment]. Ginekol Pol. 2012;83(11):871–6. Polish. PMID: 23379199.

24. Ministry of Health. Diagnosis and Management of Endometriosis in New Zealand. Wellington: Ministry of Health; 2020.
25. South African guideline for treatment of endometriosis, 2017. https://sasreg.co.za/downloads/Treatment-of-Endometriosis.pdf
26. Balshem H, Helfand M, Schunemann HJ, Oxman AD, Kunz R, Brozek J, Vist GE, Falck-Ytter Y, Meerpohl J, Norris S, Guyatt GH. GRADE guidelines: 3. Rating the quality of evidence. J Clin Epidemiol. 2011;64(4):401–6. https://doi.org/10.1016/j.jclinepi.2010.07.015.

Correction to: Endometriosis and Adenomyosis: Global Perspectives Across the Lifespan

Engin Oral

Correction to:

Endometriosis and Adenomyosis: Global Perspectives Across the Lifespan
https://doi.org/10.1007/978-3-030-97236-3

Chapter 5 in: E. Oral (ed.), Endometriosis and Adenomyosis,
https://doi.org/10.1007/978-3-030-97236-3_5
The ORCID id of the author was missed in the original publication and is provided here.
Khaleque N Khan: 0000-0002-9493-3340

The updated version of the chapters can be found at
https://doi.org/10.1007/978-3-030-97236-3_5
https://doi.org/10.1007/978-3-030-97236-3_8
https://doi.org/10.1007/978-3-030-97236-3_16
https://doi.org/10.1007/978-3-030-97236-3_23
https://doi.org/10.1007/978-3-030-97236-3_26
https://doi.org/10.1007/978-3-030-97236-3_31
https://doi.org/10.1007/978-3-030-97236-3_35
https://doi.org/10.1007/978-3-030-97236-3_36
https://doi.org/10.1007/978-3-030-97236-3_37
https://doi.org/10.1007/978-3-030-97236-3_39
https://doi.org/10.1007/978-3-030-97236-3_40
https://doi.org/10.1007/978-3-030-97236-3_42
https://doi.org/10.1007/978-3-030-97236-3_43
https://doi.org/10.1007/978-3-030-97236-3_44

E. Oral (ed.), *Endometriosis and Adenomyosis*,
https://doi.org/10.1007/978-3-030-97236-3_45

Chapter 8 in: E. Oral (ed.), Endometriosis and Adenomyosis,
https://doi.org/10.1007/978-3-030-97236-3_8
The ORCID ids of the authors were missed in the original publication and are provided here.
Jorg Keckstein: 0000-0002-3943-3300
Peter Oppelt: 0000-0003-3852-5948
Gernot Hudelist: 0000-0002-9424-2208

Chapter 16 in: E. Oral (ed.), Endometriosis and Adenomyosis,
https://doi.org/10.1007/978-3-030-97236-3_16
Dr Hanan Alsalem's name was misspelled in the initial publication as Hanan Amsalem and has been corrected in all further publications.

Chapter 23 in: E. Oral (ed.), Endometriosis and Adenomyosis,
https://doi.org/10.1007/978-3-030-97236-3_23
The ORCID ids of the authors were missed in the original publication and are provided here.
Marina Kvaskoff: 0000-0002-4557-3772
Stacey A. Missmer: 0000-0003-3147-6768

Chapter 26 in: E. Oral (ed.), Endometriosis and Adenomyosis,
https://doi.org/10.1007/978-3-030-97236-3_26
The ORCID ids of the authors were missed in the original publication and are provided here.
Maurizio N. D'Alterio: 0000-0001-9874-1488
Stefano Angioni: 0000-0002-2314-0028
Fabio Ghezzi: 0000-0003-3949-5410
Antoni Simone Laganà: 0000-0003-1543-2802

Chapter 31 in: E. Oral (ed.), Endometriosis and Adenomyosis,
https://doi.org/10.1007/978-3-030-97236-3_31
The ORCID id of the authors was missed in the original publication and is provided here.
Silvia Vannuccini: 0000-0001-5790-587X

Chapter 35 in: E. Oral (ed.), Endometriosis and Adenomyosis,
https://doi.org/10.1007/978-3-030-97236-3_35
The ORCID ids of the authors were missed in the original publication and are provided here.
Harald Krentel: 0000-0002-1238-9207
Maribel Acien: 0000-0002-6536-453X

Chapter 36 in: E. Oral (ed.), Endometriosis and Adenomyosis,
https://doi.org/10.1007/978-3-030-97236-3_36
The ORCID id of the author was missed in the original publication and is provided here.

Yasushi Hirota: 0000-0003-0241-9780

Chapter 37 in: E. Oral (ed.), Endometriosis and Adenomyosis,
https://doi.org/10.1007/978-3-030-97236-3_37
The ORCID ids of the authors were missed in the original publication and are provided here.
Jwal Banker: 0000-0001-6637-1398
Manish Banker: 0000-0001-9918-1128

Chapter 39 in: E. Oral (ed.), Endometriosis and Adenomyosis,
https://doi.org/10.1007/978-3-030-97236-3_39
The ORCID id of the author was missed in the initial publication and is provided here.
Harald Krentel: 0000-0002-1238-9207

Chapter 40 in: E. Oral (ed.), Endometriosis and Adenomyosis,
https://doi.org/10.1007/978-3-030-97236-3_40
The ORCID ids of the authors were missed in the original publication and are provided here.
Dr Hiroaki Komatsu: 0000-0002-4507-6848
Fuminori Taniguchi: 0000-0001-6922-0632
Tasuku Harada: 0000-0002-1492-7275

Chapter 42 in: E. Oral (ed.), Endometriosis and Adenomyosis,
https://doi.org/10.1007/978-3-030-97236-3_42
The ORCID ids of the authors were missed in the original publication and are provided here.
Simone Ferrero: 0000-0003-2225-5568
Fabio Barra: 0000-0003-4117-6603

Chapter 43 in: E. Oral (ed.), Endometriosis and Adenomyosis,
https://doi.org/10.1007/978-3-030-97236-3_43
The ORCID id of the author was missed in the initial publication and is provided here.
Sanjay Agarwal: 0000-0002-8046-9807

Chapter 44 in: E. Oral (ed.), Endometriosis and Adenomyosis,
https://doi.org/10.1007/978-3-030-97236-3_44
The ORCID id of the author was missed in the initial publication and is provided here.
Nura Fitnat Topbas Selcuki: 0000-0002-5749-9987

Index

E. Oral (ed.), *Endometriosis and Adenomyosis*, https://doi.org/10.1007/978-3-030-97236-3

F

G

T

U

V

W

GPSR Compliance

The European Union's (EU) General Product Safety Regulation (GPSR) is a set of rules that requires consumer products to be safe and our obligations to ensure this.

If you have any concerns about our products, you can contact us on ProductSafety@springernature.com

In case Publisher is established outside the EU, the EU authorized representative is:

Springer Nature Customer Service Center GmbH
Europaplatz 3
69115 Heidelberg, Germany

Batch number: 10732064

Printed by Printforce, the Netherlands